Diagnosis and Management of Mitochondrial Disorders

Michelangelo Mancuso
Thomas Klopstock
Editors

Diagnosis and Management of Mitochondrial Disorders

Springer

Editors
Michelangelo Mancuso
Department of Clinical and Experimental Medicine
Neurological Institute
University of Pisa
Pisa
Italy

Thomas Klopstock
Department of Neurology
Friedrich-Baur-Institute
Ludwig-Maximilians-University of Munich
Munich
Germany

ISBN 978-3-030-05516-5 ISBN 978-3-030-05517-2 (eBook)
https://doi.org/10.1007/978-3-030-05517-2

This Springer imprint is published by the registered company Springer Nature Switzerland AG
The registered company address is: Gewerbestrasse 11, 6330 Cham, Switzerland

Preface

Mitochondrial Medicine: 30 Years Old, Much to Learn

The initial spark of the "mitochondrial revolution" in medicine was the description, in 1988, of the first pathogenic mutations in mitochondrial DNA (mtDNA). Anita Harding and her team identified large-scale single deletions of mtDNA in patients with mitochondrial myopathies [1]. Soon thereafter, Doug Wallace and his team described a point mutation in the gene encoding subunit 4 of complex I in a family with Leber's hereditary optic neuropathy [2].

With the publication of this book in early 2019, we celebrate the 30th anniversary of these groundbreaking discoveries. The last 30 years have been the golden age of mitochondrial medicine, with hundreds of genes responsible for multiple genetic mitochondrial disorders being identified.

Mitochondrial diseases are now recognized as one of the most common genetic conditions worldwide, and the phenotypic expression involves all the disciplines of medicine.

We hope that we have been able to convey, with this book, the excitement that has accompanied—as it still does—the extraordinarily rapid development of mitochondrial medicine. The therapeutic era has just begun, and we are confident to see similarly exciting progress in the next few years.

It has been a great experience to serve as editors for this special book. We would like to express our special gratitude to all contributing authors for their timely and superb efforts in composing this monography.

Finally, this book is dedicated to our great mentor, Professor Salvatore "Billi" DiMauro. The enormous and still ongoing progress in our understanding of mitochondrial medicine is only possible by an intense collaboration of a team of international *mitochondriologists*, many of whom have been trained in the College of Physicians and Surgeons, Columbia University Medical Center, NY, under the guidance of Billi.

Enjoy the reading!

Pisa, Italy — Michelangelo Mancuso
Munich, Germany — Thomas Klopstock

References

1. Holt IJ, Harding AE, Morgan-Hughes JA. Deletions of muscle mitochondrial DNA in patients with mitochondrial myopathies. Nature. 1988;331(6158):717–9.
2. Wallace DC, Singh G, Lott MT, Hodge JA, Schurr TG, Lezza AM, Elsas LJ 2nd, Nikoskelainen EK. Mitochondrial DNA mutation associated with Leber's hereditary optic neuropathy. Science. 1988;242(4884):1427–30.

Contents

Mitochondrial Medicine: A Historical Point of View

Yi Shiau Ng, Salvatore DiMauro, and Doug M. Turnbull

Introduction

Mitochondria are essential double-membrane, dynamic organelles found in all nucleated cells, and they are referred as the powerhouse in cells because of their vital role in generating ATP via the oxidative phosphorylation (OXPHOS). The OXPHOS machinery is located at the inner mitochondrial membrane and comprises five enzymatic complexes, which are mitochondrial respiratory chain (complexes I to IV) and ATP synthase (complex V). The mechanism by which the passage of electrons down the respiratory chain generates ATP was described by Peter Mitchell [1], who was awarded the Nobel Prize for Chemistry in 1978. Mitochondria are also important players in multiple other cellular activities such as intrinsic apoptosis, redox, calcium handling and urea cycle.

One of the most fascinating biological features of mitochondria is that they contain extranuclear DNA materials, mitochondrial DNAs (mtDNA), which are tiny, double-stranded DNA molecules that exist in multiple copies per cell and only encode 37 genes. However, the replication and maintenance of mtDNA and almost all building blocks of mitochondria are controlled by the nuclear genome. The cross talk between the mitochondrial DNA and nucleus means that any genetic defects in either mtDNA or nuclear genome could perturb the mitochondrial functions especially the OXPHOS, consequently leading to the development of disease.

The clinical features of mitochondrial disease are very variable with high-energy demand tissues and organs such as the brain, skeletal muscle, heart, liver and optic nerves, which are particularly susceptible to the mitochondrial dysfunction. However, mitochondrial disease can affect practically any organ making the diagnosis and management challenging. Mitochondrial diseases are one of the most common groups of inherited neurogenetic disorders with a minimal prevalence of 1 in 4300 [2], comparably, if not, higher than other common neurogenetic disorders such as Charcot-Marie-Tooth neuropathy and myotonic dystrophy [3].

In this chapter, we begin with an overview of the pathological description of various mitochondrial syndromes, the biochemical classification of mitochondrial defects, followed by the era of identification of primary mtDNA mutations and discoveries of multiple nuclear genes implicated in mitochondrial disease. We also highlight the emergence of reproductive options especially mitochondrial donation in primary mtDNA disease and advancement in potential treatments (Fig. 1).

Y. S. Ng · D. M. Turnbull (✉)
Wellcome Centre for Mitochondrial Research, Institute of Neuroscience, Newcastle University, Framlington Place, Newcastle Upon Tyne, UK
e-mail: doug.turnbull@ncl.ac.uk

S. DiMauro
Houston Merritt Clinical Research Center, Columbia University, New York, NY, USA

Department of Neurology, College of Physicians and Surgeons, New York, NY, USA

M. Mancuso, T. Klopstock (eds.), *Diagnosis and Management of Mitochondrial Disorders*, https://doi.org/10.1007/978-3-030-05517-2_1

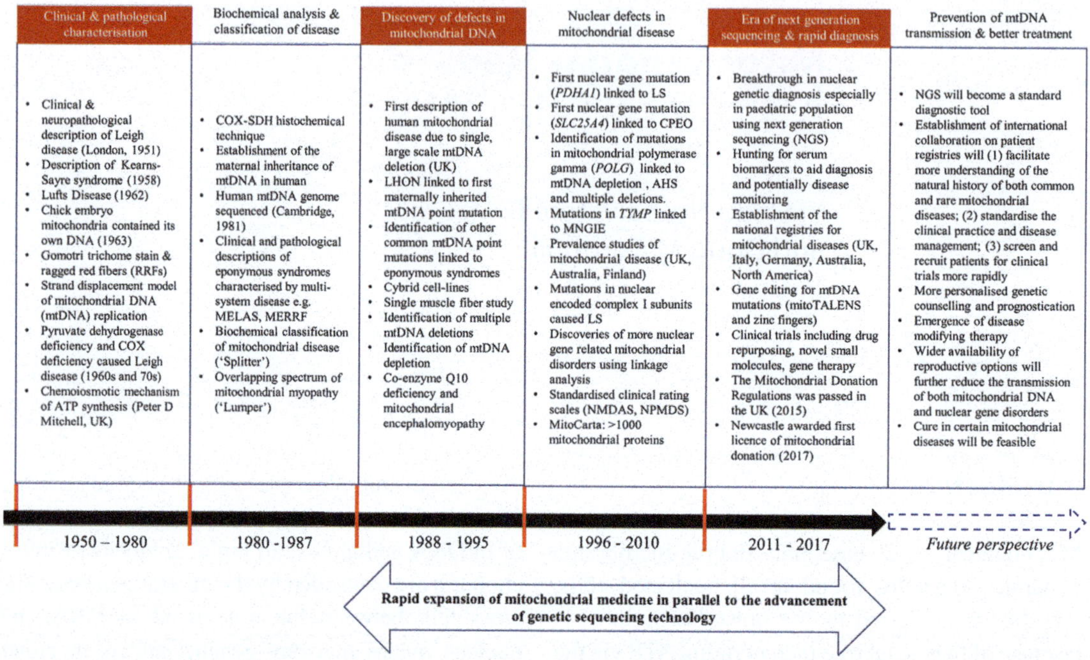

Fig. 1 Timeline summarises significant milestones and discoveries in mitochondrial disease. *AHS* Alpers-Huttenlocher syndrome, *ATP* adenosine triphosphate, *CPEO* chronic progressive external ophthalmoplegia, *COX* cytochrome c oxidase, *LHON* Leber hereditary optic neuropathy, *LS* Leigh syndrome, *MELAS* mitochondrial encephalomyopathy, lactic acidosis and stroke-like episodes, *MERRF* myoclonic epilepsy and ragged-red fibres, *mitoTALENS* mitochondrially targeted transcription activator-like effector nucleases, *MNGIE* mitochondrial neurogastrointestinal encephalopathy, *NGS* next-generation sequencing, *NMDAS* Newcastle Mitochondrial Disease Adult Scale, *NPMDS* Newcastle Paediatric Mitochondrial Disease Scale, *PDHA1* pyruvate dehydrogenase E1 alpha 1 subunit, *POLG* polymerase gamma, *SDH* succinate dehydrogenase, *SLC25A4* solute carrier family 25 member 4, *TYMP* thymidine phosphorylase

1950–1980

Leigh Syndrome

Leigh syndrome, also known as subacute necrotising encephalomyelopathy, is one of the most common presentations of mitochondrial disease among the paediatric patients with an estimated prevalence of 1 in 40,000 live births [4]. Doctor Denis Archibald Leigh (1912–1998), a talented British psychiatrist, published the first case report of clinical details and pathological findings of subacute necrotising encephalomyelopathy in London in 1951. He described a 7-month-old boy who had a normal birth and early development for 6 weeks, subsequently presented with a constellation of neurological signs and symptoms including developmental regression, poor feeding, optic atrophy and limb spasticity. A postmortem examination revealed bilateral symmetrical subacute necrotic lesions in thalami, brainstem and the posterior columns of the spinal cord with relatively sparing of the caudate and lentiform nuclei [5]. Leigh made an interesting observation that these pathological findings were very similar to patients with Wernicke's encephalopathy. The subsequent links of Leigh disease and inborn error of gluconeogenesis [6], cytochrome *c* oxidase deficiency (complex IV of respiratory chain) [7], pyruvate dehydrogenase complex deficiency [8] in the 1960s and 1970s implicated that Leigh syndrome did not result from a single molecular defect [7]. Indeed, mutations in more than 75 genes have been linked to Leigh syndrome to date [9].

Chronic Progressive External Ophthalmoplegia and Kearns-Sayre Syndrome

Chronic progressive external ophthalmoplegia (CPEO), characterised by eyelid ptosis and restricted eye movement, is now recognised as a common manifestation of mitochondrial disease (Fig. 2a) [10]. The German ophthalmologist,

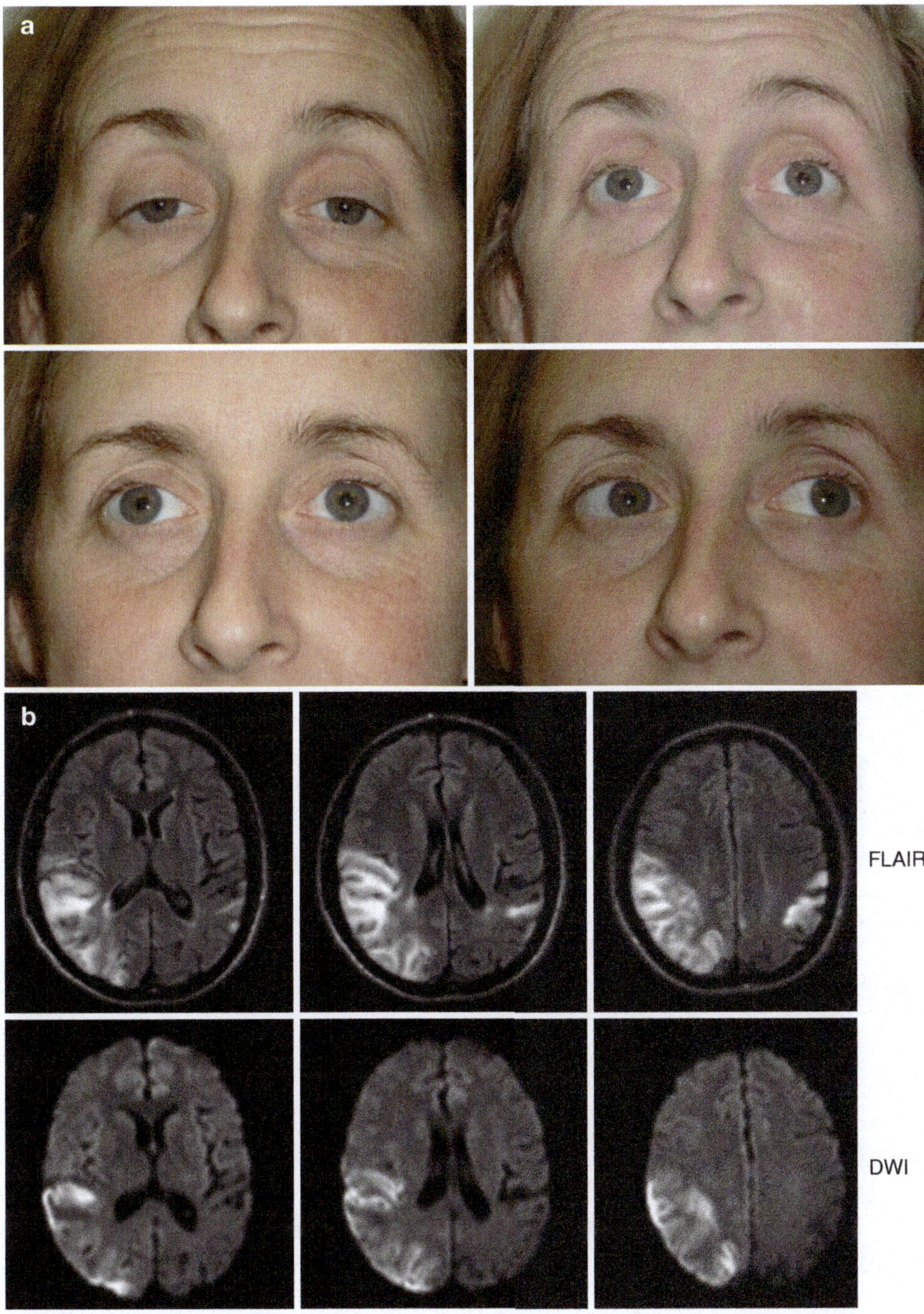

Fig. 2 (**a**) Signs of chronic progressive external ophthalmoplegia. This patient has bilateral ptosis, overactivity of frontalis, very limited upgaze, restricted abduction and adduction. (**b**) MRI head of a patient with MELAS syndrome. FLAIR sequence shows asymmetrical, bilateral stroke-like lesions with restricted diffusion involving the right temporal, parietal and occipital lobes. (**c**) Muscle biopsy. (1) A ragged-red fibre is highlighted with the modified Gomori Trichrome stain (asterisk, *); (2) COX-deficient muscle fibres exhibit pale brown colour; (3) increased SDH activities in COX-deficient fibres (darker blue); (4) sequential COX/SDH histochemistry clearly highlights the COX-deficient fibres (blue); (5) electron microscopy shows a highly abnormal mitochondrial ultrastructure. (**d**) Human mitochondrial DNA. Common point mutations including m.3243A>G, m.8344A>G, m.8993T>C/G, m.11778G>A and m.13513G>A and single, large-scale mtDNA deletion (4977 base pairs) are highlighted. (**e**) The prevalence of mitochondrial disease in an adult population of North East England. Over 75% of adult patients with mitochondrial disease are caused by a primary mtDNA defect [2]

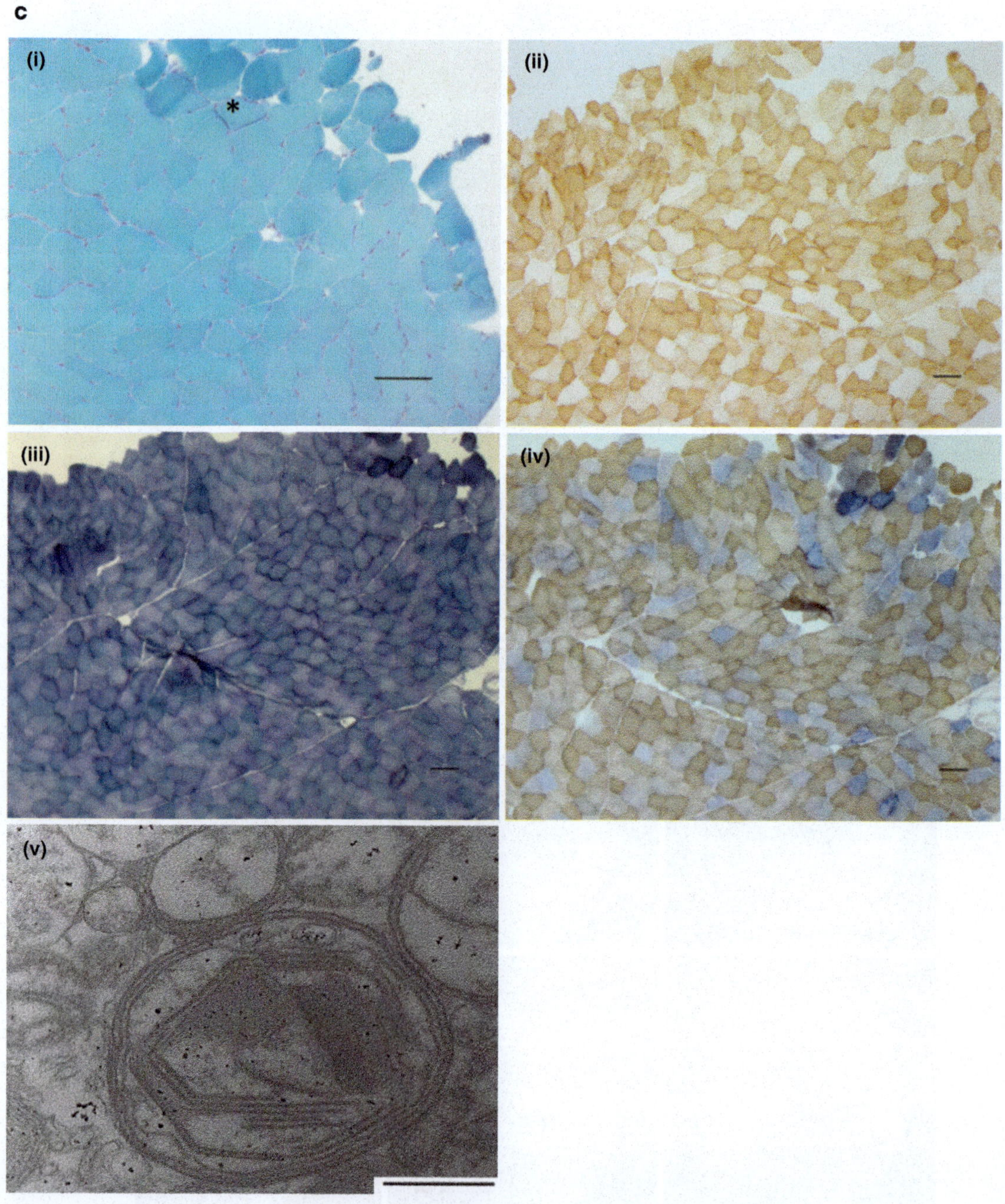

Fig. 2 (continued)

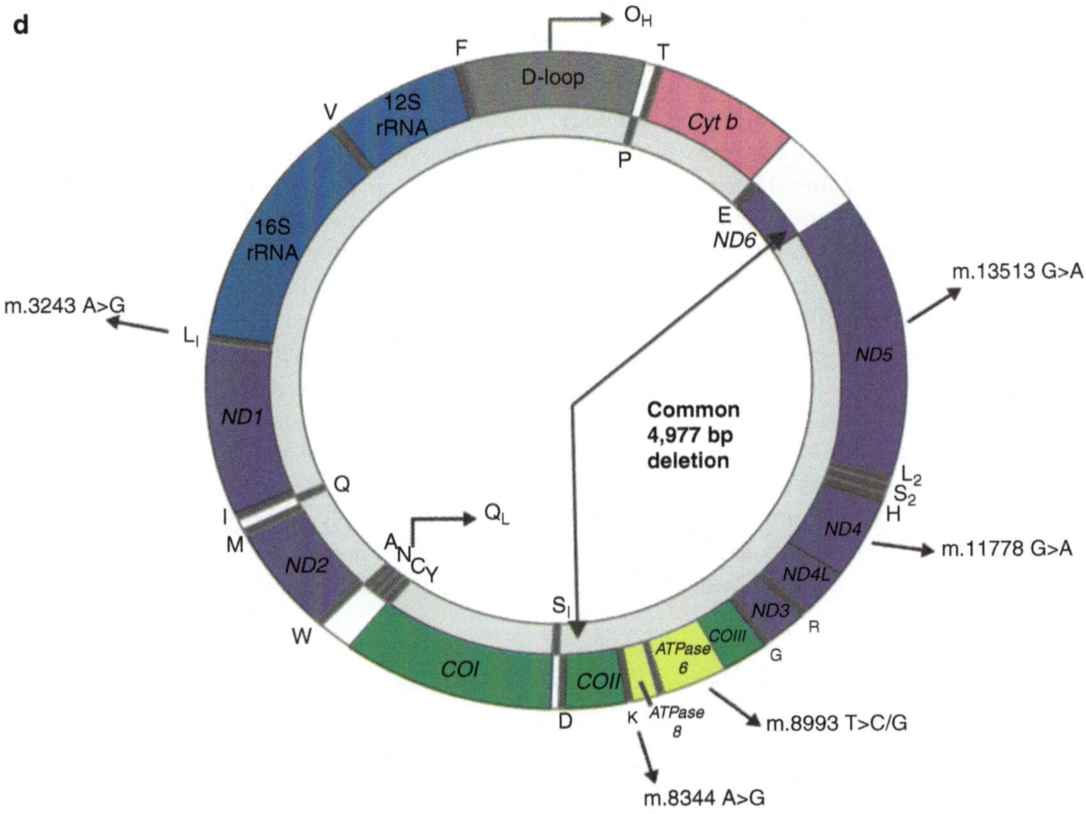

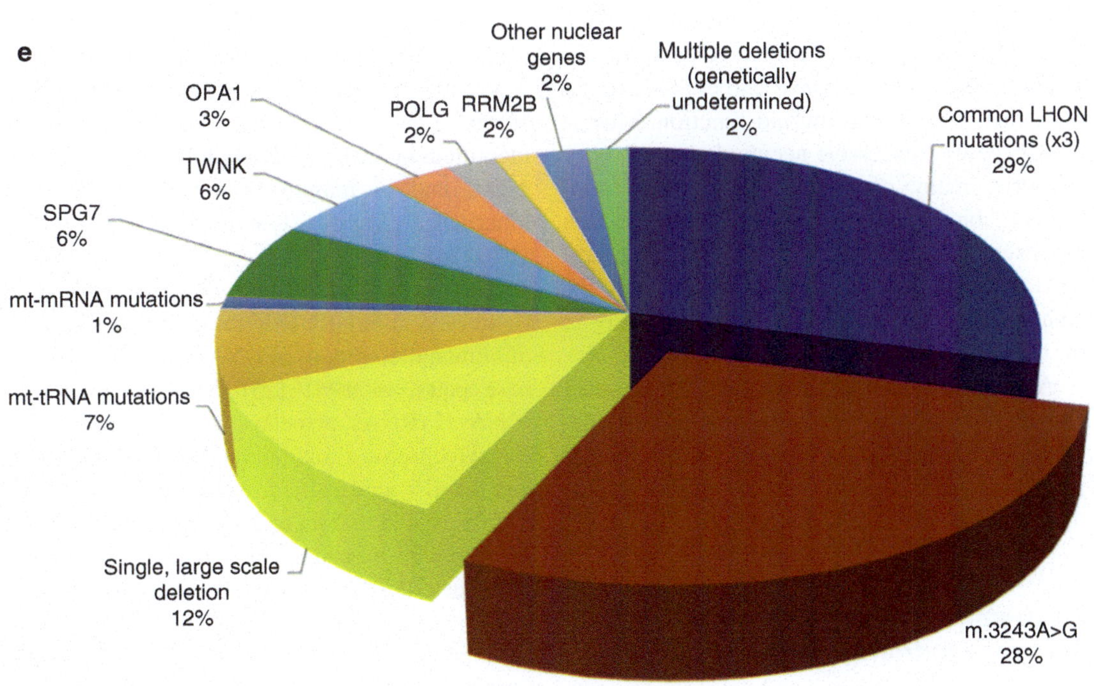

Fig. 2 (continued)

Albrecht von Graefe, described the first case in 1868, and subsequently Sir Jonathan Hutchinson reported similar cases in the English literature around 10 years later. The underlying aetiology of CPEO had been widely but incorrectly accepted as a central brainstem disorder until histopathological and electromyographic evidence of myopathy in ocular muscles of affected individuals emerged in the early 1950s. In 1958, Kearns and Sayre from the Mayo Clinic reported two cases with triad of retinitis pigmentosa, CPEO and complete heart block, and they asserted that such association represented a true clinical syndrome rather than a coincidental finding [11]; Kearns reported nine more cases and outlined the spectrum of clinical features a few years later. Moreover, Kearns also observed the lack of family history in patients affected by this syndrome.

Luft Disease

The description of Luft disease in 1962 is often regarded as the beginning of the mitochondrial medicine [12]. The patient was a Swedish woman in her 30s presented with excessive perspiration, generalised muscle weakness and elevated metabolic rate with normal thyroid function. Muscle biopsy showed excessive accumulation of mitochondria, many of which had gigantic size. Further biochemical analysis and electron microscopy (EM) studies of mitochondria isolated from skeletal muscle directly linked the pathogenesis of disease to a defect involving in the coupling of oxidative phosphorylation [13].

A second case of Luft disease—with identical clinical, muscle pathology and biochemistry features—was reported [14], but the molecular genetic defect in this unique mitochondrial myopathy remains a puzzle.

Biochemical Classification of Mitochondrial Disease

The application of EM on studying muscle biopsies led to the discoveries that structurally abnormal mitochondria were identified in myopathies after the first description of Luft disease [15]. The availability of biochemical assays led to better characterisation of myopathies caused by various metabolic defects such as carnitine deficiency [16], carnitine palmitoyltransferase (CPT) deficiency [17], pyruvate dehydrogenase deficiency [18] and cytochrome *c* oxidase deficiency (complex IV) [7, 19, 20] in the 1970s and in the early 1980s. DiMauro and colleagues proposed to broadly classify mitochondrial disease into five major groups based on different steps of metabolic pathways in mitochondria [21]. Such classification encompassed a wide range of inborn metabolic disorders, which included pyruvate dehydrogenase deficiency, glycogen storage disorders, fatty acid oxidation defects and various mitochondrial respiratory chain deficiencies [21, 22].

1980–1987

The Mapping of Human Mitochondrial DNA

The presence of extranuclear DNA in mitochondria (i.e. mitochondrial DNA) in chick embryos was first reported by Nass and Nass in 1963. Maternal inheritance of mitochondrial DNA was identified in yeast and amphibians in the late 1960s and in mammals in 1974 [23]. Such inheritance pattern was confirmed in human in 1980 [24].

Sanger and colleagues who were based in Cambridge, UK published the complete sequence of human mitochondrial DNA, which has 16,569 base pairs, in 1981 [25]. They identified 22 tRNAs, 2 rRNAs, cytochrome *b*, 3 genes encoded for cytochrome *c* oxidase (CO I-III), ATPase 6 and 8 and 7 unidentified reading frames (URFs). They revealed that these genes were organised in a very compact fashion, and the noncoding region was located in the D-loop. The seven unidentified reading frames were subsequently identified to be subunits of complex I [26, 27]. It is highly remarkable that reanalysis of the Cambridge reference sequence only identified error frequency of 0.07% nearly 20 years later [28].

1989–2012

Mitochondrial Encephalomyopathies with CoQ_{10} Deficiency

In 1989, Ogasawara and Engel discovered two sisters with lipid storage myopathy, cerebellar ataxia, seizures and recurrent myoglobinuria and profound deficiency of CoQ_{10} in muscle mitochondria [29]. In the following years, many patients were reported with muscle CoQ_{10} deficiency and variable involvement of skeletal muscle, CNS, peripheral neuropathy, nephropathy and inconsistently responsive to CoQ_{10} supplementation.

It was suggested that various aetiologies of CoQ_{10} deficiencies should be attributed to genetic defects in the long series of enzymes involved in CoQ_{10} biosynthesis: in 2006 and 2007, the first molecular defects were identified in the genes (*PDSS1*, *PDSS2* and *COQ2*) encoding the initial enzymes and causing severe infantile encephalomyopathies [30–32]. In the following years, mutations in *COQ8* explained the cause of adult-onset cerebellar ataxia, seizures, dystonia and spasticity [33–35], and several more genes have been associated with various forms of encephalomyopathies or nephropathies.

Secondary causes of CoQ_{10} deficiency have opened a new vista on ataxia, oculomotor apraxia (AOA1) due to mutations in *aprataxin (APTX)* [36] or on lipid storage myopathy due to mutations in electron-transferring flavoprotein dehydrogenase [37].

Mitochondrial Encephalomyopathy, Lactic Acidosis and Stroke-like Episodes (MELAS)

The acronym MELAS was first coined in 1984 [38], and it has become one of the most well-characterised syndromes in mitochondrial disease. Although the original case was presented at a paediatric neurology meeting in 1976, the full description of the original case of MELAS only became available 15 years later [39]. The diagnostic criteria of MELAS were proposed based on the literature review of 69 cases [39]: (1) stroke-like episode occurred before the age 40 years; (2) encephalopathy characterised by seizures, dementia or both; (3) lactic acidosis, ragged-red fibres or both; (4) normal early development; (5) recurrent headache; and (6) recurrent vomiting. Stroke-like lesions often do not confine to the vascular territories, with the predilection of occipital, parietal and temporal lobes involvement (Fig. 2b). These unique characteristics have been consistently observed in both the imaging [40–42] and neuropathological [43–46] studies. The precise pathogenesis remains debatable [47], and the leading hypotheses are angiopathy and endothelial dysfunction [48, 49], neuronal hyperexcitability [50] and inherent OXPHOS dysfunction caused combined neuronal and vascular dysfunction [44].

1988–1995

Mutations in the Mitochondrial DNA

The clear demonstration of mutations in mitochondrial DNA that was responsible for human disease only occurred in 1988: sporadic form of CPEO caused by the single, large-scale mtDNA deletion [51, 52]. In the same year, Wallace and colleagues demonstrated that Leber hereditary optic neuropathy (LHON) was caused by the maternally inherited homoplasmic mtDNA point mutation (m.11778G>A) in multiple unrelated family pedigrees for the first time [53]. Following these breakthrough discoveries, many clinical syndromes were linked to specific mtDNA mutations, such as m.8344A>G with myoclonic epilepsy and ragged-red fibres (MERRF) [54], m.3243A>G with MELAS [55], single, large-scale mtDNA deletion associated with Kearns-Sayre syndrome (KSS) [56] and Pearson syndrome [57] and other common point mutations causing LHON (Fig. 2d) [58].

Hammans and coworkers from Queen Square, London, demonstrated mtDNA mutations (m.3243A>G and m.8344A>G) were detectable in both blood and muscle and proposed to employ the molecular analysis of blood sample as a rapid screening and diagnostic tool for suspected cases in the early 1990s [59]. However, the mutant heteroplasmy level of several common point mutations such as m.3243A>G [60] and m.13513A>G has subsequently been shown to decline with time in blood, highlighting the caveat of a false-negative result by screening mtDNA mutations using blood sample alone. Other noninvasive tissues such as urine, buccal mucosa and hair follicles have since been proposed as alternative diagnostic samples to skeletal muscle and blood. Nevertheless, muscle biopsy (Fig. 2c) is important in the investigation of primary mtDNA disease, especially among individuals without apparent maternal family because single, large-scale deletion and sporadic point mutations in mtDNA can only be reliably detected in postmitotic tissues [61].

The advent of transmitochondrial cybrid cell study [62] and single muscle fibre analysis of mtDNA variant [63] have become the gold standard of ascertaining the pathogenicity of any novel mtDNA variants, given multiple polymorphisms are present in the mtDNA. The expansion of clinical spectrum associated with a given mitochondrial DNA mutation, for example, MELAS [55], MIDD [64] and CPEO [65] in patients with the m.3243A>G mutation, and genetic heterogeneity for the same clinical syndrome have been increasingly observed over time.

The mtDNA Bottleneck and Challenge in Genetic Counselling

The variations in mutant heteroplasmy level between generations are frequently observed, and the degree of variations differs between the mutations. Such observation leads to the theory of the mitochondrial genetic bottleneck, which hypothesises that only a small proportion of the maternal mitochondrial genome is transmitted to the offspring [66]. It is increasingly evident that size of bottleneck varies between the mtDNA mutations, and a recent simulation study based upon a compilation of heteroplasmy levels from family pedigrees published in the literature and unpublished data clearly demonstrated that the rate of random genetic drift varies between mutations [67]. Tighter genetic bottleneck, such as in the case of m.8993T>G/C mutation in *MTATP6*, indicates a more rapid segregation of mtDNA heteroplasmy between generations, which explains a common scenario encountered in the clinical practice that a severely affected child with very high/near homoplasmic mutant heteroplasmy born to an asymptomatic mother who carries very low mutant load [67].

1996–2010

Maintenance Defects of Mitochondrial DNA

The maintenance and replication of mtDNA are entirely dependent on machineries encoded by the nuclear genome. Defects in these machineries result in a myriad of human disease characterised by multiple deletions and/or depletion of the mtDNA copy number in postmitotic tissues [68]. Shortly after the report of sporadic, single large-scale mtDNA deletion in 1988, there was an important observation of multiple deletions in muscle biopsies and late-onset, autosomal dominant CPEO identified in several Italian families [69, 70]. The first nuclear gene reported to cause dominant, late-onset CPEO is *SLC25A4*, which encodes for the ADP/ATP translocase 1, in 2001 [71]. On the following year, a major discovery made by Van Goethem and coworkers in Belgium was the identification of dominant and recessive mutations in *POLG*, encoding for mitochondrial polymerase gamma, caused multiple deletions in mtDNA and CPEO [72]. Mutations in *POLG* have also been associated with wider phenotypic spectrum including devastating infantile-onset Alpers syndrome, ataxia neuropathy spectrum and myoclonic epilepsy, myopathy and sensory ataxia [73], Parkinsonism and premature ovarian failure [74]. The link of POLG deficiency and mitochondrial disease is significant, as highlighted by further genetic studies that the p. Trp748Ser pathogenic variant is the founder mutation of ancient European origin with the population carrier rate of 0.8% in Finland [75] whilst the p.Ala467Thr variant can be identified in 0.69% of the British population [76]. To date, at least 14 nuclear genes have been associated with multiple deletions and CPEO phenotype of mitochondrial disease [77].

The reduction of the mtDNA copy number, also known as mtDNA depletion, was recognised as a distinctive cause of severe, infantile-onset mitochondrial disorder [78, 79] around the same time as the identification of multiple deletions in mtDNA. Broadly speaking, mitochondrial depletion syndrome is associated with four major clinical phenotypes: hepatocerebral syndrome, encephaalomyopathy, pure myopathy and neurogastrointestinal involvement [80]. The underlying molecular mechanisms include impairment in the mtDNA replication (e.g. *POLG*, *POLG2* and *TWNK*) and defects in the mitochondrial deoxynucleotide (dNTP) pool regulation (e.g. *TK2*, *DGUOK*, *RRM2B* and *TYMP*) [81]. The pathogenesis of mtDNA depletion remains elusive in some genes such as *MPV17* [82].

Clinical Rating Scales for Longitudinal Study

Whilst there are subtypes of mitochondrial disease present with isolated tissue or organ involvement such as LHON [83] and hypertrophic cardiomyopathy [84], multisystem involvement is evident in many patients when their disease progresses. However, longitudinal data detailing the disease trajectory has been generally lacking, hindering the effort of developing standardised guidelines for disease surveillance, genetic counselling and patient enrolment for clinical trials. Clinical rating scales for both adult [85] and paediatric [86] patients have been developed to address these unmet needs. The Newcastle Mitochondrial Disease Adult Scale (NMDAS) has been successfully applied on modelling disease progression of single, large-scale mtDNA deletion [87].

Establishment of the Prevalence of Mitochondrial Disease

The estimated minimal birth prevalence of mitochondrial disease is 1 in 5000 in the population, based on findings derived from two separate studies performed based on North East England and South Eastern Australia populations in the early 2000s [88–90]. Studies consistently show that in adults mtDNA mutations are more prevalent, whilst autosomal recessive nuclear defects are more common in children (Fig. 2e) [91]. A subsequent study that screened over 3000 neonatal cord blood samples from sequential live births in Northern England showed that the carrier rate of common pathogenic mtDNA mutations is 1 in 200 [92]. The discrepancy between the number of mutation carriers and clinically manifesting cases reflects that many people may harbour the mutant mtDNA heteroplasmy level below the expressing threshold and remain asymptomatic throughout their life; however, the maternal transmission of mtDNA mutations may continue inconspicuously in several generations until a proband is identified clinically.

2011–2017

Revolution of Genetic Diagnosis with the Next-Generation Sequencing

There are more than 280 nuclear genes that have been associated with mitochondrial disease to date [93, 94]. It is anticipated that more disease-causing genes will be discovered in the coming years because over 1100 proteins are localised to mitochondria, according to the inventory of mammalian mitochondrial proteins, MitoCarta 2.0 [95]. The nuclear-related mitochondrial disease can be classified based upon our understanding of the protein function, secondary defects in mtDNA and downstream biochemical defects in the OXPHOS [96, 97]. Isolated complex deficiencies are usually secondary to the defects in the structural subunits or assembly factors; in stark contrast, combined mitochondrial respiratory chain deficiencies are associated with multiple genes and pathways [98].

Next-generation sequencing (NGS), a new and high-throughput technique that allows sequencing of multiple candidate genes simultaneously, is leading to a more rapid diagnosis and increase the diagnostic yield [99]. The success of whole exome sequencing (WES) in mitochondrial disease has been reported to range from 17% to 55%, depending on the patient selection criteria [100–102]. One of the greatest challenges with the NGS is to provide proof of pathogenicity for novel variants in the known genes and perhaps more so for the new genes that have not been previously linked to any disease. Segregation study of affected and unaffected family members would help to prioritise the analysis of variants of unknown significance (VUS). Detailed understanding of clinical phenotypes and identification of other affected individuals from different pedigrees are the pivotal step of validating the diagnosis [100]. Multicentre collaboration is often required to identify these patients because many of these VUS are rare. In the circumstance of private mutations for which segregation study cannot be performed, further in vitro studies such as Western blotting, mutant cell characterisation, rescue experiment and animal modelling are required [103].

Biopsies of affected tissues and biochemical measurement of these samples are invaluable when interpreting the WES findings, and they would continue to have a major role in the diagnostic workup in mitochondrial disease for the foreseeable future. However, it is also increasingly recognised that other genetics or 'acquired' neuromuscular diseases could mimic mitochondrial disease in terms of their clinical manifestations and muscle biopsy findings [104–107], again highlighting the complexity of investigating patients with evidence of 'mitochondrial dysfunction' in some cases.

Natural History and Cohort Studies

Improvement in the diagnostic strategies with the application of NGS has solved the diagnostic conundrum of many cases of mitochondrial disease. However, risk stratification and surveillance for complications, prediction of disease progression and prognostication remain extremely challenging in the clinical setting. The limitations in the longitudinal and natural history data have created significant barriers to developing medical management guidance, determining the timing of therapeutic trial and outcome measures, which are patient-centred and clinically relevant. Furthermore, more stringent patient selection would restrict the patient recruitment from a single source, and multicentre collaboration would be imperative to achieve sufficient sample size especially for randomised controlled trials (RCT) [108]. Leading mitochondrial research groups in the UK [109], Italy [110], Germany [111], the USA and Australia have established their respective national registry of mitochondrial diseases with the endeavour to elucidate the natural history of various genotypes better and prepare for patient enrolment to clinical trials since the late 2000s.

Treatment and Emerging Therapies for Mitochondrial Disease

The Cochrane review of published clinical trials concluded that there was no evidence-based treatment for mitochondrial disease in 2012 [112]. Although there remains no cure for mitochondrial disease, there are organ-specific supportive treatments [91] that could offer alleviation of symptoms (e.g. hearing aids and cochlear implant for sensorineural deafness, ptosis surgery), reduction of disease burden (e.g. pharmacological therapy for cardiomyopathy, insulin for diabetes mellitus, antiepileptic drugs for stroke-like episodes and/or seizures) and potentially life-saving treatment (e.g. solid organ transplant [113]). Targeted treatments are available for several forms of mitochondrial disorders such as allogenic haematopoietic stem cell transplant [114] and liver transplant [115] for mitochondrial neurogastrointestinal encephalopathy caused by *TYMP* mutations, supplementation of N-acetylcysteine and metronidazole for the ethylmalonic encephalopathy [91]. The dietary supplementation of vitamins and cofactors such as riboflavin, thiamine and ubiquinone has shown clinical benefits for specific groups of mitochondrial disorder [116]; however, these findings are unlikely to be validated in large-scale RCTs given the inherent small number of patients.

Idebenone, an antioxidant and inhibitor of lipid peroxidation, is the first orphan drug that was approved for the marketing authorisation by the European Medicines Agency (EMA) for patients affected by LHON in 2015, following the report of the largest, randomised controlled trial ($n = 85$) [117] and additional data derived from the expanded access programme and case record survey [118]. Advancements in the therapeutic research for LHON are prominent in recent years, especially the gene therapy using the recombinant adeno-associated virus. In vitro study [119] and early-phase clinical trials [120] have demonstrated the safety profile and observation of visual improvement, phase III, multicentre clinical trials are currently recruiting patients to confirm the therapeutic efficacy (ClinicalTrials.gov Identifier: NCT02652780, NCT03293524).

Molecular bypass therapy aiming to restore deoxyribonucleoside triphosphate (dNTP) pools [121, 122] is emerging as a novel treatment for *TK2*-related mitochondrial depletion syndrome characterised by severe myopathy. Other nuclear gene defects implicated in the nucleoside metabolism such as *RRM2B* may also benefit from the molecular bypass therapy in theory; however, neither animal nor clinical data is currently available to support its efficacy. On the other hand, several ongoing clinical trials are evaluating small molecules including novel compounds and repurposing drugs that aim to promote mitochondrial biogenesis, stabilise mitochondrial membrane or improve efficacy of scavenging reactive oxygen species [91, 98, 123]. Although small molecule therapy is generic and unlikely to be curative, it may be more cost-effective for the drug discovery and could potentially benefit more patients and have wider applications in other neurodegenerative disorders.

Zinc finger nucleases (ZFN) [124] and transcription activator-like effector nucleases (TALENS) [125] have been used experimentally to manipulate the ratio of mutant and wild-type mtDNA in cell lines and have shown an impressive reduction of mutant heteroplasmy level below the phenotypic expression threshold. Furthermore, the use of mitoTALEN has been attempted in the mouse germ line and provided proof of concept of its potential efficacy in preventing mtDNA transmission [126]. However, neither technique would be applicable to homoplasmic mtDNA mutations nor substantial reduction in the mtDNA copy number in cell lines with subsequent recovery raises a severe concern of safety in vivo.

Reproductive Options and Mitochondrial Donation

Nuclear gene-related mitochondrial disease follows the Mendelian inheritance rules, and the risk calculation of disease recurrence can be determined unequivocally. In contrast, the prediction of transmission risk is exceptionally challenging for heteroplasmic mtDNA mutations because of the random nature of mtDNA genetic bottleneck. Several reproductive options are currently available for heteroplasmic mtDNA mutations such as prenatal diagnosis and preimplantation genetic diagnosis (PGD). The success of PGD predominantly relies on selecting embryos created via in vitro fertilisation (IVF) to harbour mutation load below the threshold level expected for the individual mtDNA mutation [94]. However, these options are not appropriate for women who harbour very high mutation load or homoplasmic mutation, which have led to the innovative development of mitochondrial donation (aka mitochondrial replacement therapy).

Mitochondrial donation is an IVF-based technique that requires healthy donor oocyte and can be performed before fertilisation using metaphase II oocytes (maternal spindle transfer, MST) or after fertilisation using pronucleate stage zygotes (pronuclear transfer, PNT). Both methods result in an embryo that contains wild-type mtDNA predominantly from the donor, hence significantly reducing the risk of transmitting mutated mtDNA whilst retaining nuclear DNAs from the biological parents [94, 127]. PNT is the technique pioneered in Newcastle [128], and a recent preclinical study with the refined method has affirmed its safety profile with a note of caution that the prevention of mutated mtDNA transmission is not guaranteed [129]. In the UK, mitochondrial donation is now a feasible reproductive option in the clinical setting after the extensive scientific and ethical scrutiny of the technique, but more crucially, the law change initiated by the active campaigning participated by patient groups, general public and the scientific community [130].

Nonhuman primate and more recent preclinical data [131] using MST method have provided some encouraging results of its safety and efficacy of preventing the transmission of mtDNA mutation. A healthy baby boy was born via the MST technique performed by the US-based medical team in Mexico in 2016; the mutant heteroplasmy levels were reported to range from 2.36% to 9.23% in different tissues [132]. Whilst this news generated a global interest on the first successful attempt of mitochondrial donation in human, this causes controversies in terms of ethical and legal considerations [133, 134].

Conclusions

The field of mitochondrial medicine has grown exponentially in the last few decades. Clinical description and pathological characterisation of individual syndromes have laid a strong foundation for the discovery of underlying genetic defects and uncovered the complexities of the dual genomic control of mtDNA, mtDNA replication and maintenance. Identification of the genetic mutations will no longer be an arduous undertaking for both patients and clinicians, with the advent of high-throughput next-generation sequencing technologies and bioinformatics. Our understanding of tissue specificity related to the underlying molecular genetic defect, phenotypic heterogeneity and epigenetics will hopefully be clarified further with better modelling systems and data derived from the omic technologies [135]. International, cross-disciplinary collaborations such as sharing of genomic data [136] and the establishment of global patient registry would facilitate the elucidation of the natural history of many mitochondrial disorders, standardisation of patient care, finding better prognostic biomarkers and perhaps, more importantly, expediting patient recruitment for the increasing number of therapeutic trials. Selection of robust outcome measures [137] and innovation of trial design will be crucial to maximising the success of translating bench findings into the clinical practice but to also reduce the burden on patients. The availability of various reproductive options including mitochondrial donation and potentially other mtDNA heteroplasmy-shifting techniques will lead to the reduction of the transmission of mtDNA mutations and eventually the prevalence of mtDNA disease.

Acknowledgments Our work is supported by the Wellcome Centre for Mitochondrial Research, Newcastle University Centre for Ageing and Vitality (supported by the Biotechnology and Biological Sciences Research Council and the Medical Research Council (MRC)), the MRC Centre for Neuromuscular Disease, the MRC Centre for Translational Research in Neuromuscular Disease Mitochondrial Disease Patient Cohort (UK), the Lily Foundation, the UK National Institute for Health Research (NIHR) Biomedical Research Centre in Age and Age-Related Diseases award to the Newcastle upon Tyne Hospitals NHS Foundation Trust and UK NHS Specialist Commissioners 'Rare Mitochondrial Disorders of Adults and Children' Service. Dr. Yi Shiau Ng holds a NIHR academic clinical lectureship (CL-2016-01-003). We would like to thank Gavin Falkous for preparing the muscle biopsy for Fig. 2. We would also like to express our gratitude to Dr. Amy Vincent for the electron microscopy figure (Fig. 2c (5)) and Dr. Julie Murphy for preparing Fig. 2d (human mitochondrial DNA).

The views expressed are those of the authors and not necessarily of the NHS, the NIHR or the Department of Health.

References

1. Mitchell P. Chemiosmotic coupling in oxidative and photosynthetic phosphorylation. Biol Rev Camb Philos Soc. 1966;41(3):445–502.
2. Gorman GS, Schaefer AM, Ng Y, Gomez N, Blakely EL, Alston CL, Feeney C, Horvath R, Yu-Wai-Man P, Chinnery PF, Taylor RW, Turnbull DM, McFarland R. Prevalence of nuclear and mitochondrial DNA mutations related to adult mitochondrial disease. Ann Neurol. 2015;77(5):753–9.
3. Bargiela D, Yu-Wai-Man P, Keogh M, Horvath R, Chinnery PF. Prevalence of neurogenetic disorders in the north of England. Neurology. 2015;85(14):1195–201.
4. Rahman S, Blok RB, Dahl HH, Danks DM, Kirby DM, Chow CW, Christodoulou J, Thorburn

DR. Leigh syndrome: clinical features and biochemical and DNA abnormalities. Ann Neurol. 1996;39(3):343–51.
5. Leigh D. Subacute necrotizing encephalomyelopathy in an infant. J Neurol Neurosurg Psychiatry. 1951;14(3):216–21.
6. Hommes FA, Polman HA, Reerink JD. Leigh's encephalomyelopathy: an inborn error of gluconeogenesis. Arch Dis Child. 1968;43(230):423–6.
7. Willems JL, Monnens LA, Trijbels JM, Veerkamp JH, Meyer AE, van Dam K, van Haelst U. Leigh's encephalomyelopathy in a patient with cytochrome c oxidase deficiency in muscle tissue. Pediatrics. 1977;60(6):850–7.
8. DeVivo DC, Haymond MW, Obert KA, Nelson JS, Pagliara AS. Defective activation of the pyruvate dehydrogenase complex in subacute necrotizing encephalomyelopathy (Leigh disease). Ann Neurol. 1979;6(6):483–94.
9. Lake NJ, Compton AG, Rahman S, Thorburn DR. Leigh syndrome: one disorder, more than 75 monogenic causes. Ann Neurol. 2016;79(2):190–203.
10. Ng Y, Turnbull D. Mitochondrial disease: genetics and management. J Neurol. 2016;263:179–91.
11. Kearns TP, Sayre GP. Retinitis pigmentosa, external ophthalmoplegia, and complete heart block: unusual syndrome with histologic study in one of two cases. AMA Arch Ophthalmol. 1958;60(2):280–9.
12. Luft R. The development of mitochondrial medicine. Proc Natl Acad Sci U S A. 1994;91(19):8731–8.
13. Luft R, Ikkos D, Palmieri G, Ernster L, Afzelius B. A case of severe hypermetabolism of nonthyroid origin with a defect in the maintenance of mitochondrial respiratory control: a correlated clinical, biochemical, and morphological study. J Clin Invest. 1962;41:1776–804.
14. DiMauro S, Bonilla E, Lee CP, Schotland DL, Scarpa A, Conn H Jr, Chance B. Luft's disease. Further biochemical and ultrastructural studies of skeletal muscle in the second case. J Neurol Sci. 1976;27(2):217–32.
15. Petty RK, Harding AE, Morgan-Hughes JA. The clinical features of mitochondrial myopathy. Brain J Neurol. 1986;109(Pt 5):915–38.
16. Engel AG, Angelini C. Carnitine deficiency of human skeletal muscle with associated lipid storage myopathy: a new syndrome. Science (New York, NY). 1973;179(4076):899–902.
17. DiMauro S, DiMauro PM. Muscle carnitine palmityltransferase deficiency and myoglobinuria. Science (New York, NY). 1973;182(4115):929–31.
18. Blass JP, Avigan J, Uhlendorf BW. A defect in pyruvate decarboxylase in a child with an intermittent movement disorder. J Clin Invest. 1970;49(3):423–32.
19. Minchom PE, Dormer RL, Hughes IA, Stansbie D, Cross AR, Hendry GA, Jones OT, Johnson MA, Sherratt HS, Turnbull DM. Fatal infantile mitochondrial myopathy due to cytochrome c oxidase deficiency. J Neurol Sci. 1983;60(3):453–63.
20. Johnson MA, Turnbull DM, Dick DJ, Sherratt HS. A partial deficiency of cytochrome c oxidase in chronic progressive external ophthalmoplegia. J Neurol Sci. 1983;60(1):31–53.
21. DiMauro S, Bonilla E, Zeviani M, Nakagawa M, DeVivo DC. Mitochondrial myopathies. Ann Neurol. 1985;17(6):521–38.
22. Morgan-Hughes JA. Mitochondrial diseases. Trends Neurosci. 1986;9:15–9.
23. Hutchison CA 3rd, Newbold JE, Potter SS, Edgell MH. Maternal inheritance of mammalian mitochondrial DNA. Nature. 1974;251(5475):536–8.
24. Giles RE, Blanc H, Cann HM, Wallace DC. Maternal inheritance of human mitochondrial DNA. Proc Natl Acad Sci U S A. 1980;77(11):6715–9.
25. Anderson S, Bankier AT, Barrel BG, de Bruijn MHL, Coulson AR, Drouin J, Eperon IC, Nierlich DP, Roe BA, Sanger F. Sequence and organization of the human mitochondrial genome. Nature. 1981;290:457–65.
26. Chomyn A, Mariottini P, Cleeter MW, Ragan CI, Matsuno-Yagi A, Hatefi Y, Doolittle RF, Attardi G. Six unidentified reading frames of human mitochondrial DNA encode components of the respiratory-chain NADH dehydrogenase. Nature. 1985;314(6012):592–7.
27. Chomyn A, Cleeter MW, Ragan CI, Riley M, Doolittle RF, Attardi G. URF6, last unidentified reading frame of human mtDNA, codes for an NADH dehydrogenase subunit. Science (New York, NY). 1986;234(4776):614–8.
28. Andrews RM, Kubacka I, Chinnery PF, Lightowlers RN, Turnbull DM, Howell N. Reanalysis and revision of the Cambridge reference sequence for human mitochondrial DNA. Nat Genet. 1999;23(2):147.
29. Ogasahara S, Engel AG, Frens D, Mack D. Muscle coenzyme Q deficiency in familial mitochondrial encephalomyopathy. Proc Natl Acad Sci U S A. 1989;86(7):2379–82.
30. Mollet J, Giurgea I, Schlemmer D, Dallner G, Chretien D, Delahodde A, Bacq D, de Lonlay P, Munnich A, Rotig A. Prenyldiphosphate synthase, subunit 1 (PDSS1) and OH-benzoate polyprenyltransferase (COQ2) mutations in ubiquinone deficiency and oxidative phosphorylation disorders. J Clin Invest. 2007;117(3):765–72.
31. Lopez LC, Schuelke M, Quinzii CM, Kanki T, Rodenburg RJ, Naini A, Dimauro S, Hirano M. Leigh syndrome with nephropathy and CoQ10 deficiency due to decaprenyl diphosphate synthase subunit 2 (PDSS2) mutations. Am J Hum Genet. 2006;79(6):1125–9.
32. Quinzii C, Naini A, Salviati L, Trevisson E, Navas P, Dimauro S, Hirano M. A mutation in Para-hydroxybenzoate-polyprenyl transferase (COQ2) causes primary coenzyme Q10 deficiency. Am J Hum Genet. 2006;78(2):345–9.
33. Lagier-Tourenne C, Tazir M, Lopez LC, Quinzii CM, Assoum M, Drouot N, Busso C, Makri S, Ali-Pacha L, Benhassine T, Anheim M, Lynch DR,

Thibault C, Plewniak F, Bianchetti L, Tranchant C, Poch O, DiMauro S, Mandel JL, Barros MH, Hirano M, Koenig M. ADCK3, an ancestral kinase, is mutated in a form of recessive ataxia associated with coenzyme Q10 deficiency. Am J Hum Genet. 2008;82(3):661–72.
34. Mollet J, Delahodde A, Serre V, Chretien D, Schlemmer D, Lombes A, Boddaert N, Desguerre I, de Lonlay P, de Baulny HO, Munnich A, Rotig A. CABC1 gene mutations cause ubiquinone deficiency with cerebellar ataxia and seizures. Am J Hum Genet. 2008;82(3):623–30.
35. Horvath R, Czermin B, Gulati S, Demuth S, Houge G, Pyle A, Dineiger C, Blakely EL, Hassani A, Foley C, Brodhun M, Storm K, Kirschner J, Gorman GS, Lochmuller H, Holinski-Feder E, Taylor RW, Chinnery PF. Adult-onset cerebellar ataxia due to mutations in CABC1/ADCK3. J Neurol Neurosurg Psychiatry. 2012;83(2):174–8.
36. Quinzii CM, Kattah AG, Naini A, Akman HO, Mootha VK, DiMauro S, Hirano M. Coenzyme Q deficiency and cerebellar ataxia associated with an aprataxin mutation. Neurology. 2005;64(3):539–41.
37. Gempel K, Topaloglu H, Talim B, Schneiderat P, Schoser BG, Hans VH, Palmafy B, Kale G, Tokatli A, Quinzii C, Hirano M, Naini A, DiMauro S, Prokisch H, Lochmuller H, Horvath R. The myopathic form of coenzyme Q10 deficiency is caused by mutations in the electron-transferring-flavoprotein dehydrogenase (ETFDH) gene. Brain J Neurol. 2007;130(Pt 8):2037–44.
38. Pavlakis SG, Phillips PC, DiMauro S, De Vivo DC, Rowland LP. Mitochondrial myopathy, encephalopathy, lactic acidosis, and strokelike episodes: a distinctive clinical syndrome. Ann Neurol. 1984;16:481–8.
39. Hirano M, Ricci E, Koenigsberger MR, Defendini R, Pavlakis SG, DeVivo DC, DiMauro S, Rowland LP. Melas: an original case and clinical criteria for diagnosis. Neuromuscul Disord. 1992;2:125–35.
40. Stoquart-Elsankari S, Lehmann P, Perin B, Gondry-Jouet C, Godefroy O. MRI and diffusion-weighted imaging followup of a stroke-like event in a patient with MELAS. J Neurol. 2008;255(10):1593–5.
41. Majamaa K, Turkka J, Karppa M, Winqvist S, Hassinen IE. The common MELAS mutation A3243G in mitochondrial DNA among young patients with an occipital brain infarct. Neurology. 1997;49(5):1331–4.
42. Ito H, Mori K, Kagami S. Neuroimaging of stroke-like episodes in MELAS. Brain Dev. 2011;33(4):283–8.
43. Sparaco M, Simonati A, Cavallaro T, Bartolomei L, Grauso M, Piscioli F, Morelli L, Rizzuto N. MELAS: clinical phenotype and morphological brain abnormalities. Acta Neuropathol. 2003;106(3):202–12.
44. Gilchrist JM, Sikirica M, Stopa E, Shanske S. Adult-onset MELAS. Evidence for involvement of neurons as well as cerebral vasculature in strokelike episodes. Stroke. 1996;27(8):1420–3.
45. Betts J, Jaros E, Perry RH, Schaefer AM, Taylor RW, Abdel-All Z, Lightowlers RN, Turnbull DM. Molecular neuropathology of MELAS: level of heteroplasmy in individual neurones and evidence of extensive vascular involvement. Neuropathol Appl Neurobiol. 2006;32(4):359–73.
46. Tanahashi C, Nakayama A, Yoshida M, Ito M, Mori N, Hashizume Y. MELAS with the mitochondrial DNA 3243 point mutation: a neuropathological study. Acta Neuropathol. 2000;99(1):31–8.
47. Lax NZ, Gorman GS, Turnbull DM. Invited review: central nervous system involvement in mitochondrial disease. Neuropathol Appl Neurobiol. 2017;43(2):102–18.
48. Hasegawa H, Matsuoka T, Goto Y, Nonaka I. Strongly succinate dehydrogenase-reactive blood vessels in muscles from patients with mitochondrial myopathy, encephalopathy, lactic acidosis, and stroke-like episodes. Ann Neurol. 1991;29(6):601–5.
49. Koga Y, Akita Y, Nishioka J, Yatsuga S, Povalko N, Tanabe Y, Fujimoto S, Matsuishi T. L-arginine improves the symptoms of strokelike episodes in MELAS. Neurology. 2005;64(4):710–2.
50. Iizuka T, Sakai F, Suzuki N, Hata T, Tsukahara S, Fukuda M, Takiyama Y. Neuronal hyperexcitability in stroke-like episodes of MELAS syndrome. Neurology. 2002;59(6):816–24.
51. Holt IJ, Cooper JM, Morgan-Hughes JA, Harding AE. Deletions of muscle mitochondrial DNA. Lancet (London, England). 1988;1(8600):1462.
52. Holt IJ, Harding AE, Morgan-Hughes JA. Deletions of muscle mitochondrial DNA in patients with mitochondrial myopathies. Nature. 1988;331(6158):717–9.
53. Wallace DC, Singh G, Lott MT, Hodge JA, Schurr TG, Lezza AM, Elsas LJ 2nd, Nikoskelainen EK. Mitochondrial DNA mutation associated with Leber's hereditary optic neuropathy. Science (New York, NY). 1988;242(4884):1427–30.
54. Wallace DC, Zheng XX, Lott MT, Shoffner JM, Hodge JA, Kelley RI, Epstein CM, Hopkins LC. Familial mitochondrial encephalomyopathy (MERRF): genetic, pathophysiological, and biochemical characterization of a mitochondrial DNA disease. Cell. 1988;55(4):601–10.
55. Goto Y, Nonaka I. Horai S. a mutation in the tRNA(Leu)(UUR) gene associated with the MELAS subgroup of mitochondrial encephalomyopathies. Nature. 1990;348:651–3.
56. Zeviani M, Moraes CT, DiMauro S, Nakase H, Bonilla E, Schon EA, Rowland LP. Deletions of mitochondrial DNA in Kearns-Sayre syndrome. Neurology. 1988;38(9):1339–46.
57. Rotig A, Colonna M, Bonnefont JP, Blanche S, Fischer A, Saudubray JM, Munnich A. Mitochondrial DNA deletion in Pearson's marrow/pancreas syndrome. Lancet (London, England). 1989;1(8643):902–3.
58. Howell N, Bindoff LA, McCullough DA, Kubacka I, Poulton J, Mackey D, Taylor L, Turnbull DM. Leber hereditary optic neuropathy: identification of the

same mitochondrial ND1 mutation in six pedigrees. Am J Hum Genet. 1991;49(5):939–50.
59. Hammans SR, Sweeney MG, Brockington M, Morgan-Hughes JA, Harding AE. Mitochondrial encephalopathies: molecular genetic diagnosis from blood samples. Lancet (London, England). 1991;337(8753):1311–3.
60. Rahman S, Poulton J, Marchington D, Suomalainen A. Decrease of 3243 A→G mtDNA mutation from blood in MELAS syndrome: a longitudinal study. Am J Hum Genet. 2001;68(1):238–40.
61. Blackwood JK, Whittaker RG, Blakely EL, Alston CL, Turnbull DM, Taylor RW. The investigation and diagnosis of pathogenic mitochondrial DNA mutations in human urothelial cells. Biochem Biophys Res Commun. 2010;393(4):740–5.
62. King MP, Attardi G. Human cells lacking mtDNA: repopulation with exogenous mitochondria by complementation. Science (New York, NY). 1989;246(4929):500–3.
63. Sciacco M, Bonilla E, Schon EA, DiMauro S, Moraes CT. Distribution of wild-type and common deletion forms of mtDNA in normal and respiration-deficient muscle fibers from patients with mitochondrial myopathy. Hum Mol Genet. 1994;3(1):13–9.
64. Guillausseau PJ, Dubois-Laforgue D, Massin P, Laloi-Michelin M, Bellanné-Chantelot C, Gin H, Bertin E, Blickle JF, Bauduceau B, Bouhanick B, Cahen-Varsaux J, Casanova S, Charpentier G, Chedin P, Derrien C, Grimaldi A, Guerci B, Kaloustian E, Lorenzini F, Murat A, Olivier F, Paques M, Paquis-Flucklinger V, Tielmans A, Vincenot M, Vialettes B, Timsit J. Heterogeneity of diabetes phenotype in patients with 3243 bp mutation of mitochondrial DNA (maternally inherited diabetes and deafness or MIDD). Diabetes Metab. 2004;30(2):181–6.
65. Moraes CT, Ciacci F, Silvestri G, Shanske S, Sciacco M, Hirano M, Schon EA, Bonilla E, DiMauro S. Atypical clinical presentations associated with the MELAS mutation at position 3243 of human mitochondrial DNA. Neuromuscul Disord. 1993;3(1):43–50.
66. Stewart JB, Chinnery PF. The dynamics of mitochondrial DNA heteroplasmy: implications for human health and disease. Nat Rev Genet. 2015;16(9):530–42.
67. Wilson IJ, Carling PJ, Alston CL, Floros VI, Pyle A, Hudson G, Sallevelt SCEH, Lamperti C, Carelli V, Bindoff LA, Samuels DC, Wonnapinij P, Zeviani M, Taylor RW, Smeets HJM, Horvath R, Chinnery PF. Mitochondrial DNA sequence characteristics modulate the size of the genetic bottleneck. Hum Mol Genet. 2016;25(5):1031–41.
68. El-Hattab AW, Craigen WJ, Scaglia F. Mitochondrial DNA maintenance defects. Biochim Biophys Acta Mol Basis Dis. 2017;1863(6):1539–55.
69. Zeviani M, Servidei S, Gellera C, Bertini E, DiMauro S, DiDonato S. An autosomal dominant disorder with multiple deletions of mitochondrial DNA starting at the D-loop region. Nature. 1989;339(6222):309–11.
70. Zeviani M, Bresolin N, Gellera C, Bordoni A, Pannacci M, Amati P, Moggio M, Servidei S, Scarlato G, DiDonato S. Nucleus-driven multiple large-scale deletions of the human mitochondrial genome: a new autosomal dominant disease. Am J Hum Genet. 1990;47(6):904–14.
71. Kaukonen J, Juselius JK, Tiranti V, Kyttala A, Zeviani M, Comi GP, Keranen S, Peltonen L, Suomalainen A. Role of adenine nucleotide translocator 1 in mtDNA maintenance. Science (New York, NY). 2000;289(5480):782–5.
72. Van Goethem G, Dermaut B, Löfgren A, Martin JJ, Van Broeckhoven C. Mutation of POLG is associated with progressive external ophthalmoplegia characterized by mtDNA deletions. Nat Genet. 2001;28(3):211–2.
73. Cohen BH, Chinnery PF, Copeland WC. POLG-related disorders. 2010 Mar 16 [updated 2014 Dec 18]. In: Pagon RA, Adam MP, Ardinger HH, et al., editors. GeneReviews® [Internet]. Seattle (WA): University of Washington, Seattle. 1916. http://www.ncbi.nlm.nih.gov/books/NBK26471/.
74. Luoma P, Melberg A, Rinne JO, Kaukonen JA, Nupponen NN, Chalmers RM, Oldfors A, Rautakorpi I, Peltonen L, Majamaa K, Somer H, Suomalainen A. Parkinsonism, premature menopause, and mitochondrial DNA polymerase gamma mutations: clinical and molecular genetic study. Lancet (London, England). 2004;364(9437):875–82.
75. Hakonen AH, Heiskanen S, Juvonen V, Lappalainen I, Luoma PT, Rantamäki M, Van Goethem G, Löfgren A, Hackman P, Paetau A, Kaakkola S, Majamaa K, Varilo T, Udd B, Kääriäinen H, Bindoff LA, Suomalainen A. Mitochondrial DNA polymerase W748S mutation: a common cause of autosomal recessive ataxia with ancient European origin. Am J Hum Genet. 2005;77(3):430–41.
76. Horvath R, Hudson G, Ferrari G, Fütterer N, Ahola S, Lamantea E, Prokisch H, Lochmüller H, McFarland R, Ramesh V, Klopstock T, Freisinger P, Salvi F, Mayr JA, Santer R, Tesarova M, Zeman J, Udd B, Taylor RW, Turnbull D, Hanna M, Fialho D, Suomalainen A, Zeviani M, Chinnery PF. Phenotypic spectrum associated with mutations of the mitochondrial polymerase γ gene. Brain J Neurol. 2006;129(7):1674–84.
77. Sommerville EW, Chinnery PF, Grainne GS, Taylor RW. Adult-onset Mendelian PEO associated with mitochondrial disease. J Neuromuscul Dis. 2014;1(2):119–33.
78. Moraes CT, Shanske S, Tritschler HJ, Aprille JR, Andreetta F, Bonilla E, Schon EA, DiMauro S. mtDNA depletion with variable tissue expression: a novel genetic abnormality in mitochondrial diseases. Am J Hum Genet. 1991;48(3):492–501.
79. Ricci E, Moraes CT, Servidei S, Tonali P, Bonilla E, DiMauro S. Disorders associated with depletion of mitochondrial DNA. Brain Pathol. 1992;2(2):141–7.
80. Nogueira C, Almeida LS, Nesti C, Pezzini I, Videira A, Vilarinho L, Santorelli FM. Syndromes associated

with mitochondrial DNA depletion. Ital J Pediatr. 2014;40(1):34.

81. Suomalainen A, Isohanni P. Mitochondrial DNA depletion syndromes-many genes, common mechanisms. Neuromuscul Disord. 2010;20(7):429–37.
82. Uusimaa J, Evans J, Smith C, Butterworth A, Craig K, Ashley N, Liao C, Carver J, Diot A, Macleod L, Hargreaves I, Al-Hussaini A, Faqeih E, Asery A, Al Balwi M, Eyaid W, Al-Sunaid A, Kelly D, van Mourik I, Ball S, Jarvis J, Mulay A, Hadzic N, Samyn M, Baker A, Rahman S, Stewart H, Morris AA, Seller A, Fratter C, Taylor RW, Poulton J. Clinical, biochemical, cellular and molecular characterization of mitochondrial DNA depletion syndrome due to novel mutations in the MPV17 gene. Eur J Hum Genet. 2014;22(2):184–91.
83. Man PYW, Turnbull DM, Chinnery PF. Leber hereditary optic neuropathy. J Med Genet. 2002;39(3):162–9.
84. Taylor RW, Giordano C, Davidson MM, d'Amati G, Bain H, Hayes CM, Leonard H, Barron MJ, Casali C, Santorelli FM, Hirano M, Lightowlers RN, DiMauro S, Turnbull DM. A homoplasmic mitochondrial transfer ribonucleic acid mutation as a cause of maternally inherited hypertrophic cardiomyopathy. J Am Coll Cardiol. 2003;41(10):1786–96.
85. Schaefer AM, Phoenix C, Elson JL, McFarland R, Chinnery PF, Turnbull DM. Mitochondrial disease in adults: a scale to monitor progression and treatment. Neurology. 2006;66(12):1932–4.
86. Phoenix C, Schaefer AM, Elson JL, Morava E, Bugiani M, Uziel G, Smeitink JA, Turnbull DM, McFarland R. A scale to monitor progression and treatment of mitochondrial disease in children. Neuromuscul Disord. 2006;16(12):814–20.
87. Grady JP, Campbell G, Ratnaike T, Blakely EL, Falkous G, Nesbitt V, Schaefer AM, McNally RJ, Gorman GS, Taylor RW, Turnbull DM, McFarland R. Disease progression in patients with single, large-scale mitochondrial DNA deletions. Brain J Neurol. 2014;137(Pt 2):323–34.
88. Chinnery PF, Johnson MA, Wardell TM, Singh-Kler R, Hayes C, Brown DT, Taylor RW, Bindoff LA, Turnbull DM. The epidemiology of pathogenic mitochondrial DNA mutations. Ann Neurol. 2000;48(2):188–93.
89. Schaefer AM, McFarland R, Blakely EL, He L, Whittaker RG, Taylor RW, Chinnery PF, Turnbull DM. Prevalence of mitochondrial DNA disease in adults. Ann Neurol. 2008;63(1):35–9.
90. Skladal D, Halliday J, Thorburn DR. Minimum birth prevalence of mitochondrial respiratory chain disorders in children. Brain J Neurol. 2003;126(8):1905–12.
91. Gorman GS, Chinnery PF, DiMauro S, Hirano M, Koga Y, McFarland R, Suomalainen A, Thorburn DR, Zeviani M, Turnbull DM. Mitochondrial diseases. Nat Rev Dis Primers. 2016;2:16080.
92. Elliott HR, Samuels DC, Eden JA, Relton CL, Chinnery PF. Pathogenic mitochondrial DNA mutations are common in the general population. Am J Hum Genet. 2008;83(2):254–60.
93. Koopman WJH, Willems PHGM, Smeitink JAM. Monogenic mitochondrial disorders. N Engl J Med. 2012;366(12):1132–41.
94. Craven L, Alston CL, Taylor RW, Turnbull DM. Recent advances in mitochondrial disease. Annu Rev Genomics Hum Genet. 2017;18:257–75.
95. Calvo SE, Clauser KR, Mootha VK. MitoCarta2.0: an updated inventory of mammalian mitochondrial proteins. Nucleic Acids Res. 2016;44(D1):D1251–7.
96. Schapira AHV. Mitochondrial diseases. Lancet. 2012;379(9828):1825–34.
97. Chinnery PF, Hudson G. Mitochondrial genetics. Br Med Bull. 2013;106:135–59.
98. Lightowlers RN, Taylor RW, Turnbull DM. Mutations causing mitochondrial disease: what is new and what challenges remain? Science (New York, NY). 2015;349(6255):1494–9.
99. Tucker EJ, Compton AG, Thorburn DR. Recent advances in the genetics of mitochondrial encephalopathies. Curr Neurol Neurosci Rep. 2010;10(4):277–85.
100. Calvo SE, Compton AG, Hershman SG, Lim SC, Lieber DS, Tucker EJ, Laskowski A, Garone C, Liu S, Jaffe DB, Christodoulou J, Fletcher JM, Bruno DL, Goldblatt J, Dimauro S, Thorburn DR, Mootha VK. Molecular diagnosis of infantile mitochondrial disease with targeted next-generation sequencing. Sci Transl Med. 2012;4:118ra10.
101. Taylor RW, Pyle A, Griffin H, Blakely EL, Duff J, He L, Smertenko T, Alston CL, Neeve VC, Best A, Yarham JW, Kirschner J, Schara U, Talim B, Topaloglu H, Baric I, Holinski-Feder E, Abicht A, Czermin B, Kleinle S, Morris AA, Vassallo G, Gorman GS, Ramesh V, Turnbull DM, Santibanez-Koref M, McFarland R, Horvath R, Chinnery PF. Use of whole-exome sequencing to determine the genetic basis of multiple mitochondrial respiratory chain complex deficiencies. JAMA. 2014;312(1):68–77.
102. Ohtake A, Murayama K, Mori M, Harashima H, Yamazaki T, Tamaru S, Yamashita Y, Kishita Y, Nakachi Y, Kohda M, Tokuzawa Y, Mizuno Y, Moriyama Y, Kato H, Okazaki Y. Diagnosis and molecular basis of mitochondrial respiratory chain disorders: exome sequencing for disease gene identification. Biochim Biophys Acta. 2014;1840(4):1355–9.
103. Legati A, Reyes A, Nasca A, Invernizzi F, Lamantea E, Tiranti V, Garavaglia B, Lamperti C, Ardissone A, Moroni I, Robinson A, Ghezzi D, Zeviani M. New genes and pathomechanisms in mitochondrial disorders unraveled by NGS technologies. Biochim Biophys Acta. 2016;1857(8):1326–35.
104. Vincent AE, Rosa HS, Alston CL, Grady JP, Rygiel KA, Rocha MC, Barresi R, Taylor RW, Turnbull DM. Dysferlin mutations and mitochondrial dysfunction. Neuromuscul Disord. 2016;26(11):782–8.
105. Joshi PR, Hauburger A, Kley R, Claeys KG, Schneider I, Kress W, Stoltenburg G, Weis J,

Vorgerd M, Deschauer M, Hanisch F. Mitochondrial abnormalities in myofibrillar myopathies. Clin Neuropathol. 2014;33(2):134–42.
106. Rygiel KA, Tuppen HA, Grady JP, Vincent A, Blakely EL, Reeve AK, Taylor RW, Picard M, Miller J, Turnbull DM. Complex mitochondrial DNA rearrangements in individual cells from patients with sporadic inclusion body myositis. Nucleic Acids Res. 2016;44(11):5313–29.
107. Pyle A, Nightingale HJ, Griffin H, Abicht A, Kirschner J, Baric I, Cuk M, Douroudis K, Feder L, Kratz M, Czermin B, Kleinle S, Santibanez-Koref M, Karcagi V, Holinski-Feder E, Chinnery PF, Horvath R. Respiratory chain deficiency in nonmitochondrial disease. Neurol Genet. 2015;1(1):e6.
108. Pfeffer G, Horvath R, Klopstock T, Mootha VK, Suomalainen A, Koene S, Hirano M, Zeviani M, Bindoff LA, Yu-Wai-Man P, Hanna M, Carelli V, McFarland R, Majamaa K, Turnbull DM, Smeitink J, Chinnery PF. New treatments for mitochondrial disease-no time to drop our standards. Nat Rev Neurol. 2013;9(8):474–81.
109. Nesbitt V, Pitceathly RDS, Turnbull DM, Taylor RW, Sweeney MG, Mudanohwo EE, Rahman S, Hanna MG, McFarland R. The UK MRC mitochondrial disease patient cohort study: clinical phenotypes associated with the m.3243A>G mutation—implications for diagnosis and management. J Neurol Neurosurg Psychiatry. 2013;84(8):936–8.
110. Mancuso M, Orsucci D, Angelini C, Bertini E, Carelli V, Comi G, Donati A, Minetti C, Moggio M, Mongini T, Servidei S, Tonin P, Toscano A, Uziel G, Bruno C, Ienco E, Filosto M, Lamperti C, Catteruccia M, Moroni I, Musumeci O, Pegoraro E, Ronchi D, Santorelli F, Sauchelli D, Scarpelli M, Sciacco M, Valentino M, Vercelli L, Zeviani M, Siciliano G. The m.3243A>G mitochondrial DNA mutation and related phenotypes. A matter of gender? J Neurol. 2014;261(3):504–10.
111. Altmann J, Buchner B, Nadaj-Pakleza A, Schafer J, Jackson S, Lehmann D, Deschauer M, Kopajtich R, Lautenschlager R, Kuhn KA, Karle K, Schols L, Schulz JB, Weis J, Prokisch H, Kornblum C, Claeys KG, Klopstock T. Expanded phenotypic spectrum of the m.8344A>G "MERRF" mutation: data from the German mitoNET registry. J Neurol. 2016;263(5):961–72.
112. Pfeffer G, Majamaa K, Turnbull DM, Thorburn D, Chinnery PF. Treatment for mitochondrial disorders. Cochrane Database Syst Rev. 2012;4:Cd004426.
113. Parikh S, Karaa A, Goldstein A, Ng YS, Gorman G, Feigenbaum A, Christodoulou J, Haas R, Tarnopolsky M, Cohen BK, Dimmock D, Feyma T, Koenig MK, Mundy H, Niyazov D, Saneto RP, Wainwright MS, Wusthoff C, McFarland R, Scaglia F. Solid organ transplantation in primary mitochondrial disease: proceed with caution. Mol Genet Metab. 2016;118(3):178–84.
114. Halter JP, Michael W, Schupbach M, Mandel H, Casali C, Orchard K, Collin M, Valcarcel D, Rovelli A, Filosto M, Dotti MT, Marotta G, Pintos G, Barba P, Accarino A, Ferra C, Illa I, Beguin Y, Bakker JA, Boelens JJ, de Coo IF, Fay K, Sue CM, Nachbaur D, Zoller H, Sobreira C, Pinto Simoes B, Hammans SR, Savage D, Marti R, Chinnery PF, Elhasid R, Gratwohl A, Hirano M. Allogeneic haematopoietic stem cell transplantation for mitochondrial neurogastrointestinal encephalomyopathy. Brain J Neurol. 2015;138(Pt 10):2847–58.
115. De Giorgio R, Pironi L, Rinaldi R, Boschetti E, Caporali L, Capristo M, Casali C, Cenacchi G, Contin M, D'Angelo R, D'Errico A, Gramegna LL, Lodi R, Maresca A, Mohamed S, Morelli MC, Papa V, Tonon C, Tugnoli V, Carelli V, D'Alessandro R, Pinna AD. Liver transplantation for mitochondrial neurogastrointestinal encephalomyopathy. Ann Neurol. 2016;80(3):448–55.
116. Distelmaier F, Haack TB, Wortmann SB, Mayr JA, Prokisch H. Treatable mitochondrial diseases: cofactor metabolism and beyond. Brain J Neurol. 2017;140(2):e11.
117. Klopstock T, Yu-Wai-Man P, Dimitriadis K, Rouleau J, Heck S, Bailie M, Atawan A, Chattopadhyay S, Schubert M, Garip A, Kernt M, Petraki D, Rummey C, Leinonen M, Metz G, Griffiths PG, Meier T, Chinnery PF. A randomized placebo-controlled trial of idebenone in Leber's hereditary optic neuropathy. Brain J Neurol. 2011;134(Pt 9):2677–86.
118. Claudia BC, Klopstock T. Use of idebenone for the treatment of Leber's hereditary optic neuropathy: review of the evidence. J Inborn Errors Metab Screen. 2017:5. https://doi.org/10.1177/2326409817731112.
119. Koilkonda RD, Yu H, Chou TH, Feuer WJ, Ruggeri M, Porciatti V, Tse D, Hauswirth WW, Chiodo V, Boye SL, Lewin AS, Neuringer M, Renner L, Guy J. Safety and effects of the vector for the Leber hereditary optic neuropathy gene therapy clinical trial. JAMA Ophthalmol. 2014;132(4):409–20.
120. Yang S, Ma SQ, Wan X, He H, Pei H, Zhao MJ, Chen C, Wang DW, Dong XY, Yuan JJ, Li B. Long-term outcomes of gene therapy for the treatment of Leber's hereditary optic neuropathy. EBioMedicine. 2016;10:258–68.
121. Garone C, Garcia-Diaz B, Emmanuele V, Lopez LC, Tadesse S, Akman HO, Tanji K, Quinzii CM, Hirano M. Deoxypyrimidine monophosphate bypass therapy for thymidine kinase 2 deficiency. EMBO Mol Med. 2014;6(8):1016–27.
122. Lopez-Gomez C, Levy RJ, Sanchez-Quintero MJ, Juanola-Falgarona M, Barca E, Garcia-Diaz B, Tadesse S, Garone C, Hirano M. Deoxycytidine and deoxythymidine treatment for thymidine kinase 2 deficiency. Ann Neurol. 2017;81(5):641–52.
123. Koopman WJ, Beyrath J, Fung CW, Koene S, Rodenburg RJ, Willems PH, Smeitink JA. Mitochondrial disorders in children: toward development of small-molecule treatment strategies. EMBO Mol Med. 2016;8(4):311–27.
124. Gammage PA, Rorbach J, Vincent AI, Rebar EJ, Minczuk M. Mitochondrially targeted ZFNs for

selective degradation of pathogenic mitochondrial genomes bearing large-scale deletions or point mutations. EMBO Mol Med. 2014;6(4):458–66.
125. Bacman SR, Williams SL, Pinto M, Peralta S, Moraes CT. Specific elimination of mutant mitochondrial genomes in patient-derived cells by mitoTALENs. Nat Med. 2013;19(9):1111–3.
126. Reddy P, Ocampo A, Suzuki K, Luo J, Bacman SR, Williams SL, Sugawara A, Okamura D, Tsunekawa Y, Wu J, Lam D, Xiong X, Montserrat N, Esteban CR, Liu GH, Sancho-Martinez I, Manau D, Civico S, Cardellach F, Del Mar O'Callaghan M, Campistol J, Zhao H, Campistol JM, Moraes CT, Izpisua Belmonte JC. Selective elimination of mitochondrial mutations in the germline by genome editing. Cell. 2015;161(3):459–69.
127. Herbert M, Turnbull D. Mitochondrial donation—clearing the final regulatory hurdle in the United Kingdom. N Engl J Med. 2017;376(2):171–3.
128. Craven L, Tuppen HA, Greggains GD, Harbottle SJ, Murphy JL, Cree LM, Murdoch AP, Chinnery PF, Taylor RW, Lightowlers RN, Herbert M, Turnbull DM. Pronuclear transfer in human embryos to prevent transmission of mitochondrial DNA disease. Nature. 2010;465(7294):82–5.
129. Hyslop LA, Blakeley P, Craven L, Richardson J, Fogarty NM, Fragouli E, Lamb M, Wamaitha SE, Prathalingam N, Zhang Q, O'Keefe H, Takeda Y, Arizzi L, Alfarawati S, Tuppen HA, Irving L, Kalleas D, Choudhary M, Wells D, Murdoch AP, Turnbull DM, Niakan KK, Herbert M. Towards clinical application of pronuclear transfer to prevent mitochondrial DNA disease. Nature. 2016;534(7607):383–6.
130. Craven L, Herbert M, Murdoch A, Murphy J, Lawford Davies J, Turnbull DM. Research into policy: a brief history of mitochondrial donation. Stem Cells (Dayton, OH). 2016;34(2):265–7.
131. Kang E, Wu J, Gutierrez NM, Koski A, Tippner-Hedges R, Agaronyan K, Platero-Luengo A, Martinez-Redondo P, Ma H, Lee Y, Hayama T, Van Dyken C, Wang X, Luo S, Ahmed R, Li Y, Ji D, Kayali R, Cinnioglu C, Olson S, Jensen J, Battaglia D, Lee D, Wu D, Huang T, Wolf DP, Temiakov D, Belmonte JC, Amato P, Mitalipov S. Mitochondrial replacement in human oocytes carrying pathogenic mitochondrial DNA mutations. Nature. 2016;540(7632):270–5.
132. Zhang J, Liu H, Luo S, Lu Z, Chavez-Badiola A, Liu Z, Yang M, Merhi Z, Silber SJ, Munne S, Konstantinidis M, Wells D, Tang JJ, Huang T. Live birth derived from oocyte spindle transfer to prevent mitochondrial disease. Reprod Biomed Online. 2017;34(4):361–8.
133. Alikani M, Fauser BCJ, García-Valesco JA, Simpson JL, Johnson MH. First birth following spindle transfer for mitochondrial replacement therapy: hope and trepidation. Reprod Biomed Online. 2017;34(4):333–6.
134. Palacios-Gonzalez C, Medina-Arellano MJ. Mitochondrial replacement techniques and Mexico's rule of law: on the legality of the first maternal spindle transfer case. J Law Biosci. 2017;4(1):50–69.
135. Joyce AR, Palsson BO. The model organism as a system: integrating 'omics' data sets. Nat Rev Mol Cell Biol. 2006;7(3):198–210.
136. Falk MJ, Shen L, Gonzalez M, Leipzig J, Lott MT, Stassen AP, Diroma MA, Navarro-Gomez D, Yeske P, Bai R, Boles RG, Brilhante V, Ralph D, DaRe JT, Shelton R, Terry SF, Zhang Z, Copeland WC, van Oven M, Prokisch H, Wallace DC, Attimonelli M, Krotoski D, Zuchner S, Gai X. Mitochondrial disease sequence data resource (MSeqDR): a global grass-roots consortium to facilitate deposition, curation, annotation, and integrated analysis of genomic data for the mitochondrial disease clinical and research communities. Mol Genet Metab. 2015;114(3):388–96.
137. Mancuso M, McFarland R, Klopstock T, Hirano M. International workshop: outcome measures and clinical trial readiness in primary mitochondrial myopathies in children and adults. Consensus recommendations. Rome, Italy, 16–18 November 2016. Neuromuscul Disord. 2017;27(12):1126–37.

Mitochondria: Muscle Morphology

Monica Sciacco, Gigliola Fagiolari, Roberto Tironi, Lorenzo Peverelli, and Maurizio Moggio

Introduction

The mitochondria are the primary ATP-generating organelles in all mammalian cells and tissues, and they contain their own DNA (mtDNA) which is maternally inherited. ATP is produced via oxidative phosphorylation through five respiratory complexes located in the inner mitochondrial membrane.

These respiratory complexes are multiple polypeptide enzymes whose subunits are encoded by genes of the nuclear DNA (nDNA) and of the mtDNA. The human mitochondrial genome contains genes encoding for 13 subunits of different respiratory complexes. These include seven subunits of complex I (NADH dehydrogenase-ubiquinone oxidoreductase), one subunit of complex III (ubiquinone-cytochrome c oxidoreductase), three subunits of complex IV (COX, cytochrome c oxidase), and two subunits of complex V (ATP synthase). Mitochondria have their own transcriptional and translational machinery, but most of the proteins located within mitochondria are encoded by the nDNA, synthesized on cytoplasmic ribosomes, and subsequently imported into the mitochondria.

M. Sciacco (✉) · G. Fagiolari · R. Tironi
L. Peverelli · M. Moggio
Neuromuscular and Rare Disease Unit, Fondazione IRCCS Cà Granda Ospedale Maggiore Policlinico, Milan, Italy
e-mail: monica.sciacco@policlinico.mi.it

For this reason, any mitochondrial genetic defect can potentially affect any cell, tissue, or organ, the degree of damage and dysfunction depending on the percentage of mutated mtDNA (i.e., mtDNA point mutations and mtDNA rearrangements), on the residual quantity of mtDNA (i.e., mtDNA depletion), on the role of the mutated mitochondrial protein gene (mainly nDNA mutations), as well as on the energy requirements of the affected tissue/organ.

Indeed, mitochondrial disorders are referred to as mitochondrial encephalomyopathies to indicate that skeletal muscle and brain tissue, due to their high energy demand, are more often involved.

Given this background, skeletal muscle tissue has always been, and it still is, the most useful and extensively used target for morphological investigations. Indeed, skeletal muscle is a post-mitotic terminally differentiated tissue with only limited regenerative capacity via satellite cell transformation. This background allows to maintain a quite stable ratio between the mutant and the wild-type mtDNA and, therefore, to highlight mitochondrial dysfunction (heteroplasmy), a condition that cannot be replicated in nucleated blood cells due to selection pressure [1]. Also, skeletal muscle tissue is easily accessible and obtainable by skeletal muscle biopsy (which can be easily performed under local anesthesia even in outpatients), and it can undergo different treatments, thus becoming available for light and

M. Mancuso, T. Klopstock (eds.), *Diagnosis and Management of Mitochondrial Disorders*,
https://doi.org/10.1007/978-3-030-05517-2_2

electron microscopy studies, for biochemical investigations (respiratory chain enzyme activities), and for DNA-RNA extraction. In this regard, the possibility to parallel biochemical findings and histochemical evidence of respiratory chain defects at single-fiber level represents an added value. Histological, histochemical, and ultrastructural alterations seen in skeletal muscle tissue affected with mitochondrial disorders are quite unique and mostly pathognomonic compared with the relatively nonspecific changes detectable in other tissues applying the same techniques [2, 3].

Light Microscopy Studies

The most exhaustive methods to visualize normal and pathological mitochondria on frozen tissue sections are the modified Gomori trichrome (MGT) and hematoxylin eosin (HE) histological stains and the histochemical methods for the demonstration of oxidative enzyme activity. More specifically, enzyme cytochemistry for the activity of succinate dehydrogenase (SDH) and cytochrome c oxidase (COX) can be considered the most reliable histochemical methods for both the correct visualization of normal mitochondria and the interpretation of the mitochondrial alterations affecting skeletal muscle [4].

Fifty years after its description, the most informative cytochemical alteration in skeletal muscle is still the ragged-red fiber (RRFs), observed on frozen tissue sections stained with the trichrome method of Engel and Cunningham (Fig. 1) [5]. It is called ragged-red because of the reddish appearance of the trichrome-stained muscle fiber following subsarcolemmal and/or intermyofibrillar proliferation of the mitochondria. The red staining is due to the strong affinity of chromotrome-2R, a lipophilic constituent of the MGT, and sphingomyelin, a complex phospholipid highly represented in mitochondrial membranes [6]. The fibers harboring abnormal mitochondria are most often type I myofibers, whose metabolism is highly oxidative; these fibers may also contain increased numbers of lipid droplets which accounts for the presence of fibers with increased lipid contents seen using histochemical methods for lipid identification (oil red, Nile red) (Fig. 2a). However, since non-mitochondrial fiber degeneration or accumulation of materials other than mitochondria may sometimes mimic RRFs formation, the application of oxidative enzyme stains is always required to confirm the nature of any suspected mitochondrial proliferation inside muscle fibers.

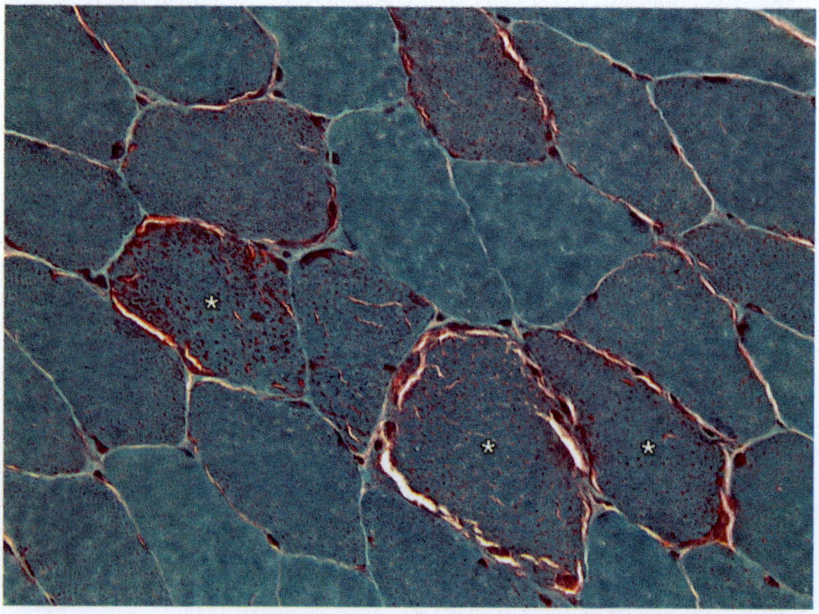

Fig. 1 RRFs (40×) modified trichrome method of Engel and Cunningham (MGT): Ragged-red fibers (asterisks) indicating proliferation of mitochondria

Succinate Dehydrogenase

Succinate dehydrogenase (SDH) is the enzyme that catalyzes the conversion of succinate to fumarate in the tricarboxylic acid cycle. It consists of two large and two smaller subunits which form complex II of the mitochondrial respiratory chain [7, 8]. Complex II is the only component of the respiratory chain whose subunits are all encoded by the nuclear genome, and this is why SDH histochemistry is extremely helpful to detect any variation in mitochondria distribution in muscle fibers, no matter which alteration affects the mtDNA. It is the most sensitive and specific stain for mitochondrial proliferation in muscle fibers and confirmation of mitochondrial dysfunction.

In normal muscle sections, histochemistry for detection of SDH activity shows two populations of fibers resulting in a checkerboard pattern. Type II fibers, which rely on glycolytic metabolism,

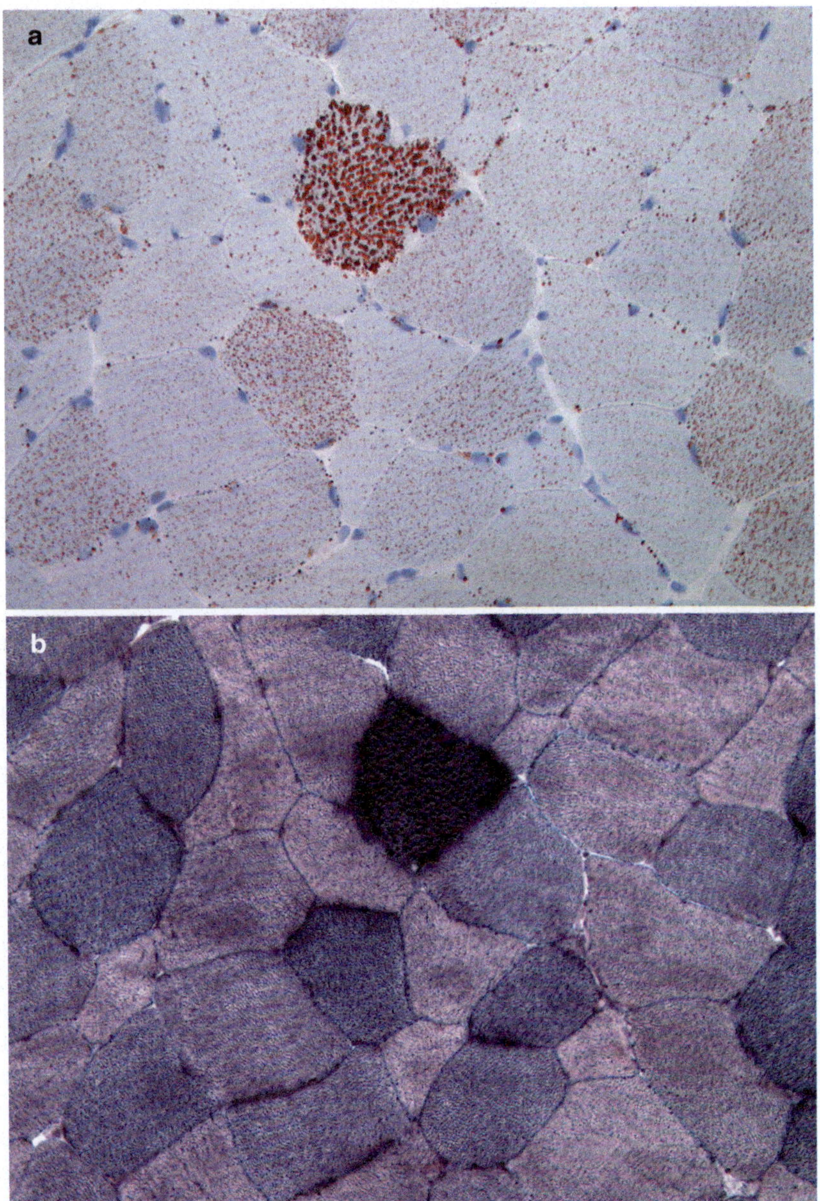

Fig. 2 Increased lipid contents in a fiber harboring abnormal mitochondrial proliferation (40×). Increased lipid droplets (**a**: oil-red-O) in a COX-negative fiber with increased mitochondria proliferation (**b**, SDH; **c**, COX-SDH)

Fig. 2 (continued)

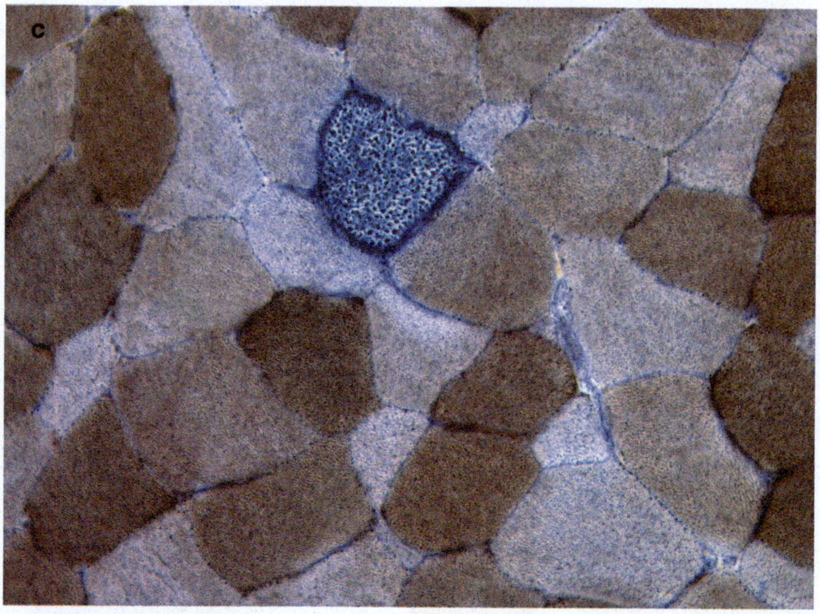

show a light blue network-like stain, whereas type I fibers, whose metabolism is highly oxidative and therefore contain more mitochondria, show a darker mitochondrial network. In samples with pathological proliferation of mitochondria (RRFs), the RRFs show an intense blue SDH reaction reflecting the distribution of the mitochondria within the fiber (ragged-blue fibers). This compensatory proliferation of mitochondria is associated with most mtDNA defects (deletions, tRNA point mutations, and depletion), as well as with defects of nDNA interfering with mitochondrial function.

RRFs are seen in defects affecting mitochondrial protein synthesis (mtDNA rearrangements and point mutations), being more frequently observed in MELAS, MERRF, and KSS and, to a lower extent, in CPEO [9, 10]. RRFs are usually absent in defects in mitochondrial protein-coding genes (LHON, NARP), though few RRFs may be seen in myopathic forms with isolated defects of complexes I, III, and IV due to mutations in mtDNA genes encoding ND subunits, cytochrome b, and COX subunits, respectively [9]. RRFs are also present in myopathic forms of mtDNA depletion syndromes [11], and also, along with lipid storage, they characterize myopathic and encephalomyopathic forms of primary CoQ10 deficiency [12].

Also, specific diseases like MELAS may show strongly SDH-reactive blood vessels (SSVs), a manifestation due to the microangiopathy which is associated with the CNS lesions, but which is evident in extra-CNS tissues as well [13].

In addition, SDH histochemistry is helpful for the diagnosis of diseases associated with complex II deficiency. In these cases, SDH activity is lacking in muscle tissue [14, 15].

Cytochrome c Oxidase

Cytochrome c oxidase (COX), or complex IV of the respiratory chain, is a multiple polypeptide enzyme composed of 13 subunits. The three largest subunits (CO I, CO II, and CO III) are encoded by mtDNA and confer the catalytic and proton-pumping activities to the enzyme. The ten smaller subunits are encoded by nDNA and are thought to provide tissue specificity by adjusting the enzymatic activity to the metabolic demands of the different tissues [16]. This peculiar COX genetic background accounts for the utility of COX histochemistry and immunocytochemistry for the investigation and the diagnosis of mitochondrial encephalomyopathies at both light and electron microscopy levels [17, 18].

As in the case of SDH, staining of normal muscle for COX activity also shows a checkerboard pattern. Type I fibers stain darker due to their mainly oxidative metabolism and more abundant mitochondrial content, and type II fibers show a finer and less intensely stained mitochondrial network.

The application of COX histochemistry to the investigation of mitochondrial disorders has been extremely relevant for the study of their pathogenesis. The activity can be absent or reduced in skeletal muscle fibers, the distribution being diffuse or in scattered fibers depending on the molecular defect and on the patient's age. The "COX-deficient fiber" is the histochemical signature of most mitochondrial disorders and represents the earliest evidence of mitochondrial dysfunction in most patients with mtDNA deletions or point mutations. It is most often associated with mitochondrial proliferation (i.e., RRFs/increased SDH activity) (Fig. 3). The fact that most RRFs are COX-negative, but not all COX-negative fibers are also RRFs, indicates that the histochemical defect precedes compensatory mitochondrial proliferation [18, 19]. Also,

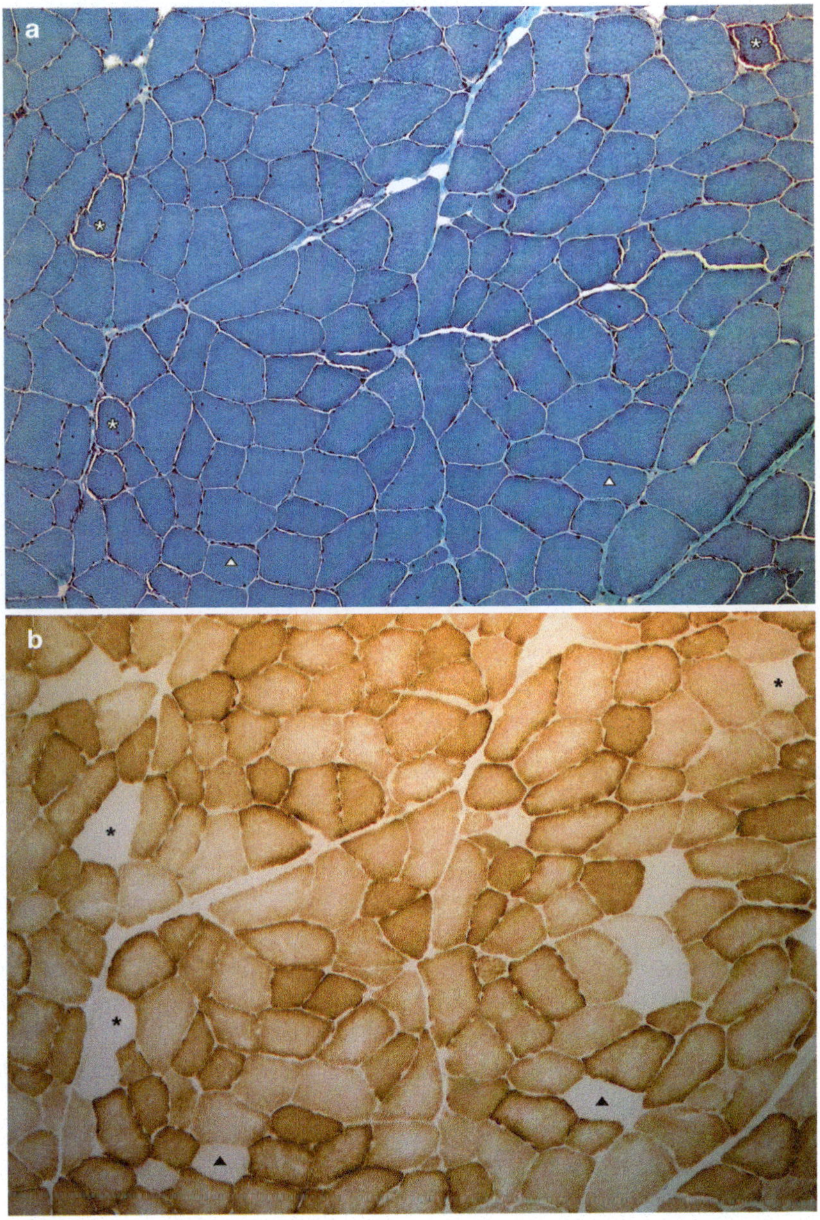

Fig. 3 COX deficiency and RRFs, **a–d** serial sections (10×). (**a**) MGT showing few RRFs (asterisks). (**b**) COX activity is lacking in the RRFs (asterisks) and in some fibers with still normal appearance at MGT (**a**, arrowheads). (**c**) SDH activity is increased in the RRFs indicating mitochondria proliferation (asterisks). (**d**) Double COX-SDH stain confirms the presence of COX-deficient fibers (blue, arrowheads). The RRFs appear dark-blue, indicating mitochondrial proliferation (asterisks)

Fig. 3 (continued)

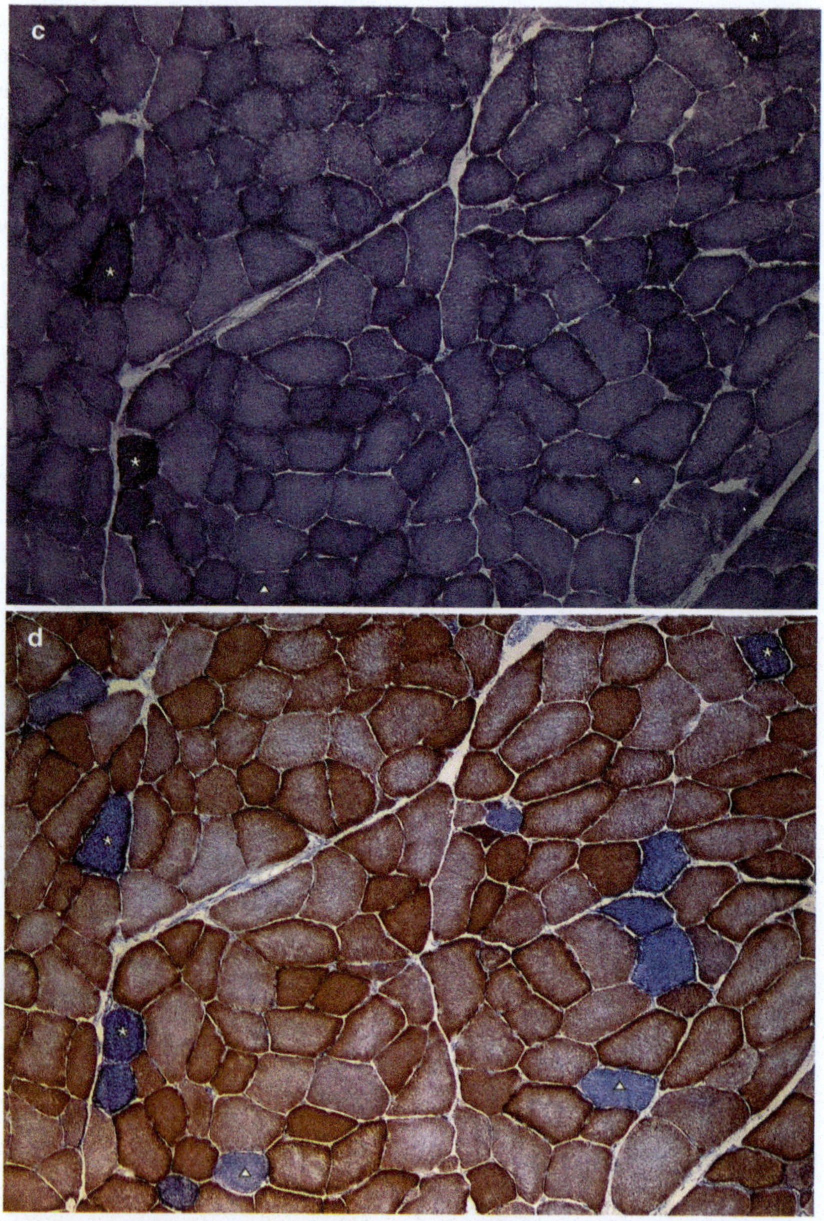

the presence of COX deficiency is extremely helpful to identify patients with mitochondrial disorders not associated with mitochondrial proliferation (normal SDH), i.e., some mutations affecting COX subunits (Fig. 4).

In patients harboring mtDNA mutations affecting mitochondrial protein synthesis (rearrangements and point mutations in mitochondrial tRNA or ribosomal RNA genes) or, rarely, mtDNA-encoded COX subunits, the mosaic distribution of COX-deficient and COX-positive fibers is an indicator of the heteroplasmic nature of the genetic defects [1, 20, 21]. A similar mosaic pattern is seen in skeletal muscle samples from patients with defects in mtDNA maintenance, especially cases of PEO with multiple mtDNA deletions, due to overlapping influences of mitochondrial and Mendelian genetics [21–23]. In contrast, Mendelian disorders due to mutations in COX assembly factors, i.e., Leigh syndrome caused by SURF1 mutations, show diffuse COX deficiency [24, 25]. A diffuse and generalized COX deficiency, possibly associated with the evidence of COX-negative RRFs, is observed in infants with depletion of muscle mtDNA or with either the fatal or the benign infantile COX deficiency [26].

In some cases, however, muscle histochemistry shows the presence of SDH-intense fibers

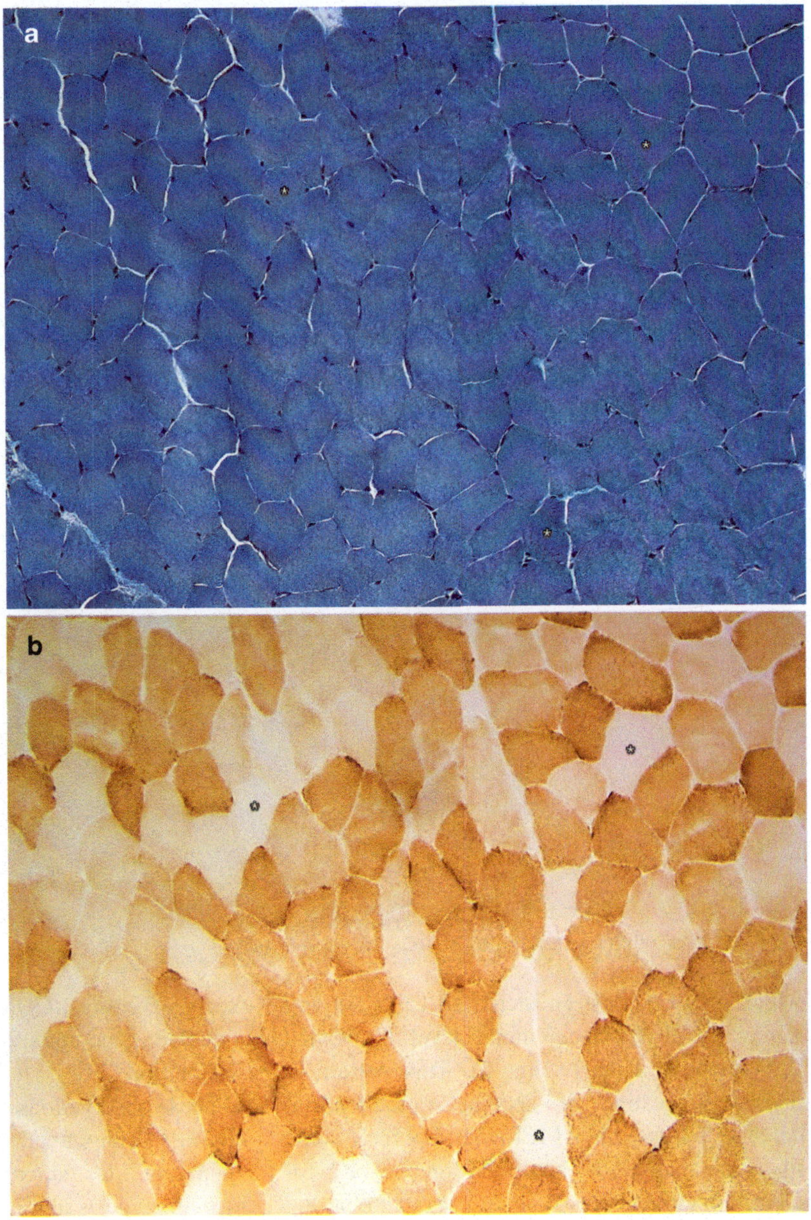

Fig. 4 Isolated COX deficiency, **a–d** serial sections (10×). MGT (**a**) is normal, but several fibers show reduced or absent COX activity (**b**, some COX-negative fibers indicated with asterisks). SDH activity (**c**) is not increased in COX-negative/COX-deficient fibers indicating lack of mitochondrial proliferation as confirmed by double COX-SDH stain (**d**)

Fig. 4 (continued)

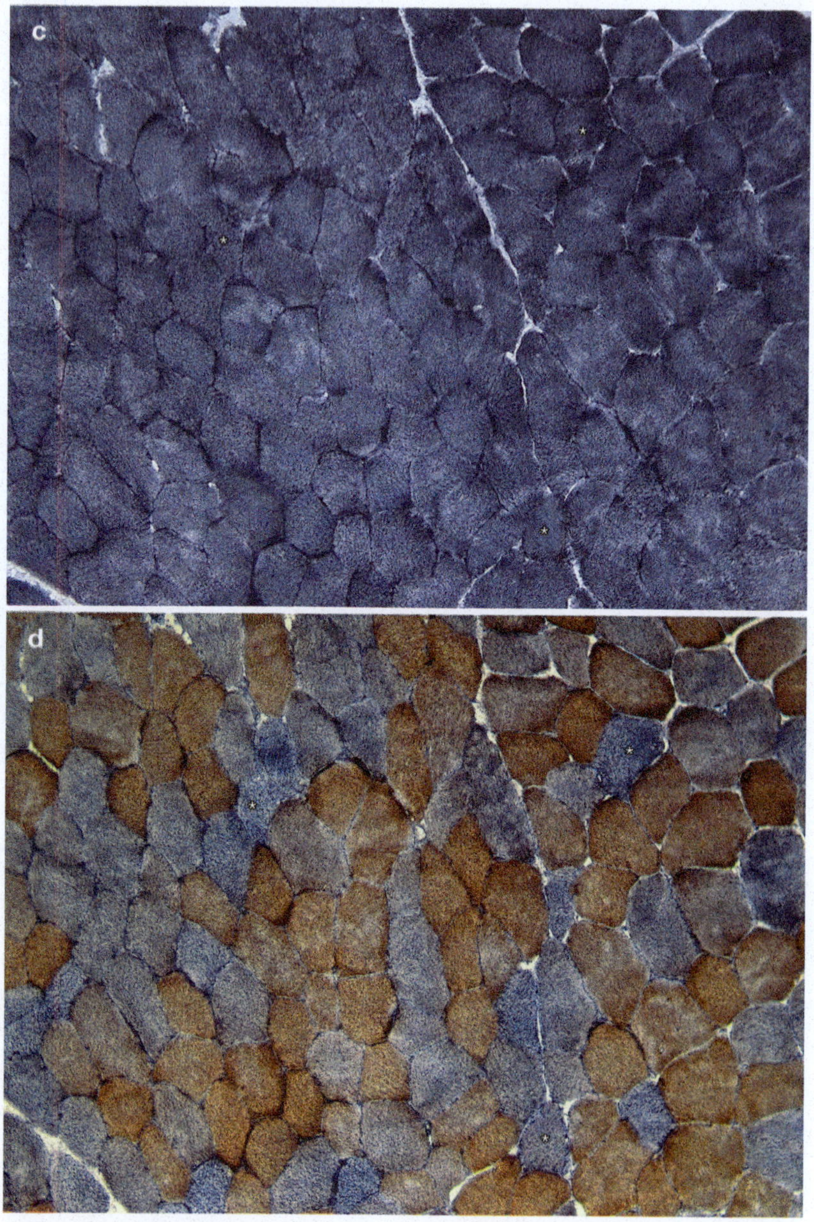

which also manifest an increased COX activity especially at subsarcolemmal level (so called COX-positive RRFs) (Fig. 5). This pattern is highly suggestive of specific mitochondrial defects, for example MELAS, in which some fibers are both COX- and SDH-intense, or cytochrome b defects, in which all fibers with strong SDH activity are also COX-positive. Similar patterns can be seen in mutations in certain mtDNA protein-encoding genes (e.g., ND mutations), except, of course, COX genes, and in mutations in nuclear gene mutations causing mitochondrial dysfunction [27].

These observations indicate that cytochemical studies in mitochondrial disorders can provide significant information about both the nature and the pathogenesis of mitochondrial disorders. As a consequence, they provide useful clues as to which molecular testing is needed to provide a specific diagnosis.

SDH-COX Double Stain

An extremely useful method to easily detect and highlight COX-negative fibers is to stain the same section for COX and SDH activities [2, 28]. In samples from patients with COX deficiency, this double stain shows a mosaic of brown (COX-positive) and blue (COX-negative) fibers, and, if RRFs are also present, they appear more intensely bluish. In patients affected with MELAS (due to tRNA-Leu point mutation), muscle biopsies can show both COX-negative and COX-positive RRFs. In the latter case, COX activity tends to be decreased in the center of the fibers but typically preserved and intense in the subsarcolemmal regions.

Also, SDH-COX double-stain technique has proven extremely useful for studies on longitudinal muscle sections. Indeed, examination of longitudinal double-stained cryostat sections has demonstrated that COX deficiency and

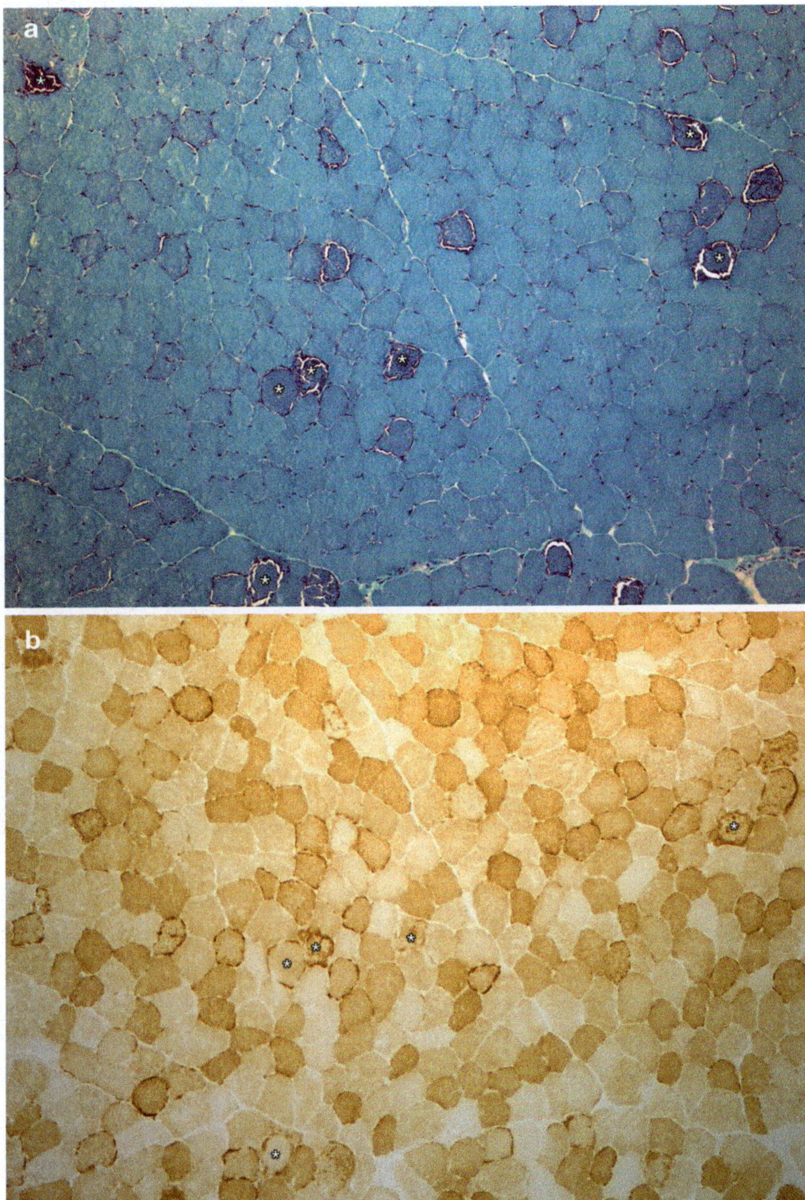

Fig. 5 MELAS (10×). (**a**) MGT showing several RRFs (some indicated with asterisks). (**b**) COX activity is increased at subsarcolemmal level in some RRFs (asterisks). (**c**) SDH activity is increased in the RRFs indicating mitochondria proliferation (asterisks). (**d**) Double COX-SDH stain confirms the presence of RRFs (asterisks)

Fig. 5 (continued)

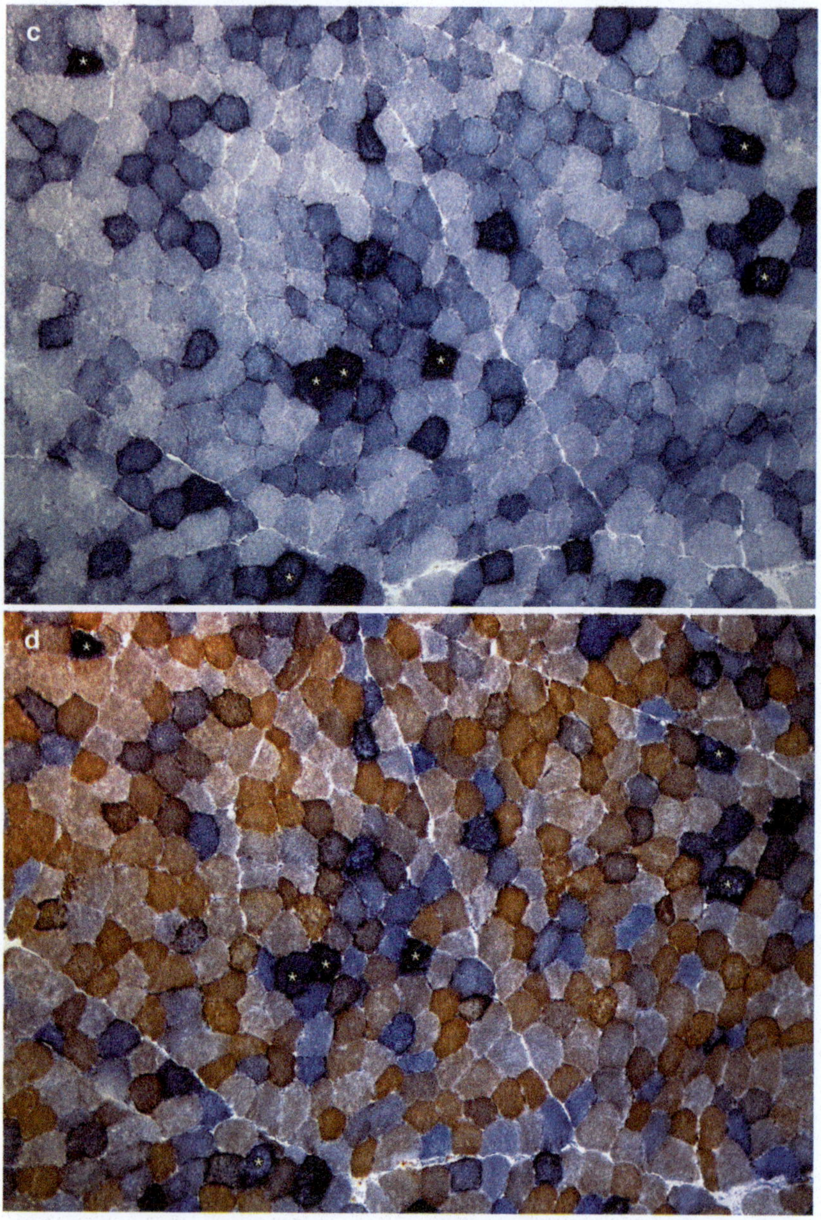

mitochondria proliferation (RRFs) are segmentally distributed over the length of the muscle fiber. There is a direct correlation between deficient oxidative phosphorylation and the segmental changes, thus confirming that COX deficiency and abnormal proliferation of mitochondria are secondary to defective respiratory chain function (Larsson and Oldfors 2001) (Fig. 6).

This histochemical method has proven quite relevant for the development of pathogenetic studies aiming at studying the distribution of mutated mtDNA molecules at single muscle fiber level in patients affected with mtDNA deletions or point mutations. These studies have been carried out by single-fiber PCR-based methods consisting in the amplification of DNA extracted from microdissected single-fiber segments.

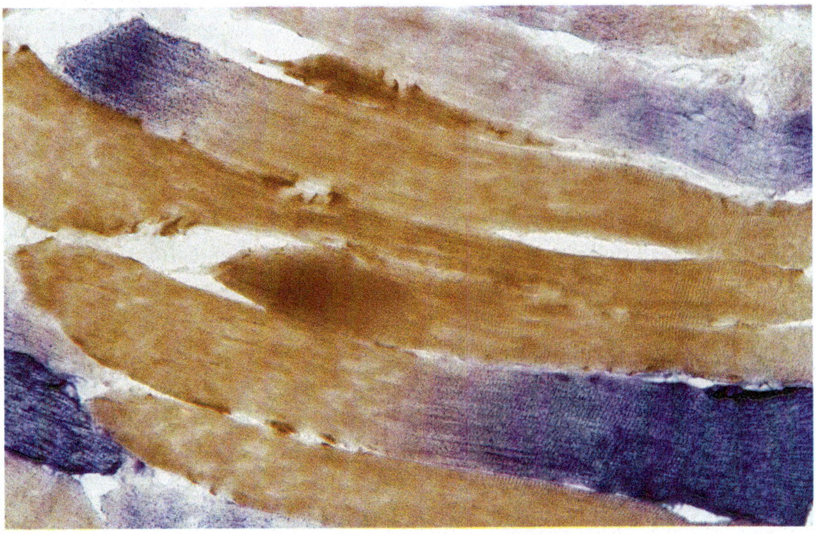

Fig. 6 Longitudinal cryostat section double-stained for COX and SDH (40×). COX deficiency and mitochondria proliferation (RRFs) are segmentally distributed over the length of the muscle fiber

All these studies have demonstrated that phenotypically affected fibers contain much higher amounts of either deleted or point-mutated mtDNA molecules compared with normal (COX-positive) muscle fibers and that the amount of defective molecules is directly proportional to the severity of the fiber phenotype. More specifically, these studies have indicated that a threshold ratio between mutated and wtDNA must be achieved before a respiration impairment is observed in skeletal muscle [29–31].

This threshold is quite variable depending on the mutation type, and in skeletal muscle, it can be as high as over 90% for tRNA point mutations, whereas it tends to be lower (70–80%) in large-scale mtDNA deletion [29, 32]. In addition, the mutation load in polypeptide-coding genes can determine the clinical phenotype, namely, the same mutation can be responsible for different diseases depending on the percentage of mutated mtDNA. For example, the m.8993TtoG mutation in the ATP synthase 6 (ATP6) gene manifests as maternally inherited Leigh's syndrome (MILS) at mutation loads above 90% and with neuropathy, ataxia, and retinitis pigmentosa (NARP) in the 70–90% range. By contrast, patients with 70% mutation in a tRNA will rarely display overt disease [33].

Myopathology of Pediatric Mitochondrial Disorders

Pediatric presentations of mitochondrial disorders are often more difficult to define than adult forms. Neonatal or early infantile diseases often manifest with severe progressive encephalomyopathy, with multi-organ involvement such as cardiomyopathy or hepatopathy and myopathic involvement suggested by hypotonia, muscle weakness, wasting, and arthrogryposis [34–37]. Over 90% of pediatric patients carry mutations in their nuclear genes causing defective OXPHOS [38]. This explains why the typical mosaic of COX-positive and RRFs/COX-negative fibers is an uncommon finding in infantile muscle biopsies. In biopsies of these patients, RRFs and/or COX-negative fibers were demonstrated in 89% of biopsies with mtDNA mutations, but only in 17% of biopsies without detectable mtDNA mutations in a large series of 117 children with mitochondrial disorders [39].

Typical examples of diffuse infantile COX deficiency in skeletal muscle are the fatal infantile COX deficiency, also affecting the heart and brain, which is linked to autosomal recessive mutations in COX assembly factors (SCO2, COX15, COA5, and COA6) [40–43] and the severe, but reversible, infantile mitochondrial myopathy with COX deficiency caused by a homoplasmic mutation in mitochondrial tRNAGlu. The latter form can be associated with the presence of RRFs in muscle biopsy [44, 45]. The biopsy features in reversible and irreversible, fatal COX deficiency in the neonatal period are identical, and in both conditions, the histochemical defect is restricted to extrafusal myofibers, sparing intrafusal muscle fibers and vascular smooth muscle [45–48].

RRFs and COX-negative fibers, along with increased lipid content, are frequently observed in skeletal muscle samples from children with mtDNA depletion syndromes secondary to defects in nuclear genes involved in mtDNA maintenance and in CoQ10 deficiency [35]. In the majority of cases, COX-deficient fibers prevail over RRFs, and they may be the only abnormal finding in muscle biopsies (Fig. 7a, b) [49] suggesting that the compensatory proliferative response may develop over time to form RRFs. In neonates, there may be no detectable light microscopic abnormalities [50], and, in addition, the small size of fibers in biopsies from neonates and infants may make the morphological

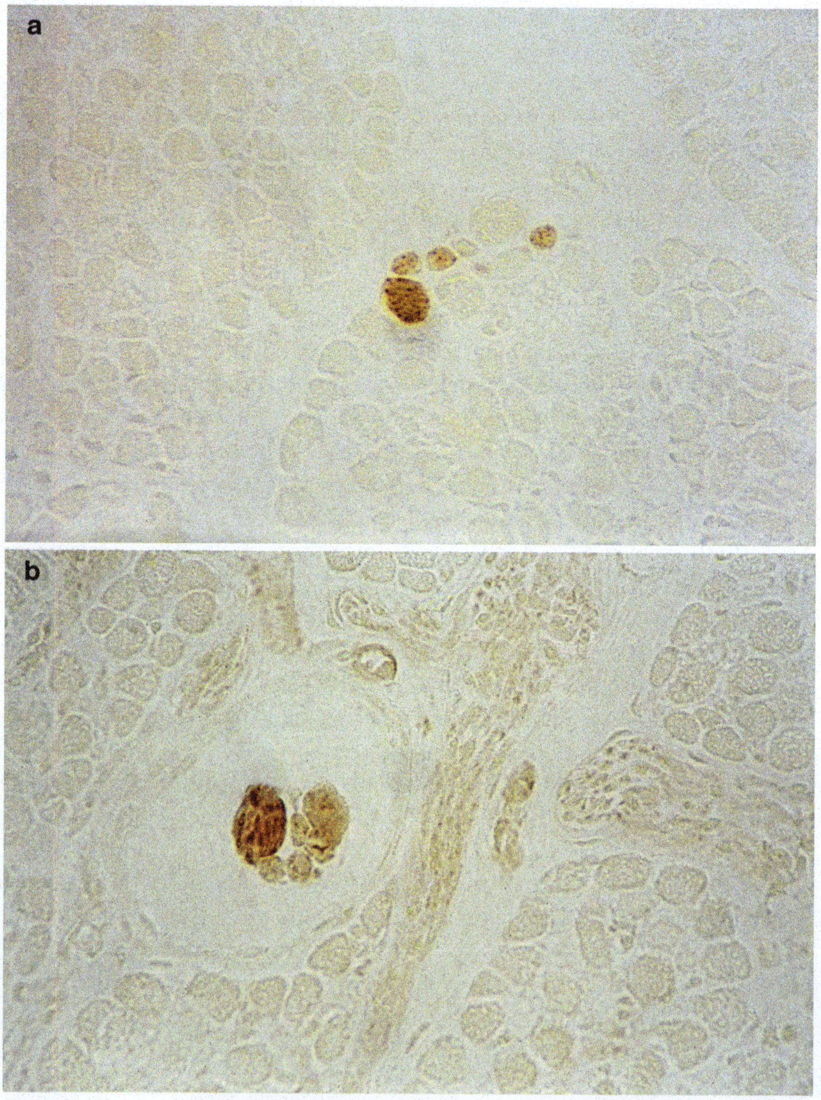

Fig. 7 MtDNA depletion. (**a–b**) (10×) Very severe COX deficiency in a case of mtDNA depletion. COX activity is preserved only in scattered muscle fibers (**a**) and in a neuromuscular spindle (**b**). (**c–d**) (40×) Immunolocalization of DNA. In normal muscle, anti-DNA antibodies stain both nuclei and mitochondrial network (**c**). In case of mitochondrial DNA depletion, only nuclear DNA is detected (**d**)

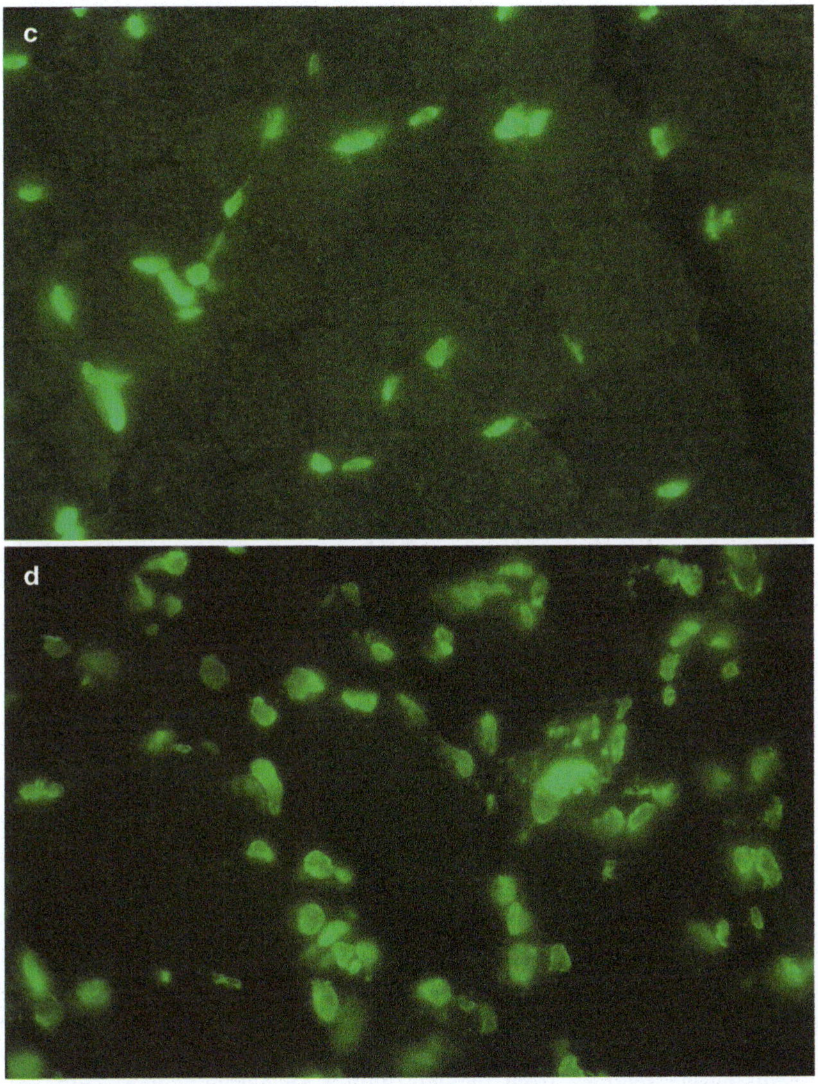

Fig. 7 (continued)

abnormalities harder to recognize. It has been suggested that SDH-positive subsarcolemmal mitochondrial aggregates (SSMA) representing a milder form of mitochondrial proliferation are more prevalent in pediatric mitochondrial disorders [20].

Immunocytochemistry

Immunocytochemistry has a relevant role in the study of mitochondrial disorders because it allows the detection of specific proteins in single cells, and it is therefore the method of choice to study the expression of both mtDNA and nDNA genes in mitochondria of small and heterogeneous tissue samples.

Several immunological probes are available to perform immunocytochemical studies of mitochondria on frozen tissue sections. These include antibodies directed against mtDNA- and nDNA-encoded subunits of the respiratory chain complexes and antibodies against DNA that allow the detection of mtDNA. The availability of these has made it possible to study the expression of these peptides in COX-deficient RRFs from patients with deletions and depletion of mtDNA [19, 51].

There are several immunocytochemical methods for the study of mitochondria on tissue sections. These include enzyme-linked methods (peroxidase, alkaline phosphatase, and glucose oxidase) and methods based on the application of fluorochromes [52]. We favor the use of fluorochromes because they allow for the direct visualization of the antigen-antibody binding sites and because they are more suitable for double-labeling experiments on frozen tissue sections. Double-labeling studies allow the visualization of two different probes in the same mitochondrion/mitochondria and in the same plane of section, thus eliminating the biases that can arise from studies made on serial sections.

Immunolocalization of Nuclear DNA- and Mitochondrial DNA-Encoded Subunits of Respiratory Chain

Routinely, polyclonal antibodies against two mtDNA-encoded peptides, subunit 2 of COX (COX-II) and subunit 1 of complex I (ND-1), are used as probes for mtDNA-encoded proteins, whereas a monoclonal antibody against the nDNA-encoded subunit IV of COX (COX-IV) is used as probe for nDNA-encoded mitochondrial protein.

Using muscle sections from normal samples, a checkerboard pattern resembling the one described for histochemistry is usually observed, type I fibers appearing brighter due to their higher mitochondria content.

In muscle sections from patients with KSS harboring an mtDNA macrodeletion, all subunits are normally present in nonaffected fibers. Conversely, in COX-deficient RRFs, we have found lack or marked reduction of mtDNA-encoded subunits associated with normal immunostain with antibodies directed against the nDNA-encoded COX-IV subunit. Because the defective mtDNA subunits were seen even with mtDNA deletions not involving the genes for these subunits, it can be concluded that the mitochondrial genome functions as a single genetic unit rather than a series of individual genes [19]. Most probably, the deletion eliminates essential tRNA genes that are required for mitochondrial translation of all 13 mtDNA-encoded subunits of the respiratory chain [53, 54]. Consequently, a deletion anywhere in the mitochondrial genome can affect translation of all genes [19, 55].

Immunolocalization of Mitochondrial DNA

Immunological probes against mtDNA and nDNA subunits can be also applied to the study of children with mtDNA depletion [26]. Muscle histochemistry of these patients shows a mosaic of COX-positive and COX-negative fibers, numerous RRFs, and severe lipid storage. COX-deficient RRFs from these patients shows marked mtDNA depletion which accounts for the immunocytological lack or marked reduction of mtDNA-encoded subunits associated with normal or increased immunostain for nDNA-encoded COX-IV, similar to what was observed in patients with KSS and mtDNA deletions. Depletion of mtDNA in some fibers can be so severe that mitochondria contain less than one copy of mtDNA per mitochondrion [26, 51, 56–58].

Another useful immunocytochemical approach is represented by the use of antibodies against DNA [59] which serves as an alternative method to in situ hybridization for the studies of localization and distribution of mtDNA in normal and pathological conditions [26]. The method has the main advantages that both mitochondrial and nuclear DNA are detected simultaneously at the single cell level and that the nuclear signal can be used as an internal control. In normal muscle, these antibodies stain both nuclei and mitochondrial network (Fig. 7c, d).

In patients with depletion of mtDNA, the nuclei stain normally, but there is lack or marked reduction of the particulate cytoplasmic stain of mitochondria (Fig. 7c, d). In contrast, the cytoplasmic stain is enhanced in RRFs from patients with other mitochondrial myopathies. This approach in conjunction with in situ hybridization has facilitated the diagnosis of mtDNA depletion [26, 51, 59].

Electron Microscopy

The first description of mitochondrial ultrastructure in human skeletal muscle dates back to the 1960s [60–62].

Mitochondria are double membrane organelles whose size and shape, the latter oscillating between tubular and spherical, are determined by the interaction between fusion and fission processes (see below/before). They are endowed with an inner and an outer mitochondrial membrane (IMM and OMM, respectively). The space between the two membranes is called intermembrane space, whereas the core, surrounded by the IMM, is known as mitochondrial matrix. The IMM bends inward toward the matrix to form a series of tubular invaginations called cristae. In normal mitochondria, the matrix is a single space which contains enzymes involved in biochemical and biosynthetic processes, as well as several copies of the mitochondrial genome.

Pathological modifications of mitochondria at electron microscopy examination can affect their number as well as their shape and size. Indeed, one of the hallmarks in mitochondrial disorders is the proliferation of abnormally shaped and enlarged mitochondria in both subsarcolemmal and intermyofibrillar spaces. Affected mitochondria can be as big as 3–4 sarcomeres in length.

The changes in mitochondria shape and size are often the ultimate expression of pathological modifications of the organelle structure which ultimately results in a loss of their function.

More specifically, abnormal mitochondrial ultrastructure, particularly modifications of the highly conserved IMM cristae, where a number of OXPHOS enzymes are located, alters the efficiency of the mitochondrial machinery which implies the existence of a correlation between mitochondrial ultrastructure and function. Understanding the mechanisms underlying modifications of mitochondrial ultrastructure and related functions may help elucidate the pathophysiology of human mitochondrial diseases [63].

The main alterations observed in mitochondrial structures in patients affected with mitochondrial disorders are the following:

Paracrystalline (Parking Lot) Inclusions (PCIs)

PCIs present as rigid rectangular or square-shaped crystals consisting of stacked sheets arranged with regular geometrical periodicity either obliquely or in parallel to the length of the inclusions. They can occupy both the intracristae and the intermembrane mitochondrial space causing the disruption of IMM and OMM. They commonly occur in fibers with mitochondrial proliferation and are more prevalent in mitochondria located in the subsarcolemmal region though they can also affect mitochondria in the intermyofibrillar space (Fig. 8).

Cristae Modifications

In affected mitochondria, cristae may undergo linearization of their membrane and become abnormally shaped (giant mitochondria), more often angular or variously geometric. Linear cristae segments show enhanced electron density or electrondense inclusions, suggesting the presence of large molecular weight proteins and/or substantial change in membrane lipid composition. Also, cristae may lose their physiological interspace and be arranged in concentric cristae compartments free of fenestration which give mitochondria an "onion-like" shape (Fig. 9).

In all these cases, the IMM loses its regular shape, characterized by periodical invaginations (cristae), which reflects mitochondria loss of function.

The ultimate expression of cristae disruption is represented by mitochondrial compartmentalization which consists in the formation of membrane-bound submitochondrial compartments located in the mitochondrial matrix either centrally or close to the IMM. In both cases, these electrondense structures, usually round-shaped, cause the loss of the normal cristae structure and of the cristae-IMM junction. 3-D studies on mitochondria have shown that these compartments have no connection with the OMM (review). Submitochondrial compartmentalization could be the product of partial fusion processes among mitochondria due to OMM fusion without concomitant IMM fusion. Thus, the result is a single expanded mitochondrion containing multiple matrix spaces belonging to the original smaller mitochondria [64].

Parallel to this, focal distensions of the OMM can be observed with associated release of mitochondrial matrix content into the cytoplasm.

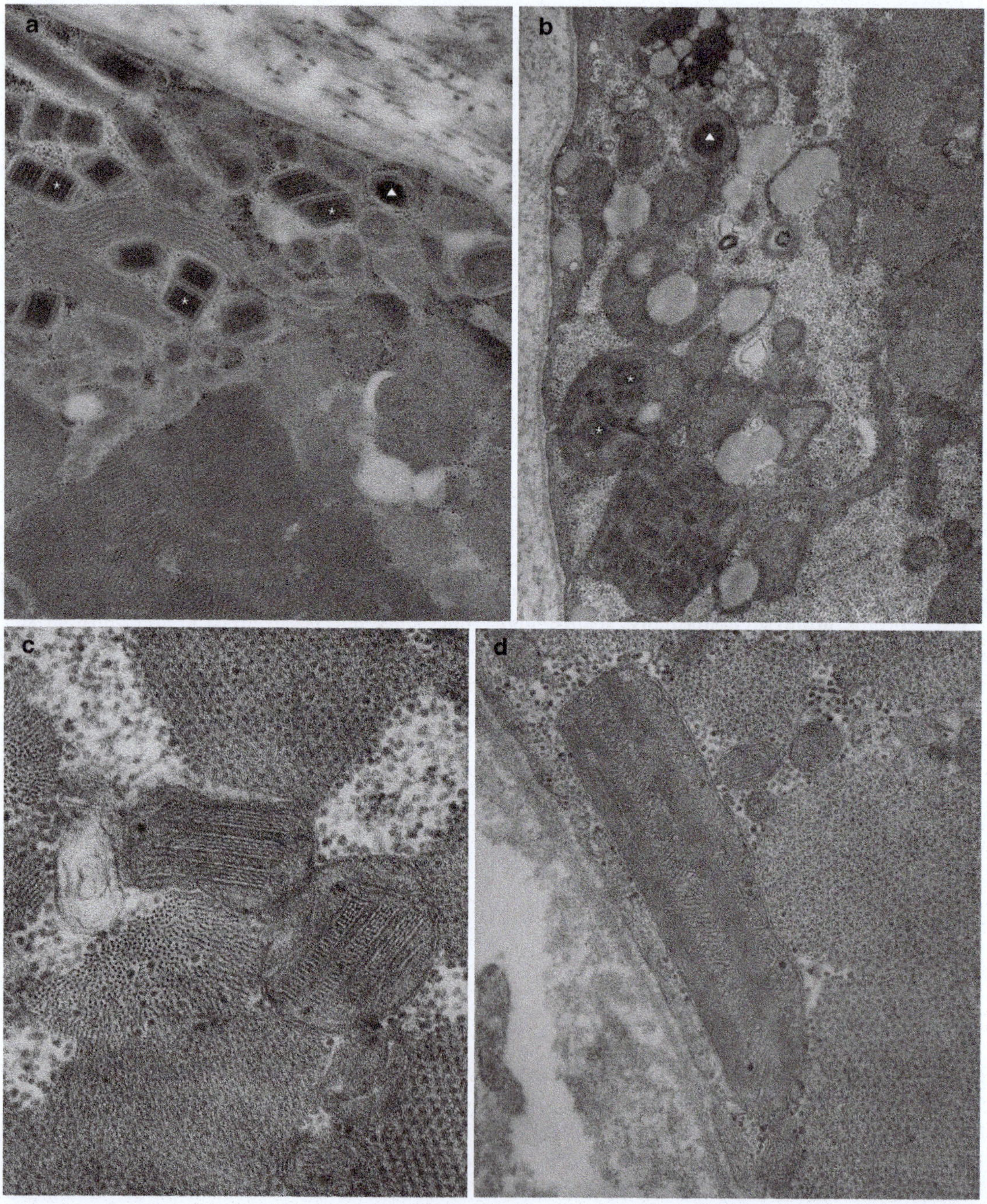

Fig. 8 RRFs. (**a**–**b**) Mitochondria proliferation in RRFs. Mitochondria often contain paracrystalline (asterisks) and globular (arrowhead) osmophilic inclusions [**a** 12000×; **b** 6000×]. (**c**–**d**) Isolated abnormally shaped mitochondria with paracrystalline inclusions [**c**–**d** 30000×]

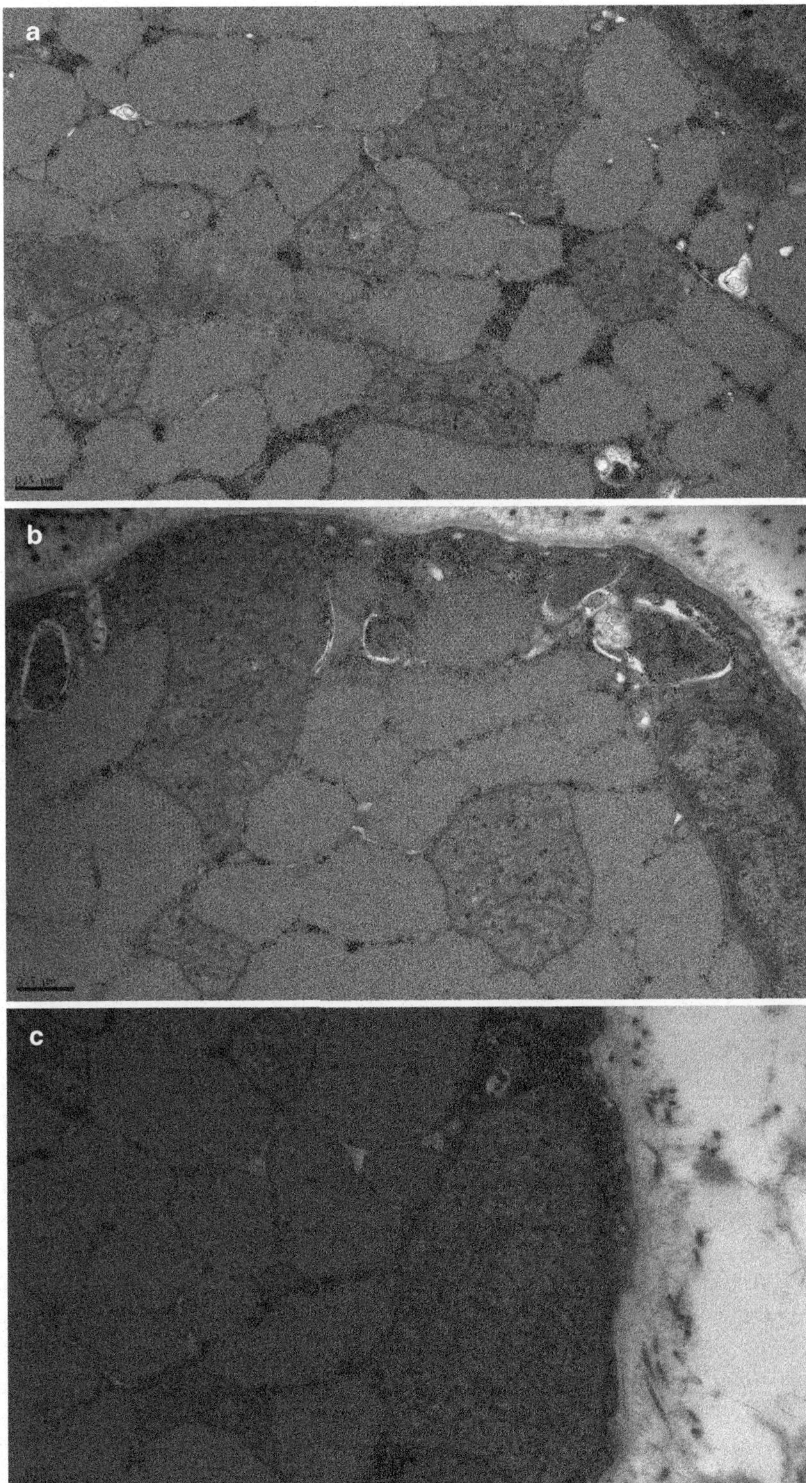

Fig. 9 Giant mitochondria. (**a**–**c**) Isolated giant mitochondria with disarray and abnormal shape of the cristae. One giant mitochondrion (**d**) contains paracrystalline inclusions and shows parallel arrangement of the cristae [**a** 25000×; **b** 30000×; **c** 30000; **d** 20000×]

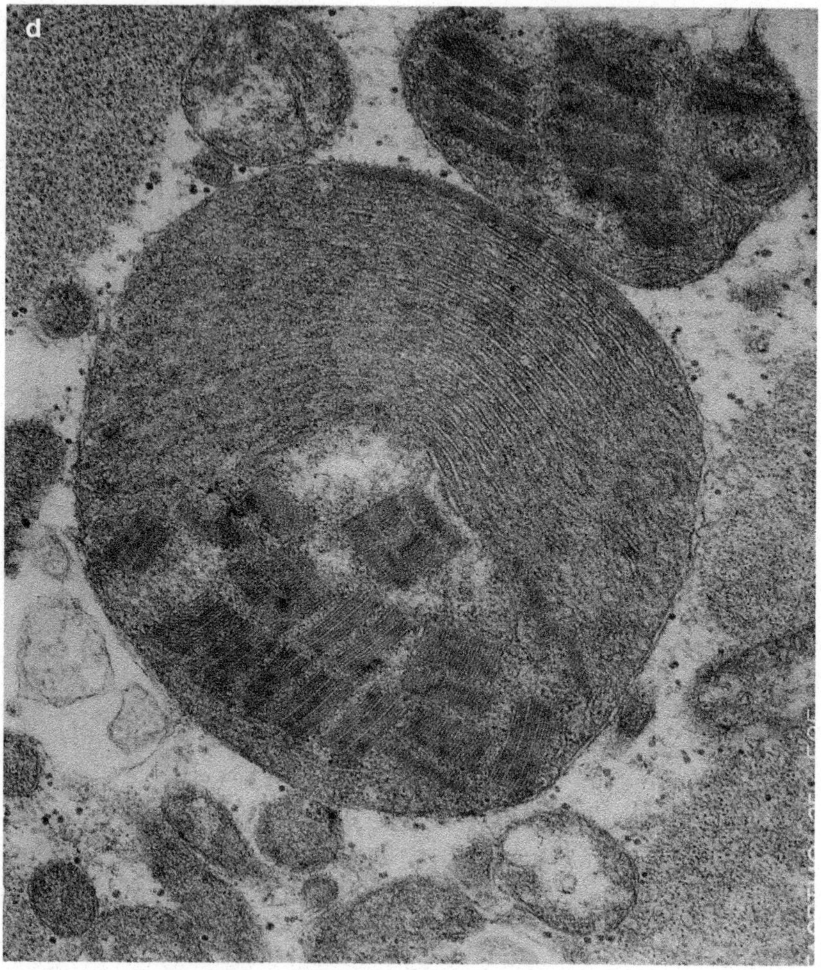

Fig. 9 (continued)

Mitochondria Hyperbranching

Mitochondria elongation or hyperbranching is the result of an unbalance between fission and fusion, more specifically of an increased fusion vs. a lack of fission. In vitro studies [65–67] have demonstrated that mitochondria hyperbranching is directly proportional to the mutational load and/or to the age process which would make hyperbranching an indicator of mitochondrial dysfunction.

Fission and Fusion

As it has already been said, mitochondria are central to several vital cell functions, more specifically ATP generation via OXPHOS, regulation of programmed cell death, calcium homeostasis, fatty acid oxidation and nuclear gene expression, biosynthesis of heme complexes, and release of immunogenic pro-inflammatory molecules. For this reason, mitochondria need to be highly dynamic cellular organelles, with the ability to change size, shape, position, and, consequently, function, over the course of a few seconds to meet the physiological needs of the cell.

These changes mainly depend on their ability to undergo the processes of fission, i.e., the division of a single mitochondrion into two or more independent organelles, and fusion, meant as the ability of fusing together forming a single closed network [68]. These actions occur simultaneously and continuously in many cell types under the regulation of specific proteins which act on mitochondrial membranes and organelle interactions.

In detail, the scission of the membrane is carried out by dynamin, a mechanical enzyme that forms tight spirals around the neck of vesicles to constrict and then cleave them off. Dynamin is a GTPase that provides the mechanical forces required for organelle division by using the energy from GTP hydrolysis. Many of the proteins involved in mitochondrial fission and fusion are members of the dynamin GTPase protein family.

Also, changes in the biophysical properties of lipids in mitochondrial membranes are now being seen as another aspect in the regulation of organelle morphology [69]. The appearance of mitochondria within cells is a result of the balance between the forces of fission and fusion, a slight increase in one or the other being enough to change the organelle morphology [70].

Mitochondrial fission and fusion are critical events in a number of cellular processes, and removal of either one can compromise the long-term viability of the cell (Fig. 10).

Mitochondrial Morphology as a Tool for Basic Research and Treatment Implications

Muscle immunohistochemistry and ultrastructure have recently proven very useful in a series of experimental in vivo studies focusing on possible treatments for mitochondrial disorders. So far, there are no effective treatments for mitochondrial disorders, and clinical management is mostly based on treating complications. Stimulation of mitochondriogenesis and MRC activity is one of the strategies that have been proposed to correct OXPHOS failure leading to these conditions. More specifically, great attention has been given to the potential treatment implications of two systems, PPARs and AMPK/PGC-1a, known to increase mitochondrial aerobic metabolism, acting on genes related to mitochondrial bioenergetic pathways.

The hypothesis has been tested by activating the homeostatic pathways of these two systems on three recombinant mouse models characterized by defective cytochrome c oxidase (COX) activity: a knockout (KO) mouse for Surf1, a knockout/knockin mouse for Sco2, and a muscle-restricted KO mouse for Cox15. The study demonstrated that treatment with the AMPK agonist AICAR leads to partial correction of COX deficiency in all three models associated with

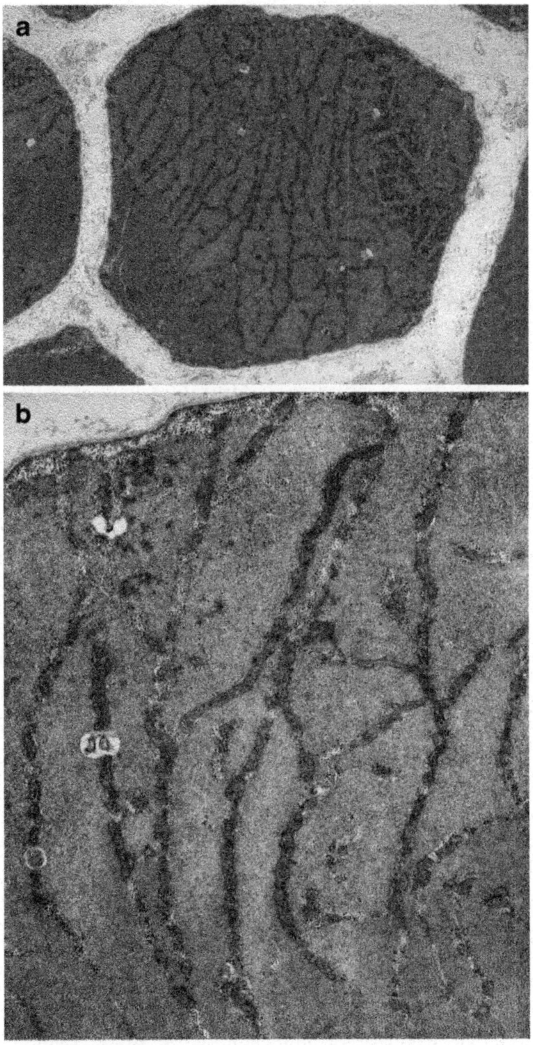

Fig. 10 Fusion-fission. (**a–c**) Mitochondrial network is mainly defined by mitochondrial ramifications without interruptions [**a** 4400×; **b** 7000×; **c** 20000×]. (**d**) Two connecting mitochondria 30,000×

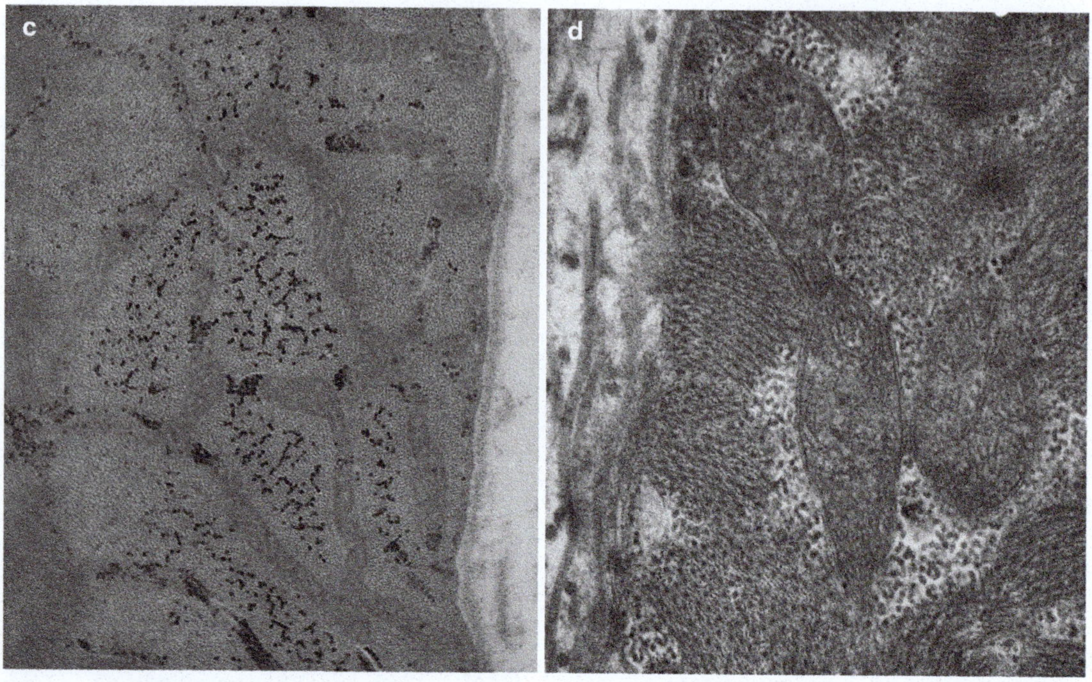

Fig. 10 (continued)

reduction of abnormal mitochondria at ultrastructural level [71].

Also histochemical reactions for COX performed on different tissues, including skeletal muscle, from mouse models affected with ethylmalonic encephalopathy have helped elucidate the mechanism of COX deficiency in this autosomal recessive, fatal infantile disorder characterized by accumulation of toxic sulfide (H2S) in mammalian tissues and caused by mutations in ETHE1, a gene encoding a mitochondrial sulfur dioxygenase [72].

References

1. Bourgeois JM, Tarnopolsky MA. Pathology of skeletal muscle in mitochondrial disorders. Mitochondrion. 2004;4:441–52.
2. Sciacco M, Bonilla E. Cytochemistry and immunocytochemistry of mitochondria in tissue sections. Methods Enzymol. 1996;264:509–21.
3. Phadke R. Myopathology of adult and paediatric mitochondrial diseases. J Clin Med. 2017;6(7):E64. https://doi.org/10.3390/jcm6070064.
4. Bonilla E, Sciacco M, Tanji K, Sparaco M, Petruzzella V, Moraes CT. New morphological approaches to the study of mitochondrial encephalomyopathies. Brain Pathol. 1992;2:1.13–9.
5. Engel WK, Cunningham GG. Neurology. 1963;13:919.
6. Sarnat HB, Marín-García J. Pathology of mitochondrial encephalomyopathies. Can J Neurol Sci. 2005;32:152–66.
7. Hatefi Y. The mitochondrial electron transport and oxidative phosphorylation system. Annu Rev Biochem. 1985;54:1015–69.
8. Beinert H. Recent developments in the field of iron-sulfur proteins. FASEB J. 1990;4(8):2483–91.
9. Shoffner JM, Lott MT, Lezza AMS, Seibel P, Ballinger SW, Wallace DC. Myoclonic epilepsy and ragged-red fiber disease (MERRF) is associated with a mitochondrial DNA tRNALVs mutation. Cell. 1990;61:931–7.
10. Kobayashi Y, Momoi MY, Tominaga K, Nihei K, Yanagisawa M, Kagawa Y. A point mutation in the mitochondrial tRNALeu(uUR) gene in MELAS (mitochondrial myopathy, encephalopathy, lactic acidosis and stroke-like episodes). Biochem Biophys Res Cornm. 1990;173(81):6–822.
11. El-Hattab AW, Scaglia F. Mitochondrial DNA depletion syndromes: review and updates of genetic basis, manifestations, and therapeutic options. Neurotherapeutics. 2013;10:186–98.
12. Quinzii CM, DiMauro S, Hirano M. Human coenzyme Q10 deficiency. Neurochem Res. 2007;32:723–7.
13. Naini A, Kaufmann P, Shanske S, Engelstad K, De Vivo DC, Schon EA. Hypocitrullinemia in patients with MELAS: an insight into the "MELAS paradox". J Neurol Sci. 2005;229–230:187–93.

14. Garavaglia C, Antozzi F, Girotti D, Peluchetti M, Rimoldi MZ, DiDonato S. Neurology. 1990;40(Suppl. 1):294.
15. Hailer RG, Henriksson KG, Jorfeldt L, Hultman E, Wibom R, Sahlin K, Areskog NH, Gunder M, Ayyad K, Blomquist CG, Hall RE, Thuillier P, Kennaway NG, Lewis SF. J Clin Invest. 1991;88:1197.
16. Kadenbach B, Kuhn-Nentwig L, Buge U. Evolution of a regulatory enzyme: cytochrome-c oxidase (complex IV) book chapter. Curr Topics Bioenergetics. 1987;15:113–61.
17. Bonilla E, Schotland DL, DiMauro S, Aldover B. J Ultrastruct Res. 1975;51:404.
18. Johnson MA, Turnbull DM, Dick DJ, Sherrat HSA. A partial deficiency of cytochrome c oxidase in chronic progressive external ophthalmoplegia. J Neurol Sci. 1983;60(1):31–53.
19. Mita S, Schmidt B, Schon EA, DiMauro S, Bonilla E. Detection of "deleted" mitochondrial genomes in cytochrome c oxidase-deficient muscle fibers of a patient with Kearns-Sayre syndrome. Proc Natl Acad Sci U S A. 1989;86:9509–9513 19.
20. Haas RH, Parikh S, Falk MJ, Saneto RP, Wolf NI, Darin N, Wong LJ, Cohen BH, Naviaux RK, Mitochondrial Medicine Society's Committee on Diagnosis. The in-depth evaluation of suspected mitochondrial disease. Mol Genet Metab. 2008;94:16–37.
21. DiMauro S, Schon EA, Carelli V, Hirano M. The clinical maze of mitochondrial neurology. Nat Rev Neurol. 2013;9:429–44.
22. Kornblum C, Nicholls TJ, Haack TB, Schöler S, Peeva V, Danhauser K, Hallmann K, Zsurka G, Rorbach J, Iuso A, et al. Loss-of-function mutations in MGME1 impair mtDNA replication and cause multisystemic mitochondrial disease. Nat Genet. 2013;45:214–9.
23. Ronchi D, Garone C, Bordoni A, Gutierrez Rios P, Calvo SE, Ripolone M, Ranieri M, Rizzuti M, Villa L, Magri F, et al. Next-generation sequencing reveals DGUOK mutations in adult patients with mitochondrial DNA multiple deletions. Brain. 2012;135:3404–15.
24. Sue CM, Karadimas C, Checcarelli N, Tanji K, Papadopoulou LC, Pallotti F, Guo FL, Shanske S, Hirano M, De Vivo DC, et al. Differential features of patients with mutations in two COX assembly genes, SURF-1 and SCO2. Ann Neurol. 2000;589–595:47.
25. Teraoka M, Yokoyama Y, Ninomiya S, Inoue C, Yamashita S, Seino Y. Two novel mutations of SURF1 in Leigh syndrome with cytochrome c oxidase deficiency. Hum Genet. 1999;105:560–3.
26. Tritschler HJ, Andreetta F, Moraes CT, Bonilla E, Arnaudo E, Danon MJ, Glass S, Zalaya EM, Vamos E, Shanske S, Kadenbach B, DiMauro S, Schon EA. Mitochondrial myopathy of childhood with depletion of mitochondrial DNA. Neurology. 1992;42:209–17.
27. Mitochondrial medicine DiMauro Gavidson 2005.
28. DiMauro S, Bonilla E, Lombes A, Shanske S, Minetti C, Moraes CT. Mitochondrial encephalomyopathies. Neurol Clin. 1990;8:483–506.
29. Sciacco M, Bonilla E, Schon EA, DiMauro S, Moraes CT. Distribution of wild-type and common deletion forms of mtDNA in normal and respiration-deficient muscle fibers from patients with mitochondrial myopathy. Hum Mol Genet. 1994;3:13–9.
30. Petruzzella V, Moraes CT, Sano MC, Bonilla E, DiMauro S, Schon EA. Extremely high levels of mutant mtDNAs co-localize with cytochrome c oxidase-negative ragged-red fibers in patients harboring a point mutation at nt 3243. Hum Mol Genet. 1994 Mar;3(3):449–54.
31. Silvestri G, Rana M, Odoardi F, Modoni A, Paris E, Papacci M, Tonali P, Servidei S. Single-fiber PCR in MELAS(3243) patients: correlations between intratissue distribution and phenotypic expression of the mtDNA(A3243G) genotype. Am J Med Genet. 2000;94(3):201–6.
32. Yoneda M, Miyatake T, Attardi G. Heteroplasmic mitochondrial tRNA(Lys) mutation and its complementation in MERRF patient-derived mitochondrial transformants. Muscle Nerve. 1995;3:S95–S101.
33. Schon EA, DiMauro S, Hirano M. Human mitochondrial DNA: roles of inherited and somatic mutations. Nat Rev Genet. 2012;13:878–90.
34. Tulinius M, Oldfors A. Neonatal muscular manifestations in mitochondrial disorders. Semin Fetal Neonatal Med. 2011;16:229–35.
35. Nascimento A, Ortez C, Jou C, O'Callaghan M, Ramos F, Garcia-Cazorla A. Neuromuscular manifestations in mitochondrial diseases in children. Semin Pediatr Neurol. 2016;23:290–305.
36. Koenig MK. Presentation and diagnosis of mitochondrial disorders in children. Pediatr Neurol. 2008;38:305–13.
37. Goldstein AC, Bhatia P, Vento JM. Mitochondrial disease in childhood: nuclear encoded. Neurotherapeutics. 2013;10:212–26.
38. Taylor RW, Schaefer AM, Barron MJ, McFarland R, Turnbull DM. The diagnosis of mitochondrial muscle disease. Neuromuscul Disord. 2004;14:237–45.
39. Lamont PJ, Surtees R, Woodward CE, Leonard JV, Wood NW, Harding AE. Clinical and laboratory findings in referrals for mitochondrial DNA analysis. Arch Dis Child. 1998;79:22–7.
40. Papadopoulou LC, Sue CM, Davidson MM, Tanji K, Nishino I, Sadlock JE, Krishna S, Walker W, Selby J, Glerum DM, et al. Fatal infantile cardioencephalomyopathy with COX deficiency and mutations in SCO2, a COX assembly gene. Nat Genet. 1999;23:333–7.
41. Alfadhel M, Lillquist YP, Waters PJ, Sinclair G, Struys E, McFadden D, Hendson G, Hyams L, Shoffner J, Vallance HD. Infantile cardioencephalopathy due to a COX15 gene defect: report and review. Am J Med Genet A. 2011;155:840–4.
42. Huigsloot M, Nijtmans LG, Szklarczyk R, Baars MJ, van den Brand MA, Hendriksfranssen MG, van den Heuvel LP, Smeitink JA, Huynen MA, Rodenburg RJ. A mutation in C2orf64 causes impaired cytochrome c oxidase assembly and mitochondrial cardiomyopathy. Am J Hum Genet. 2011;88:488–93.

43. Ghosh A, Trivedi PP, Timbalia SA, Griffin AT, Rahn JJ, Chan SS, Gohil VM. Copper supplementation restores cytochrome c oxidase assembly defect in a mitochondrial disease model of COA6 deficiency. Hum Mol Genet. 2014;23:3596–606.
44. DiMauro S, Nicholson JF, Hays AP, Eastwood AB, Papadimitriou A, Koenigsberger R, DeVivo DC. Benign infantile mitochondrial myopathy due to reversible cytochrome c oxidase deficiency. Ann Neurol. 1983;14:226–34.
45. Horvath R, Kemp JP, Tuppen HA, Hudson G, Oldfors A, Marie SK, Moslemi AR, Servidei S, Holme E, Shanske S, et al. Molecular basis of infantile reversible cytochrome c oxidase deficiency myopathy. Brain. 2009;132:3165–74.
46. Boczonadi V, Bansagi B, Horvath R. Reversible infantile mitochondrial diseases. J Inherit Metab Dis. 2015;38:427–35.
47. Bresolin N, Zeviani M, Bonilla E, Miller RH, Leech RW, Shanske S, Nakagawa M, DiMauro S. Fatal infantile cytochrome C oxidase deficiency: decrease of immunologically detectable enzyme in muscle. Neurology. 1985;35:802–12.
48. DiMauro S, Lombes A, Nakase H, Mita S, Fabrizi GM, Tritschler HJ, Bonilla E, Miranda AF, De Vivo DC, Schon EA. Cytochrome c oxidase deficiency. Pediatr Res. 1990;28:536–41.
49. Yamamoto M, Koga Y, Ohtaki E, Nonaka I. Focal cytochrome c oxidase deficiency in various neuromuscular diseases. J Neurol Sci. 1989;91:207–13.
50. Gire C, Girard N, Nicaise C, Einaudi MA, Montfort MF, Dejode JM. Clinical features and neuroradiological findings of mitochondrial pathology in six neonates. Childs Nerv Syst. 2002;18:621–8.
51. Moraes CT, Shanske S, Tritschler HJ, Aprille JR, Andreetta F, Bonilla E, Schon EA, DiMauro S. Mitochondrial DNA depletion with variable tissue expression: a novel genetic abnormality in mitochondrial diseases. Am J Hum Genet. 1991;48:492–501.
52. Reisner HM, Wick MR. In: Wick MR, Siegal GP, editors. Monoclonal antibodies in diagnostic immunohistochernistry. New York and Basel: Dekker; 1988. p. 1.
53. Nakase H, Moraes CT, Rizzuto R, Lombes A, DiMauro S, Schon EA. Am J Hum Genet. 1990;46:418.
54. Moraes CT, Ricci E, Petruzzella V, Shanske S, DiMauro S, Schon EA, Bonilla E. Nat Genet. 1992;1:359.
55. Ricci E, Andreetta F, Moraes CT, Minetti C, Schon EA, DiMauro S, Bonilla E. Immunodeficiency of mtDNA encoded proteins in muscle from patients with deletion-mutation-depletion of mtDNA. Neurology ISuppfl. 1991;1:208.
56. Bogenhagen D, Clayton DA. The number of mitochondrial DNA genomes in mouse and human HeLa cells. J Biol Chem. 1974;249(7991–7995):31.
57. Shmookler-Reis RJ, Goldstein S. Mitochondrial DNA in mortal and immortal human cells. J Biol Chem. 1983;258(9078–9085):32.
58. Robin ED, Wong R. Mitochondrial DNA molecules and virtual number of mitochondria per cell in mammalian cells. J Cell Physiol. 1988;136:507–13.
59. Andreetta F, Tritschler HJ, Schon EA, Bonilla E. Localization of mitochondrial DNA using immunological probes: a new approach for the study of mitochondrial myopathies. J Neurol Sci. 1991;105: 88–92.
60. Van Wijngaarden GK, Bethlem J, Meijer AE, Hulsmann WC, Feltkamp CA. Skeletal muscle disease with abnormal mitochondria. Brain. 1967;90: 577–92.
61. Price HM, Gordon GR, Munsat TL, Pearson CM. Myopathy with atypical mitochondria in type I skeletal muscle fibers. A histochemical and ultrastructural study. J Neuropathol Exp Neurol. 1967;26:475–97.
62. Hulsmann WC, Bethlem J, Meijer AE, Fleury P, Schellens JP. Myopathy with abnormal structure and function of muscle mitochondria. J Neurol Neurosurg Psychiatry. 1967;30:519–25.
63. Cogliati S, Enriquez JA, Scorrano L. Mitochondrial cristae: where beauty meets functionality. Trends Biochem Sci. 2016;41(3):261–73.
64. Zick M, Rabl R, Reichert AS. Cristae formation—linking ultrastructure and function of mitochondria. Biochim Biophys Acta. 2009;1793:5–19.
65. Picard M, et al. Progressive increase in mtDNA 3243A > G heteroplasmy causes abrupt transcriptional reprogramming. Proc Natl Acad Sci U S A. 2014;111:E4033–42.
66. Shutt TE, McBride HM. Staying cool in difficult times: mitochondrial dynamics, quality control and the stress response. Biochim Biophys Acta. 2013;1833: 417–24.
67. Leduc-Gaudet JP, et al. Mitochondrial morphology is altered in atrophied skeletal muscle of aged mice. Oncotarget. 2015;6:17923–37.
68. Suen D-F, Norris KL, Youle RJ. Mitochondrial dynamics and apoptosis. Genes Dev. 2008;22:1577–90.
69. Devay RM, Dominguez-Ramirez L, Lackner LL, Hoppins S, Stahlberg H, Nunnari J. Coassembly of Mgm1 isoforms requires cardiolipin and mediates mitochondrial inner membrane fusion. J Cell Biol. 2009;186:793–803.
70. Sesaki H, Jensen RE. Division versus fusion: Dnm1p and Fzo1p antagonistically regulate mitochondrial shape. J Cell Biol. 1999;149:699–706.
71. Viscomi C, Bottani E, Civiletto G, Cerutti R, Moggio M, Fagiolari G, Schon EA, Lamperti C, Zeviani M. In vivo correction of COX deficiency by activation of the AMPK/PGC-1α axis. Cell Metab. 2011;14(1):80–90. https://doi.org/10.1016/j.cmet.2011.04.011.
72. Di Meo I, Fagiolari G, Prelle A, Viscomi C, Zeviani M, Tiranti V. Chronic exposure to sulfide causes accelerated degradation of cytochrome c oxidase in ethylmalonic encephalopathy. Antioxid Redox Signal. 2011;15(2):353–62. https://doi.org/10.1089/ars.2010.3520.

Mitochondrial Disease Genetics

Laura S. Kremer, Elizabeth M. McCormick,
Holger Prokisch, and Marni J. Falk

Introduction

Primary mitochondrial disease represents a broad and highly diverse group of genetic conditions that share in common impaired energy production [1]. Clinical manifestations of primary mitochondrial disease are varied and range from isolated involvement of nearly any organ at any age to multi-organ involvement that can be lethal in the neonatal period.

Mitochondria are subcellular cytoplasmic organelles with an inner and outer membrane, between which is an intermembrane space. The mitochondrial matrix lies within the inner mitochondrial membrane, which is highly rugated to form cristae on which oxidative phosphorylation (OXPHOS) occurs that transfers nutrient energy as electrons in the presence of oxygen to generate chemical energy in the form of adenosine triphosphate (ATP). This process of aerobic respiration occurs within the five complexes of the respiratory chain (RC), each of which has multiple protein subunits that must be properly assembled. Thirteen of these subunits are encoded for by mitochondrial DNA, which form the core structure of RC complexes I, III, IV, and V. All remaining RC subunits in all five complexes are encoded by nuclear genes and imported into the mitochondria. Beyond energy production, mitochondria are vital to a host of other cellular functions including regulating diverse aspects of intermediary metabolism, calcium homeostasis, and programmed cell death (apoptosis). Each mitochondrion is comprised of more than 1500 proteins, which are all nuclear encoded except for the 13 RC complex subunits encoded by mtDNA. These proteins were inventoried and experimentally confirmed first in 2008 [2] and later updated in 2016 [3], in compendia known as MitoCarta and MitoCarta 2.0, respectively.

Laura S. Kremer and Elizabeth M. McCormick contributed equally to this work.

L. S. Kremer · H. Prokisch (✉)
Institute of Human Genetics, Technische Universität München, Munich, Germany

Institute of Human Genetics, Helmholtz Zentrum München, Munich, Germany
e-mail: prokisch@helmholtz-muenchen.de

E. M. McCormick
Mitochondrial Medicine Frontier Program, Division of Human Genetics, Department of Pediatrics, Children's Hospital of Philadelphia, Philadelphia, PA, USA

M. J. Falk (✉)
Mitochondrial Medicine Frontier Program, Division of Human Genetics, Department of Pediatrics, Children's Hospital of Philadelphia, Philadelphia, PA, USA

Department of Pediatrics, Perelman School of Medicine, Philadelphia, PA, USA
e-mail: falkm@email.chop.edu

M. Mancuso, T. Klopstock (eds.), *Diagnosis and Management of Mitochondrial Disorders*,
https://doi.org/10.1007/978-3-030-05517-2_3

Primary mitochondrial disease is caused by pathogenic variants in mtDNA or nDNA, with any inheritance pattern possible. More than 350 genes have now been identified in which mutations cause primary mitochondrial disease [4, 5], primarily involving genes that encode mitochondria-localized proteins or factors that regulate mitochondria, with functions ranging from OXPHOS subunits, assembly factors, metabolic enzymes or cofactors, mtDNA maintenance, transcription, translation, and replication, quality control, mitochondrial import, and a range of other processes that ultimately affect chemical energy production. This chapter focuses on mitochondrial disease genetics, providing an overview of genetic etiologies underlying primary mitochondrial disease, reviewing the approach to identifying and confirming genetic etiologies of primary mitochondrial disease, and summarizing the current state of genomic variant curation and deposition as it relates to primary mitochondrial disease.

Genetic Etiologies of Primary Mitochondrial Disease

Primary mitochondrial disease may be caused by pathogenic variants in either mtDNA or nDNA with considerable phenotypic overlap among the many genetic etiologies.

mtDNA Causes of Mitochondrial Disease

Mitochondrial DNA is located within mitochondria attached to the inner mitochondrial membrane. It is a small, circular genome of only 16,569 base pairs that has 37 genes. Thirteen of these are protein-coding genes. The remaining 24 genes encode RNA needed for synthesis of the protein-coding mtDNA genes, including 2 rRNAs and 22 tRNAs. mtDNA also has a small noncoding, hypervariable D-loop region that is important in the regulation of mtDNA genome transcription and replication.

The mtDNA genome has several unique properties, including the following: (1) Multiple copies of mtDNA are present per mitochondrion, with many mitochondria present per cell, leading to quantitative genetics. Thus, a mtDNA mutation can be present only in a portion of the genomes in a given cell or tissue (a state termed heteroplasmy) or in all copies (a state termed homoplasmy). (2) The mtDNA genome undergoes continuous and autonomous replication, which is not related to the cell cycle. (3) mtDNA genes do not undergo splicing as genes are transcribed in polycistronic transcripts without introns [6]. (4) Mitochondria are highly dynamic organelles that continually undergo fission and fusion with nearby mitochondria to enable mitochondrial and mtDNA repair and maintenance. (5) mtDNA has a higher mutation rate than nuclear DNA, accumulating mutations at low levels with age. (6) Certain fixed (homoplasmic) mtDNA variants occur together to form haplogroups, which are inherited through the oocyte and used to track maternal lineages and human population migrations. The clinical significance of these unique aspects of mtDNA is discussed in greater detail below.

Up to 80% of primary mitochondrial disease in adults [1] and up to 25% of primary mitochondrial disease in children are caused by pathogenic variants in mtDNA [7]. More than 300 pathogenic variants have now been identified in the mitochondrial genome (https://www.mitomap.org). Pathogenic variants in protein-coding mtDNA genes can result in an isolated RC complex deficiency, although multiple RC complex deficiencies can also occur since the RC exists in supercomplexes between the individual complexes. Pathogenic variants in a MT-tRNA gene tend to cause multiple RC complex deficiencies since they impair all 13 protein-coding genes from being effectively translated into subunits of complexes I, III, IV, and V of the RC.

Primary mitochondrial disease may also result from large mitochondrial DNA deletions, which are often heteroplasmic and may cause different clinical syndromes depending on in which tissue(s) they occur. A "common" five kilobase (5 kb) deletion of the mtDNA genome is frequently seen, although pathogenic deletions may be highly variable and range in size from 1 to 10 kb [8].

Heteroplasmy and threshold effect. Within a mitochondrion, cell, or tissue, a mixture of copies of mtDNA genomes with and without a particular genomic variant may exist, a phenomenon known as heteroplasmy. Heteroplasmy levels of a particular variant can differ among tissues in the same individual and among family members and change over time. For some pathogenic variants, the level of heteroplasmy must exceed a certain threshold to cause disease manifestations, a phenomenon known as threshold effect. While this level is often deemed above 70–80% for severe clinical disease manifestations, this may vary greatly by mutation and is difficult to assess in non-accessible tissues such as the retina, heart, or brain. The specific manifestations of some disorders may also be very variable at low, middle, or high heteroplasmy levels, as is most commonly demonstrated for m.3243A>G mutation that at low levels below 10% causes maternally inherited diabetes and deafness, at moderate levels may cause mitochondrial encephalopathy lactic acidosis, and stroke-like episodes (MELAS) or a variety of multi-system problems, and at very high levels above 90% may cause pediatric-onset Leigh syndrome.

Maternal inheritance of mtDNA. mtDNA is exclusively maternally inherited through the oocyte [9, 10]. Given the phenomenon of heteroplasmy and a genetic bottleneck that occurs between the specific mtDNA genomes present in an oocyte (with hundreds of thousands of mitochondria) and the cell that will form the embryo (with only a few hundred mitochondria), each offspring may have very different heteroplasmy levels both from their mother and then between their different organs in which those inherited mtDNA mutant genomes may segregate over time. Pathogenic mtDNA mutations may also arise de novo in an oocyte or embryo, although confirming that a variant arose de novo is technically difficult since it may only be present in the mother's germline and not in her somatic cells.

Therefore, testing in multiple maternal tissues must be undertaken before concluding a variant occurred de novo in an affected individual. Standard sequencing techniques that were commonly utilized in the past, such as Sanger sequencing, would not reliably detect heteroplasmy levels below 50%, so that failure to detect a mutation was not confirmation that it was not biologically present in the mother at low levels. Further, a given mtDNA variant may not be present in certain tissues in the mother, such as blood, but present in other tissues such as muscle, skin fibroblasts, or urine epithelial cells.

Haplogroups. In the mitochondrial genome, there exist single nucleotide polymorphisms (SNPs) that arise and become fixed in a population over time [11]. These variants comprise a haplogroup, which are the background sequence of the mtDNA genome that becomes passed down the matrilineal line through generations and allows for tracing of ancestral origins and population migration. The presence of haplogroups may complicate mtDNA variant interpretation, as some pathogenic variants appear more closely associated with certain haplogroups, and certain haplogroups may modulate the penetrance or spectrum of phenotypic manifestations for some pathogenic mtDNA variants [12, 13].

Interestingly, the rare haplogroup of the original mtDNA reference sequence that is widely used for mtDNA sequence data interpretation has provided further complications. The widely used reference sequence is rCRS, or the revised Cambridge Reference Sequence, which does not represent the original human "mitochondrial eve" from which all haplogroups evolved but rather was obtained from the first person who had their mtDNA genome sequenced and represents a rare haplogroup. Therefore, a homoplasmic nucleotide variation identified at a certain position from this reference may not be a disease-causing mutation but rather reflect an individual's varying ethnic origins from the reference with different haplogroup background.

Clinical syndrome associations. Several pathogenic mtDNA variants have been classically associated with clinical syndromes. These clinical syndromes were characterized in the late 1980s and early 1990s before thorough understanding of the full range of genetic etiologies, and the wide spectrum of potential disease manifestations was fully appreciated [14].

MELAS has classically been associated with several mtDNA variants, most commonly including m.3243A>G in MT-tRNA(Leu-UUR). However, only 10% of individuals who carry m.3243A>G manifest with classical MELAS, while individuals with very high levels of this mutation (<90–95%) may present with Leigh syndrome and with very low levels of this mutation (<10%) manifest with mitochondrial inherited diabetes and deafness (MIDD) [15]. Other individuals may have a range of non-specific symptoms such as fatigue, headaches, renal failure, or exercise intolerance. Indeed, the m.3243A>G mutation is thought to account for 1% of all diabetes mellitus [16]. Other classical mtDNA point mutation syndromes include myoclonic epilepsy with ragged red fibers syndrome (MERRF) caused by *MT-tRNA(LYS)* m.8344A>G mutation, neuropathy, ataxia, and retinitis pigmentosa (NARP) caused by the *MT-ATP6* m.8993T>G mutation, and Leber's hereditary optic neuropathy (LHON) that results from mutations in mtDNA genes encoding complex I subunits of which m.3460G>A in *MT-ND1*, m.11778G>A in *MT-ND4*, and m.14484T>C in *MT-ND6* are the most common. Given the widely variable levels of heteroplasmy in different patients and range of potential symptom involvement, pre-defined clinical syndromes can complicate genetic counseling and recognition of a genetic etiology and prognosis. Many affected individuals do not meet all criteria pre-defined in these syndromes or may meet some criteria from multiple clinical syndromes. Indeed, mitochondrial disease patients each have an average of 16 major medical problems, regardless of age [17].

Heteroplasmic mtDNA large deletions or duplications have been associated with a spectrum of clinical syndromes. These may include (1) Pearson syndrome occurring in early childhood that involves transfusion-dependent sideroblastic anemia and exocrine pancreatic dysfunction; (2) Kearns-Sayre syndrome (KSS) that is characterized by chronic progressive external ophthalmoplegia (CPEO), retinal dystrophy prior to age 20 years, and one of several additional features (cardiac conduction block, ataxia, or elevated (>100 mg/dL) cerebrospinal fluid protein concentration); and (3) CPEO that may be isolated when involving eye muscle paralysis with ptosis or "plus" when associated with extraocular symptoms such as general myopathy, exercise intolerance, hearing loss, and cataracts, among other features.

Given the broad overlap in these clinical syndromes, improved understanding that single genetic etiologies may cause a spectrum of disease manifestations and the increasing requirement of defined molecular genetic etiology for clinical trial eligibility, strict definitions of clinically defined syndromes are becoming less essential than careful phenotyping of specific symptoms and outcomes present in individuals with distinct genetic disorders.

Classes of mtDNA Genes

Protein-coding mtDNA genes. Seven of the 13 protein-coding genes in the mitochondrial genome encode complex I subunits (*MT-ND1*, *MT-ND2*, *MT-ND3*, *MT-ND4*, *MT-ND5*, *MT-ND6*, and *MT-ND4L*), 1 encodes a complex III subunit (*MT-CYB*), 3 encode complex IV subunits (*MT-CO1*, *MT-CO2*, and *MT-CO3*), and 2 encode complex V subunits (*MT-ATP6* and *MT-ATP8*). As there are no mtDNA encoded subunits in complex II, detection of complex II deficiency would indicate a likely nuclear gene etiology.

Many pathogenic variants have been identified in the protein-coding mtDNA genes, including variants that have been associated with Leber's hereditary optic neuropathy or LHON. Three pathogenic variants are thought to cause 90–95% of LHON in most ethnicities, m.3460G>A in *MT-ND1*, m.11778G>A in *MT-ND4*, and m.14484T>C in *MT-ND6*. LHON is characterized by painless subacute vision loss that typically occurs in the second to third decade in one eye, followed within weeks to months by the same pattern of vision loss in the other eye. Most pathogenic mtDNA variants causing LHON are highly heteroplasmic or even homoplasmic. Interestingly, only 50% of males and 10% of females develop vision loss, with penetrance increased by exposures such as smoking or by hormonal levels [18]. Although classically considered an isolated ophthalmologic disorder, many individuals with these pathogenic variants may develop additional multisystemic concerns, such as fatigue, exercise intolerance, cardiac problems, and a range of neurologic problems including myopathy, neuropathy, and brain MRI abnormalities extending to Leigh syndrome at high heteroplasmy levels in some cases.

MT-tRNA genes. Twenty-two genes in the mitochondrial genome encode for human mitochondrial transfer RNAs, or MT-tRNAs, essential in the translation of the 13 protein-coding genes. Pathogenic variants in these MT-tRNAs impair the synthesis of mtDNA genome-encoded RC subunits, resulting in deficient energy production.

Several classical primary mitochondrial diseases are caused by pathogenic missense variants in mt-tRNAs, namely, MELAS caused by m.3243A>G in MT-tRNA(leu-UUR) and MERRF caused by the m.8344A>G variant in MT-tRNA(lys) that accounts for more than 80% of those with features consistent with MERRF. MERRF is classically characterized by four key features: myoclonus, epilepsy, ataxia, and ragged red fibers seen on muscle biopsy, although additional features commonly seen include lipomas, hearing loss, myopathy, neuropathy, and optic atrophy.

MT-rRNA genes. Two genes in the mitochondrial genome code for ribosomal RNAs or rRNAs. *MT-RNR1* encodes for mitochondrial 12S rRNA and *MT-RNR2* encoding for mitochondrial 16S rRNA. The m.1555A>G variant in *MT-RNR1* is associated with non-syndromic sensorineural hearing loss that can be induced by aminoglycoside exposure or can occur without exposure later in life, although other phenotypes including optic neuropathy or neurologic disease have been reported [19, 20].

Family member testing. No guidelines exist for testing unaffected siblings of individuals with pathogenic mtDNA variants nor is there consensus regarding medical management recommendations for a pre-symptomatic individual with a pathogenic mtDNA variant. Genetic testing may therefore be useful to prevent risk factors that may precipitate disease manifestations or transmission of disease to future offspring but may also provoke anxiety if a pathogenic variant is identified in a seemingly healthy individual.

While both genders may be affected by mtDNA diseases, mtDNA disease may only be passed on through the female germline (oocytes). Therefore, adult female relatives through the maternal germline of individuals with known mtDNA pathogenic variants should be informed of their risk to harbor and pass on that mutation to their offspring and be offered carrier testing for that mtDNA mutation. Siblings of affected individuals under the age of 18 may undergo cardiac evaluation if the variant is present and/or started on preventive medicines if found to be at high risk for certain manifestations; genetic testing to determine whether pediatric age siblings also carry the pathogenic mtDNA mutation known in their family should be carefully considered based on whether there may be pediatric-onset of symptoms or preventative measures that could be taken to reduce their risk of penetrance or severity of mitochondrial disease.

Distinct from definite pathogenic variants, when considering the potential pathogenicity of a mtDNA variant of uncertain significance (VUS) identified in a patient with suspected mitochondrial disease, testing healthy siblings or maternal family members to determine whether and at what level they carry that same variant may provide additional evidence to accurately assess its pathogenicity. Detecting the mtDNA variant at higher heteroplasmic or homoplasmic levels in healthy family members would markedly decrease suspicion that the variant is causal of the index patient's symptoms. However, it may not be able to fully exclude the pathogenicity of the variant given variable expressivity and inability to test certain inaccessible tissues that may be affected in a given individual, such as the heart or brain. Of note, most pathogenic variants are present in heteroplasmy, whereas most homoplasmic variants fixed in all individuals in a given family tend to be indicative of rare haplogroups and benign.

Prenatal testing. Until recently, prenatal testing and prevention of transmission have been limited for women with mtDNA pathogenic variants. Amniocentesis and chorionic villus sampling (CVS) may not always provide accurate assessments of mutation load given they are looking at placental or discarded cells, making it challenging to accurately predict clinical outcomes or disease severity in resultant offspring [21]. Technical challenges also relate to poorly reliable and poorly sensitive heteroplasmy quantitation methods, which have recently improved with massively parallel sequencing technologies.

Prenatal implantation diagnosis, or PGD, is increasingly recognized to be a feasible option for some families with known pathogenic mtDNA mutations. Healthy children stemming from pregnancies with mutation loads ranging from 5% to 18% have been reported; however, not all cycles generate an embryo with such low heteroplasmy levels [22]. Further, mutation levels may become enriched in some tissues or with some mutations between the time of embryo sampling and birth, and it is difficult to determine if any perhaps less-severe medical symptoms might develop over time across the life span of the resulting individual in whom the pathogenic mtDNA mutation was identified at a low level as an embryo.

Mitochondrial replacement techniques (MRT) aim to not just identify embryos with low-level heteroplasmy for pathogenic mutations but to actively reduce the chances of transmission of mtDNA pathogenic variants from the mother by replacing the mutant mitochondria with that of a healthy unrelated donor egg that does not harbor that mtDNA mutation. MRT may be performed either by metaphase spindle transfer in oocytes (a technique that transfers the intended mother's nuclear genome into a donor oocyte whose nucleus was removed) or pronuclear transfer in early zygotes (a technique that transfers the pronucleus from the intended parents' fertilized oocyte within 1 day of fertilization into a donor oocyte that has been fertilized with the same father's sperm and then at the same early stage had its pronuclei removed). Pronuclear transfer was legally approved in 2017 by the UK Parliament to be performed at selected sites with initial licenses for the first clinical cases to be performed in 2017 [23]. However, legal hurdles to clinical research evaluation of the safety and efficacy of MRT by any method remain in place in other countries, including the United States where further research into these options has been prohibited since 2016 [24].

Nuclear DNA Causes of Mitochondrial Disease

Pathogenic variants in nuclear genes causing primary mitochondrial disease may be inherited in any Mendelian inheritance pattern including autosomal dominant, autosomal recessive, and X-linked.

Inheritance of Nuclear Gene Causes of Mitochondrial Disease

Autosomal dominant. Primary mitochondrial diseases inherited in an autosomal dominant manner are more likely to be adult-onset [25], although childhood-onset certainly may occur particularly including de novo dominant disorders that involve severe neurologic manifestations such as epilepsy. Pathogenic mutations in genes inherited in an autosomal dominant manner cause disease when present on just one allele of a given gene, which can be inherited or occur de novo. An individual with an autosomal dominant disorder has a 50% (1 in 2) likelihood of passing the pathogenic mutation onto his or her offspring. The clinical manifestations may vary greatly between individuals in a given family for autosomal dominant disorders due to variable expressivity and thus be difficult to predict for one's offspring.

Autosomal recessive. The majority of pediatric-onset primary mitochondrial diseases result from pathogenic variants in genes inherited in an autosomal recessive manner. Here, a pathogenic variant must be present on both alleles of a given gene to cause clinical disease manifestations. An individual with a pathogenic variant present in the homozygous state (same variant present on each allele of a given gene) or in a compound heterozygous state (different variants, one on each allele of a given gene) will pass on one of their pathogenic mutations to each offspring. However, the chances his or her offspring would be affected depend on the affected or carrier status of the individual's partner, who would have to carry a pathogenic mutation in the same gene and then also pass this variant on in order for their offspring to be clinically affected with the disease. Affected individuals with pathogenic mutations in a gene inherited in an autosomal recessive manner hence inherited one mutation from each carrier parent. Carriers are individuals who have a pathogenic mutation on only one copy of a gene inherited in an autosomal recessive manner with no pathogenic variants on their other allele and therefore are typically healthy or unaffected with that specific disease condition. Rarely, pathogenic variants in autosomal recessive genes occur de novo or may result from a chromosomal copy number alteration (deletion) involving that gene region. Two carriers have a 25% (1 in 4) chance of having a child affected with the condition. Unaffected full siblings of affected individuals have a 67% (2 in 3) chance of being a carrier. Siblings of carriers are each at 50% (1 in 2) chance of also carrying that disease allele.

X-linked. Primary mitochondrial disease can be caused by pathogenic mutations in genes located on the X chromosome. Males with an X-linked pathogenic variant will be clinically affected, whereas females with a pathogenic mutation on one copy of their X chromosome will most typically be unaffected carriers. However, the presence of skewed X-inactivation in females can result in a female with X-linked disease manifestations. Male offspring of female carriers for an X-linked disorder will have a 50% (1 in 2) chance of being affected, while female offspring will have a 50% (1 in 2) chance of being a carrier (with possibility to be affected if X-inactivation is skewed). Male offspring of affected males with an X-linked disorder will be unaffected, while female offspring will be carriers (with possibility to be affected if X-inactivation is skewed).

Prenatal testing. Prenatal testing for pathogenic variants in nuclear genes associated with primary mitochondrial disease is readily available in most reproductive endocrinology clinics, including amniocentesis and chorionic villus sampling as described above. These techniques are highly reliable for nuclear gene disorders, which are not subject to variable heteroplasmy levels as occur for mtDNA gene disorders. Reliable clinical techniques also are readily available to prevent transmission of primary mitochondrial disease caused by nuclear gene pathogenic variants, including in vitro fertilization (IVF) followed by preimplantation genetic diagnosis (PGD). This testing is now routinely performed in many institutions worldwide when definitely pathogenic variants are detected. However, many laboratories and institutions are hesitant to proceed with clinical diagnostic testing for variants of uncertain significance, often necessitating functional validation of novel or unknown variants first be performed, as discussed later in this chapter.

Classes of nDNA Genes that Cause Primary Mitochondrial Disease

Pathogenic variants in nuclear genes cause primary mitochondrial disease by impairing the function of the protein product encoded by a given gene. Genes important for mitochondrial structure and function code for a variety of protein products, including respiratory chain enzyme complex subunits or assembly factors, cofactors, mtDNA translation machinery and enzymes, mtDNA maintenance factor, mitochondrial import channels, and mitochondrial fission and fusion, and many others.

Respiratory chain subunits and assembly factors. The nuclear genome encodes all subunits that comprise the mitochondrial RC with the exception of 13 encoded by mtDNA. nDNA genes also encode for all assembly factors needed to assemble the RC complexes, serve as cofactors, and properly orient the complexes within the inner mitochondrial membrane. Complexes I, II, III, and IV shuttle electrons from reducing equivalents derived from nutrient metabolism to molecular oxygen. Complexes I, III, and IV also pump protons from the mitochondrial matrix across the mitochondrial inner membrane into the intermembrane space, creating a charge separation or potential difference that is used to power complex V to generate chemical energy in the form of adenosine triphosphate (ATP) within the mitochondrial matrix.

Complex I. Complex I, or nicotinamide adenine dinucleotide (NADH):ubiquinone oxidoreductase, has 45 subunits, 38 of which are encoded by nDNA. Collectively, they move electrons from NADH to ubiquinone (CoQ10) [26]. Approximately 15 assembly factors important for complex I have now been identified, including *ACAD9*, *FOXRED1*, *TIMMDC1*, and *TMEM126B* [27]. Phenotypes associated with complex I deficiency due to mutations in complex I subunit genes or assembly factors are diverse and may include Leigh syndrome, cardiomyopathy, neurologic problems, and renal failure. Age of onset may range from neonatal- or childhood-onset severe or even fatal phenotypes to adult-onset conditions with a relatively more mild course. Most complex I diseases are inherited in an autosomal recessive manner, although two are X-linked (*NDUFA1* and *NDUFB11*).

Complex II. Complex II, or succinate-ubiquinone oxidoreductase, is comprised of four nuclear-encoded subunits (*SDHA*, *SDHB*, *SDHC*, and *SDHD*). Complex II transfers electrons from succinate and $FADH_2$ generated in the tricarboxylic acid (TCA) cycle to ubiquinone [28]. Homozygous or compound heterozygous pathogenic variants in *SDHA*, *SDHB*, and *SDHD* have been shown to cause primary mitochondrial disease characterized by Leigh or Leigh-like syndrome, either with or without additional organ system involvement [29]. Single pathogenic variants inherited in an autosomal dominant manner in these genes are also causal for hereditary paragangliomas with cancer predisposition [30]. Several complex II assembly factors have also been identified, including *SDHAF1* that has been associated with autosomal recessive complex II deficiency and leukoencephalopathy [31, 32] and *SDHAF2* that has been associated with autosomal dominant hereditary paragangliomas [33].

Complex III. Complex III, or ubiquinol-ferrocytochrome c oxidoreductase, has 11 subunits, 10 of which are nuclear-encoded. Complex III oxidizes CoQ10 and transfers electrons to cytochrome c. Pathogenic variants in several structural subunits (*UQCRB*, *UQCRQ*, *UQCRC2*, and *CYC1*) and assembly factors (*BCS1L*, *LYRM7*, *UQCC2*, and *UQCC3*) have now been associated with complex III deficiency. Various phenotypes may be seen consistent with primary mitochondrial disease including both hypoglycemia and hyperglycemia, hepatomegaly and other liver involvement, Leigh syndrome and other neurologic abnormalities, renal tubular acidosis, and episodic metabolic decompensation [34].

Complex IV. Complex IV, or cytochrome c oxidase, is comprised of 13 structural subunits, 10 of which are encoded by nuclear DNA. Complex IV transfers electrons from cytochrome c to the final electron acceptor, oxygen [35]. Unlike the other RC complexes, the majority of disease-causing mutations in nDNA genes known to cause complex IV deficiency occur not in structural subunits but rather in assembly factors such as *SURF1*, *SCO1*, and *SCO2*. Pathogenic mutations in complex IV assembly factors have been associated with multiple clinical presentations including Leigh syndrome and cardiomyopathy [27].

Complex V. Complex V, or ATP synthase, is comprised of at least 15 subunits, 13 of which are nuclear encoded. Complex V dissipates the electrochemical gradient established by complexes I through IV of the electron transport chain to generate ATP. Pathogenic mutations have been identified in several nuclear-encoded complex V subunits (*ATP5A1*, *ATP5E*, *USMG5*) and assembly factors (*TMEM70*, *ATPAF2*), with disease phenotypes ranging from Leigh syndrome to cardiomyopathy [36, 37].

mtDNA genome maintenance. mtDNA replicates continuously, a process that requires incorporation of deoxynucleotide triphosphates (dNTPs) and error repair. Defects in this process lead to accumulation of multiple deletions and/or mtDNA depletion, which ultimately prevent proper incorporation of mtDNA-encoded subunits into the five complexes of the RC and impair energy production.

Polymerase gamma, encoded by the nuclear gene *POLG*, is the only mtDNA polymerase, responsible for both mtDNA replication and repair. Pathogenic *POLG* mutations have been associated with a spectrum of medical problems ranging from isolated chronic progressive external ophthalmoplegia (CPEO) on the relatively mild end to early-onset Leigh syndrome or Alpers-Huttenlocher syndrome that involves liver failure and early death on the severe end. *POLG* disease may be inherited in either autosomal recessive or dominant fashion, although it is rare that carrier parents of affected children will themselves have disease manifestations. Several clinically useful tools have been developed to aid in *POLG* variant interpretation. These include the *POLG* variant database [38] (https://tools.niehs.nih.gov//polg/), which expertly catalogs and visualizes variant pathogenicity, as well as the *POLG* variant server prediction tool, which predicts clinical consequences of *POLG* variants alone and in combination based on their location within distinct gene region clusters [39].

Twinkle (encoded by the nuclear gene *TWNK*) is the mtDNA genome helicase, which allows for mtDNA strand unwinding and separation as is necessary for its replication. CPEO plus is a common clinical manifestation of *TWNK* mutations that are inherited in an autosomal dominant manner. Infantile-onset spinocerebellar ataxia and epilepsy are caused by *TWNK* pathogenic variants inherited in an autosomal recessive manner [40, 41]. Of note, protein products of many other nuclear genes are important for mtDNA replication, and pathogenic variants in these genes have also been demonstrated to cause primary mitochondrial disease [42].

mtDNA replication requires access to a continuous pool of nucleotides (dNTPs), which may be converted to deoxynucleosides in the mitochondrial matrix or be imported from the cytosol. Several nuclear-encoded enzymes are vital in the conversion process of adenine, guanine, uridine, and thymidine nucleotides necessary for mtDNA replication, including *TK2*, *DGUOK*, *SUCLG1*, *SUCLA2*, *ABAT*, *TYMP*, and *RRM2B*. Several nuclear-encoded protein products are important for importing dNTPs from the cytosol, including *SLC25A4*, *AGK*, and *MPV17*. Affected individuals with pathogenic variants in these genes typically present in early childhood (although mitochondrial neurogastrointestinal encephalopathy (MNGIE) that results from pathogenic mutations in *TYMP* typically has onset in adulthood), with multi-organ system involvement including predominantly neurologic, hepatic, or myopathic phenotypes [43]. Although these conditions may be clinically devastating, therapies to replenish mitochondrial dNTP pools are currently under active clinical investigation, most notably involving at this time *TK2*-related disorders [44].

mtDNA translation. The 13 protein-coding mtDNA genes must undergo transcription and translation within mitochondria to generate RC protein subunits. The mitochondrion therefore requires its own machinery where these 13 polypeptides are synthesized by mitochondrial ribosomes. Nuclear genes encode for many integral components of this mitochondrial transcription and translation process, with several classes of nuclear genes involved in this process now having been associated with mitochondrial diseases. These include (1) *TFAM*, which encodes for a mitochondrial transcription factor having important roles in mtDNA replication, transcription, and packaging into nucleoids. Pathogenic variants in *TFAM* result in liver failure in infancy [45]. (2) Nuclear genes encode each of the mitochondrial aminoacyl-tRNA synthetases (mt-ARSs) necessary to charge the MT-tRNAs. Mutations in many of these genes have now been shown to cause a wide spectrum of mitochondrial diseases with varying phenotypes ranging from severe neurologic disease to liver disease and failure to thrive [46]. (3) Nuclear-encoded mitochondrial ribosomal subunit proteins have also been recognized to cause primary mitochondrial disease. Pathogenic variants have been identified in many different subunits of small (MRPS) and large (MRPL) mitochondrial ribosomes [47]. (4) Translation factors important in translation activation (*TACO1*), elongation (*GFM1*), and release of newly made proteins (*C12ORF65*) have all now been found to harbor disease-causing mutations with a range of clinical features stemming from multiple RC deficiencies from neurologic disease to vision loss or liver problems [48–50].

Mitochondrial fission and fusion. Mitochondria are constantly moving, undergoing fission and fusion with nearby mitochondria as part of their normal life cycle to allow for mixing and repair of mtDNA genomes and proteins. The fission and fusion processes are regulated by nuclear genes, including *OPA1*, *MFN1*, and *MFN2*, important in mitochondrial membrane fusion and *DNM1L* and *MIEF2* necessary for mitochondrial fission. Peripheral neuropathy and optic neuropathy are predominant phenotypes of this group of disorders, as mitochondrial clumping occurs when mitochondria cannot divide and fuse, thereby preventing mitochondria from traveling along the long axons of nerves to where they are needed to support neurotransmission.

Identifying and Confirming Molecular Causes of Primary Mitochondrial Disease

Remarkably, pathogenic variants in more than 350 genes have now been associated with primary mitochondrial disease, with at least one or two new gene causes identified each month for the past decade. Extensive phenotypic overlap exists across these many distinct genetic etiologies. In most instances, it is impossible to predict a definitive genetic etiology based solely on phenotype. Pleiotropy is common, where, for example, the m.3243A>G mutation may be causal of diverse phenotypes including MELAS, diabetes mellitus, hearing loss, CPEO, and Leigh syndrome [15]. Allelic heterogeneity is extensive, where a wide range of pathogenic mutations is common in many genes such as *ACAD9*, in which there have been more than 70 reported patients worldwide representing the most frequently encountered nuclear-encoded complex I disease gene, with symptoms ranging from encephalopathy to cardiomyopathy [51]. Locus heterogeneity is also very common, where there is often strong overlap of the clinical phenotypes between different disease loci. For example, Leigh syndrome and Leigh-like syndrome can result from mutations in more than 90 genes in either nuclear or mtDNA genome [52]. Given this extensive genetic heterogeneity with generally poor genotype-phenotype correlations, a comprehensive untargeted diagnostic approach is required to properly diagnose primary mitochondrial disease. To this end, diagnostic testing options have rapidly evolved over the past decade to now include whole exome sequencing (WES), whole genome sequencing (WGS), RNA sequencing (RNA-seq), and genome-wide single nucleotide polymorphism (SNP) microarray analysis (see section "Genomic Testing Technical Specifications" for detailed descriptions of test methods, analytic considerations, and diagnostic limitations).

Efficient but comprehensive molecular diagnostics are prerequisite for individuals with suspected primary mitochondrial disease, as the underlying genetic etiology can guide specific therapeutic regimes, obviate the need for further and potentially more invasive testing, and enable patient stratification for clinical treatment trials that facilitates development of novel treatment regimes. Additionally, confirming the precise molecular etiology allows for appropriate genetic counseling and consideration of prenatal testing options for family members and offspring of affected individuals.

Given the decreased cost and increased utility of minimally invasive genetic diagnostic testing [14], this has now become the first-line diagnostic testing option for primary mitochondrial disease [53, 54], with more invasive testing options only being pursued when this testing is unrevealing. Whole exome sequencing is increasingly used as a first tier diagnostic test for primary mitochondrial disease, especially when mtDNA genome sequencing is either normal or concurrently performed for the same total testing cost.

Genomic sequencing. WES has revolutionized molecular diagnostics and over the past 6 years has become readily implemented into routine diagnostic workflows. For individuals with suspected mitochondrial disorders, this has led to a shift away from clinical reliance on invasive histological, immunohistochemical, and biochemical investigations of muscle biopsy specimens that have long been the gold standard means to diagnose mitochondrial disorders, toward less invasive genetic diagnostic testing in blood being the first-tier test [14, 55]. WES of nuclear genes has tripled to quadrupled the diagnostic yield for suspected mitochondrial disease with dramatic reduction in the time to reach a definitive diagnosis from years or decades to now weeks or months, although a diagnostic gap does remain for some individuals. Across a broad range of complex disorders, approximately half of the patients in stratified cohorts and about one-third of those in heterogeneous cohorts receive a clear molecular diagnosis by WES. Specifically in the case of primary mitochondrial disease, a success rate of 53% was reported by Taylor et al. for a highly stratified patient cohort [56]. Wortmann et al. achieved 39% diagnostic yield for a heterogeneous group of suspected mitochondrial disease patients through WES alone, with improvement to a 57% yield upon taking into account additional biochemical, histochemical, clinical, and neurologic information [57]. 43% of the cases were diagnosed in a Japanese cohort published by Ohtake et al. [58], which is similar to the experience at the Institute of Human Genetics in Munich, where approximately half of 1500 suspected mitochondrial disease patients from European and Middle Eastern origins receive a definitive genetic diagnosis. Depending on the a priori likelihood of mitochondrial disease and extent of biochemical confirmation performed prior to pursuit of exome sequencing, some groups have achieved higher diagnostic yields on the order of 70%.

Inconclusive WES may result from a range of causes. These include insufficient sequence capture to include or sufficiently cover the causative variant in a given individual or the informatics failure to recognize and prioritize the causative variant from the available data. The former category includes all noncoding variants, as WES by design sequences solely the coding genome regions, but on some designs or capture methodologies, coding variants may not be adequately covered. This can largely be overcome by performing whole genome sequencing (WGS), which achieves more complete coverage of all genomic regions without requiring specific regions to be initially enriched for analysis. Interestingly, WGS usually does not resolve the failure to identify the pathogenic variant when missed by WES. The challenge in interpreting WGS data stems both from a vast number of variants identified by WGS are noncoding single nucleotide variants (about 60,000 per genome) as compared to protein-affecting rare variants (only 475 variants with minor allele frequency (MAF) < 0.005 per genome) and limited understanding of the clinical relevance of the noncoding genome that renders successful variant prioritization highly challenging [59].

Although classically considered in testing for neurodevelopmental disabilities and congenital malformations, genome-wide SNP microarray analysis remains an important diagnostic tool to detect chromosomal deletions or duplications of varying size at millions of sites across the nuclear genome. As with any other Mendelian disorder, nuclear gene-based mitochondrial diseases may be caused by a copy number change that includes a nuclear gene associated with primary mitochondrial disease.

Variant prioritization in large-scale sequence data. WES analysis yields between 20,000 and 23,000 coding variants on average per individual, whereas WGS yields three million variants per individual [60–62]. When considering only protein-altering variants for WES analysis, 12,000–14,000 variants still remain. To identify the pathogenic variant among this large number of variants, careful and sophisticated variant evaluation is required. The American College of Medical Genetics 2015 variant curation guidelines proposed a classification scheme of variants into five categories, namely, "pathogenic," "likely pathogenic," "uncertain significance," "likely benign," and "benign," using evidence derived from population data, computational and predictive data, functional data, segregation data, de novo data, allelic data, as well as other databases and data [63]. In compliance with these recommendations, variants in massively parallel exome or genome datasets are first filtered for their frequency in a control population, which can be a large in-house database as well as publically available databases such as gnomAD [64]. The ACMG suggest assuming a MAF cutoff representing the prevalence of a given disease. Such prevalence data are often unknown, however, so instead others provide a bottom-up approach using frequencies of causative variants in the ExAC database to calculate a disease-specific cutoff [65]. For mitochondrial disorders, a very stringent filter of a 0.1% MAF cutoff is typically applied, since only one mitochondrial disease-associated gene, *MTFMT*, is reported to harbor a more frequently detected pathogenic variant [66].

The variants can further be filtered by considering allelic data and familial pedigree information. For most childhood-onset mitochondrial diseases, autosomal recessive inheritance can be suspected to limit consideration only to bi-allelic variants [67]. In the setting of consanguinity, a homozygous pathogenic mutation is likely. Autosomal dominant mutations should be suspected in some mitochondrial disease scenarios such as adult-onset PEO and KSS. In families where males related to each other via a female are affected, X-linked inheritance can be assumed. Regarding de novo mutations, only very few pathogenic de novo mutations in nuclear DNA have been described, while conversely, mtDNA deletions are mostly sporadic [67–69]. Using a frequency and allele filter together yields on average rare, bi-allelic variants in about 5–25 genes per individual and heterozygous variants in about 125–250 genes per individual. Trio sequencing (of proband and both parents) further results in the identification of 1.6 de novo variants on average per index patient. The remaining variants can subsequently be screened for reported disease associations in public databases as ClinVar [70] or the Human Gene Mutation Database (HGMD) [71]. In the majority of cases, however, no known pathogenic variants will be revealed, requiring that novel variants be evaluated using computational and predictive data. Indeed, 85% of sequence variants in ClinVar were deposited by single submitters, indicating the rarity of most pathogenic variants [65]. To prioritize novel variants, it can be informative to identify novel variants in genes already associated with mitochondrial disease or in novel disease genes encoding mitochondrial proteins. Additionally, the predicted effect of the variant on the protein level (e.g., loss-of-function, missense, etc.) should to be considered. Further clues can be derived from statistical means, conservation and prediction scores, as well as experimental data reported in the literature. Exome data reanalysis at a later time can also be a helpful strategy, with an estimated 10% improved diagnostic yield reported from research-based functional analyses and exome data reanalysis, due to improved general knowledge, as in the case of mitochondrial disease where an average of 22 novel disease genes have been identified per year since 2012 [5, 72–75].

Recently, functional evidence derived from RNAseq-based transcriptome profiling has proven useful to further judge variants of unknown significance (VUS), which are defined as WES or WGS variants for which the association with a disease is unclear. RNAseq data provides a comprehensive view on variants resulting in RNA transcript alterations. A systematic genome-wide analysis revealed there occurs a median of one aberrant expression, five aberrant splicing, and six mono-allelic expression (MAE) events per patient, respectively [76]. This low number of detected events per dataset enables ready manual examination to facilitate identification of pathogenic coding and noncoding variants. The utility of RNAseq for pathogenic variant identification was exemplified for *COL6A1*, when a recurrent de novo intronic pathogenic variant was identified [77]. RNAseq enables the immediate probing of the impact of coding as well as noncoding variants on RNA abundance and sequence.

The pathogenicity of novel variants, especially in genes not previously associated with a given disease, needs to be further evaluated and with functional analyses and/or statistical means that require identification of additional unrelated cases. Since it is now well-recognized that up to 20% of suspected mitochondrial diseases are actually non-mitochondrial genetic disorders [57], it is important to evaluate the entire exome and not restrict focus to mitochondrial disease genes only in the clinical interpretation. It is also important to recognize that up to 5% of all suspected inherited disease patients actually have more than one gene disorder [78].

Variant validation. To provide a firm molecular diagnosis, validation of the likely pathogenic variant is mandatory [79]. First, sequencing errors and sample mix-ups should be excluded by performing Sanger sequencing on a second, independent sample from the individual. Validation of VUS requires further confirmatory steps. As outlined by the ACMG, variant segregation as expected with presumed inheritance pattern in the family needs to be confirmed, as the presence of segregation is a strong indicator for pathogenicity [63]. Eventually, final evidence for the validation of the pathogenicity can be derived from functional studies, which are extremely powerful, or the identification of multiple unrelated patients who share both a causal mutation or disease gene and a distinct clinical phenotype.

Frequently employed techniques for the functional investigation into the effect of a variant on mRNA and protein stability include quantitative real-time PCR or RNASeq for RNA and Western blot analysis or quantitative proteomics for proteins. For functional studies in the field of mitochondrial or metabolic disorders, one can further exploit detectable biochemical and metabolic phenotypes. For example, biochemical assays for the measurement of the oxygen consumption rate, the measurement of the activity of the RC complex enzyme activities, assays tailored to the known function(s) of a protein under investigation, as well as metabolite investigations can provide crucial evidence to demonstrate the pathogenicity of a suspect allele. Often, such phenotypes are detectable in patient-derived fibroblasts, such that collecting and biobanking fibroblasts represent an invaluable resource for validation of VUS [80]. These personalized cellular models provide a useful platform in which to evaluate the functional effects of protein or gene rescue of the biochemical or metabolic phenotype, such as by lentiviral-mediated re-expression of a wild-type copy of the gene or metabolic supplementation assays, to ultimately demonstrate the pathogenicity of a candidate variant affecting that protein or process [79, 81]. Due to the limited availability of patient specimens, yeast models can present a valid alternative, which allows fast and relatively easy modeling of patient-specific variants and investigations of variant effects, which is particularly powerful if the gene is essential [82].

Identification of additional patients harboring mutations in the same gene represents an obvious challenge inherent in the field of rare disorders. Joining efforts by developing international registries currently approached by a Pan-European consortium (GENOMIT.eu) and platforms like GeneMatcher [83], Genesis [84], or the Matchmaker Exchange [85] represent essential resources for the global genomic community that has already strongly demonstrated their vast utility and potential.

mtDNA genome sequencing. mtDNA genome sequencing remains an important diagnostic tool for primary mitochondrial disease, although the phenomenon of heteroplasmy brings unique caveats. Care must be taken by clinicians both when ordering and reviewing results from mtDNA genome sequencing. The sequencing technique employed is extremely important to consider, as techniques such as Sanger sequencing will not reliably detect heteroplasmy levels below 50%. Therefore, a normal Sanger sequencing result does not mean a pathogenic variant is not present in a given individual, but rather only that it is not present in that sample above 50% heteroplasmy. Next-generation sequencing (NGS) is the gold standard for mtDNA sequencing, which depending on technological factors can reliably detect heteroplasmy levels down to 1.5%. Care must also be taken when considering what tissues were tested. Some mtDNA variants and deletions are only present in certain tissues, such as the muscle. Therefore, if a mtDNA disorder is suspected, the muscle or the relevant symptomatic tissue (such as the liver) should be tested.

Blood testing offers a minimally invasive way to obtain a useful sample for testing, although blood heteroplasmy levels for some well-characterized variants such as m.3243A>G are known to decrease with age even as the patient's disease severity increases and heteroplasmy levels rise in other tissues. Urine sample heteroplasmy testing offers a noninvasive way to obtain and test urine epithelial cells, although obtaining sufficient cells to perform diagnostic testing can be challenging in children and there may be variable urine heteroplasmy levels even in the same person [86]. Buccal testing offers another noninvasive option, and heteroplasmy levels in a patient's fibroblasts can be readily evaluated when a skin biopsy has been performed.

Confirming a novel mtDNA variant as pathogenic and causative of an individual's presentation may be complex. Transmitochondrial cybrid cell line studies are useful in this regard. Transmitochondrial cybrids are generated by merging cell lines with a given mtDNA variant with a cell line lacking mtDNA. Since the nuclear background is controlled for, the effects of mtDNA variants can then be functionally assessed in the cybrid lines by means such as electron transport chain enzyme analysis or polarography [87].

ACMG guidelines exist to aid in and standardize the assessment of nuclear DNA variants [63]. However, there are limitations in applying these guidelines to mtDNA variant assessment as they do not address issues such as heteroplasmy, threshold effect, and haplogroups. Careful consideration of mtDNA variant curation guidelines in light of the ACMG general guidelines has now been addressed by the MSeqDR-ClinGen mitochondrial DNA working group (manuscript in preparation).

Consistency in identifying and laboratory reporting of mtDNA variants is crucial to standardize diagnosis. If one clinical laboratory reports a mtDNA variant to be present in an individual while another laboratory does not, the clinician is left unclear whether the initial variant was absent in the tissue tested by the second lab or if the variant was not reported because it was interpreted to be benign. These two scenarios have drastically different management implications for the patient, since demonstrating a variant to be present at homoplasmy in several tissues reduces suspicion for its pathogenicity (although exceptions exist, as for the LHON mtDNA-encoded complex I subunit variants) while having a variant absent in one tissue and present at high heteroplasmy or homoplasmy in another tissue would raise suspicion for its pathogenicity in that individual. Furthermore, a clinician with less experience in primary mitochondrial disease and mtDNA genetics may inherently assume one scenario over the other, causing them to provide misleading information to the affected individual and incorrectly base management recommendations on false assumptions.

Mitochondrial Genome Variant Curation and Deposition

Variant curation. Many bioinformatics tools exist to facilitate variant curation. The Mitochondrial Disease Sequence Data Resource, MSeqDR, is a central and organized hub for primary mitochondrial disease knowledge that enables variant assessment in both genomes [88–91]. Within MSeqDR is MSeqDR-LSDB, a locus-specific database which houses gene and variant information for more than 1500 genes relevant to mitochondrial function. MSeqDR also curates updated data from several sources including ClinVar [70] and MITOMAP [92]. Tools specific for MT-tRNA variant interpretation are also readily available, including Mitotip [93] and HmtVAR [94, 95]. Efforts are underway to facilitate expert curation of both nuclear and mtDNA genes associated with primary mitochondrial disease as part of the Clinical Genome Resource project, or ClinGen [96]. mvTOOLs is a useful tool to automatically annotate extensive knowledge about mtDNA variants [91]. MSeqDR also has a host of tools to facilitate submission by individuals or expert panels of variants and variant pathogenicity assertions [90].

Genomic Testing Technical Specifications

Whole Exome Sequencing (WES)

WES is an unbiased method to detect both previously characterized and novel disease-associated genes. WES is the massively parallel sequencing of the 2% exonic, or protein-coding regions, of the genome [61]. As the exonic regions are predicted to contain 85% of the Mendelian disease-causing variants, WES is a cost-effective comprehensive strategy applicable in large scale [97], as technical cost can be as low as several hundred dollars depending on volume, although clinical diagnostic costs are typically tenfold higher. WES was only introduced in 2009, and the first mitochondrial disease gene identified by WES occurred just 1 year later, after which it quickly developed to become the gold standard of molecular diagnostics. Around 300 novel disease-associated genes across all fields are now identified by WES every year [98, 99]. Importantly, the breakthrough of WES reflects a synergistic improvement of sequencing technology as well as the development of bioinformatics pipelines for sequence alignment, variant calling and annotation, and filtering strategies [100–102].

WES Methodology. Performing WES analysis starts with shearing of an individual's genomic DNA (gDNA) into small fragments. While gDNA and mtDNA can be derived from any tissue, mtDNA mutation load may differ between tissues. If not specifically targeted for enrichment, mtDNA coverage is about 50-fold, which is sufficient to detect most pathogenic variants and initiate tissue-specific studies; however, targeted enrichment can be performed by capture or long-range qPCR methods to substantially increase mtDNA genome coverage to improve the sensitivity and reliability of low-level heteroplasmy detection [103, 104]. Adaptors are ligated to the fragments, and the exonic regions are selectively captured by in-solution enrichment using biotinylated oligonucleotide baits. Commercial enrichment kits differing in bait type (DNA and RNA), bait length, and captured regions are offered from various companies (e.g., Agilent (SureSelect Human AllExon Kit), Illumina (TruSeq Exome Enrichment Kit), and Roche (Nimblegen SeqCap EZ Exome), where a comparison of technologic platforms is described in [105–107]). Baits are subsequently pulled down by magnetic streptavidin beads, and then hybridized fragments are amplified by PCR. Eventually, enriched and amplified sequences are subjected to massively parallel sequencing.

WES Analysis. To detect variants from the raw WES data, sophisticated bioinformatic processing is required. First, the short sequence reads stored in the FASTQ file are aligned to a reference genome, for example, using the Burrows-Wheeler Alignment (BWA) tool. Subsequently, single nucleotide variants (SNVs) and small insertions and deletions of 1–10 bp (indels) are called between the input and reference sequences. In principle, such variant calling simply calculates the proportion of bases differing from the reference at a given position. A variant is deemed to be heterozygous if it is present in a proportion of reads ranging roughly between 20% and 80%, depending on the coverage and quality of the underlying reads. If the proportion is higher than 80%, the variant is called as homozygous. However, this simplified picture does not take into consideration base quality, mapping quality, or neighboring bases; hence, more sophisticated models were developed. The recently developed GATK HaplotypeCaller outperforms other variant callers for detecting SNVs and indels [108], by first determining regions that vary from the reference, so-called active regions and then performing de novo assembly of all possible haplotypes within that active region [109]. Subsequently, a per-read likelihood of a given haplotype is derived by aligning each individual read to all possible haplotypes and then determining the most likely genotype by calculating a per-read likelihood of an allele for each variant site. As WES is a short-read sequencing technology, it is challenging to use this approach to call larger variants, such as structural variants and copy number variants (CNVs) that range in size from 1 base pair to several megabases. Different strategies have been developed for CNV detection (read depth, split-read, paired-end assembly, and a combination approach) [110, 111]. A particularly suitable option among these is read depth, which compares the normalized read depth of a given chromosomal window (such as exon), in a given sample to the expected read depth in that window as determined by a statistical model. For example, the CNV caller ExomDepth uses a Hidden Markov Model to compare exons of one sample against those of around ten control samples.

Despite high sensitivity when compared to other tools, a high false-positive rate remains, requiring caution be used when evaluating CNV or indel results in WES data. Following variant calling, variants are filtered for quality and minimal read depth and annotated with supplementary information. Frequently used annotation tools are ANNOVAR [112], SnpEff [113], or customized in-house tools to annotate each variant with its genomic coordinates as exonic, intergenic, intronic, splice site, 3'-UTR, or 5'-UTR. Based on the mRNA sequence, exonic variants can be further annotated with the predicted consequence of the variant on the protein sequence, including synonymous, non-synonymous, frameshift, stop-gain, or stop-loss. To ease variant interpretation, pathogenicity scores as provided by, e.g., CADD [114], MutationTaster [115], PolyPhen-2 [116], and SIFT [117, 118] and frequency information derived from comprehensive database like ExAC and gnomAD need to be taken into account. Further considerations for variant annotation were provided by 2015 consensus guidelines from the American College of Medical Genetics and Genomics (ACMG) and the Association of Molecular Pathology (AMP) [63].

WES Limitations. While the most evident shortcoming of WES is that it neglects noncoding sequence variants, one also needs to be aware of the coding region detection caveats of WES. One pitfall is our lack of complete understanding of the coding genome regions, with new genomic regions steadily being identified as exonic. As the design of the baits of the enrichments kits are based on the current understanding of the exome, only known exonic regions are included and captured. A second challenge is the varying efficiency with which baits capture their intended targets. Indeed, some regions escape complete capture. Furthermore, even though an exonic region might be captured, the coverage of that fragment might be adversely affected by PCR amplification and enrichment. Despite great efforts of the enrichment kit manufacturers, the latest version of the Agilent SureSelect kit (SureSelect Human All Exon V7), for example, covers 99.3% of RefSeq genes. Investigating the performance of clinical exome sequencing, the ACMG found that 6 of 56 investigated actionable disease genes had 1 exon insufficiently covered, while more than half of known HGMD variant locations in 7 genes showed inadequate coverage [119]. In a different study, 7% of exons of genes known to be associated with neuropathy were covered insufficiently, and 2% of exons in these genes were completely missed [120]. In addition to technical limitations, the analytical steps of sequence alignment, variant calling, and annotation may be error prone. Repeat sequence regions and homopolymers pose particular challenges to predictive tools. While the caveat of calling indels was largely resolved by the development of the GATK HaplotypeCaller, the detection of CNVs in WES data, especially in repetitive regions, remains nontrivial. Finally, our incomplete understanding of genes and transcripts limits the proper annotation of the genomic location and functional impact of WES variants.

Whole Genome Sequencing (WGS)

Due to steadily decreasing sequencing costs, it is now becoming feasible to perform whole genome sequencing (WGS) instead of WES. WGS achieves almost complete coverage of the whole genome. Additionally, WGS library preparation does not require exon capture or PCR amplification, which often introduces bias. In addition, WGS provides more even sequence coverage that strongly facilitates CNV detection and markedly enriches capture of mtDNA genomes relative to nuclear genomes to allow for highly sensitive heteroplasmy detection.

WGS Methodology and Sequence Analysis. Similarly as for WES methodology, WGS is initiated by shearing gDNA into small fragments. Libraries can be prepared using different commercially available kits. For example, using the Illumina TruSeq DNA PCR-Free Library Prep Kit, gDNA fragments are subsequently hybridized to paramagnetic beads and ligated to adapters, after which massively parallel sequencing is performed. Similarly as for WES workflows, raw WGS reads are aligned to a reference, followed by variant calling, filtering, and annotation.

WGS Limitations. One important aspect to consider when performing WGS is the sizable amount of data and variants generated. Furthermore, WGS fails to achieve complete coverage of the whole genome. Analytical shortages mentioned for WES remain equally applicable to WGS, including challenge with analyzing repetitive sequences other than CNV. Finally, our poor understanding of noncoding genome regions renders variant annotation extremely challenging in regard to assessing their functional effects.

RNA Sequencing (RNA-seq)

RNA sequencing (RNA-seq) describes sequencing of the entire transcriptome. It is becoming an important addition to WES and WGS as it enables complementation of genomic sequence data with functional expression evidence. RNA-seq permits the immediate probing of the impact of variants, both coding and noncoding, on RNA abundance and sequence [76]. One important observation can be assessing expression outliers to detect impaired gene expression, which can result from coding variants or noncoding variants in regulatory regions like promoters, enhancers, and suppressors. Expression outliers may not only be caused by reduced transcription but also by RNA degradation through nonsense-mediated decay (NMD). A second possible finding unique to RNA-seq is the detection of aberrant splicing caused by variants in splice sites or splice motifs, which often cause the generation of a premature stop codon to provoke NMD that would be detected as an expression outlier. A third phenomenon evident at the RNA level is mono-allelic expression (MAE). MAE arises if only one allele is impacted by aberrant expression or aberrant splicing, while the other allele expressed. While the best-known case of MAE is the widely studied phenomenon of X chromosome inactivation, an increasing number of autosomal genes are now known to show random MAE expression [121]. Importantly, diseases associated with MAE in such genes do not follow standard Mendelian patterns of inheritance.

RNA-seq Methodology. Unlike DNA, RNA is a compendium of several subspecies including ribosomal (rRNA), messenger (mRNA), transfer (tRNA), and microRNA. Many different protocols have been established to investigate these respective RNA species. Here, we focus on mRNA sequencing. Using the commonly employed Illumina TruSeq RNA Library preparation protocol, an input of 0.1–1 μg of high-quality total RNA (having RNA integrity number (RIN) above 8) is required. This kit is compatible with RNA from different human tissue sources (TruSeq® RNA Sample Preparation v2 Guide (Illumina)). Initially, mRNAs are purified by poly(A) selection, after which RNA is fragmented and reverse transcribed into cDNA. Subsequently, cDNA molecules are then end repaired and A-tailed to facilitate adapter ligation. The library is PCR enriched and further subjected to quality control and quantification. Libraries from different samples are pooled in equimolar amounts, and massively parallel sequencing is performed.

RNA-seq Analysis. To compute expression outliers, statistical testing can be performed on Z-scores, a measure of fold-change that accounts for inter-sample variance [76]. To detect aberrant splicing, algorithms for splicing quantitative trait loci (QTLs) can be adapted; however, these often lack assessment of statistical significance or rely on arbitrary manual corrections for confounders [76]. Novel splice sites are identified by comparing each splicing event in a given sample against all other samples. To investigate MAE, filtering for heterozygous rare single nucleotide variants (SNVs) that were called by WES or WGS in the same sample and are covered with more than 10 RNA-seq reads can be performed. SNVs are considered to have MAE if more than 80% of the reads are harbored by the respective variant with a Hochberg adjusted P-value smaller than 0.05 [76].

RNA-seq Limitations. A major caveat of RNA-seq analysis is tissue-specific gene expression. Indeed, it is not biologically possible to obtain comprehensive analysis of the entire transcriptome by investigating solely one or potentially even several tissues. Hence, pathogenic events may be missed if sequencing is not performed in the clinically affected tissue, which is however often the case. No systematic study has been performed to determine whether disease-causing variants cluster in specific tissues, although expression of 68% of disease genes listed in OMIM was seen in patient-derived fibroblasts which are usually not the primarily affected tissue [122]. Importantly, RNA-seq analysis on patient-derived fibroblasts has been shown to successfully enable molecular diagnosis in suspected mitochondrial disease patients [76]. Prediction tools used to analyze RNA alterations remain error prone, particularly those that detect the extremely complex phenomenon of alternative splicing. RNA-seq statistical analysis models remain under development, and threshold values need to be better defined, which are expected to improve diagnostic yield from RNA-seq in the near future [123].

Conclusion

Mitochondrial disease genetics is a rapidly expanding field facilitated by the continual refinement and increased uptake of sensitive and comprehensive genomic sequencing methodologies, bioinformatics resources, and expert curation. Increasing understanding of mitochondrial biology and mitochondrial disease pathophysiology is enabling novel approaches to mitochondrial disease treatment, bringing the promise of personalized therapies tailored to specific molecular disorders and/or disease mechanisms.

References

1. Gorman GS, Chinnery PF, DiMauro S, Hirano M, Koga Y, McFarland R, et al. Mitochondrial diseases. Nat Rev Dis Primers. 2016;2:16080.
2. Pagliarini DJ, Calvo SE, Chang B, Sheth SA, Vafai SB, Ong SE, et al. A mitochondrial protein compendium elucidates complex I disease biology. Cell. 2008;134(1):112–23.
3. Calvo SE, Clauser KR, Mootha VK. MitoCarta2.0: an updated inventory of mammalian mitochondrial proteins. Nucleic Acids Res. 2016;44(D1):D1251–7.
4. Rahman J, Rahman S. Mitochondrial medicine in the omics era. Lancet. 2018;391(10139):2560–74.
5. Frazier AE, Thorburn DR, Compton AG. Mitochondrial energy generation disorders: genes, mechanisms and clues to pathology. J Biol Chem. 2017;
6. Anderson S, Bankier AT, Barrell BG, de Bruijn MH, Coulson AR, Drouin J, et al. Sequence and organization of the human mitochondrial genome. Nature. 1981;290(5806):457–65.
7. Thorburn DR. Mitochondrial disorders: prevalence, myths and advances. J Inherit Metab Dis. 2004;27(3):349–62.
8. DiMauro S, Hirano M. Mitochondrial DNA deletion syndromes. In: Adam MP, Ardinger HH, Pagon RA, Wallace SE, Bean LJH, Stephens K, et al., editors. GeneReviews((R)). Seattle (WA): University of Washington; 1993.
9. Egger J, Wilson J. Mitochondrial inheritance in a mitochondrially mediated disease. N Engl J Med. 1983;309(3):142–6.
10. Giles RE, Blanc H, Cann HM, Wallace DC. Maternal inheritance of human mitochondrial DNA. Proc Natl Acad Sci U S A. 1980;77(11):6715–9.
11. Brown MD, Torroni A, Reckord CL, Wallace DC. Phylogenetic analysis of Leber's hereditary optic neuropathy mitochondrial DNA's indicates multiple independent occurrences of the common mutations. Hum Mutat. 1995;6(4):311–25.
12. Wei W, Gomez-Duran A, Hudson G, Chinnery PF. Background sequence characteristics influence the occurrence and severity of disease-causing mtDNA mutations. PLoS Genet. 2017;13(12):e1007126.
13. Hudson G, Carelli V, Spruijt L, Gerards M, Mowbray C, Achilli A, et al. Clinical expression of Leber hereditary optic neuropathy is affected by the mitochondrial DNA-haplogroup background. Am J Hum Genet. 2007;81(2):228–33.
14. McCormick E, Place E, Falk MJ. Molecular genetic testing for mitochondrial disease: from one generation to the next. Neurotherapeutics. 2013;10(2):251–61.
15. Nesbitt V, Pitceathly RD, Turnbull DM, Taylor RW, Sweeney MG, Mudanohwo EE, et al. The UK MRC mitochondrial disease patient cohort study: clinical phenotypes associated with the m.3243A>G mutation—implications for diagnosis and management. J Neurol Neurosurg Psychiatry. 2013;84(8):936–8.
16. Murphy R, Turnbull DM, Walker M, Hattersley AT. Clinical features, diagnosis and management of maternally inherited diabetes and deafness (MIDD) associated with the 3243A>G mitochondrial point mutation. Diabet Med. 2008;25(4):383–99.
17. Zolkipli-Cunningham Z, Xiao R, Stoddart A, McCormick EM, Holberts A, Burrill N, et al. Mitochondrial disease patient motivations and barriers to participate in clinical trials. PLoS One. 2018;13(5):e0197513.

18. Caporali L, Maresca A, Capristo M, Del Dotto V, Tagliavini F, Valentino ML, et al. Incomplete penetrance in mitochondrial optic neuropathies. Mitochondrion. 2017;36:130–7.
19. Rahman S, Ecob R, Costello H, Sweeney MG, Duncan AJ, Pearce K, et al. Hearing in 44-45 year olds with m.1555A>G, a genetic mutation predisposing to aminoglycoside-induced deafness: a population based cohort study. BMJ Open. 2012;2:e000411.
20. Khan NA, Govindaraj P, Jyothi V, Meena AK, Thangaraj K. Co-occurrence of m.1555A>G and m.11778G>A mitochondrial DNA mutations in two Indian families with strikingly different clinical penetrance of Leber hereditary optic neuropathy. Mol Vis. 2013;19:1282–9.
21. Vachin P, Adda-Herzog E, Chalouhi G, Elie C, Rio M, Rondeau S, et al. Segregation of mitochondrial DNA mutations in the human placenta: implication for prenatal diagnosis of mtDNA disorders. J Med Genet. 2018;55(2):131–6.
22. Smeets HJ, Sallevelt SC, Dreesen JC, de Die-Smulders CE, de Coo IF. Preventing the transmission of mitochondrial DNA disorders using prenatal or preimplantation genetic diagnosis. Ann N Y Acad Sci. 2015;1350:29–36.
23. Herbert M, Turnbull D. Mitochondrial donation—clearing the final regulatory hurdle in the United Kingdom. N Engl J Med. 2017;376(2):171–3.
24. Falk MJ, Decherney A, Kahn JP. Mitochondrial replacement techniques-implications for the clinical community. N Engl J Med. 2016;374(12):1103–6.
25. Chinnery PF. Mitochondrial disease in adults: what's old and what's new? EMBO Mol Med. 2015;7(12):1503–12.
26. Formosa LE, Dibley MG, Stroud DA, Ryan MT. Building a complex complex: assembly of mitochondrial respiratory chain complex I. Semin Cell Dev Biol. 2018;76:154–62.
27. Ghezzi D, Zeviani M. Human diseases associated with defects in assembly of OXPHOS complexes. Essays Biochem. 2018;62(3):271–86.
28. Jain-Ghai S, Cameron JM, Al Maawali A, Blaser S, MacKay N, Robinson B, et al. Complex II deficiency-a case report and review of the literature. Am J Med Genet A. 2013;161A(2):285–94.
29. Renkema GH, Wortmann SB, Smeets RJ, Venselaar H, Antoine M, Visser G, et al. SDHA mutations causing a multisystem mitochondrial disease: novel mutations and genetic overlap with hereditary tumors. Eur J Hum Genet. 2015;23(2):202–9.
30. Kirmani S, Young WF. Hereditary paraganglioma-pheochromocytoma syndromes. In: Adam MP, Ardinger HH, Pagon RA, Wallace SE, Bean LJH, Stephens K, et al., editors. GeneReviews((R)). Seattle (WA): University of Washington; 1993.
31. Ghezzi D, Goffrini P, Uziel G, Horvath R, Klopstock T, Lochmuller H, et al. SDHAF1, encoding a LYR complex-II specific assembly factor, is mutated in SDH-defective infantile leukoencephalopathy. Nat Genet. 2009;41(6):654–6.
32. Ohlenbusch A, Edvardson S, Skorpen J, Bjornstad A, Saada A, Elpeleg O, et al. Leukoencephalopathy with accumulated succinate is indicative of SDHAF1 related complex II deficiency. Orphanet J Rare Dis. 2012;7:69.
33. Hao HX, Khalimonchuk O, Schraders M, Dephoure N, Bayley JP, Kunst H, et al. SDH5, a gene required for flavination of succinate dehydrogenase, is mutated in paraganglioma. Science. 2009;325(5944):1139–42.
34. Fernandez-Vizarra E, Zeviani M. Nuclear gene mutations as the cause of mitochondrial complex III deficiency. Front Genet. 2015;6:134.
35. Shoubridge EA. Cytochrome c oxidase deficiency. Am J Med Genet. 2001;106(1):46–52.
36. Hejzlarova K, Mracek T, Vrbacky M, Kaplanova V, Karbanova V, Nuskova H, et al. Nuclear genetic defects of mitochondrial ATP synthase. Physiol Res. 2014;63(Suppl 1):S57–71.
37. Barca E, Ganetzky RD, Potluri P, Juanola-Falgarona M, Gai X, Li D, et al. USMG5 Ashkenazi Jewish founder mutation impairs mitochondrial complex V dimerization and ATP synthesis. Hum Mol Genet. 2018;27(19):3305–12.
38. Longley MJ, Graziewicz MA, Bienstock RJ, Copeland WC. Consequences of mutations in human DNA polymerase gamma. Gene. 2005;354:125–31.
39. Nurminen A, Farnum GA, Kaguni LS. Pathogenicity in POLG syndromes: DNA polymerase gamma pathogenicity prediction server and database. BBA Clin. 2017;7:147–56.
40. Spelbrink JN, Li FY, Tiranti V, Nikali K, Yuan QP, Tariq M, et al. Human mitochondrial DNA deletions associated with mutations in the gene encoding twinkle, a phage T7 gene 4-like protein localized in mitochondria. Nat Genet. 2001;28(3):223–31.
41. Young MJ, Copeland WC. Human mitochondrial DNA replication machinery and disease. Curr Opin Genet Dev. 2016;38:52–62.
42. Almannai M, El-Hattab AW, Scaglia F. Mitochondrial DNA replication: clinical syndromes. Essays Biochem. 2018;62(3):297–308.
43. El-Hattab AW, Scaglia F. Mitochondrial DNA depletion syndromes: review and updates of genetic basis, manifestations, and therapeutic options. Neurotherapeutics. 2013;10(2):186–98.
44. Lopez-Gomez C, Levy RJ, Sanchez-Quintero MJ, Juanola-Falgarona M, Barca E, Garcia-Diaz B, et al. Deoxycytidine and Deoxythymidine treatment for thymidine kinase 2 deficiency. Ann Neurol. 2017;81(5):641–52.
45. Stiles AR, Simon MT, Stover A, Eftekharian S, Khanlou N, Wang HL, et al. Mutations in TFAM, encoding mitochondrial transcription factor a, cause neonatal liver failure associated with mtDNA depletion. Mol Genet Metab. 2016;119(1–2):91–9.

46. Fuchs SA, Schene IF, Kok G, Jansen JM, Nikkels PGJ, van Gassen KLI, et al. Aminoacyl-tRNA synthetase deficiencies in search of common themes. Genet Med. 2018;
47. Lake NJ, Webb BD, Stroud DA, Richman TR, Ruzzenente B, Compton AG, et al. Biallelic mutations in MRPS34 lead to instability of the small mitoribosomal subunit and leigh syndrome. Am J Hum Genet. 2018;102(4):713.
48. Seeger J, Schrank B, Pyle A, Stucka R, Lorcher U, Muller-Ziermann S, et al. Clinical and neuropathological findings in patients with TACO1 mutations. Neuromuscul Disord. 2010;20(11):720–4.
49. Spiegel R, Mandel H, Saada A, Lerer I, Burger A, Shaag A, et al. Delineation of C12orf65-related phenotypes: a genotype-phenotype relationship. Eur J Hum Genet. 2014;22(8):1019–25.
50. Galmiche L, Serre V, Beinat M, Zossou R, Assouline Z, Lebre AS, et al. Toward genotype phenotype correlations in GFM1 mutations. Mitochondrion. 2012;12(2):242–7.
51. Repp BM, Mastantuono E, Alston CL, Schiff M, Haack TB, Rotig A, et al. Clinical, biochemical and genetic spectrum of 70 patients with ACAD9 deficiency: is riboflavin supplementation effective? Orphanet J Rare Dis. 2018;13(1):120.
52. Lake NJ, Compton AG, Rahman S, Thorburn DR. Leigh syndrome: one disorder, more than 75 monogenic causes. Ann Neurol. 2016;79(2): 190–203.
53. Parikh S, Goldstein A, Koenig MK, Scaglia F, Enns GM, Saneto R, et al. Diagnosis and management of mitochondrial disease: a consensus statement from the mitochondrial medicine society. Genet Med. 2015;17(9):689–701.
54. Parikh S, Goldstein A, Karaa A, Koenig MK, Anselm I, Brunel-Guitton C, et al. Patient care standards for primary mitochondrial disease: a consensus statement from the mitochondrial medicine society. Genet Med. 2017;19(12):1380.
55. Stenton SL, Prokisch H. Advancing genomic approaches to the molecular diagnosis of mitochondrial disease. Essays Biochem. 2018;62(3):399–408.
56. Taylor RW, Pyle A, Griffin H, Blakely EL, Duff J, He L, et al. Use of whole-exome sequencing to determine the genetic basis of multiple mitochondrial respiratory chain complex deficiencies. JAMA. 2014;312(1):68–77.
57. Wortmann SB, Koolen DA, Smeitink JA, van den Heuvel L, Rodenburg RJ. Whole exome sequencing of suspected mitochondrial patients in clinical practice. J Inherit Metab Dis. 2015;38(3):437–43.
58. Ohtake A, Murayama K, Mori M, Harashima H, Yamazaki T, Tamaru S, et al. Diagnosis and molecular basis of mitochondrial respiratory chain disorders: exome sequencing for disease gene identification. Biochim Biophys Acta. 2014;1840(4):1355–9.
59. Consortium GP, Auton A, Brooks LD, Durbin RM, Garrison EP, Kang HM, et al. A global reference for human genetic variation. Nature. 2015;526:68–74.
60. Wieland T. Next-generation sequencing data analysis [Dissertation]. Diss. Technische Universität München. 2015. http://nbn-resolving.de/urn/resolver.pl?urn:nbn:de:bvb:91-diss-20151111-1244253-1-6.
61. Bamshad MJ, Ng SB, Bigham AW, Tabor HK, Emond MJ, Nickerson DA, et al. Exome sequencing as a tool for Mendelian disease gene discovery. Nat Rev Genet. 2011;12(11):745–55.
62. Genomes Project C, Abecasis GR, Auton A, Brooks LD, DePristo MA, Durbin RM, et al. An integrated map of genetic variation from 1,092 human genomes. Nature. 2012;491(7422):56–65.
63. Richards S, Aziz N, Bale S, Bick D, Das S, Gastier-Foster J, et al. Standards and guidelines for the interpretation of sequence variants: a joint consensus recommendation of the American College of Medical Genetics and Genomics and the Association for Molecular Pathology. Genet Med. 2015;17(5):405–24.
64. Lek M, Karczewski KJ, Minikel EV, Samocha KE, Banks E, Fennell T, et al. Analysis of protein-coding genetic variation in 60,706 humans. Nature. 2016;536:285–91.
65. Kobayashi Y, Yang S, Nykamp K, Garcia J, Lincoln SE, Topper SE. Pathogenic variant burden in the ExAC database: an empirical approach to evaluating population data for clinical variant interpretation. Genome Med. 2017;9(1):13.
66. Haack TB, Gorza M, Danhauser K, Mayr JA, Haberberger B, Wieland T, et al. Phenotypic spectrum of eleven patients and five novel MTFMT mutations identified by exome sequencing and candidate gene screening. Mol Genet Metab. 2014;111(3):342–52.
67. Chinnery PF. Mitochondrial disorders overview. In: Pagon RA, Adam MP, Ardinger HH, Wallace SE, Amemiya A, Bean LJH, et al., editors. GeneReviews(R). Seattle (WA): University of Washington; 1993.
68. Alston CL, Rocha MC, Lax NZ, Turnbull DM, Taylor RW. The genetics and pathology of mitochondrial disease. J Pathol. 2017;241:236–50.
69. Thompson K, Majd H, Dallabona C, Reinson K, King MS, Alston CL, et al. Recurrent de novo dominant mutations in SLC25A4 cause severe early-onset mitochondrial disease and loss of mitochondrial DNA copy number. Am J Hum Genet. 2016;99(6):1405.
70. Landrum MJ, Lee JM, Riley GR, Jang W, Rubinstein WS, Church DM, et al. ClinVar: public archive of relationships among sequence variation and human phenotype. Nucleic Acids Res. 2014;42(Database issue):D980–5.
71. Stenson PD, Ball EV, Mort M, Phillips AD, Shiel JA, Thomas NS, et al. Human gene mutation database (HGMD): 2003 update. Hum Mutat. 2003;21(6):577–81.
72. Al-Murshedi F, Meftah D, Scott P. Underdiagnoses resulting from variant misinterpretation: time for systematic reanalysis of whole exome data? Eur J Med Genet. 2018;

73. Nambot S, Thevenon J, Kuentz P, Duffourd Y, Tisserant E, Bruel AL, et al. Clinical whole-exome sequencing for the diagnosis of rare disorders with congenital anomalies and/or intellectual disability: substantial interest of prospective annual reanalysis. Genet Med. 2018;20(6):645–54.
74. Eldomery MK, Coban-Akdemir Z, Harel T, Rosenfeld JA, Gambin T, Stray-Pedersen A, et al. Lessons learned from additional research analyses of unsolved clinical exome cases. Genome Med. 2017;9(1):26.
75. Wenger AM, Guturu H, Bernstein JA, Bejerano G. Systematic reanalysis of clinical exome data yields additional diagnoses: implications for providers. Genet Med. 2017;19(2):209–14.
76. Kremer LS, Bader DM, Mertes C, Kopajtich R, Pichler G, Iuso A, et al. Genetic diagnosis of Mendelian disorders via RNA sequencing. Nat Commun. 2017;8:15824.
77. Cummings BB, Marshall JL, Tukiainen T, Lek M, Donkervoort S, Foley AR, et al. Improving genetic diagnosis in Mendelian disease with transcriptome sequencing. Sci Transl Med. 2017;9(386):eaal5209.
78. Balci TB, Hartley T, Xi Y, Dyment DA, Beaulieu CL, Bernier FP, et al. Debunking Occam's razor: diagnosing multiple genetic diseases in families by whole-exome sequencing. Clin Genet. 2017;92(3):281–9.
79. Haack TB, Danhauser K, Haberberger B, Hoser J, Strecker V, Boehm D, et al. Exome sequencing identifies ACAD9 mutations as a cause of complex I deficiency. Nat Genet. 2010;42(12):1131–4.
80. Saada A. Mitochondria: mitochondrial OXPHOS (dys) function ex vivo-the use of primary fibroblasts. Int J Biochem Cell Biol. 2014;48:60–5.
81. Kremer LS, Prokisch H. Identification of disease-causing mutations by functional complementation of patient-derived fibroblast cell lines. Methods Mol Biol. 2017;1567:391–406.
82. Lasserre JP, Dautant A, Aiyar RS, Kucharczyk R, Glatigny A, Tribouillard-Tanvier D, et al. Yeast as a system for modeling mitochondrial disease mechanisms and discovering therapies. Dis Model Mech. 2015;8(6):509–26.
83. Sobreira N, Schiettecatte F, Valle D, Hamosh A. GeneMatcher: a matching tool for connecting investigators with an interest in the same gene. Hum Mutat. 2015;36(10):928–30.
84. Gonzalez M, Falk MJ, Gai X, Postrel R, Schule R, Zuchner S. Innovative genomic collaboration using the GENESIS (GEM.App) platform. Hum Mutat. 2015;36(10):950–6.
85. Sobreira NLM, Arachchi H, Buske OJ, Chong JX, Hutton B, Foreman J, et al. Matchmaker exchange. Curr Protoc Hum Genet. 2017;95:9.31.1–9.31.15.
86. Grady JP, Pickett SJ, Ng YS, Alston CL, Blakely EL, Hardy SA, et al. mtDNA heteroplasmy level and copy number indicate disease burden in m.3243A>G mitochondrial disease. EMBO Mol Med. 2018;10(6):e8262.
87. Wilkins HM, Carl SM, Swerdlow RH. Cytoplasmic hybrid (cybrid) cell lines as a practical model for mitochondriopathies. Redox Biol. 2014;2:619–31.
88. Falk MJ, Shen L, Gonzalez M, Leipzig J, Lott MT, Stassen AP, et al. Mitochondrial disease sequence data resource (MSeqDR): a global grass-roots consortium to facilitate deposition, curation, annotation, and integrated analysis of genomic data for the mitochondrial disease clinical and research communities. Mol Genet Metab. 2015;114(3):388–96.
89. Falk MJ, Shen L, Gai X. From case studies to community knowledge base: MSeqDR provides a platform for the curation and genomic analysis of mitochondrial diseases. Cold Spring Harb Mol Case Stud. 2016;2(3):a001065.
90. Shen L, Diroma MA, Gonzalez M, Navarro-Gomez D, Leipzig J, Lott MT, et al. MSeqDR: a centralized knowledge repository and bioinformatics web resource to facilitate genomic investigations in mitochondrial disease. Hum Mutat. 2016;37(6):540–8.
91. Shen L, Attimonelli M, Bai R, Lott MT, Wallace DC, Falk MJ, et al. MSeqDR mvTool: a mitochondrial DNA web and API resource for comprehensive variant annotation, universal nomenclature collation, and reference genome conversion. Hum Mutat. 2018;39(6):806–10.
92. Lott MT, Leipzig JN, Derbeneva O, Xie HM, Chalkia D, Sarmady M, et al. mtDNA variation and analysis using mitomap and mitomaster. Curr Protoc Bioinformatics. 2013;44:1.23.1–26.
93. Sonney S, Leipzig J, Lott MT, Zhang S, Procaccio V, Wallace DC, et al. Predicting the pathogenicity of novel variants in mitochondrial tRNA with MitoTIP. PLoS Comput Biol. 2017;13(12):e1005867.
94. Santorsola M, Calabrese C, Girolimetti G, Diroma MA, Gasparre G, Attimonelli M. A multi-parametric workflow for the prioritization of mitochondrial DNA variants of clinical interest. Hum Genet. 2016;135(1):121–36.
95. Clima R, Preste R, Calabrese C, Diroma MA, Santorsola M, Scioscia G, et al. HmtDB 2016: data update, a better performing query system and human mitochondrial DNA haplogroup predictor. Nucleic Acids Res. 2017;45(D1):D698–706.
96. Rehm HL, Berg JS, Brooks LD, Bustamante CD, Evans JP, Landrum MJ, et al. ClinGen-the clinical genome resource. N Engl J Med. 2015;372(23):2235–42.
97. Majewski J, Schwartzentruber J, Lalonde E, Montpetit A, Jabado N. What can exome sequencing do for you? J Med Genet. 2011;48(9):580–9.
98. Cooper DN, Chen JM, Ball EV, Howells K, Mort M, Phillips AD, et al. Genes, mutations, and human inherited disease at the dawn of the age of personalized genomics. Hum Mutat. 2010;31(6):631–55.
99. Haack TB, Haberberger B, Frisch E-M, Wieland T, Iuso A, Gorza M, et al. Molecular diagnosis in mitochondrial complex I deficiency using exome sequencing. J Med Genet. 2012;49:277–83.

100. Li H, Durbin R. Fast and accurate short read alignment with burrows-wheeler transform. Bioinformatics. 2009;25(14):1754–60.
101. Li H. A statistical framework for SNP calling, mutation discovery, association mapping and population genetical parameter estimation from sequencing data. Bioinformatics. 2011;27(21):2987–93.
102. Li H, Handsaker B, Wysoker A, Fennell T, Ruan J, Homer N, et al. The sequence alignment/map format and SAMtools. Bioinformatics. 2009;25(16):2078–9.
103. Falk MJ, Pierce EA, Consugar M, Xie MH, Guadalupe M, Hardy O, et al. Mitochondrial disease genetic diagnostics: optimized whole-exome analysis for all MitoCarta nuclear genes and the mitochondrial genome. Discov Med. 2012;14(79):389–99.
104. Zhang W, Cui H, Wong LJ. Comprehensive one-step molecular analyses of mitochondrial genome by massively parallel sequencing. Clin Chem. 2012;58(9):1322–31.
105. Sulonen AM, Ellonen P, Almusa H, Lepisto M, Eldfors S, Hannula S, et al. Comparison of solution-based exome capture methods for next generation sequencing. Genome Biol. 2011;12(9):R94.
106. Warr A, Robert C, Hume D, Archibald A, Deeb N, Watson M. Exome sequencing: current and future perspectives. G3 (Bethesda). 2015;5(8):1543–50.
107. Mamanova L, Coffey AJ, Scott CE, Kozarewa I, Turner EH, Kumar A, et al. Target-enrichment strategies for next-generation sequencing. Nat Methods. 2010;7(2):111–8.
108. Hwang S, Kim E, Lee I, Marcotte EM. Systematic comparison of variant calling pipelines using gold standard personal exome variants. Sci Rep. 2015;5:17875.
109. McKenna A, Hanna M, Banks E, Sivachenko A, Cibulskis K, Kernytsky A, et al. The genome analysis toolkit: a MapReduce framework for analyzing next-generation DNA sequencing data. Genome Res. 2010;20(9):1297–303.
110. Tan R, Wang Y, Kleinstein SE, Liu Y, Zhu X, Guo H, et al. An evaluation of copy number variation detection tools from whole-exome sequencing data. Hum Mutat. 2014;35(7):899–907.
111. Medvedev P, Stanciu M, Brudno M. Computational methods for discovering structural variation with next-generation sequencing. Nat Methods. 2009;6(11 Suppl):S13–20.
112. Wang K, Li M, Hakonarson H. ANNOVAR: functional annotation of genetic variants from high-throughput sequencing data. Nucleic Acids Res. 2010;38(16):e164.
113. Cingolani P, Platts A, Wang le L, Coon M, Nguyen T, Wang L, et al. A program for annotating and predicting the effects of single nucleotide polymorphisms, SnpEff: SNPs in the genome of Drosophila melanogaster strain w1118; iso-2; iso-3. Fly (Austin). 2012;6(2):80–92.
114. Kircher M, Witten DM, Jain P, O'Roak BJ, Cooper GM, Shendure J. A general framework for estimating the relative pathogenicity of human genetic variants. Nat Genet. 2014;46(3):310–5.
115. Schwarz JM, Rodelsperger C, Schuelke M, Seelow D. MutationTaster evaluates disease-causing potential of sequence alterations. Nat Methods. 2010;7(8):575–6.
116. Adzhubei IA, Schmidt S, Peshkin L, Ramensky VE, Gerasimova A, Bork P, et al. A method and server for predicting damaging missense mutations. Nat Methods. 2010;7(4):248–9.
117. Ng PC, Henikoff S. SIFT: predicting amino acid changes that affect protein function. Nucleic Acids Res. 2003;31(13):3812–4.
118. Kumar P, Henikoff S, Ng PC. Predicting the effects of coding non-synonymous variants on protein function using the SIFT algorithm. Nat Protoc. 2009;4(7):1073–81.
119. Park JY, Clark P, Londin E, Sponziello M, Kricka LJ, Fortina P. Clinical exome performance for reporting secondary genetic findings. Clin Chem. 2015;61(1):213–20.
120. Klein CJ, Middha S, Duan X, Wu Y, Litchy WJ, Gu W, et al. Application of whole exome sequencing in undiagnosed inherited polyneuropathies. J Neurol Neurosurg Psychiatry. 2014;85(11):1265–72.
121. Eckersley-Maslin MA, Spector DL. Random monoallelic expression: regulating gene expression one allele at a time. Trends Genet. 2014;30:237–44.
122. Kremer LS, Wortmann SB, Prokisch H. "Transcriptomics": molecular diagnosis of inborn errors of metabolism via RNA-sequencing. J Inherit Metab Dis. 2018;41(3):525–32.
123. Brechtmann F, Matuseviciute A, Mertes C, Yepez VA, Avsec Z, Herzog M, et al. OUTRIDER: a statistical method for detecting aberrantly expressed genes in RNA sequencing data. Am J Hum Genet. 2018;103(6):907–17.

Epidemiology of Mitochondrial Disease

Andrew Schaefer, Albert Lim, and Grainne Gorman

Introduction

Like the clinical findings and pathology, the epidemiology of a disease is an integral part of its basic description [1]. It seeks to define the disease in question, in relation to the population at risk. It therefore requires the study of both the sick and the healthy, requiring access to as well as the understanding of both. The nature of mitochondrial disease presents several obstacles in achieving this goal. Clinical heterogeneity of mitochondrial disease surpasses any known inherited disorder. This is partially explained by the reliance of all tissues, with the one exception of erythrocytes, on the intracellular energy production provided by the mitochondria contained within their cytoplasm. Heteroplasmy of mitochondrial DNA (mtDNA) mutations accounts for further phenotypic variability because of variable biochemical phenotypes between these tissues. This aspect of mitochondrial disease remains poorly understood however, with several examples of homoplasmic mutation causing tissue-specific disease. Clinical presentations might therefore be restricted to a single tissue, such as optic neuropathy in Leber's hereditary optic neuropathy (LHON), sensory neural deafness due to the m.1555A>G mutation or cardiomyopathy due to the m.4300A>G mutation [2–5]. In each case there are numerous possible aetiologies, and a high level of clinical suspicion is required to diagnose mitochondrial disease as only specific genetic testing or in some cases resort to invasive muscle biopsy will confirm the diagnosis. In other cases the presence of several relatively common disorders might not be interpreted as a pattern of mitochondrial disease, but instead a coincidence. For example, a patient with what appears to be age-related hearing loss might also have diabetes, renal disease and left ventricular hypertrophy. Each disorder is relatively common, especially in later life, and the presence of diabetes may predispose to renal and cardiac disease. Each can also be a feature of the m.3243A>G mutation and only a high level of clinical suspicion and specific molecular genetic investigation will reveal this.

A. Schaefer (✉) · A. Lim · G. Gorman
NHS Highly Specialised Services for Rare Mitochondrial Disorders and Wellcome Trust Centre for Mitochondrial Research, Newcastle University, Newcastle Upon Tyne, UK
e-mail: Andrew.Schaefer@nuth.nhs.uk

What Do We Include as 'Primary Mitochondrial Disease'?

Primary mitochondrial disease refers to a heterogeneous group of genetic disorders resulting from abnormal oxidative phosphorylation, including the electron transfer chain (ETC) and leading to defective cellular energy production in the form of adenosine triphosphate (ATP) [6] (Table 1).

M. Mancuso, T. Klopstock (eds.), *Diagnosis and Management of Mitochondrial Disorders*,
https://doi.org/10.1007/978-3-030-05517-2_4

Table 1 Prevalence of adult and paediatric mitochondrial disease (including pathogenic mutations of both the mitochondrial and nuclear genomes) [6]

Age range (years)	Prevalence/100,000 (95% confidence interval)	Region	References	PMID
0–6	8.9 (5.3–14.0)	Western Sweden	Darin et al. [16]	11261513
0–10	15 (9.8–21)	Centro region of Portugal	Diogo et al. [15]	19380071
0–16	4.7 (2.8–7.6)	Western Sweden	Darin et al. [16]	11261513
0–16	6.2 (4.5–8.4)	South Eastern Australia	Skladal et al. [8]	12805096
0–16	71 (32–136)	Families of Lebanese ancestry in South Eastern Australia	Skladal et al. [8]	12805096
0–18	7.5 (5–10)	North West Spain	Castro-Gago et al. [17]	16504790
0–18	~12	Northern Finland	Uusimaa et al. [18]	10699115
"Childhood"	~11	Ireland	Ryan et al. [20]	17144232
"Childhood"	~10	Japan	Yamazaki et al. [19]	24266892
Adults (>16)	12.5 (11.1–14.1)	North East England (clinically affected)	Gorman et al. [14, 124]	25652200
Adults (>16)	23.0 (14.6–34.5)	North East England (clinically affected + at risk)	Gorman et al. [14, 124]	25652200

What Obstacles Are There to the Epidemiology Study of Mitochondrial Disease?

The rapid increase in our understanding of the genetic basis of mitochondrial disorders, over the last three decades, has promoted more accurate and timely diagnosis, and has advanced endeavours to truly estimate the prevalence of mitochondrial disease. Meticulous epidemiological evaluation encounters many challenges in mitochondrial disease not least due to the capricious genotype-phenotype correlates and expanding and often disparate clinical features. These factors are exacerbated by the complexity of referral pathways and diagnostic algorithms, age of onset, defined inclusion criteria, effects of genetic founder mutations and inherent aspects of mitochondrial genetics including population bottlenecks that individually or cumulatively contribute to both the under- or over-representation of specific mtDNA- or nuclear-related mitochondrial diseases [7, 8]. For example, the most common cause of adult-onset mtDNA-related mitochondrial disease is due to the m.3243A>G mutation (in *MT-TL1*). However, the original epidemiology studies reported that the frequency of the m.3243A>G mutation in association with diabetes was highly variable, ranging from 0.13% to up to 60% [9, 10]. These preliminary studies were superseded by the first population-based study of the m.3243A>G mutation, in northern Ostrobothnia, Finland [11]. A minimum point prevalence of disease due to m.3243A>G alone was estimated to be 5.7 per 100,000 (mutation prevalence including carriers 16.3 per 100,000). A subsequent UK-based population-based study of all forms of mtDNA diseases [12] estimated that 6.6 per 100,000 suffered mtDNA-related disease (mutation prevalence including carriers 12.5 cases per 100,000). The marked disparity between these studies most likely relates to ascertainment bias and study design (population studies versus cohort studies of affected individuals) and, in part, composition of populations under investigation. The most detailed prevalence of adults with mitochondrial disease estimates is from a cohort study in the North East of England [13, 14], which suggests that some of the original prevalence figures represented a significant underestimate, with a revised prevalence rate of adult mitochondrial disease determined as closer to 9.6 cases per 100,000 individuals caused by mutations in mtDNA and 12.5 per 100,000 (1 in 8000) individuals caused by pathogenic mutations of both mt and nuclear (n) genomes. Conservative estimates of the combined prevalence of both mtDNA and nDNA mutations were 23 per 100,000 (1 in 4300) (Table 2).

Table 2 Prevalence estimates for affected adults and at-risk adults and children with mitochondrial disease (NE England) [14]

Mutation	Prevalence in affected adults/ 100,000 (95% CI)	Prevalence in at-risk adults and children/ 100,000 (95% CI)
Single mtDNA deletion[a]	1.5 (1.0–2.1)	0
Primary LHON mutations[b]	3.7 (2.9–4.6)	4.4 (3.7–5.3)
mt-tRNA mutations[c]	4.3 (3.5–5.3)	6.3 (5.4–7.4)
mt-mRNA mutations	0.1 (0.0–0.4)	0.1 (0.0–0.3)
mtDNA (total)	9.6 (8.3–11.0)	10.8 (9.6–12.2)
Nuclear gene defects	2.9 (2.2–3.7)	5.9 (5.0–6.9)
Total	12.5 (11.1–14.1)	23 (14.6–34.5)

[a]Sporadic mutations
[b]Three common LHON mutations (m. m.3460G>A, *MT-ND1*, m.11778G>A, *MT-ND4* m.14484T>C, *MT-ND6*)
[c]Including (but not limited to) m.3243A>G, *MT-TL1:* affected adults 3.5 (2.7–4.4); at-risk adults and children 4.4 (3.7–5.3) × 10^{-5} and m.8344A>G, *MT-TK:* affected adults 0.2 (0.1–0.5); at-risk adults and children 0.5 (0.2–0.8)

While intrinsic difficulties are still acknowledged in relation to the diagnosis of adult mitochondrial disease, defining children with primary mitochondrial disorders is unquestionably more onerous. This was, in part, historically due to the often conspicuous absence of classic syndromic findings, limited useful laboratory tests and lack of consensus on abnormal results. With the advancement in diagnostic technologies and acumen, it has become readily apparent that the majority of mitochondrial disorders in children are precipitated by (n)DNA mutations. Conservative estimates would now suggest that only 20–25% of childhood-onset mitochondrial disorders are caused by mtDNA mutations. Currently, the prevalence of childhood-onset mitochondrial disorders has been predicted to range from 5 to 15 cases per 10,000 [8, 15–20]. The substantial variation in prevalence rates may be not only attributable to study design (particularly affected by age ranges and diagnostic algorithms), but also due to the presence of genetic founder mutations. For example, Leigh syndrome (LS), the most common paediatric manifestation of mitochondrial disease, is a progressive neurodegenerative disorder, caused by >75 pathogenic mutations in both mt and nDNA. LS has been reported on average in ~2.5 cases per 100,000 births; yet it is tenfold higher in Saguenay-Lac-St-Jean, Canada, due to a founder mutation in *LRPPRC* [21, 22]. Similarly, due to the spread of single ancient European founders in *POLG*, this is now recognised as one of the most common causes of childhood-onset recessive mitochondrial disorders, through Europe, the USA, New Zealand and Australia. Increased prevalence rates in discrete populations with high consanguinity may also impact prevalence rates as exemplified in Australian-Lebanese and Irish travelling communities [8, 20] of higher rates of autosomal recessive childhood-onset mitochondrial diseases.

Epidemiology Studies

Population-Based Studies of mtDNA Mutations

The natural starting point when discussing the epidemiology of mitochondrial disorders is to consider the prevalence of pathogenic mutations within the general population. It is an attractive strategy to take a random sample of the general population and screen relevant tissues for all known pathogenic mutations. Of course the logistics of that are somewhat more challenging, particularly when one considers the vast genetic heterogeneity of the mitochondrial disorders. Historically this has simply not been a viable strategy, even when restricting studies to mtDNA alone. Screening of the entire mitochondrial genome used to be a laborious and expensive task, but as with all gene-based diagnostic technologies, this is becoming both easier and more affordable. Nevertheless, no true population-based prevalence studies have yet been performed using whole-genome sequencing, whether analysing either the mitochondrial or nuclear genome or both. Instead, existing studies have screened for individual mtDNA mutations within cohorts felt to be representative of the general population.

Molecular epidemiological studies of mtDNA disease became a possibility with the identification of single, large-scale mtDNA deletions in patients with mitochondrial myopathy [23, 24], and in Kearns-Sayre syndrome [25]. These publications were accompanied by the first description of mtDNA point mutations causing disease in patients with LHON [2]. Shortly afterwards single, large-scale mtDNA deletions were described in chronic progressive external ophthalmoplegia (CPEO) [26] and the m.3243A>G and m.8344A>G mutations were described as the underlying aetiologies in MELAS [27] and MERRF [28] syndromes, respectively. The subsequent two decades saw a near-exponential increase in the identification of mtDNA mutations associated with disease and there are now over 250 recognised pathogenic mutations to consider. The distinction between disease and asymptomatic carriage of a pathogenic mutation should be highlighted however, as it is common in the available literature for these terms to become blurred, and for prevalence figures for either category to be used interchangeably. This is a particularly important distinction in mtDNA mutations, where disease penetrance can be highly variable due to heteroplasmy and idiosyncrasies of individual mutations.

In 2007, the population prevalence of the m.3243A>G mutation (in *MT-TL1*) had been estimated much higher than previously reported in up to 1 in 236 cases per 100,000 individuals (0.24%, 95% CI 0.10–0.49%, equivalent of 1400) in an Australian-Caucasian-based study. All individuals were originally recruited to the Blue Mountains Eye and Hearing Studies (BMES and BMHS) [29]. Importantly these were not patient cohorts, but instead a population-based representative sample of almost exclusively white Caucasians (99%), within two suburban areas west of Sydney. mtDNA haplogroup analysis confirmed the study population to be similar to those observed in Europe [30]. Participants (n = 2954; 57% women; mean age 66.4 years) were non-institutionalised permanent residents aged 49 years or older, identified by door-to-door census of two suburban postcode areas between 1991 and 1999. Between 82% and 85% agreed to take part in the two studies. Only seven participants (n = 6 women; n = 5, age ≥70 years) tested positive for the m.3243A>G mutation (0.24%). All were oligo-symptomatic with mild-to-moderate hearing loss. Unfortunately, mtDNA heteroplasmy levels were not reported, but all positive results were identified from mtDNA extraction from hair follicles with all seven corresponding blood-derived DNA samples being negative for the m.3243A>G mutation. In an ageing population the failure to identify the m.3243A>G mutation in blood is not surprising, as studies have shown a steady decrease in blood-derived mtDNA heteroplasmy levels over time (~2.3%/year) [31, 32]. The lack of heteroplasmy data does however make it difficult to know whether the m.3243A>G mutation was present at levels that might be expected to cause disease, or whether the hearing loss identified merely represented senile presbycusis.

A follow-up, prospective study of the same Blue Mountains Hearing Study cohort (n = 2856) estimated the prevalence of the m.1555A>G mutation in the same study group [33]. This mtDNA mutation, located in the 12S ribosomal RNA gene, is known to cause sensorineural hearing loss, especially in the context of exposure to aminoglycoside antibiotics. Six of the study participants were found to carry homoplasmic m.1555A>G mutations, correlating to a prevalence of 0.21% (95% CI, 0.08–0.46) or ~1:500 of the Caucasian population. All six subjects had evidence of hearing loss in at least one ear, and in three carriers mean auditory thresholds were significantly higher than in the general population. None of the subjects reported exposure to aminoglycosides. In the same issue of the New England Journal of Medicine, an English group reported similar prevalence estimates for the m.1555A>G mutation, analysing mtDNA from children of the Avon Longitudinal Study of Parents and Children (ALSPAC) birth cohort [34]. Similar to the BMES and BMHS studies, approximately 85% of eligible subjects consented to the study and were typical of a Caucasian population of European background. The numbers were larger, with 9371 children being tested. Eighteen were found to be homoplasmic for the m.1555A>G mutation. This represents 0.19% of the population, or 1 in 520. None had received aminoglycosides and none showed signs of deafness when tested at the age of 7–9 years.

In 2011, a study in Iowa screened 703 former patients from a neonatal intensive care unit (admitted predominantly due to prematurity), and 1473 anonymised adult samples from the hospital's blood centre—deemed to represent the local population. Results for the m.1555A>G mutation were comparable in the two cohorts (0.23% and 0.2%, respectively) and mirrored the findings in the earlier studies [35].

A very similar study was performed in the same year in Taiwan, offering prevalence figures for a non-European population [36]. One thousand and seventeen consecutive newborns in a tertiary hospital were screened for four genes commonly associated with deafness in the Taiwanese population. One newborn (0.1%) was found to carry a homoplasmic m.1555A>G mutation. In comparison, two mutated alleles (either homozygous or compound heterozygous) in the non-mitochondrial GJB2 gene were found in 1.7% of those screened, and no homozygous mutations (0%) were found in the SLC26A4 gene. The consanguinity rates were not stated.

The near-identical prevalence figures from these Australian, English and North American studies support their legitimacy. Prevalence in Asian populations may be lower but still significant. The prevalence rates identified between these studies are comparable for both infancy and old age, implying a negligible effect of the m.1555A>G mutation on life expectancy.

The study by Vandebona et al. also suggests that in the absence of aminoglycoside exposure the m.1555A>G mutation may at most be expected to contribute to the spectrum of age-related hearing loss. This is somewhat at odds with a much more prominent phenotype described elsewhere in the literature [37–39] but these studies investigated disease rather than population-based cohorts and serve to highlight the pitfalls of assuming that both are directly comparable. Studies of disease cohorts are discussed later in this chapter. What is apparent is that the penetrance of the m.1555A>G mutation, as with other homoplasmic mutations, is not complete and in many cases requires further study.

The fourth study requiring discussion in this section reported a minimum prevalence of 1 in 200 live births for the carriage of pathogenic mtDNA mutations [40]. In this study the authors screened 3168 sequential cord blood and matched maternal blood samples for 10 known pathogenic mtDNA mutations: m.1555A>G, m.3243A>G, m.3460G>A, m.7445A>G, m.8344A>G, m.8993T>G, m.11778G>A, m.13513G>A, m.14459G>A and m.14484T>C. Samples were taken from newborns in North Cumbria in the UK, with participation rates similar to the previous studies described above (just over 80%). Fifteen (0.54%, 95% CI = 0.30–0.89%) offspring were identified to harbour an mtDNA mutation. Only five of the ten mtDNA mutations screened were identified. Four individuals carried the m.3243A>G mutation, at heteroplasmy levels of 0.5%, 1.7%, 10.2% and 32.7%, respectively. Three participants tested positive for the m.11778G>A mutation (heteroplasmy 56.5%, 74.8% and 100%); three participants the m.3460G>A mutation (heteroplasmy 12.9%, 18.4% and 42.5%); and a further three participants the m.14484T>C mutation (heteroplasmy 89.1%, and two siblings both carrying 100%). Two patients carried the m.1555A>G mutation but at surprisingly low levels of heteroplasmy—4.4% for each subject. Although the penetrance of the m.1555A>G and the three common LHON mutations is incomplete, disease usually occurs in the context of mtDNA homoplasmy [5]. Eight of the 11 subjects harbouring these mtDNA mutations may reasonably be considered to have a very low likelihood of developing mitochondrial disease throughout their lifetimes. The correlation of blood mtDNA heteroplasmy with clinical phenotype in the 3243A>G mutation is less well defined, but nevertheless it is unlikely that the two subjects carrying <2% heteroplasmy are at significant risk of developing mitochondrial disease either [41].

This study is therefore an interesting insight into the prevalence of these 10 mtDNA mutations within a typical Caucasian population, but the low levels of mtDNA heteroplasmy identified in 10 of 15 subjects raise questions as to its relevance to healthcare provision for clinically manifesting disease. In this study, the distribution of the three common LHON mutations was equal. In disease-based cohorts in the North East of England 60% of LHON cases harbour the m.11778A>G mutation. The discrepancy between the respective prevalence rates for the three common LHON mutations in this study and those identified in clinical cohorts may reflect both the contribution of mutation load and penetrance to clinically relevant disease [13, 14, 42]. The prevalence of the m.3243A>G mutation was less than that reported in the Australian-based population study by Manwaring et al. (0.14% vs. 0.24%) but the reason for that is not clear. Heteroplasmy levels were not reported in the Australian study so they too may have included mtDNA mutation loads below that expected to cause disease. It would have been expected that levels as low as 2–3% would have been expected to be identified in that study. The relative lack of the m.1555A>G mutation (and the absence of mtDNA homoplasmy) in this study is harder to explain. The mutation was present in 0.07% of the population. This is at odds with the data provided by both Vandebona et al. and Bitner-Glindlicz et al. in 2009, where prevalence rates were virtually identical at 0.21% and 0.19%, respectively, and they identified homoplasmic levels of mutation in all cases. It should be noted however that Elliott et al. set out to identify mtDNA mutations within an unselected population, rather than intending to identify disease. They also looked to clarify the *de novo* mutation rate by analysing matched maternal blood samples. 0.00107% of live births harboured a mutation not detected in the mother's blood, providing an estimate of the *de novo* mutation rate but this estimate must be interpreted with caution. Only 8 of the 15 positive cases were accompanied by matched maternal samples and the data related to these paired samples were not provided in detail. mtDNA mutations were not detectable in the blood of three mothers, the child of one harbouring the m.11778G>A mutation, and the children of two mothers harbouring the m.3243A>G mutation. In this case the details of these pairings are important, as although the m.11778G>A mutation appears highly likely to have occurred as a *de novo* mutation, that assertion is more difficult to prove in the case of the m.3243A>G mutations as all four positive carriers harbour relatively low levels of mtDNA heteroplasmy, two of which are already on the boundaries of the diagnostic test's sensitivity. Because the levels of the m.3243A>G mutation in blood are known to decrease by ~2.3%/year, it would seem reasonable to assume that birth levels of the m.3243A>G mutation in the blood of those mothers might no longer be detectable using these methods had their own birth levels been similar, or in at least two of the cases even higher than their offspring.

Prevalence of Mitochondrial Disease Within Defined Geographic Populations

Another epidemiological approach is to document all clinically manifesting mitochondrial diseases within a defined population, and hence to determine the prevalence of disease, rather than simply the potential for disease as identified by the studies described above. If ascertainment is both full and accurate, this is potentially more helpful in planning current healthcare resource implications as pathogenic mtDNA mutations in particular may have impaired clinical penetrance, either due to low levels of heteroplasmy and high thresholds for clinical expression (e.g. the m.8993T>G/C mutations) or in some cases impaired penetrance despite homoplasmy of the mutated mtDNA species (e.g. LHON mutations).

Determining the point prevalence of mitochondrial disease is highly reliant on accurate ascertainment within a stable and well-defined population. This relies on patient motivation, access to medical services, well-established referral routes, existing infrastructure and expertise to optimise accurate diagnosis. For all of these reasons, studies of this nature are rare. Those that exist are generally accepting of their own limitations, usually stating a minimum point prevalence of disease because of strict molecular genetic diagnostic criteria and inevitable underestimation of cases because of unidentified oligosymptomatic or misdiagnosed individuals within the population (Table 1).

The first study of this type was conducted in the province of Northern Ostrobothnia in Northern Finland, but looked only at disease occurring as a result of the m.3243A>G mutation [11]. In Scandinavian countries, generally stable populations with reliable census data and well-established state-funded healthcare systems provide an inviting backdrop to studies of this type. This study screened hospital records for recognised phenotypes such as deafness, diabetes or epilepsy, and the presence of a maternal family history based on results from a postal questionnaire. Screens for other phenotypes such as cardiomyopathy or suggestive cerebral imaging were also used. Blood samples were then screened for the m.3243A>G mutation. Majamaa and colleagues detected a prevalence of clinically affected individuals with the m.3243A>G mutation of 5.71 in 100,000. Prior to this study the authors were aware of five pedigrees affected by this mutation. Adopting this technique of screening hospital records, they not only identified additional individuals within these five pedigrees but also identified five more pedigrees that were previously undiagnosed. Assuming maternal first-degree relatives of verified mutation carriers to be obligate carriers, they estimated a minimum point prevalence of the m.3243A>G mutation within this population to be 16.3 per 100,000.

More extensive studies have been carried out in a similarly stable population in the North East of England. These studies took advantage of established referral pathways to a tertiary neurology centre with molecular genetic and clinical expertise in mitochondrial disease.

These studies initially reported prevalence rates for the most common mtDNA mutations. The first of these reported a total prevalence of disease due to mtDNA mutations of 6.57 per 100,000 [12]. Prevalence of the m.3243A>G mutation was only 1.41 per 100,000 however, less than one-tenth of the figure reported in Finland. Taking into account the newly diagnosed patients from existing pedigrees in the Finnish study, the subsequent British study in 2008 utilised fastidious family tracing to identify not only clinically affected individuals but also asymptomatic carriers and oligosymptomatic patients in the same geographic area [13]. This probably accounts for the higher prevalence rates identified in maternally inherited mtDNA mutations, but near-identical figures for sporadic single, large-scale deletions of the mtDNA. Ongoing development of the Highly Specialised Service for Mitochondrial Disease in Newcastle and associated increased awareness of mitochondrial disease in referring hospitals and non-neurological specialities are also likely to have contributed to this increase. In this study, the authors reported a conservative estimate of the prevalence of the m.3243A>G mutation (restricted to those affected, carrying the mutation, and first-degree maternal relatives) at over five times higher than the earlier study, at 7.69 per 100,000. This highlights the potential risk of underestimation that exists in this sort of study, but also the positive influence of increased awareness, clear referral routes and effective family tracing. Another important finding from this study was the clarification of transmission risks for maternal relatives from those carrying common mtDNA mutations. First-degree relatives of those carrying the m.3243A>G mutation had positive genetic testing in 82% of cases. This dropped to 75% in those with no evidence of disease. The study demonstrated no significant variation in the frequency of positive results among mothers, siblings or children of an affected individual or among the first-, second- and third-degree relatives who requested predictive genetic testing. Transmission rates for m.8344A>G and m.14709T>C were even higher. Similar testing in the earlier Finnish study reported identical transmission rates for the m.3243A>G mutation [11].

Finally, a further study was performed in the North East of England, on this occasion taking advantage of advances in diagnostic techniques to include mitochondrial disease due to nuclear DNA mutations [14] (Table 2). This remains the most comprehensive study of its type. Overall, the prevalence of all pathogenic mutations in both nDNA and mtDNA is 23 per 100,000 or 1 in 4300. The prevalence of patients clinically affected as a result of these mutations was 12.5 per 100,000, making mitochondrial disease the most common inherited neuromuscular disorder in adults. Disease due to nDNA mutations made up less than one-quarter of disease (2.9 per 100,000). Prevalence rates for mtDNA mutations remained comparable to the earlier study in 2008 [13] reflecting the relative stability of mtDNA prevalence both geographically and over time.

Prevalence of mtDNA Mutations Within Defined Disease Cohorts

Since the first mtDNA mutations were identified it has been a natural progression to screen existing disease cohorts for mutations that have been described in association with that particular phenotype. Deafness and diabetes have been studied extensively, in part because of the prevalence of the m.3243A>G mutation within the population and its strong association with a phenotype of maternally inherited deafness and diabetes (MIDD) [13, 14, 43]. Such studies are also aided by clear definitions of disease, and an existing infrastructure for such studies using well-defined referral routes and patient cohorts within established audiology and diabetes clinics. There is also an inherent risk of ascertainment bias, however, with a tendency for more severe cases to be referred for an expert opinion, and perhaps for the more difficult cases, or those with a positive family history, to be kept under review.

Diabetes

Diabetes mellitus is well recognised within mitochondrial phenotypes and is the most common endocrine manifestation of mitochondrial disease. In most scenarios, diabetes is considered an endpoint in the diagnostic process, rather than a potential component of a more expansive syndrome, so appreciation of its place in mitochondrial phenotypes is important if a diagnosis is to be made. The importance of pattern recognition in achieving a genetic diagnosis is key, but for the m.3243A>G mutation the main features are presenile sensorineural hearing loss, a low BMI despite other features suggesting type 2 diabetes, and a maternal family history of diabetes and deafness. Impaired penetrance of disease (due to lower levels of heteroplasmy) often means that the family history may be patchy and it is common for some family members to appear unaffected. Although often considered a hallmark of mitochondrial disease, the prevalence of diabetes in most forms of mitochondrial disease is no higher than 10–12% as compared with prevalence in the general population of approximately 4.45% [43]. It is well recognised in mitochondrial disease because of the MIDD phenotype associated with the m.3243A>G *MTTL1* mutation and the fact that this is the most prevalent of all pathogenic mtDNA or nuclear DNA mutations [14]. Within a cohort of clinically affected individuals carrying the m.3243A>G mutation in the North East of England, 38% had diabetes as part of their clinical phenotype [44]. Within that North East cohort, the m.3243A>G mutation is the most common cause of mitochondrial disease with a prevalence of 3.5×10^{-5} [14]. These data however are dependent on clear and well-defined referral routes to minimise the loss of clinically affected individuals with the defined cohort. Another approach is to take unrefined diabetic populations and screen these cohorts for the mutation in question. Potential pitfalls exist here too, as not all patients with diabetes are diagnosed, not all attend specialist clinics, and the presence of comorbidities such as cognitive impairment, dementia or severe disability might reduce the likelihood of referral or attendance. Conversely, patients referred to specialist clinics may not represent the true cross section of disease, perhaps favouring more severe or difficult cases, those with comorbidities, or possibly those of 'interest' to an academic department because of multisystem disease or an extended pedigree.

Numerous studies have now been performed in these cohorts, primarily in Europe and Japan. Among the larger of those studies, prevalence of the m.3243A>G mutation in reportedly unselected diabetic populations varies between 0 and 2.8% [45–63]. Maassen et al. reported in 2004 that a random screen of 1400 blood samples sent in for HbA1C determinations in the Leiden region of the Netherlands identified that 1.3% of these samples were positive for the m.3243A>G mutation. Taking into account the age-related reduction of m.3243A>G mutation levels in blood-derived DNA samples, it is possible that this may represent a slight underestimate [61].

Understandably, investigators have looked to improve the diagnostic yield by applying diagnostic filters to these cohorts. The presence of sensorineural hearing loss, neuromuscular disease, end-stage renal disease and/or a maternal family history were all found to increase the likelihood of mitochondrial disease when screening diabetic populations [9, 48, 60, 62–68]. Crispim et al. investigated a Brazilian cohort consisting of 407 patients with 'classical' type 2 diabetes and a further 38 patients who were very strictly selected for features of MIDD. In this multicentre trial, 344 patients were Caucasian and 101 African-Brazilian. Blood-derived DNA was screened for ten reported mtDNA mutations including the m.3243A>G mutation, and a further five mtDNA variants included after these were identified by sequencing in the MIDD group. The m.3243A>G mutation was identified in 0.45% of the 'classical' group, but 5.26% of the MIDD group. Mutations and variants were identified in 2.45% of the 'classical' type 2 diabetes group, but 36.84% of the strictly defined MIDD group.

Diabetes may also feature prominently in a number of other mtDNA mutations (e.g. m.14709T>C, m.8344A>G mutation), but the overall prevalence of these mutations is low and has a much smaller contribution to diabetic cohorts than the m.3243A>G mutation. In routine clinical practice, and therefore many cohort studies, a self-fulfilling prophecy is likely to exist as well, as low diagnostic yields and prohibitive costs discourage a search for rarer mtDNA mutations, possibly creating a wider gap in recorded prevalence figures for 'common' and 'rare' mutations. Many maternal diabetic lineages might be screened for the common m.3243A>G mutation, but relatively few will be put forward for full mtDNA sequencing.

Of these 'rarer' mtDNA mutations, the m.8296A>G *MTTK* gene mutation was identified in 0.9% unrelated Japanese patients with diabetes, and 2.3% with diabetes and deafness [69]. The m.14577T>C *MTND6* mutation, associated with isolated complex I deficiency, was found in 0.79% unrelated Japanese patients with diabetes [70]. The m.14709T>C mutation [71–73] may cause up to 13% of mitochondrial diabetes in the North East of England despite representing only 2% of all mtDNA mutations in that cohort [13, 44]. Of patients carrying the m.14709T>C mutation in that cohort, over 50% (7 of 13) had diabetes, suggesting that the genotype-phenotype correlation with diabetes mellitus is even stronger for the m.14709T>C mutation than the much more prevalent m.3243A>G mutation [44]. Reported to be homoplasmic in some patients, the m.14709T>C mutation typically produces a proximal myopathy, cerebellar ataxia and diabetes mellitus [74].

A number of other mtDNA and nDNA mutations are known to have an increased risk of diabetes, but estimations of this frequency are only available from cohorts of mitochondrial disease within specialist centres, as opposed to genetic screening of unselected diabetic cohorts. Whittaker et al. reported diabetes to affect just over 10% (3 of 29) of MERRF patients carrying the m.8344A>G mutation in a clinical cohort [44]. Mancuso et al. reported on a cohort of 42 patients carrying the m.8344A>G mutation, identified in a multicentre, retrospective, database-based study (Nation-wide Italian Collaborative Network of Mitochondrial Diseases). Within this group diabetes was also documented in approximately 12% of patients (4 of 34) [75]. Single, large-scale mtDNA deletions cause diabetes in 11% (6 of 55 patients) of patients with CPEO and Kearns-Sayre syndrome in the North East of England [44]. An earlier paper reviewing existing case reports of KSS reported the prevalence of diabetes to be 13% (29 of 226) but not all cases had genetic confirmation of a deleted mitochondrial genome [76].

The appreciation of the role of nuclear maintenance genes in mitochondrial pathogenesis continues to expand, but the inherent difficulties in achieving a genetic diagnosis means that clinical cohorts are not yet as well established as those for the m.3243A>G mutation, for example. However, diabetes has been reported in 11% of adult CPEO phenotypes with recessive *POLG* mutations [77]. Studies of other maintenance genes have failed to show an increased prevalence of diabetes as compared to the general population. In adult-onset PEO due to *RRM2B* mutations, only 4.5% (1 of 22 in this cohort) had diabetes [78]. Diabetes was not a feature of recessive *TWNK* gene mutations or of OPA1 pedigrees [79, 80].

Rare reports exist of diabetes in association with many of the reported pathogenic mtDNA mutations. One has to be careful in interpreting these as diabetes is relatively common in the general population, is widely acknowledged as a mitochondrial phenotype, and therefore is often expected to be so, even where age, lifestyle and body mass index offer reasonable explanation for impaired glucose tolerance. In some mtDNA mutations, however, diabetes is not considered part of the established phenotype. This group includes the m.8993T>C mutation which is associated with the maternally inherited Leigh syndrome (MILS) phenotype [81] and mtDNA mutations causing LHON [82–85].

Deafness

Deafness, or more specifically sensorineural hearing loss, has long been considered a hallmark of mitochondrial disease. The genotype-phenotype correlation with the prevalent m.3243A>G mutation is even stronger than it is for diabetes, and can progress with age such that more severely affected individuals require cochlear implants to retain any level of useful hearing. Hearing loss is common among many mtDNA mutations as part of a broader phenotype and in the m.1555A>G mutation represents the sole manifestation of disease, especially in carriers exposed to aminoglycoside antibiotics [3, 86, 87]. Attempts to clarify the prevalence of the m.1555A>G mutation in a number of populations have been driven, in part, by the desire to assess the feasibility of instigating screening programmes to identify patients, and children in particular, at risk of aminoglycoside-induced deafness (AID). We have already discussed how the m.3243A>G and m.1555A>G mutations have been identified in up to 1 in 400 and 1 in 500 of the population, respectively, in both Australian and UK population-based screening studies [30, 34]. Prevalence figures for the m.1555A>G vary greatly between, but also within, geographically distinct populations with documented hearing loss. This likely reflects study design and differences in case ascertainment in many studies. Prevalence rates in most non-Spanish-European studies vary between 0.38% and 3.6% [86–94]. Much like prevalence studies in diabetic populations, adding filters to the selection process increases yield. In the case of the m.1555A>G mutation, screening cohorts with a family history of deafness, or AID, predictably tends to produce higher prevalence rates. An Italian study reported a higher prevalence of 5.38% but was more focussed on AID cases. In China, prevalence figures range from 1.85% to 13.33%, with studies of familial hearing loss or high rates of AID producing the higher figures of 11.68%, 12% and 13.33% [95–101].

Studies from South Korea, Taiwan, Indonesia and Mongolia report rates of 0.88%, 3.17%, 5.33% and 7.7%, respectively [102–105]. South Korean cases were isolated presentations without any family history, whereas the Mongolian cases were identified by screening students at the only residential School for Deaf and Blind in Mongolia. Family history is not discussed, but might be expected to be higher in this setting. In a study of Moroccan patients, Nahili et al. screened for the m.1555A>G mutation in patients with congenital, non-syndromic, sensorineural hearing loss [38]. The study included 80 sporadic cases, 84 unrelated familial cases and 100 normal hearing controls. The presence of a homoplasmic m.1555A>G mutation was identified in three of the familial cases but none of the sporadic cases or normal controls. This represents 3.6% of the familial cases screened. In 2014, Yano et al. screened Japanese deafness cohorts using whole-mtDNA screening. Cohort 1 comprised 254 patients with a maternal inheritance pattern of deafness and Cohort 2 was made up of 140 patients with predominantly sporadic or recessive inheritance patterns. The m.1555A>G and m.3243A>G mutations were found in 9% and 4%, respectively, in Cohort 1: the Cohort with maternal inheritance. Neither was found in Cohort 2 [106].

In Spain, studies focussing on familial hearing loss produce rates considerably higher than elsewhere, ranging from 15.6% to 20% in those cohorts [37, 107, 108]. The reasons for this are unclear. It is tempting to postulate that widespread aminoglycoside usage and a heightened awareness of AID may have influenced referral patterns in certain catchment areas. It seems clear however that this was not felt to be the case by the authors. Del Castillo et al. report that of 649 unrelated Spanish families enrolled in their study, the only filter applied was that each family had at least two affected members, but did not specify maternal inheritance or AID. These families had already come to medical attention through some means however, and it is difficult to quantify how much influence that might have over the composition of that 'familial cohort'. Interestingly, Torroni et al. performed a phylogenetic analysis of mtDNA haplogroups in 50 unrelated Spanish families. This suggested that the m.1555A>G mutation was not a result of a single major founder event, but instead may be caused by 30 independent mutational events, occurring in mtDNA haplogroups which are common in all European populations [109].

Optic Neuropathy

Leber's hereditary optic neuropathy (LHON) occurs as a result of three common mutations in over 90% of affected patients. The m.11778G>A, m.14484T>C and m.3460G>A (usually in that order) make up the bulk of this disease. Studies in the North East of England identified 82 individuals with LHON and those alive at the midpoint of 1998 made up a minimum point prevalence of 3.22 per 100,000. Through pedigree analysis a point prevalence of LHON mutations (not disease) was estimated to be 11.82 per 100,000 [42]. The m.11778G>A, m.14484T>C and m.3460G>A mutations were subsequently identified in 55%, 8% and 37% of individuals, respectively, in a larger prevalence study [14]. Despite the disease being associated in most cases with homoplasmy of the mutated mtDNA species, LHON exhibits a reduced penetrance and a marked male predominance of disease. Males have a 50% lifetime risk whereas females are affected in only 10% of cases. Risks to maternal relatives are slightly lower on average [110].

Studies from different populations show slightly different representation. The most dramatic example of this is the predominance of the m.14484T>C in French-Canadian subjects where 86% of cases carry this mutation [7]. Subsequent studies have shown that this is due to a founder affect [111], and genealogical reconstructions identified a female founder, born in France, and married in Quebec City in 1669 [112].

Similar overall prevalence figures for LHON have been described in European populations [113, 114]. Throughout Europe, the m.11778G>A is reported to represent between 36% and 77% of LHON cases, but the m.14484T>C is seen more frequently than the m.3460G>A mutation in the remainder of cases [115–117].

In Asian populations, the m.11778G>A mutation is also most prevalent. The m.3460G>A mutation appears under-represented as compared to European populations. As a proportion of LHON cases, one Japanese study identified the m.11778G>A mutation in 87% of LHON cases [118]. Korean, Chinese and Indian studies report 56%, 35% and 28%, respectively [119–122]. Another Indian study reports only 8.9% however, reminding us of the marked variability between many studies [123]. Study design, potential ascertainment biases and founder effects need to be considered carefully when interpreting the available literature. In LHON, the phenotype and causative mutations are relatively well defined.

Despite that advantage (as compared to many mitochondrial disorders), reduced penetrance in families is likely to contribute to underdiagnosis. Male predominance and reduced penetrance make genetic counselling in LHON extremely complex but highlight the need for detailed epidemiological studies to provide guidance.

Conclusion

Mitochondrial disease is a modern disorder in terms of its phenotypic definitions, genetic classification and increasing recognition over the last three decades. Compared to stroke, Parkinson's disease or multiple sclerosis, our appreciation of mitochondrial disease is in its infancy; yet existing science has acted as a catalyst to our understanding and has allowed a precocious accrual of knowledge in a relatively short period of time. Since the first mtDNA mutations were identified in 1988, our knowledge and understanding of these rare and heterogeneous disorders have blossomed, with much of our understanding coming from scientific advances, accrued clinical expertise and successive epidemiological studies. Acknowledgement of the cumulative prevalence of rare disorders under a common 'umbrella heading' has been key in facilitating improved recognition, research and resource provision for a progressive and disabling group of disorders. Not only has our appreciation of disease prevalence improved, but we now also have a better understanding of the prevalence of those mutations within our society that predispose to disease. This has allowed a clearer estimate of those at risk from mitochondrial disease in subsequent generations. Estimates of potential disease burden and poor outcomes in some of the most severe mtDNA mutations have supported efforts to establish effective reproductive options for women with mtDNA disease [124]. The development of expert centres and highly specialised services in many countries has been instrumental to the accurate epidemiological study of the mitochondrial disorders worldwide. Cohort studies have promoted a keener understanding of disease phenotypes and natural history, as well as paving the way for robust and adequately powered clinical studies, an area that has been sadly lacking in previous years [125]. Development of a comprehensive clinical rating scale has allowed more detailed study of the natural history of the mitochondrial disorders, and in turn has supported endeavours to facilitate those studies, including treatment trials, by providing objective and clinically meaningful outcome measures [126].

Our understanding of the mitochondrial disorders is still, at best, in its early adolescence. There are many questions that remain unanswered, not least the explanation for the varied clinical phenotypes seen even within the same pedigree. Well-designed epidemiological studies have been vital to our advances so far, and are likely to play an integral role in furthering our future efforts in this field.

References

1. Rose G, Barker DJ. What is epidemiology? Br Med J. 1978;2(6140):803–4.
2. Wallace D, Singh G, Lott M, et al. Mitochondrial DNA mutation associated with Leber's hereditary optic neuropathy. Science. 1988;242(4884):1427–30. https://doi.org/10.1126/science.3201231.
3. Prezant TR, Agapian JV, Bohlman MC, et al. Mitochondrial ribosomal RNA mutation associated with both antibiotic-induced and non-syndromic deafness. Nat Genet. 1993;4(3):289–94. https://doi.org/10.1038/ng0793-289.
4. Taylor RW, Giordano C, Davidson MM, et al. A homoplasmic mitochondrial transfer ribonucleic acid mutation as a cause of maternally inherited hypertrophic cardiomyopathy. J Am Coll Cardiol. 2003;41(10):1786–96.
5. Yu-Wai-Man P, Chinnery PF. Leber hereditary optic neuropathy. In: Adam MP, Ardinger HH, Pagon RA, et al., editors. GeneReviews((R)). Seattle, WA: University of Washington; 1993.
6. Gorman GS, Chinnery PF, DiMauro S, et al. Mitochondrial diseases. Nat Rev Dis Primers. 2016;2:16080. https://doi.org/10.1038/nrdp.2016.80.
7. Macmillan C, Kirkham T, Fu K, et al. Pedigree analysis of French Canadian families with T14484C Leber's hereditary optic neuropathy. Neurology. 1998;50(2):417–22. https://doi.org/10.1212/wnl.50.2.417.
8. Skladal D, Halliday J, Thorburn DR. Minimum birth prevalence of mitochondrial respiratory chain disorders in children. Brain J Neurol. 2003;126(Pt 8):1905–12. https://doi.org/10.1093/brain/awg170.

9. Newkirk JE, Taylor RW, Howell N, et al. Maternally inherited diabetes and deafness: prevalence in a hospital diabetic population. Diabet Med. 1997;14(6):457–60. https://doi.org/10.1002/(sici)1096-9136(199706)14:6<457::aid-dia372>3.3.co;2-n.
10. Kadowaki T, Kadowaki H, Mori Y, et al. A subtype of diabetes mellitus associated with a mutation of mitochondrial DNA. N Engl J Med. 1994;330(14):962–8. https://doi.org/10.1056/nejm199404073301403.
11. Majamaa K, Moilanen JS, Uimonen S, et al. Epidemiology of A3243G, the mutation for mitochondrial encephalomyopathy, lactic acidosis, and stroke-like episodes: prevalence of the mutation in an adult population. Am J Hum Genet. 1998;63(2):447–54. https://doi.org/10.1086/301959.
12. Chinnery PF, Johnson MA, Wardell TM, et al. The epidemiology of pathogenic mitochondrial DNA mutations. Ann Neurol. 2000;48(2):188–93. https://doi.org/10.1002/1531-8249(200008)48:2<188::aid-ana8>3.3.co;2-g.
13. Schaefer AM, McFarland R, Blakely EL, et al. Prevalence of mitochondrial DNA disease in adults. Ann Neurol. 2008;63(1):35–9. https://doi.org/10.1002/ana.21217.
14. Gorman GS, Schaefer AM, Ng Y, et al. Prevalence of nuclear and mitochondrial DNA mutations related to adult mitochondrial disease. Ann Neurol. 2015;77(5):753–9. https://doi.org/10.1002/ana.24362.
15. Diogo L, Grazina M, Garcia P, et al. Pediatric mitochondrial respiratory chain disorders in the Centro region of Portugal. Pediatr Neurol. 2009;40(5):351–6. https://doi.org/10.1016/j.pediatrneurol.2008.11.012.
16. Darin N, Oldfors A, Moslemi AR, et al. The incidence of mitochondrial encephalomyopathies in childhood: clinical features and morphological, biochemical, and DNA abnormalities. Ann Neurol. 2001;49(3):377–83.
17. Castro-Gago M, Blanco-Barca MO, Campos-Gonzalez Y, et al. Epidemiology of pediatric mitochondrial respiratory chain disorders in northwest Spain. Pediatr Neurol. 2006;34(3):204–11. https://doi.org/10.1016/j.pediatrneurol.2005.07.011.
18. Uusimaa J, Remes AM, Rantala H, et al. Childhood encephalopathies and myopathies: a prospective study in a defined population to assess the frequency of mitochondrial disorders. Pediatrics. 2000;105(3 Pt 1):598–603.
19. Yamazaki T, Murayama K, Compton AG, et al. Molecular diagnosis of mitochondrial respiratory chain disorders in Japan: focusing on mitochondrial DNA depletion syndrome. Pediatr Int. 2014;56(2):180–7. https://doi.org/10.1111/ped.12249.
20. Ryan E, King MD, Rustin P, et al. Mitochondrial cytopathies, phenotypic heterogeneity and a high incidence. Ir Med J. 2006;99(9):262–4.
21. Debray FG, Morin C, Janvier A, et al. LRPPRC mutations cause a phenotypically distinct form of Leigh syndrome with cytochrome c oxidase deficiency. J Med Genet. 2011;48(3):183–9. https://doi.org/10.1136/jmg.2010.081976.
22. Lake NJ, Compton AG, Rahman S, et al. Leigh syndrome: one disorder, more than 75 monogenic causes. Ann Neurol. 2016;79(2):190–203. https://doi.org/10.1002/ana.24551.
23. Holt IJ, Cooper JM, Morgan-Hughes JA, et al. Deletions of muscle mitochondrial DNA. Lancet. 1988;1(8600):1462.
24. Holt IJ, Harding AE, Morgan-Hughes JA. Deletions of muscle mitochondrial DNA in patients with mitochondrial myopathies. Nature. 1988;331(6158):717–9. https://doi.org/10.1038/331717a0.
25. Zeviani M, Moraes CT, DiMauro S, et al. Deletions of mitochondrial DNA in Kearns-Sayre syndrome. Neurology. 1988;38(9):1339–46.
26. Moraes CT, DiMauro S, Zeviani M, et al. Mitochondrial DNA deletions in progressive external ophthalmoplegia and Kearns-Sayre syndrome. N Engl J Med. 1989;320(20):1293–9. https://doi.org/10.1056/NEJM198905183202001.
27. Goto YI, Nonaka I, Horai S. A mutation in the tRNALeu(UUR) gene associated with the MELAS subgroup of mitochondrial encephalomyopathies. Nature. 1990;348(6302):651–3. https://doi.org/10.1038/348651a0.
28. Shoffner JM, Lott MT, Lezza AMS, et al. Myoclonic epilepsy and ragged-red fiber disease (MERRF) is associated with a mitochondrial DNA tRNALys mutation. Cell. 1990;61(6):931–7. https://doi.org/10.1016/0092-8674(90)90059-n.
29. Manwaring N, Jones MM, Wang JJ, et al. Mitochondrial DNA haplogroups and age-related hearing loss. Arch Otolaryngol Head Neck Surg. 2007;133(9):929–33. https://doi.org/10.1001/archotol.133.9.929.
30. Manwaring N, Jones MM, Wang JJ, et al. Prevalence of mitochondrial DNA haplogroups in an Australian population. Intern Med J. 2006;36(8):530–3. https://doi.org/10.1111/j.1445-5994.2006.01118.x.
31. Rahman S, Poulton J, Marchington D, et al. Decrease of 3243 A-->G mtDNA mutation from blood in MELAS syndrome: a longitudinal study. Am J Hum Genet. 2001;68(1):238–40. https://doi.org/10.1086/316930.
32. Sue CM, Quigley A, Katsabanis S, et al. Detection of MELAS A3243G point mutation in muscle, blood and hair follicles. J Neurol Sci. 1998;161(1):36–9.
33. Vandebona H, Mitchell P, Manwaring N, et al. Prevalence of mitochondrial 1555A→G mutation in adults of European descent. N Engl J Med. 2009;360(6):642–4. https://doi.org/10.1056/nejmc0806397.
34. Bitner-Glindzicz M, Pembrey M, Duncan A, et al. Prevalence of mitochondrial 1555A→G mutation in European children. N Engl J Med. 2009;360(6):640–2. https://doi.org/10.1056/nejmc0806396.

35. Ealy M, Lynch KA, Meyer NC, et al. The prevalence of mitochondrial mutations associated with aminoglycoside-induced sensorineural hearing loss in an NICU population. Laryngoscope. 2011;121(6):1184–6. https://doi.org/10.1002/lary.21778.
36. Wu C-C, Hung C-C, Lin S-Y, et al. Newborn genetic screening for hearing impairment: a preliminary study at a tertiary center. PLoS One. 2011;6(7):e22314. https://doi.org/10.1371/journal.pone.0022314.
37. Estivill X, Govea N, Barcelo E, et al. Familial progressive sensorineural deafness is mainly due to the mtDNA A1555G mutation and is enhanced by treatment of aminoglycosides. Am J Hum Genet. 1998;62(1):27–35.
38. Nahili H, Charif M, Boulouiz R, et al. Prevalence of the mitochondrial A 1555G mutation in Moroccan patients with non-syndromic hearing loss. Int J Pediatr Otorhinolaryngol. 2010;74(9):1071–4. https://doi.org/10.1016/j.ijporl.2010.06.008.
39. Tang X, Yang L, Zhu Y, et al. Very low penetrance of hearing loss in seven Han Chinese pedigrees carrying the deafness-associated 12S rRNA A1555G mutation. Gene. 2007;393(1–2):11–9. https://doi.org/10.1016/j.gene.2007.01.001.
40. Elliott HR, Samuels DC, Eden JA, et al. Pathogenic mitochondrial DNA mutations are common in the general population. Am J Hum Genet. 2008;83(2):254–60. https://doi.org/10.1016/j.ajhg.2008.07.004.
41. Grady JP, Pickett SJ, Ng YS, et al. mtDNA heteroplasmy level and copy number indicate disease burden in m.3243A>G mitochondrial disease. EMBO Mol Med. 2018;10(6):e8262. https://doi.org/10.15252/emmm.201708262.
42. Yu-Wai-Man P, Griffiths PG, Brown DT, et al. The epidemiology of Leber hereditary optic neuropathy in the North East of England. Am J Hum Genet. 2003;72(2):333–9. https://doi.org/10.1086/346066.
43. Schaefer AM, Walker M, Turnbull DM, et al. Endocrine disorders in mitochondrial disease. Mol Cell Endocrinol. 2013;379(1–2):2–11. https://doi.org/10.1016/j.mce.2013.06.004.
44. Whittaker RG, Schaefer AM, McFarland R, et al. Prevalence and progression of diabetes in mitochondrial disease. Diabetologia. 2007;50(10):2085–9. https://doi.org/10.1007/s00125-007-0779-9.
45. Vionnet N, Passa P, Froguel P. Prevalence of mitochondrial gene mutations in families with diabetes mellitus. Lancet. 1993;342(8884):1429–30.
46. Katagiri H, Asano T, Ishihara H, et al. Mitochondrial diabetes mellitus: prevalence and clinical characterization of diabetes due to mitochondrial tRNA(Leu(UUR)) gene mutation in Japanese patients. Diabetologia. 1994;37(5):504–10.
47. Otabe S, Sakura H, Shimokawa K, et al. The high prevalence of the diabetic patients with a mutation in the mitochondrial gene in Japan. J Clin Endocrinol Metab. 1994;79(3):768–71. https://doi.org/10.1210/jcem.79.3.8077358.
48. t Hart LM, Lemkes HH, Heine RJ, et al. Prevalence of maternally inherited diabetes and deafness in diabetic populations in The Netherlands. Diabetologia. 1994;37(11):1169–70.
49. Kishimoto M, Hashiramoto M, Kanda F, et al. Mitochondrial mutation in diabetic patient with gastrointestinal symptoms. Lancet. 1995;345(8947):452.
50. Odawara M, Asano M, Yamashita K. Mitochondrial gene mutations that affect the binding of the termination factor and their prevalence among Japanese diabetes mellitus. Nucleic Acids Symp Ser. 1995;34:237–8.
51. Uchigata Y, Mizota M, Yanagisawa K, et al. Large-scale study of an A-to-G transition at position 3243 of the mitochondrial gene and IDDM in Japanese patients. Diabetologia. 1996;39(2):245–6.
52. Abad MM, Cotter PD, Fodor FH, et al. Screening for the mitochondrial DNA A3243G mutation in children with insulin-dependent diabetes mellitus. Metab Clin Exp. 1997;46(4):445–9.
53. Saker PJ, Hattersley AT, Barrow B, et al. UKPDS 21: low prevalence of the mitochondrial transfer RNA gene (tRNA(Leu(UUR))) mutation at position 3243bp in UK Caucasian type 2 diabetic patients. Diabet Med. 1997;14(1):42–5. https://doi.org/10.1002/(SICI)1096-9136(199701)14:1<42::AID-DIA295>3.0.CO;2-T.
54. Tsukuda K, Suzuki Y, Kameoka K, et al. Screening of patients with maternally transmitted diabetes for mitochondrial gene mutations in the tRNA[Leu(UUR)] region. Diabet Med. 1997;14(12):1032–7. https://doi.org/10.1002/(SICI)1096-9136(199712)14:12<1032::AID-DIA504>3.0.CO;2-Y.
55. Holmes-Walker DJ, Mitchell P, Boyages SC. Does mitochondrial genome mutation in subjects with maternally inherited diabetes and deafness decrease severity of diabetic retinopathy? Diabet Med. 1998;15(11):946–52. https://doi.org/10.1002/(SICI)1096-9136(1998110)15:11<946::AID-DIA707>3.0.CO;2-L.
56. Lehto M, Wipemo C, Ivarsson SA, et al. High frequency of mutations in MODY and mitochondrial genes in Scandinavian patients with familial early-onset diabetes. Diabetologia. 1999;42(9):1131–7. https://doi.org/10.1007/s001250051281.
57. Matsuura N, Suzuki S, Yokota Y, et al. The prevalence of mitochondrial gene mutations in childhood diabetes in Japan. J Pediatr Endocrinol Metab. 1999;12(1):27–30.
58. Malecki M, Klupa T, Wanic K, et al. Search for mitochondrial A3243G tRNA(Leu) mutation in polish patients with type 2 diabetes mellitus. Med Sci Monit. 2001;7(2):246–50.
59. Ohkubo K, Yamano A, Nagashima M, et al. Mitochondrial gene mutations in the

tRNA(Leu(UUR)) region and diabetes: prevalence and clinical phenotypes in Japan. Clin Chem. 2001;47(9):1641–8.

60. Suzuki S, Oka Y, Kadowaki T, et al. Clinical features of diabetes mellitus with the mitochondrial DNA 3243 (A-G) mutation in Japanese: maternal inheritance and mitochondria-related complications. Diabetes Res Clin Pract. 2003;59(3):207–17.
61. Maassen JA, Lm TH, Van Essen E, et al. Mitochondrial diabetes: molecular mechanisms and clinical presentation. Diabetes. 2004;53(Suppl 1):S103–9.
62. Crispim D, Estivalet AA, Roisenberg I, et al. Prevalence of 15 mitochondrial DNA mutations among type 2 diabetic patients with or without clinical characteristics of maternally inherited diabetes and deafness. Arq Bras Endocrinol Metabol. 2008;52(8):1228–35.
63. Murphy R, Turnbull DM, Walker M, et al. Clinical features, diagnosis and management of maternally inherited diabetes and deafness (MIDD) associated with the 3243A>G mitochondrial point mutation. Diabet Med. 2008;25(4):383–99. https://doi.org/10.1111/j.1464-5491.2008.02359.x.
64. Majamaa K, Turkka J, Karppa M, et al. The common MELAS mutation A3243G in mitochondrial DNA among young patients with an occipital brain infarct. Neurology. 1997;49(5):1331–4.
65. Smith PR, Bain SC, Good PA, et al. Pigmentary retinal dystrophy and the syndrome of maternally inherited diabetes and deafness caused by the mitochondrial DNA 3243 tRNA(Leu) A to G mutation. Ophthalmology. 1999;106(6):1101–8. https://doi.org/10.1016/s0161-6420(99)90244-0.
66. Ng MC, Yeung VT, Chow CC, et al. Mitochondrial DNA A3243G mutation in patients with early- or late-onset type 2 diabetes mellitus in Hong Kong Chinese. Clin Endocrinol. 2000;52(5):557–64.
67. Iwasaki N, Babazono T, Tsuchiya K, et al. Prevalence of A-to-G mutation at nucleotide 3243 of the mitochondrial tRNA(Leu(UUR)) gene in Japanese patients with diabetes mellitus and end stage renal disease. J Hum Genet. 2001;46(6):330–4. https://doi.org/10.1007/s100380170068.
68. Klemm T, Neumann S, Trulzsch B, et al. Search for mitochondrial DNA mutation at position 3243 in German patients with a positive family history of maternal diabetes mellitus. Exp Clin Endocrinol Diabetes. 2001;109(5):283–7. https://doi.org/10.1055/s-2001-16348.
69. Kameoka K, Isotani H, Tanaka K, et al. Impaired insulin secretion in Japanese diabetic subjects with an A-to-G mutation at nucleotide 8296 of the mitochondrial DNA in tRNA(Lys). Diabetes Care. 1998;21(11):2034–5.
70. Tawata M, Hayashi JI, Isobe K, et al. A new mitochondrial DNA mutation at 14577 T/C is probably a major pathogenic mutation for maternally inherited type 2 diabetes. Diabetes. 2000;49(7):1269–72.
71. Hanna MG, Nelson I, Sweeney MG, et al. Congenital encephalomyopathy and adult-onset myopathy and diabetes mellitus: different phenotypic associations of a new heteroplasmic mtDNA tRNA glutamic acid mutation. Am J Hum Genet. 1995;56(5):1026–33.
72. Vialettes BH, Paquis-Flucklinger V, Pelissier JF, et al. Phenotypic expression of diabetes secondary to a T14709C mutation of mitochondrial DNA. Comparison with MIDD syndrome (A3243G mutation): a case report. Diabetes Care. 1997;20(11):1731–7.
73. Choo-Kang AT, Lynn S, Taylor GA, et al. Defining the importance of mitochondrial gene defects in maternally inherited diabetes by sequencing the entire mitochondrial genome. Diabetes. 2002;51(7):2317–20.
74. McFarland R, Schaefer AM, Gardner JL, et al. Familial myopathy: new insights into the T14709C mitochondrial tRNA mutation. Ann Neurol. 2004;55(4):478–84. https://doi.org/10.1002/ana.20004.
75. Mancuso M, Orsucci D, Angelini C, et al. Phenotypic heterogeneity of the 8344A>G mtDNA "MERRF" mutation. Neurology. 2013;80(22):2049–54. https://doi.org/10.1212/WNL.0b013e318294b44c.
76. Harvey JN, Barnett D. Endocrine dysfunction in Kearns-Sayre syndrome. Clin Endocrinol. 1992;37(1):97–103.
77. Horvath R, Hudson G, Ferrari G, et al. Phenotypic spectrum associated with mutations of the mitochondrial polymerase gamma gene. Brain J Neurol. 2006;129(Pt 7):1674–84. https://doi.org/10.1093/brain/awl088.
78. Pitceathly RDS, Smith C, Fratter C, et al. Adults with RRM2B-related mitochondrial disease have distinct clinical and molecular characteristics. Brain J Neurol. 2012;135(11):3392–403. https://doi.org/10.1093/brain/aws231.
79. Lonnqvist T, Paetau A, Valanne L, et al. Recessive twinkle mutations cause severe epileptic encephalopathy. Brain J Neurol. 2009;132(Pt 6):1553–62. https://doi.org/10.1093/brain/awp045.
80. Yu-Wai-Man P, Griffiths PG, Gorman GS, et al. Multi-system neurological disease is common in patients with OPA1 mutations. Brain J Neurol. 2010;133(Pt 3):771–86. https://doi.org/10.1093/brain/awq007.
81. Nagashima T, Mori M, Katayama K, et al. Adult Leigh syndrome with mitochondrial DNA mutation at 8993. Acta Neuropathol. 1999;97(4):416–22.
82. Newman NJ, Lott MT, Wallace DC. The clinical characteristics of pedigrees of Leber's hereditary optic neuropathy with the 11778 mutation. Am J Ophthalmol. 1991;111(6):750–62.
83. DuBois LG, Feldon SE. Evidence for a metabolic trigger for Leber's hereditary optic neuropathy. A case report. J Clin Neuroophthalmol. 1992;12(1):15–6.

84. Pilz D, Quarrell OW, Jones EW. Mitochondrial mutation commonly associated with Leber's hereditary optic neuropathy observed in a patient with Wolfram syndrome (DIDMOAD). J Med Genet. 1994;31(4):328–30.
85. Cole A, Dutton GN. Leber's hereditary optic neuropathy and maturity onset diabetes mellitus: is there a metabolic association. Br J Ophthalmol. 2000;84(4):439–40.
86. Jacobs HT, Hutchin TP, Kappi T, et al. Mitochondrial DNA mutations in patients with postlingual, nonsyndromic hearing impairment. Eur J Hum Genet. 2005;13(1):26–33. https://doi.org/10.1038/sj.ejhg.5201250.
87. Lehtonen MS, Uimonen S, Hassinen IE, et al. Frequency of mitochondrial DNA point mutations among patients with familial sensorineural hearing impairment. Eur J Hum Genet. 2000;8(4):315–8. https://doi.org/10.1038/sj.ejhg.5200455.
88. Häkli S, Luotonen M, Sorri M, et al. Mutations in the two ribosomal RNA genes in mitochondrial DNA among Finnish children with hearing impairment. BMC Med Genet. 2015;16(1):3. https://doi.org/10.1186/s12881-015-0145-6.
89. Kokotas H, Grigoriadou M, Korres GS, et al. Detection of deafness-causing mutations in the greek mitochondrial genome. Dis Markers. 2011;30(6):283–9. https://doi.org/10.1155/2011/350987.
90. Rydzanicz M, Wróbel M, Cywińska K, et al. Screening of the general polish population for deafness-associated mutations in mitochondrial 12S rRNA and tRNASer(UCN) genes. Genet Test Mol Biomarkers. 2009;13(2):167–72. https://doi.org/10.1089/gtmb.2008.0098.
91. Konings A, Van Camp G, Goethals A, et al. Mutation analysis of mitochondrial DNA 12SrRNA and tRNASer(UCN) genes in non-syndromic hearing loss patients. Mitochondrion. 2008;8(5–6):377–82. https://doi.org/10.1016/j.mito.2008.08.001.
92. OStergaard E, Montserrat-Sentis B, Gronskov K, et al. The A1555G mtDNA mutation in Danish hearing-impaired patients: frequency and clinical signs. Clin Genet. 2002;62(4):303–5.
93. Kupka S, Braun S, Aberle S, et al. Frequencies of GJB2 mutations in German control individuals and patients showing sporadic non-syndromic hearing impairment. Hum Mutat. 2002;20(1):77–8. https://doi.org/10.1002/humu.9044.
94. Rydzanicz M, Wrobel M, Pollak A, et al. Mutation analysis of mitochondrial 12S rRNA gene in Polish patients with non-syndromic and aminoglycoside-induced hearing loss. Biochem Biophys Res Commun. 2010;395(1):116–21. https://doi.org/10.1016/j.bbrc.2010.03.149.
95. Jiang Y, Huang S, Deng T, et al. Mutation Spectrum of common deafness-causing genes in patients with non-syndromic deafness in the Xiamen area, China. PLoS One. 2015;10(8):e0135088. https://doi.org/10.1371/journal.pone.0135088.
96. Du W, Cheng J, Ding H, et al. A rapid method for simultaneous multi-gene mutation screening in children with nonsyndromic hearing loss. Genomics. 2014;104(4):264–70. https://doi.org/10.1016/j.ygeno.2014.07.009.
97. Li Q, Ji Y, Han B, et al. Comparative study of mutation spectrums of MT-RNR1 m.1555A>G, GJB2, and SLC26A4 between familial and sporadic patients with nonsyndromic sensorineural hearing loss in Chinese Han. Chin Med J. 2014;127(18):3233–7.
98. Chen G, He F, Fu S, et al. GJB2 and mitochondrial DNA 1555A>G mutations in students with hearing loss in the Hubei Province of China. Int J Pediatr Otorhinolaryngol. 2011;75(9):1156–9. https://doi.org/10.1016/j.ijporl.2011.06.011.
99. Yuan Y, You Y, Huang D, et al. Comprehensive molecular etiology analysis of nonsyndromic hearing impairment from typical areas in China. J Transl Med. 2009;7(1):79. https://doi.org/10.1186/1479-5876-7-79.
100. Guo Y-F, Guo Y-F, Liu X-W, et al. GJB2, SLC26A4 and mitochondrial DNA A1555G mutations in prelingual deafness in Northern Chinese subjects. Acta Otolaryngol. 2008;128(3):297–303. https://doi.org/10.1080/00016480701767382.
101. Li Z, Li R, Chen J, et al. Mutational analysis of the mitochondrial 12S rRNA gene in Chinese pediatric subjects with aminoglycoside-induced and non-syndromic hearing loss. Hum Genet. 2005;117(1):9–15. https://doi.org/10.1007/s00439-005-1276-1.
102. Wu C-C, Chiu Y-H, Chen P-J, et al. Prevalence and clinical features of the mitochondrial m.1555A>G mutation in Taiwanese patients with idiopathic sensorineural hearing loss and association of haplogroup F with low penetrance in three families. Ear Hear. 2007;28(3):332–42. https://doi.org/10.1097/aud.0b013e318047941e.
103. Bae JW, Lee KY, Choi SY, et al. Molecular analysis of mitochondrial gene mutations in Korean patients with nonsyndromic hearing loss. Int J Mol Med. 2008;22(2):175–80.
104. Malik SG, Pieter N, Sudoyo H, et al. Prevalence of the mitochondrial DNA A1555G mutation in sensorineural deafness patients in island Southeast Asia. J Hum Genet. 2003;48(9):480–3. https://doi.org/10.1007/s10038-003-0056-9.
105. Pandya A, Xia XJ, Erdenetungalag R, et al. Heterogenous point mutations in the mitochondrial tRNA Ser(UCN) precursor coexisting with the A1555G mutation in deaf students from Mongolia. Am J Hum Genet. 1999;65(6):1803–6. https://doi.org/10.1086/302658.
106. Yano T, Nishio SY, Usami S, et al. Frequency of mitochondrial mutations in non-syndromic hearing loss as well as possibly responsible variants found by whole mitochondrial genome screening. J Hum Genet. 2014;59(2):100–6. https://doi.org/10.1038/jhg.2013.128.

107. del Castillo FJ, Rodriguez-Ballesteros M, Martin Y, et al. Heteroplasmy for the 1555A>G mutation in the mitochondrial 12S rRNA gene in six Spanish families with non-syndromic hearing loss. J Med Genet. 2003;40(8):632–6.
108. Ballana E, Morales E, Rabionet R, et al. Mitochondrial 12S rRNA gene mutations affect RNA secondary structure and lead to variable penetrance in hearing impairment. Biochem Biophys Res Commun. 2006;341(4):950–7. https://doi.org/10.1016/j.bbrc.2006.01.049.
109. Torroni A, Cruciani F, Rengo C, et al. The A1555G mutation in the 12S rRNA gene of human mtDNA: recurrent origins and founder events in families affected by sensorineural deafness. Am J Hum Genet. 1999;65(5):1349–58. https://doi.org/10.1086/302642.
110. Yu-Wai-Man P, Chinnery PF. Leber hereditary optic neuropathy—therapeutic challenges and early promise. Taiwan J Ophthalmol. 2011;1(1):12–5. https://doi.org/10.1016/j.tjo.2011.09.001.
111. Macmillan C, Johns TA, Fu K, et al. Predominance of the T14484C mutation in French-Canadian families with Leber hereditary optic neuropathy is due to a founder effect. Am J Hum Genet. 2000;66(1):332–5. https://doi.org/10.1086/302716.
112. Laberge AM, Jomphe M, Houde L, et al. A "Fille du Roy" introduced the T14484C Leber hereditary optic neuropathy mutation in French Canadians. Am J Hum Genet. 2005;77(2):313–7. https://doi.org/10.1086/432491.
113. Spruijt L, Kolbach DN, de Coo RF, et al. Influence of mutation type on clinical expression of Leber hereditary optic neuropathy. Am J Ophthalmol. 2006;141(4):676–82. https://doi.org/10.1016/j.ajo.2005.11.007.
114. Puomila A, Hamalainen P, Kivioja S, et al. Epidemiology and penetrance of Leber hereditary optic neuropathy in Finland. Eur J Hum Genet. 2007;15(10):1079–89. https://doi.org/10.1038/sj.ejhg.5201828.
115. Carelli V, Achilli A, Valentino ML, et al. Haplogroup effects and recombination of mitochondrial DNA: novel clues from the analysis of Leber hereditary optic neuropathy pedigrees. Am J Hum Genet. 2006;78(4):564–74. https://doi.org/10.1086/501236.
116. Howell N, Herrnstadt C, Shults C, et al. Low penetrance of the 14484 LHON mutation when it arises in a non-haplogroup J mtDNA background. Am J Med Genet A. 2003;119A(2):147–51. https://doi.org/10.1002/ajmg.a.20135.
117. Huoponen K, Lamminen T, Juvonen V, et al. The spectrum of mitochondrial DNA mutations in families with Leber hereditary optic neuroretinopathy. Hum Genet. 1993;92(4):379–84.
118. Mashima Y, Yamada K, Wakakura M, et al. Spectrum of pathogenic mitochondrial DNA mutations and clinical features in Japanese families with Leber's hereditary optic neuropathy. Curr Eye Res. 1998;17(4):403–8.
119. Kim JY, Hwang JM, Chang BL, et al. Spectrum of the mitochondrial DNA mutations of Leber's hereditary optic neuropathy in Koreans. J Neurol. 2003;250(3):278–81. https://doi.org/10.1007/s00415-003-0985-4.
120. Jiang P, Liang M, Zhang J, et al. Prevalence of mitochondrial ND4 mutations in 1281 Han Chinese subjects with Leber's hereditary optic neuropathy. Invest Ophthalmol Vis Sci. 2015;56(8):4778–88. https://doi.org/10.1167/iovs.14-16158.
121. Jia X, Li S, Xiao X, et al. Molecular epidemiology of mtDNA mutations in 903 Chinese families suspected with Leber hereditary optic neuropathy. J Hum Genet. 2006;51(10):851–6. https://doi.org/10.1007/s10038-006-0032-2.
122. Mishra A, Devi S, Saxena R, et al. Frequency of primary mutations of Leber's hereditary optic neuropathy patients in North Indian population. Indian J Ophthalmol. 2017;65(11):1156–60. https://doi.org/10.4103/ijo.IJO_380_17.
123. Sundaresan P, Kumar SM, Thompson S, et al. Reduced frequency of known mutations in a cohort of LHON patients from India. Ophthalmic Genet. 2010;31(4):196–9. https://doi.org/10.3109/13816810.2010.510818.
124. Gorman GS, Grady JP, Turnbull DM. Mitochondrial donation—how many women could benefit? N Engl J Med. 2015;372(9):885–7. https://doi.org/10.1056/NEJMc1500960.
125. Nesbitt V, Pitceathly RD, Turnbull DM, et al. The UK MRC mitochondrial disease patient cohort study: clinical phenotypes associated with the m.3243A>G mutation—implications for diagnosis and management. J Neurol Neurosurg Psychiatry. 2013;84(8):936–8. https://doi.org/10.1136/jnnp-2012-303528.
126. Schaefer AM, Phoenix C, Elson JL, et al. Mitochondrial disease in adults: a scale to monitor progression and treatment. Neurology. 2006;66(12):1932–4. https://doi.org/10.1212/01.wnl.0000219759.72195.41.

Mitochondrial Encephalomyopathy, Lactic Acidosis, and Stroke-Like Episodes (MELAS)

Amy Goldstein and Serenella Servidei

Introduction

Mitochondrial encephalomyopathy, lactic acidosis, and stroke-like episodes, also known as MELAS (MIM 540000), is a primary mitochondrial disease caused by pathogenic variants within the mitochondrial genome (mtDNA). While the majority of patients (~80%) have the common MELAS pathogenic variant m.3243A>G, the number of genotypes causing the MELAS phenotype continues to expand and may include nuclear genes (nDNA) as well. The experienced clinician may recognize the clinical scenario of a child or young adult who presents with a prolonged yet subacute history of failure to thrive, short stature, neurobehavioral issues, hirsutism, sensorineural hearing loss, and then with a physiological stressor (illness, fasting/dehydration, surgery) has a stroke-like episode in a nonvascular distribution of the brain and symptoms of seizures, headache, vomiting, altered mental status, hemiparesis, and/or cortical blindness. The diagnosis of MELAS brings to attention not only that patient but all potentially affected maternal family members. Subsequently, the affected person may develop intractable epilepsy, dementia, fatigue and exercise intolerance (myopathy), recurrent headaches, diabetes, gastrointestinal dysmotility, and cardiac involvement. Recurrent stroke-like episodes lead to cortical and cerebellar atrophy with evolution to permanent disability due to weakness, hemiparesis, and cortical visual impairment. Disease onset is during childhood with symptoms arising between 2 and 10 years old. Diagnosis is made both clinically and with laboratory testing including genetic confirmation of pathogenic variants.

A. Goldstein (✉)
Division of Human Genetics, Department of Pediatrics, Children's Hospital of Philadelphia, Philadelphia, PA, USA

S. Servidei
Institute of Neurology, Catholic University of the Sacred Heart, Rome, Italy

Clinical Diagnosis

MELAS was first described as a "neurodegenerative disease caused by the decreased ability of cells to produce sufficient energy in the form of ATP" [1] and subsequently associated with the pathogenic variant in the mitochondrial genome at position 3243 (m.3243A>G), which codes for tRNA-leucine (MT-TL1) [2–4]. The pathogenic variant impairs mitochondrial translational RNA, protein synthesis, and complexes of the electron transport chain (ETC) and ultimately disrupts oxidative phosphorylation and ATP synthesis. The addition genotypes in mtDNA affect other translational RNAs and cause similar pathophysiology.

Clinical diagnostic criteria for MELAS were published in 1992: (1) stroke-like episodes before age 40 years, (2) encephalopathy with seizures

M. Mancuso, T. Klopstock (eds.), *Diagnosis and Management of Mitochondrial Disorders*,
https://doi.org/10.1007/978-3-030-05517-2_5

and/or dementia, and (3) mitochondrial myopathy (weakness, fatigue, poor endurance, exercise intolerance) and, in addition to 2/3 of the following criteria, (1) normal early psychomotor development, (2) recurrent headache, and (3) recurrent vomiting. Laboratory criteria include lactic acidosis and/or ragged red fibers (RRFs) on muscle biopsy [5].

Updated criteria were proposed by the MELAS Study Group in 2011 [6] and divided into definitive vs. suspicious MELAS based on two categories (A and B). Definitive MELAS requires two from Category A and two from Category B (total of four items or more), and suspicious MELAS requires one from Category A and two from Category B (at least three items). Category A includes clinical findings of stroke-like episodes: (1) headache with vomiting, (2) seizure, (3) hemiplegia, (4) cortical blindness or hemianopsia, and (5) acute focal lesion observed via brain imaging (CT and/or MRI). Category B includes evidence of mitochondrial dysfunction: (1) High lactate levels in plasma and/or cerebrospinal fluid (CSF) or deficiency of mitochondrial-related enzyme activities (lactate of 2 mmol/L (18 mg/dl) or more; lactate in plasma at rest or in CSF) and/or deficiency in ETC; pyruvate-related, tricyclic acid cycle (TCA)-related enzymes or lipid metabolism-related enzymes in somatic/muscle cells); and (2) mitochondrial abnormalities in muscle biopsy, including ragged red fibers (RRF) on modified Gomori trichrome and/or strongly SDH-reactive vessels (SSVs) on succinate dehydrogenase (SDH) stain; cytochrome C oxidase (COX) negative fibers or abnormal mitochondria on electron microscopy.

Clinical Symptoms

MELAS is a multisystem disorder and symptoms typically begin in childhood. Early development is usually normal, and short stature is common. First onset of symptoms is frequently between 2 and 10 years old, with some having delayed onset between ages 10 and 40 years; onset of symptoms before 2 years or after 40 years is uncommon. The most common *initial symptoms* are seizures, recurrent headaches, poor appetite, failure to thrive, recurrent vomiting, muscle weakness, short stature, stroke-like episodes, sensorineural hearing loss, exercise intolerance, visual symptoms, and developmental delay. Nearly 100% of cases have stroke-like episodes, with intermittent symptoms of headache, vomiting, and new focal neurological signs such as cortical blindness or hemiplegia, typically presenting after a stressor such as surgery or infection [7].

The most common *ongoing symptoms* of MELAS are seizures, headaches, poor appetite, and recurrent vomiting. Neurological symptoms include stroke-like episodes, seizures (including epilepsia partialis continua), hemiparesis, cortical blindness, and/or altered mental status. Though the stroke-like episodes (SLEs) are potentially reversible, the recurrence of SLEs and the progressive brain atrophy can cause permanent difficulties with motor, vision, and/or cognitive abilities. Migraine headaches are frequently associated with stroke-like episodes. Additional characteristic symptoms of MELAS include exercise intolerance, limb weakness, hemianopsia, nausea, vomiting, hearing loss, learning disability, basal ganglia calcifications, myoclonus, heart failure, Wolff-Parkinson-White syndrome or other cardiac conduction block, diabetes, and nephropathy.

In a series of 31 patients affected by MELAS whom were longitudinally followed in the natural history study at the Columbia University Medical Center, the incidence of symptoms were exercise intolerance (93%), seizures (90%), gastrointestinal disturbance (90%), hearing loss (70%), night blindness (44%), ptosis (41%), growth failure (40%), diabetes (39%), hirsutism (25%), school difficulties (51%), motor delay (39%), perinatal difficulties (34%), need for special education (34%), and speech delay (28%) [8]. In another review of 110 MELAS patients, the frequency of major symptoms were exercise intolerance (100%), symptom onset before age 40 years (99%), seizures (96%) lactic acidosis (94%), dementia (90%), limb weakness (89%), hemiparesis (83%), short stature (82%), hemianopia (79%), headache (77%), nausea and vomiting (77%), onset before age 20 years (76%), hearing loss

(75%), learning disabilities (60%), myoclonus (38%), cerebellar ataxia (33%), episodic coma (20%), optic atrophy (20%), congestive heart failure (18%), pigmentary retinopathy (16%), Wolff-Parkinson-White (14%), progressive external ophthalmoplegia (PEO) (13%), cardiac conduction block (6%), and diabetes (5%) [9].

Review of Symptoms by Organ System

Central Nervous System Involvement

Central nervous system involvement includes stroke-like episodes, epilepsy, migraine headaches, encephalopathy, and cognitive decline or dementia. Less common neurological manifestations are myoclonus and ataxia [10]. Neurobehavioral manifestations include mood disorders (major depression or anxiety), dementia, psychosis, and autistic-like features [11]. Cognitive impairment and progressive decline are common and are characterized by global neuropsychological deficits, with changes in attention, executive function, visual perception, and construction, which correlate with presence and extent of cerebral atrophy on MRI [12].

Stroke-Like Episodes (SLEs)

SLEs manifest in young patients without cardiovascular risk factors and are frequently associated with epileptic seizures and/or migraine. Visual field defects (hemianopsia) or positive visual symptoms (from elementary to complex visual hallucinations) are significantly more frequent than motor deficits. Moreover, compared with vascular strokes, there is higher incidence of bilateral clinical symptoms such as cortical blindness or auditory agnosia [13]. Acute neuropsychiatric symptoms, confusion and behavioral changes, are also commonly observed. Frequency of, and interval between, SLEs varies widely and cannot be predicted. Hearing loss and/or diabetes are common pre-existing clinical manifestations.

Stroke-like episodes need to be differentiated from vascular ischemic stroke [14] and require a different management. They occur repeatedly at different times and regions moving from the temporal toward the surrounding parietal and occipital cortex and spread slowly over a few weeks up to several months after the initial symptoms [15]. On conventional magnetic resonance imaging (MRI), stroke-like lesions (SLLs) affect preferentially the cortical gyri and do not respect the vascular territories of major cerebral arteries or border zones [16, 17]. Lesions appear as large T2-bright areas in supratentorial cortical and subcortical regions with nonvascular distribution and migrational behavior. Lesions are bright on diffusion-weighted imaging (DWI), with mixed pattern of increased (vasogenic edema) and restricted (cytotoxic edema) diffusion on ADC maps since the early stages (Fig. 1). However, there are several controversies in the features of SLLs on DWI. More recent studies demonstrated, during the acute phase, a pattern of acute DWI hyperintensity with decreased ADC, prevalent in the cortex regions, and increased ADC in most affected subcortical white matter [18]. In contrast with the typical hypoperfusion in acute vascular stroke, in the affected areas of MELAS patients, there is no reduction in regional cerebral blood flow, with several studies demonstrating instead normal or even increased perfusion [19, 20], perhaps related to metabolic stress-induced lactic acidosis and consequential vasodilation and/or damage to vascular musculature and vasoparalysis or as a compensatory mechanism in the attempt to provide more oxygen supply to energy-depleted neurons [21]. Angiography shows absence of larger vessel pathology and arterial obstruction. Some lesions with time may turn into pseudolaminar necrosis, gyral contrast enhancement, gliosis, and atrophy. Proton MR spectroscopy (MRS) demonstrates an abnormally elevated lactate peak, due to the mitochondrial dysfunction, and reduction of the N-acetyl aspartate (NAA) peak, indicating neuronal loss, *both in affected and non-affected areas*, and in CSF (voxels placed over the ventricles) (Fig. 1).

Pathophysiology of stroke-like events is still debated but is likely due to the combination of

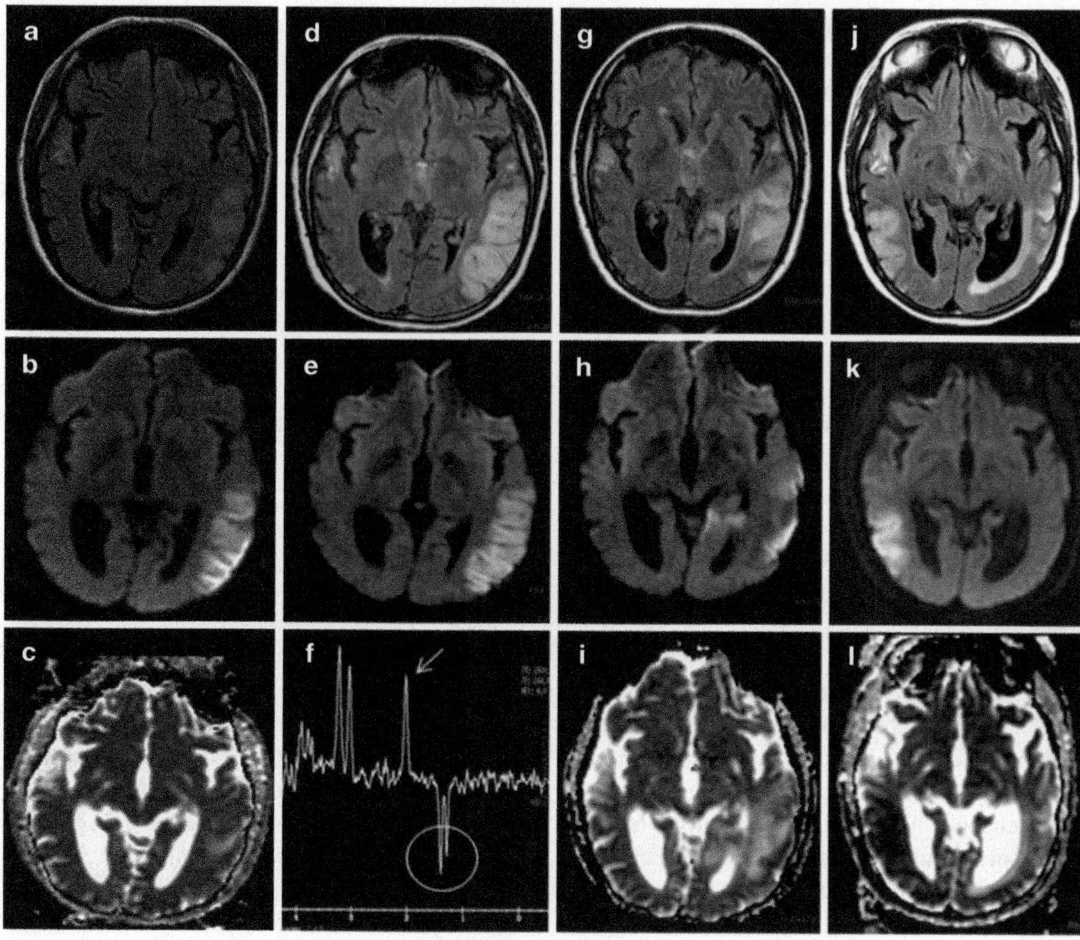

Fig. 1 Stroke-like lesions (SLLs) are bright on T2 FLAIR (**a**, **d**, **g**, **j**) and DWI (**b**, **e**, **h**, **k**) with mixed pattern of increased (vasogenic edema) (increased signal on **c**, **i**) and restricted (cytotoxic edema) diffusion (**l**) with darker lesion over right temporo-occipital area) on ADC maps. MRS (**f**) shows reduced NAA peak (arrow) as well as a lactate doublet (circled)

several factors [16]; (1) an "ischemic" mechanism based on a mitochondrial microangiopathy, with accumulation of abnormal mitochondria and reduced cytochrome C oxidase (COX) activity in the smooth muscle and endothelial cells of the pial arterioles and small arteries of the brain, with a mutation load (heteroplasmy) even more elevated in vessels than in neurons [22]; (2) a primarily metabolic mechanism sustained by neuronal energetic dysfunction (mitochondrial cytopathy theory), the toxic effect of lactic acid and vasogenic edema as the result of increased capillary permeability due to mitochondrial respiratory failure of cerebral artery endothelium and reduction of pH [23]; and (3) a nonischemic neurovascular cellular mechanism with neuronal hyperexcitability, energy failure of group of neuronal cells, and inability of the defective mitochondria to respond adequately to periods of high metabolic demand. The second and third mechanisms are strictly interconnected, as mitochondrial dysfunction of the capillary endothelium contributes to functional impairment of the blood-brain barrier and may in turn lower the threshold of neuronal excitability by changing ion homeostasis, causing or sustaining epileptic activity [23]. In support to this third mechanism, paroxysmal events are common at the onset of SLEs, as are migrainous attacks, focal (mainly motor) or generalized seizures, or status epilepticus, conditions all with high-energy requirements. Epilepsy in particular influences overall morbidity and mortality, with rapid deterioration after periods of persistent seizure activity, severe neuronal energy deprivation, neuronal injury, and cell death.

It is still unclear why temporoparietal and occipital regions are the preferred targets in MELAS. No correlation in fact has been demonstrated with the heteroplasmy level of mutated mtDNA genomes, and in brain autopsies of MELAS patients, no significant regional variability of percentage of m.3243A>G mutation between affected and intact areas, nor among gray matter, white matter, and deep subcortical nuclei [22] with the highest proportion of mutated mtDNA, present in the walls of the leptomeningeal and cortical blood vessels in all brain regions.

Another interesting hypothesis is that in analogy to migraine attacks, SLEs and migraine may share a similar mechanism: the "Cortical Spread Depression," a wave of cortical depolarization that originates in the middle-posterior areas triggered by neuronal hyperexcitability. Another interesting peculiarity is that symmetric brain regions are often affected by single or successive relapses, maybe because they are structurally and neurochemically similar [13].

In the series of patients enrolled in the Italian Registry of Mitochondrial patients, among the 133 patients harboring the m.3243A>G variant, male gender seems to represent a risk factor for the development of stroke-like episodes [24]; this observation however was not confirmed in another study [25].

SLEs in MELAS due to m.3243A>G need to be differentiated from SLEs in other mitochondrial diseases. *POLG* (polymerase gamma 1) is the second most common mitochondrial disorder in which SLEs may manifest. In both MELAS- and *POLG*-related encephalopathies, the lesions are spreading and show a predilection for occipital lobe. However, parietal and temporal involvements are more common in MELAS, while thalamic and prefrontal cortical lesions are more frequently seen in *POLG*. Calcification in the caudate, lentiform nuclei, and dentate nuclei is frequently observed in MELAS, but not in *POLG*-encephalopathies. Moreover in brain-affected areas on ADC map, only cytotoxic edema is present in *POLG*-related disorders, and on brain MRS, a lactate peak is present in the affected brain regions but absent in the normal regions, in contrast with what is seen in MELAS patients where a lactate peak is visible even in radiographically unaffected areas. Furthermore, although seizures are common, it appears unlikely that epileptic activity in *POLG* is the primary mechanism behind the stroke-like lesion expansion or clinical progression. Finally, no mitochondrial microangiopathy is present in *POLG*-encephalopathies, and no cytochrome oxidase negative/succinate dehydrogenase reactive vessels were found in the brains at autopsy [26].

Paroxysmal Events

Seizures commonly occur during stroke-like episodes and may result in epilepsia partialis continua or other focal seizures, generalized tonic-clonic seizures and myoclonic seizures, with status epilepticus in about 20% of cases. Migraines may have complicated features such as vision loss and/or hemiparesis and may be seen in association with new stroke-like episodes.

Seizures manifest in up to 96% and headache in 77% of individuals with full MELAS syndrome (Di Mauro and Hirano, GeneReviews, last update [9]). Seizure semiology and electroencephalography abnormalities do not have syndrome-specific characteristics, but focal motor is far more frequent than generalized seizures [27, 28]. Prolonged focal seizures can progress to secondarily generalized seizures. Epilepsia partialis continua, complex partial status epilepticus with cognitive symptoms, occipital status epilepticus with visual hallucinations, and nonconvulsive status epilepticus are all described in association with stroke-like episodes [27].

Migraine headaches occur in the majority of affected individuals and are often severe during the acute phase of the stroke. Repeated episodes of migraine are one of the most frequent symptoms. Headache is sometimes the only clinical feature in oligosymptomatic maternal relatives of patients with MELAS [29, 30].

Epilepsy in particular influences morbidity and mortality with deterioration after periods of persistent seizure activity, consequent neuronal energy deprivation, severe neuronal injury, and cell death. Seizures are not always present, but ongoing seizure activity represents a treatable factor in the acute stroke-like episode and requires rapid and aggressive intervention. Increased metabolic demand due to seizure activity may perpetuate the focal metabolic crisis and worsen neuronal loss and subsequent neurological outcomes [15, 23].

Peripheral Nervous System Involvement

Muscle involvement includes myopathy with fatigue and exercise intolerance, muscle wasting, and ragged red fibers on muscle biopsy. In the GeneReviews survey, exercise intolerance was present in 100% out of 110 patients with full MELAS syndrome, limb weakness in 89%, and PEO in 13% (Di Mauro and Hirano, GeneReviews last update [9]). However, in most of the other large series, the frequency of myopathy and neuropathy was defined in the whole cohort of m.3243A>G mutation carriers independent of clinical phenotype. Karrpa et al. studied the presence of clinically manifest myopathy in 50 patients harboring the m.3243A>G mutation and found that was present in 50% of patients, including mild to moderate limb weakness, ptosis, and ophthalmoplegia, presenting most commonly in the fifth decade [31]. In other studies, exercise intolerance was present in 41–90% of the patients, PEO in 25–35%, and muscle weakness in 40–89% [24, 32, 33].

In the literature, the occurrence of neuropathy varies widely between 22% and 77% [33] and up to 92% of the patients [34]. Neuropathy does not correlate with diabetes, is mostly a sensory axonal neuropathy, may not present much in terms of clinical symptoms, and in a minority of patients is a distal sensory-motor axonal neuropathy.

Hearing and Vision

Sensorineural hearing loss in MELAS is typically early onset, progressive, and bilateral and can be found not only in the index patient but in maternal relatives, especially in combination with diabetes (maternally inherited diabetes and deafness, known as MIDD, is a clinical phenotype also associated with pathogenic variants in m.3243A>G). Hearing impairment occurs in 71–77% of patients [33].

Visual symptoms may include cortical blindness and/or hemianopsia from stroke-like episodes affecting the visual cortex and optic pathways but may also include ophthalmoplegia, pigmentary retinopathy, optic atrophy, and bilateral cataracts.

Gastrointestinal Manifestations

Gastrointestinal (GI) symptoms include GI dysmotility and pseudo-obstruction as well as cyclic vomiting [35, 36]. GI dysmotility may represent a severe complication in mitochondrial encephalomyopathies [37–39]. Chronic intestinal pseudo-obstruction (CIPO) was detected in 13% of 226 adult patients with genetically determined m.3243A>G-related mitochondrial diseases, among which 14 had history of SLEs [38, 39]. The mechanism of paralytic ileus in MELAS is not fully understood, and both a myenteric plexus neuropathy and a visceral myopathy have been postulated [36]. In line with the second hypothesis, Betts et al. [40] demonstrated a severe cytochrome C oxidase deficiency in the intestinal smooth muscle cells in the whole gastrointestinal tract. Thus, pathophysiology of intestinal pseudo-obstruction in these patients might be related to energy metabolism imbalance similar to the brain in stroke-like episodes [37]. Accordingly, in the Ng series, eight patients presented acutely with severe CIPO and a concomitant acute SLE, leading the authors to speculate on an additional centrally mediated mechanism [38, 39]. In spite of the pathological mechanisms, however, early recognition of gastrointestinal dysmotility is mandatory to promptly introduce adequate medical therapies, including feeding therapies and/or total parental nutrition, and to avoid life-threating CIPO and unnecessary surgical interventions.

Endocrinopathies

Endocrinopathies seen in MELAS include mitochondrial diabetes, hypothyroidism, growth hormone deficiency, and adrenal insufficiency. General features include short stature, failure to thrive, thin body habitus, and hirsutism.

Diabetes mellitus is a common endocrine feature of patients with mitochondrial disease and in particular with the m.3243A>G mutation. It may be a manifestation of MELAS or may be part of the phenotype of maternally inherited diabetes and deafness (MIDD).

The frequency of various endocrinopathies was reported by Al-Gadi et al. in 91 patients with m.3243A>G mutation from the NAMDC (North American Mitochondrial Disease Consortium) registry: diabetes mellitus 31.9%, abnormal growth and sexual maturation 50%, and hypothyroidism 12.2% [41].

Cardiovascular Involvement

Cardiovascular issues include arrhythmias such as Wolff-Parkinson-White or other conduction abnormalities, in addition to structural lesions including left ventricular/biventricular hypertrophy and dysfunction, which may progress to heart failure [42–44]. Cardiac disease in patients with mitochondrial disease may progress insidiously and rarely causes symptoms until advanced in severity. Hypertrophic remodeling is the dominant pattern of cardiomyopathy, and the probability of progression to ventricular dilatation and heart failure is high. Dilated cardiomyopathy is rarer than the hypertrophic phenotype; restrictive cardiomyopathy and left ventricular noncompaction are very rare presentations [45]. Conduction defects such as preexcitation (Wolff-Parkinson-White syndrome), AV-conduction defects, or intraventricular conduction defects are also reported. The most frequent conduction defect is Wolff-Parkinson-White syndrome. Patients with m.3243A>G mutation are at highest risk of MACE (Major Adverse Cardiac Event), with 14% incidence, mainly associated with decompensated HF [46]. Some asymptomatic relatives have had acute onset cardiac arrhythmia and sudden death [38, 39].

Renal Involvement

Renal manifestations of MELAS syndrome include Fanconi proximal tubulopathy, proteinuria, and focal segmental glomerulosclerosis [47].

Additional Phenotypes Associated with m.3243A>G

Clinical syndromes classically associated with the phenotypic expression of the m.3243A>G mutation include MELAS, maternally inherited deafness and diabetes (MIDD), and chronic progressive external ophthalmoplegia (PEO). Nonsyndromic phenotypes include hypertrophic cardiomyopathy, cluster headaches, ataxia, pancreatitis, subacute dementia, and myoclonus with ragged red fibers. All the described manifestations may be part of the full MELAS syndrome, may be isolated, or may be grouped in specific sub-phenotypes. In this regard, Nesbitt et al. [29] recently reported a cohort of 129 individuals from 83 unrelated families carrying the m.3243A>G mtDNA mutation, only 10% of patients manifested a classical MELAS phenotype; instead 30% had MIDD, 6% MELAS/MIDD, 2% MELAS/PEO, and 5% MIDD/PEO overlap syndromes; 6% had PEO and other features not consistent with recognized syndrome, 3% isolated sensorineural hearing loss, and 28% showed a variety of symptoms not fitting a classic phenotype; 9% remained asymptomatic [29]. In the most recent review [25], the more common symptoms of m.3243A>G include sensorineural hearing loss, gastrointestinal symptoms, neuropsychiatric symptoms, diabetes, migraine headache, and ataxia; seizures affected 25%, and stroke-like episodes affected 17%. Contrary to previous reports, the age of onset and heteroplasmy levels did not correlate with phenotype. Surprisingly, hearing impairment, diabetes, and encephalopathy showed the strongest associations, but the highest heritability was estimated for psychiatric involvement and moderate for cognition, ataxia, migraine, and hearing impairment. With these results, the authors supported the idea of nuclear genetic factors influencing clinical outcomes and phenotypic expression.

Laboratory Testing and Diagnostic Clues

Laboratory Diagnosis

Serum creatine kinase level is only mildly elevated in most patients. Lactic acidosis (in blood and CSF) is typical for MELAS and may be severe, although overall have low sensitivity and specificity as in most mitochondrial disorders. Increased lactate in the CSF, detectable by 1H-MRS or lumbar puncture, is a frequent finding in patients and oligosymptomatic carriers and correlates with neuropsychological and neurologic impairment [48].

Muscle Biopsy

The histopathological hallmarks of mitochondrial diseases, including MELAS, are the presence of mitochondrial proliferation as classic ragged red fibers (RRFs) on modified Gomori trichrome stain. RRFs strongly react with succinate dehydrogenase (SDH, complex II of the respiratory chain) ("ragged blue" fibers), with SDH being a good histological and enzymatic marker of mitochondrial abundance because complex II is encoded entirely by nuclear genes [49]. However, in contrast to what is observed in most other mtDNA-related genetic disorders, in which RRFs are COX-negative (COX, complex IV of the respiratory chain), in classical MELAS patients, there is normal reactivity for COX, i.e., they are COX-positive staining [50]. On the other hand, MELAS patients with clinically symptomatic myopathy may also show COX-negative RRFs or a variable COX negativity, likely related to the uneven distribution of mutated genomes with higher concentration in COX-deficient fibers that are roughly proportional to the severity of the myopathy [51]. Characteristically, blood vessels in MELAS also show hyperreactivity for SDH. These so-called SSVs (strongly SDH-reactive vessels) are the expression of the microangiopathy with mitochondrial proliferation that occurs not only in muscle fibers but also, as in the brain, in smooth muscle and endothelial cells of arterial walls [52].

Although strongly suggestive of MELAS, SSVs can be found also in other mitochondrial disorders but are absent in muscle biopsies of patients with *POLG*-encephalopathies and SLEs [26].

Biochemical analysis in frozen muscle tissue or cultured fibroblasts by spectrophotometric assays of the complexes of the respiratory chain (RC) may be normal or show deficiencies in complexes I, III, and IV.

Neurophysiology

Electromyography (*EMG*) may show a myopathic process. Neuropathy is a common manifestation, and accurate nerve conduction velocity (*NCV*) should be performed even in absence of symptoms, as asymptomatic sensory axonal neuropathy is the most frequent neuropathy [34, 53]. NCV typically shows axonal or, less frequently, mixed axonal and demyelinating neuropathy.

EEG does not have specific MELAS patterns and may show focal or multifocal epileptiform activity associated with focal or generalized slowing. Periodic lateralized epileptiform discharges can be seen in association with prolonged seizures and SLEs [27].

Neuroimaging

The neuroradiological hallmarks of MELAS are the stroke-like lesions (SLLs), acute and slowly spreading lesions involving mostly occipital and temporal-parietal lobes (Fig. 1). The affected areas do not correspond to vascular territories and involve cortex and juxtacortical white matter. Lesions may spread over days, weeks, and even months or go to the contralateral side (skipping lesions) after the acute episode. Areas of DWI hyperintensity show ADC map consistent with a mixed vasogenic and cytotoxic edema (for more details, see the earlier paragraph on SLEs).

The most severe lesions develop into cortical pseudolaminar necrosis, gyral contrast enhancement, gliosis, and atrophy that correlate with disease progression. The gyral necrosis may cause partial gyral signal suppression on T2/FLAIR sequences, the so-called black toenail sign due to its radiographic appearance [54].

Laminar cortical necrosis, expression of the severe parenchymal loss probably related to the irreversible cortical energy failure, is another typical neuroradiological feature of MELAS, and mitochondrial diseases are the third common cause of laminar necrosis after cerebral ischemia and hypoxia [55].

Deep gray matter changes are mainly subcortical involving caudate nuclei, globus pallidus, putamen, pulvinar of thalamus, and dentate nucleus of cerebellum. Microcalcifications in vessel walls and sidero-calcific deposits have been also shown to occur in the putamen and globus pallidus [17].

Small lacunar infarcts may also occur mainly in the frontal deep white matter, periventricular area, and bilateral ganglia [18].

Brain atrophy is present in the majority of MELAS patients and accentuated in the cerebellum [56]. Severe cerebral atrophy is mostly seen in patients with a relatively early onset and long duration of illness or accompanying the end stage of the disease [57]. Cerebellar atrophy is also common, mainly manifested as dilation of posterior cistern.

Brain atrophy far more exceeds the extension of the SLLs (Fig. 2), and interesting studies by Tsujikawa et al. using voxel-based morphometry with magnetic resonance imaging demonstrated

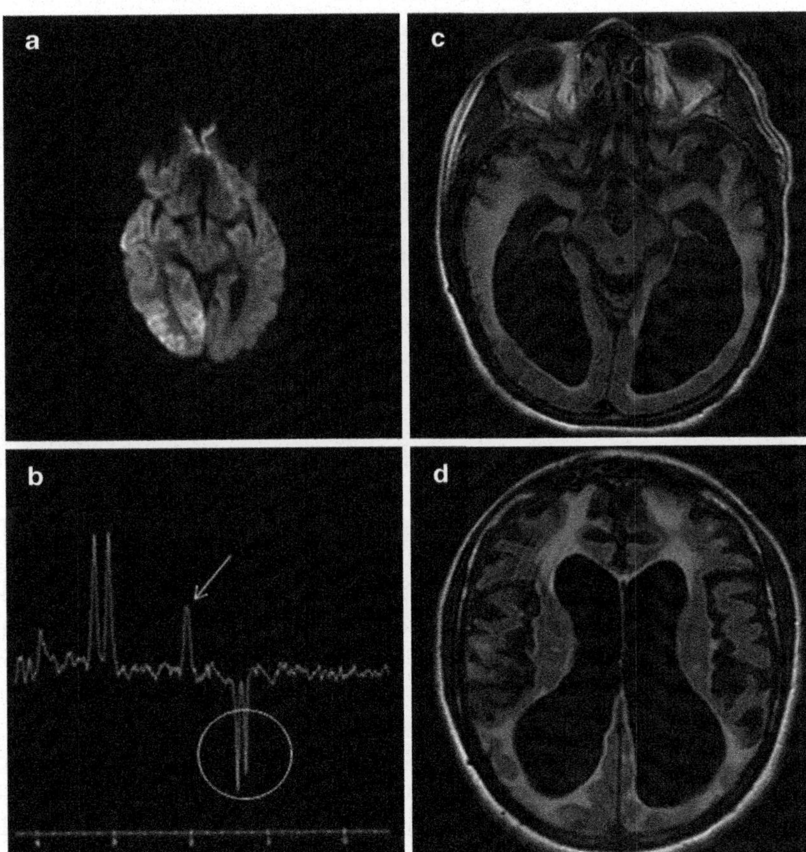

Fig. 2 Stroke-like lesions (SLLs) are shown by DWI (**a**). T2 FLAIR demonstrates both cerebral atrophy (marked ventriculomegaly) as well as increased signal of the white matter (**c**, **d**). MRS demonstrates lactate peak (**b**)

in four MELAS patients significant gray matter (GM) volume reductions in the left superior parietal lobule (SPL), right precuneus, right middle temporal gyrus (MTG), and bilateral posterior lobes of the cerebellum. The areas of GM volume reduction were beyond the regions of previous SLLs. The same patients showed also significant white matter (WM) volume reductions in the bilateral or unilateral temporal sub-gyral regions, which instead were included in the regions of previous SLLs. Furthermore, five oligosymptomatic carriers also show variable and less extensive reductions in the left SPL, right precuneus, right MTG, and bilateral posterior lobes of the cerebellum, but not of the WM. The authors suggested that the similar pattern of GM volume reduction both in patients and in carriers indicates a common vulnerability of specific brain regions, independently from SLLs [58].

Neuropathology studies on postmortem tissues confirm the severe atrophy demonstrated by MRI. The MELAS brain is in fact much smaller than controls, and brain weight is reduced by an average of 18% [59]. Neuropathological changes associated with stroke-like episodes demonstrate cortical necrosis affecting the occipital, temporal, and parietal lobes, extensive neuronal loss, microvacuole formation, and gliosis [22, 59]. At the level of cerebellar cortex are also evident numerous areas of necrosis and extreme neuronal loss affecting Purkinje cells and granule cells [59].

Neuroradiology and neuropathological studies clearly show that neuronal cell loss can occur via two different mechanisms: acute events, such as in stroke-like lesions, and a global, protracted loss of cells that occur independently from SLLs and often starting even before.

1H-magnetic resonance spectroscopy (MRS) in SLLs shows decrease in N-acetylaspartate (NAA) that reflect a loss or impairment of neurons and an increase in lactate (Figs. 1 and 2). Lactate peak is evident not only in the area of the acute stroke-like lesion but also in "unaffected" brain and can be detected in CSF. MRS has been used to follow disease course and progression, and an elevated lactate peak has been associated with increased severity and reduced survival [8, 60]. 1H-MRS has also been proposed as possible biomarker to identify carriers at risk of developing the MELAS phenotype [61].

Genetic Testing for MELAS

Pathogenic variants in mitochondrial DNA cause MELAS, and although >80% of MELAS is due to the common m.3243A>G variant, more than 30 other genes have been reported to lead to the MELAS phenotype. In addition to the m.3243A>G variant, which accounts for approximately 80% of MELAS, the next most common variants include m.3271T>C in MT-TL1 (7.5%), m.3253A>G in MT-TL1 (5%), and m.13513G>A in MT-ND5 (15%) (see Table 1) [9]. Testing can be done in blood leukocytes, but due to tissue heteroplasmy, the mutation is not always detectable in blood, and alternative tissue must be tested. Buccal swab, hair follicles, urine sediment, and muscle biopsy are alternatives; urine sediment has been found to be an excellent accessible tissue for testing if enough DNA can be extracted from epithelial cells [62, 63]. The blood heteroplasmy level decreases about 1.4% per year, and therefore testing more than one tissue type is recommended, especially in the adult population [64].

Family History

When taking a family history for an individual with MELAS, especially the m.3243A>G genotype, it is important for the clinician to illicit specific symptoms regarding matrilineal relatives. Family members may have lower levels of heteroplasmy and have mild (oligosymptomatic) or no symptoms and be unaware of the possibility of this genetic syndrome. Specific phenotypes that may be seen within one family include maternally inherited diabetes and deafness (MIDD), progressive external ophthalmoplegia (PEO), as well as MERRF(myoclonic epilepsy with ragged red fibers)/MELAS overlap

Table 1 Pathogenic variants reported in MELAS (modified from GeneReviews)

% of affected individuals	Mitochondrial DNA nucleotide change	Gene	Protein amino acid change	References
~80%	m.3243A>G	*MT-TL1*	No protein translated	[2]
~<10%	m.3271T>C			[65]
<5%	m.3252A>G			[66]
Rare	m.3291T>C			[67]
	m.3256C>T			[68]
	m.3260A>G			[69]
	m.583G>A	*MT-TF*		[70]
	m.1642G>A	*MT-TV*		[71]
	m.1644G>A			[72]
	m.4332G>A	*MT-TQ*		[73]
	m.5521G>A	*MT-TW*		[74]
	m.5814A>G	*MT-TC*		[75]
	m.7512T>C	*MT-TS1*		[76]
	m.12146A>G	*MT-TL2*		[77]
	m.12299A>C			[78]
	m.8316T>C	*MT-TK*		[79]
	m.8296A>G	*MT-TK*		[80]
	m.3481G>A	*MT-ND1*	p.Gln59Lys	[81]
	m.3697G>A	*MT-ND1*	p.Gly131Ser	[82]
	m.3946G>A	*MT-ND1*	p.Gln214Lys	[82]
	m.3949T>C	*MT-ND1*	p.Tyr215His	[82]
	m.7023G>A	*MT-CO2*	p.Val374Met	[83]
	m.9957T>C	*MT-CO3*	p.Phe251Leu	[84]
<10%	m.13513G>A	MT-ND5	p.Asp393Asn	[85]
Rare	m.12770A>G		p.Glu145Gly	[86]
	m.13042G>A		p.Ala236Thr	[87]
	m.13084A>T		p.Ser250Cys	[88]
	m.13514A>G		p.Asp393Gly	[89]
	m.13528A>G		p.Thr398Ala	[90]
	m.14453G>A	*MT-ND6*	p.Ala74Val	[91]
	m.14787delTTAA (4-bp del)	*MT-CYB*	p.Ile14Thrfs	[92]
	m.14864T>C		p.Cys40Arg	[93]

syndrome and MELAS/Leigh overlap syndrome [3, 94]. In addition, due to tissue-specific heteroplasmy, it is possible to see isolated hypertrophic cardiomyopathy, cluster headaches, pancreatitis, subacute dementia, and myoclonus. Some asymptomatic relatives have had acute onset cardiac arrhythmia and sudden death [38, 39]. Within a single family, the phenotypes can vary widely on the spectrum of symptoms. The variation is due to tissue heteroplasmy levels and mitochondrial DNA copy number [95]. In addition, nuclear genes may play a role in phenotypic heterogeneity [25].

Natural History of MELAS

Several retrospective and prospective natural history studies have been published in regard to MELAS, mainly the m.3243A>G pathogenic variant. MELAS is known to be a progressive disorder, with episodic deterioration due to recurrent stroke-like episodes. In 2006, 33 adults were reported who had been followed for 3 years and found to have progressive sensorineural hearing loss, left ventricular hypertrophy, and EEG abnormalities [96]. In 2011, Kaufmann et al. described 31 individuals with MELAS and

54 carrier relatives, who were followed over 10 years. Those with MELAS had neurological decline and an increased rate of death, compared to their carrier relatives [8]. From the time of first focal neurological symptoms, the survival time was about 17 years, with 22% deaths prior to age 18. Symptom severity was correlated to higher lactate levels as well as childhood onset of disease. In 2012, the MELAS Study Group in Japan published their prospective natural history study of 96 people over 5 years. 20% died within 7 years from the diagnosis of MELAS. Common symptoms in adults included hearing loss, cortical vision loss, and diabetes in addition to stroke-like episodes, seizure, and headache. Short stature was reported in childhood-onset disease [6]. In 2013, a retrospective analysis of 41 people with m.3243A>G reviewed over 5 years had onset between ages 24 and 40 years old, with symptoms including sensorineural hearing loss, myopathy, cognitive impairment, neuropathy, ophthalmoplegia, diabetes, and stroke-like episodes. Cardiac manifestations included left ventricular hypertrophy and/or left ventricular dysfunction (n = 18), Wolff-Parkinson-White (n = 7), conduction system disease (n = 4), and atrial fibrillation (n = 1). Cardiac disease was responsible for morbidity and mortality with three deaths, six hospitalizations for severe heart failure, and one heart transplant [97]. Major Adverse Cardiac Event has a 4% incidence, mainly associated with decompensated heart failure [46]. Besides cardiac, other causes of death are multi-organ failure, ketoacidosis, cardiac arrest after prolonged seizure [98], intestinal pseudo-obstruction in occasion or not with SLEs [38, 39, 57], aspiration pneumonia and sepsis, and cardiorespiratory failure. All the patients at the end stage of the disease have a severe and diffuse brain atrophy [57]. Another large published cohort of m.3243A>G families was published in 2013 by Nesbitt et al., reporting on 129 patients from 83 unrelated families in the Mitochondrial Disease Patient Cohort Study, UK. Within this well-phenotyped cohort, 10% have classic MELAS, 30% MIDD, 6% MELAS/MIDD overlap, 6% with CPEO, 2% MELAS/CPEO, 5% MIDD/CPEO, 4% SNHL, and 28% variety of other symptoms not fitting one of these phenotypes. In the most recent patient cohort reported by Pickett et al. [25], the authors reported more common symptoms of m.3243A>G include SNHL, GI symptoms, neuropsychiatric symptoms, diabetes, migraine headache, and ataxia. Seizures affected 25% and stroke-like episodes 17%. The age of onset and % heteroplasmy level of the mutation did not correlate with the clinical phenotype.

MELAS Treatment

As for most of mitochondrial disorders, there are currently no specific chronic treatments with proven efficacy. Various "cocktails" of antioxidants, vitamins, and cofactors are currently used in mitochondrial disease, including Coenzyme Q10 (CoQ10), idebenone, riboflavin, thiamine, folic acid, L-carnitine, alpha-lipoic acid, vitamin E, and creatine monohydrate. CoQ10 supplementation stimulates the functioning of the electron transport chain with improvement of muscle weakness and exercise intolerance and reduction of lactate level [99]. A combination therapy with creatine monohydrate, CoQ10, and lipoic acid also resulted in similar results [100]. Idebenone, an analog of CoQ_{10} that crosses the blood-brain barrier more efficiently, has also been reported as beneficial in anecdotal reports [101]. All these natural compounds are safe, but no consistent dosing, length of treatment, or which outcomes to follow are currently available. Some medications have shown side effects, such as dichloroacetate (DCA), used to lower serum lactate by activating the pyruvate dehydrogenase enzyme, which yielded no clinical improvement and resulted in a partially irreversible toxic neuropathy in MELAS m.3243A>G patients [53, 102]. Moreover, the 2012 Cochrane review on treatment of mitochondrial diseases confirmed that dichloroacetate should not be used because of the high incidence of potentially irreversible side effects and concluded that there is currently no clear evidence on the use of any of the drugs examined [103]. However, in the recent consensus conference "Nutritional Interventions in

Primary Mitochondrial Disorders: Developing an Evidence Base" [104], an agreement was achieved, using the Delphi consensus methodology on the following points, among others, that can be adopted for the MELAS patients: (1) CoQ10 should be administered to most patients with a diagnosis of mitochondrial disease, and not exclusively for the primary CoQ10 deficiency. (2) Alpha-lipoic acid and riboflavin are the only other supplements that obtained a certain degree of agreement. (3) Folinic acid may be considered in patients with CNS manifestations due to occurrence of secondary cerebral folate deficiency. (4) L-carnitine should only be administered when there is documented carnitine deficiency. (5) It is prudent to correct nutrient deficiency states. Particular attention should be paid to this last point because common features in these patients are cachexia, failure to thrive, low body mass index, reduced food intake or absorption due to gastrointestinal or endocrinological problems, easy fatigue, and early satiety. Thus, it is extremely important to avoid prolonged fasting and consume adequate nutrients and calories. Further studies need to be completed on specific dietary recommendations for mitochondrial disease.

Stroke-Like Episodes

There are no approved medications proven effective in the treatment of stroke-like episodes, but benefit from L-arginine has been suggested by multiple authors on the basis of small and non-blinded trials; however, additional collaborative randomized double-blind placebo controlled trials are still needed to confirm the L-arginine benefit.

In 2005, Koga et al. published "L-arginine improves the symptoms of strokelike episodes in MELAS," based on the hypothesis that the episodes are caused by impaired vasodilation and improved with L-arginine as a nitric oxide precursor. By administering oral arginine (open label), the frequency and severity of stroke-like episodes were reduced [105]. The authors later evaluated endothelial function in patients with MELAS via flow-mediated vasodilation (FMD) and found a decrease compared to controls, which improved after L-arginine therapy [106].

Nitric oxide deficiency in MELAS patients was established, leading to symptoms including the stroke-like episodes, myopathy, diabetes, and lactic acidosis. The NO deficiency is caused by endothelial dysfunction, sequestration by cytochrome C oxidase, shunting into reactive nitrogen species, and decreased availability of citrulline and arginine (NO precursors). Treatment has been proposed with both citrulline and arginine to increase nitric oxide production [107]. Using stable isotope infusion, El-Hattab et al. [108] assessed nitric oxide metabolism in children with MELAS and found a lower NO synthesis rate which was increased with arginine and citrulline supplementation. More recently, Ohasawa proposed taurine as add on therapy in MELAS patients, and in small open-label trial, taurine supplementations further reduced the number of SLEs in most patients already under-treatment with arginine and or Coenzyme Q10 [109]. Based on the available data and despite the lack of a randomized controlled trial using arginine or citrulline vs. placebo, the Mitochondrial Medicine Society published recommendations using arginine for acute stroke as well as for stroke prevention in 2016 [110]. During the acute episode, suggested dose for intravenous L-arginine is 0.5 g/kg given once per day for 3–5 days (ideally when symptoms resolve). The therapy should be started preferentially within 3 h of symptom onset. Blood pressure, glucose, and CO_2 should be monitored to watch for side effects of hypotension, hypoglycemia, and acidosis (as arginine is as arginine HCl). As prophylactic management, oral arginine is given as 0.3 g/kg divided TID. However, in absence of large, blinded, controlled trials, these recommendations are not universally accepted nor practiced. Evaluation of treatment efficacy is in fact difficult in small group of patients affected by a rare disorder, as MELAS, in which data on natural history are lacking. SLEs are unpredictable in time and frequency, show variable degrees of spontaneous resolution, and tend to reduce in the course of the disease. Moreover, despite the low serum NO, most studies demonstrate hyperemia and hyperperfusion in SLE areas which increase as the disease progresses [21, 111], raising the question as to whether low NO and arginine levels are instead the consequence of chronic vascular dilatation [112]. Based on this data, some authors have used corticosteroids, with good clinical response, to counteract the effect of hyperperfusion that leads to apoptotic neuronal death due to the progression from vasogenic to cytotoxic edema [21, 112]. Authors in fact hypothesize that hyperperfusion is a compensatory mechanism to increase oxygen supply and nutrients to dysfunctional neurons that are unable to meet their metabolic demands. Steroids help to stabilize the blood-brain barrier, reducing the vasogenic edema and the progression to widespread cytotoxic edema. Steroids are firstly used in intravenous high dose and then slowly tapered to a maintenance dose [21, 112].

Acetyl salicylic acid and other blood thinners are not indicated in these patients.

The proper management of SLEs includes prompt and effective treatment of seizures and a strict control of lactic acidosis, diabetes, gastrointestinal dysmotility, and any potential precipitating factors such as infection, dehydration, hyponatremia, fasting, surgery, and other physiological stressors, in addition to medications which may cause lactic acidosis such as metformin and propofol.

Epilepsy

Early treatment of epilepsy and good control of interictal seizures may improve the prognosis of the disease. Patients have a predisposition for prolonged seizures or status epilepticus, and most of the patients experienced more than one episode of status epilepticus [27]. All patients need more than one drug, and about 20% the patients show a drug-resistant epilepsy [28]. Although seizures may respond to conventional anticonvulsants, the choice of antiepileptic drugs is complicated because of the potential mitochondrial toxicity associated with the most common AEDs, including valproic acid, carbamazepine, oxcarbazepine, phenytoin, and phenobarbital. In particular, valproic acid is an effective anticonvulsant for partial and generalized seizures and myoclonus; however, it should be avoided because it inhibits carnitine uptake, potentially exacerbating fatigability, lactic acidosis, and hyperammonemia and may trigger MELAS manifestations [33]. Carbamazepine and oxcarbazepine may cause side effects such as hyponatremia and leukopenia. Lorazepam (and all benzodiazepines), lamotrigine, and levetiracetam are effective and well tolerated. In addition to antiepileptic action, levetiracetam and lamotrigine may act on myoclonus and have neuroprotective effects. Lacosamide is safe and effective as adjunctive therapy, especially in the treatment of refractory epilepsy in MELAS [113].

The treatment of generalized tonic-clonic status epilepticus should be treated in accordance with the existing guidelines, with the exception of the sodium valproate that should be avoided due to potential severe toxic effects.

Treatment of Comorbidities

Symptoms of *gastrointestinal dysmotility* need a careful surveillance and treatment to prevent chronic intestinal pseudo-obstruction (CIPO) [37–39]. Correct management of the symptoms requires an appropriate and balanced diet, good hydration, and the use of osmotic laxatives, antibiotics as pro-motility agents (erythromycin), and other prokinetic medications such as pyridostigmine or prucalopride, a high affinity 5-HT4 receptor agonist that is safe even in long-term therapy [37]. In the case of ileus, it is important to avoid unnecessary surgery that is associated with poor outcome [38, 39]; parenteral nutrition or intravenous fluids are given while providing gut rest, avoidance of lactated Ringer's solution, and if necessary decompressive colonoscopy is in general sufficient to control the acute manifestations.

In the case of severe *dysphagia* or prominent cachexia, a percutaneous endoscopic gastroenterostomy (PEG), gastrostomy tube (G tube) or, if needed, a jejunal tube (J tube) should be considered to deliver enteral nutrition.

Individuals with MELAS who have *diabetes* are typically thin, with mid-adult onset. Although individuals initially respond to diet, then to oral hypoglycemic agents, they rapidly develop insulin dependence. Hemoglobin A1Cs are typically higher, with high fasting blood glucose levels. However, they may also be very sensitive to insulin, and if not eating well due to nausea or early satiety, caution must be taken with preprandial insulin and an unfinished meal in order to avoid hypoglycemia [114].

Cardiac manifestations can be treated with standard pharmacologic therapy, but some patients cannot tolerate beta-blockers. Others may improve by treating comorbidities such as chronic headache or other symptoms of dysautonomia. Some MELAS patients may progress to cardiomyopathy and need more frequent studies.

Patients with clinically manifest myopathy and *respiratory insufficiency* may require nocturnal or continuous noninvasive or invasive ventilation and aggressive pulmonary toilet with chest physiotherapy and cough assist.

In those with ptosis and ophthalmoplegia, *surgical management of ptosis may be indicated* to avoid visual impairment and secondary complications, such as postural problems, neck pain, and headache.

Hearing loss can benefit of appropriate hearing devices and, if needed, cochlear implants [115].

General Recommendations

Patients should have sufficient sleep and should perform, if possible, regular aerobic activity below the maximum limit. They should be advised to avoid fasting, dehydration, exercise stress, emotional stress, extreme cold, extreme heat, alcohol, nicotine, and infectious diseases. They should receive standard vaccinations, including yearly pneumococcal and influenza vaccines.

Genetic Counseling

MELAS is caused by mitochondrial DNA pathogenic variants; men cannot pass these down to their offspring. Women may pass the mutation to their offspring in unpredictable and with a wide spectrum of heteroplasmy. Women with mitochondrial disease may have increased symptoms and complications during pregnancy [116]. Reproductive options include preimplantation genetics, testing during the pregnancy with amniocentesis or chorionic villus sampling, but may not yield accurate results. Mitochondrial replacement therapies are controversial but may help prevent transmission of the mtDNA pathogenic variant while allowing a woman to have her own genetically related child [117].

References

1. Pavlakis SG, Phillips PC, DiMauro S, De Vivo DC, Rowland LP. Mitochondrial myopathy, encephalopathy, lactic acidosis, and strokelike episodes: a distinctive clinical syndrome. Ann Neurol. 1984;16(4):481–8.
2. Goto Y, Nonaka I, Horai S. A mutation in the tRNA(Leu)(UUR) gene associated with the MELAS subgroup of mitochondrial encephalomyopathies. Nature. 1990;348(6302):651–3.
3. Scaglia F, Northrop JL. The mitochondrial myopathy encephalopathy, lactic acidosis with stroke-like episodes (MELAS) syndrome: a review of treatment options. CNS Drugs. 2006;20(6):443–64. Review. Erratum in: CNS Drugs. 2008;22(1):81
4. Kami K, Fujita Y, Igarashi S, Koike S, Sugawara S, Ikeda S, Sato N, Ito M, Tanaka M, Tomita M, Soga T. Metabolomic profiling rationalized pyruvate efficacy in cybrid cells harboring MELAS mitochondrial DNA mutations. Mitochondrion. 2012;12(6):644–53. https://doi.org/10.1016/j.mito.2012.07.113.
5. Hirano M, Ricci E, Koenigsberger MR, Defendini R, Pavlakis SG, DeVivo DC, DiMauro S, Rowland LP. Melas: an original case and clinical criteria for diagnosis. Neuromuscul Disord. 1992;2(2):125–35. Review
6. Yatsuga S, Povalko N, Nishioka J, Katayama K, Kakimoto N, Matsuishi T, Kakuma T, Koga Y, Taro Matsuoka for MELAS Study Group in Japan. MELAS: a nationwide prospective cohort study of 96 patients in Japan. Biochim Biophys Acta. 2012;1820(5):619–24.

7. Goodfellow JA, Dani K, Stewart W, Santosh C, McLean J, Mulhern S, Razvi S. Mitochondrial myopathy, encephalopathy, lactic acidosis and stroke-like episodes: an important cause of stroke in young people. Postgrad Med J. 2012;88(1040):326–34.
8. Kaufmann P, Engelstad K, Wei Y, Kulikova R, Oskoui M, Sproule DM, Battista V, Koenigsberger DY, Pascual JM, Shanske S, Sano M, Mao X, Hirano M, Shungu DC, Dimauro S, De Vivo DC. Natural history of MELAS associated with mitochondrial DNA m.3243A>G genotype. Neurology. 2011;77(22):1965–71.
9. DiMauro S, Hirano M. MELAS. 2001 Feb 27 [Updated 2013 Nov 21] 2013. In: Adam MP, Ardinger HH, Pagon RA, et al., editors. GeneReviews® [Internet]. Seattle (WA): University of Washington, Seattle; 1993–2018. https://www.ncbi.nlm.nih.gov/books/NBK1233/.
10. Petruzzella V, Zoccolella S, Amati A, Torraco A, Lamberti P, Carnicella F, Serlenga L, Papa S. Cerebellar ataxia as atypical manifestation of the 3243A>G MELAS mutation. Clin Genet. 2004;65:64–5.
11. Anglin RE, Garside SL, Tarnopolsky MA, Mazurek MF, Rosebush PI. The psychiatric manifestations of mitochondrial disorders: a case and review of the literature. J Clin Psychiatry. 2012;73:506–12.
12. Kraya T, Neumann L, Paelecke-Habermann Y, Deschauer M, Stoevesandt D, Zierz S, Watzke S. Cognitive impairment, clinical severity and MRI changes in MELAS syndrome. Mitochondrion. 2019;44:53–7.
13. Miceli G, Conti G, Cianfoni A, Di Giacopo R, Zampetti P, Servidei S. Acute auditory agnosia as the presenting hearing disorder in MELAS. Neurol Sci. 2008;29(6):459–62.
14. Kolb SJ, Costello F, Lee AG, et al. Distinguishing ischemic stroke from the stroke-like lesions of MELAS using apparent diffusion coefficient mapping. J Neurol Sci. 2003;216:11–5.
15. Iizuka T, Sakai F, Kan S, Suzuki N. Slowly progressive spread of the stroke-like lesions in MELAS. Neurology. 2003;61:1238–44.
16. Ito H, Mori K, Kagami S. Neuroimaging of stroke-like episodes in MELAS. Brain and Development. 2011;33(4):283–8.
17. Malhotra K, Liebeskind DS. Imaging of MELAS. Curr Pain Headache Rep. 2016;20(9):54.
18. Xu W, Wen J, Sun C, Cao J, Li Y, Geng D. Conventional and diffusional magnetic resonance imaging. Features of mitochondrial encephalomyopathy, lactic acidosis, and stroke-like episodes in Chinese patients: a study of 40 cases. J Comput Assist Tomogr. 2018;42(4):510–6.
19. Ooiwa Y, Uematsu Y, Terada T, Nakai K, Itakura T, Komai N, et al. Cerebral blood flow in mitochondrial myopathy, encephalopathy, lactic acidosis, and strokelike episodes. Stroke. 1993;24:304–9.
20. Kim JH, Lim MK, Jeon TY, Rha JH, Eo H, Yoo SY, Shu CH. Diffusion and perfusion characteristics of MELAS (mitochondrial myopathy, encephalopathy, lactic acidosis, and stroke-like episode) in thirteen patients. Korean J Radiol. 2011;12(1):15–24.
21. Walcott BP, Edlow BL, Xia Z, Kahle KT, Nahed BV, Schmahmann JD. Steroid responsive A3243G mutation MELAS. Clinical and radiographic evidence for regional hyperperfusion leading to neuronal loss. Neurologist. 2012;18:159–70.
22. Betts J, Jaros E, Perry RH, Schaefer AM, Taylor RW, Abdel-All Z, et al. Molecular neuropathology of MELAS: level of heteroplasmy in individual neurones and evidence of extensive vascular involvement. Neuropathol Appl Neurobiol. 2006;32(4):359–73.
23. Iizuka T, Sakai F. Pathogenesis of stroke-like episodes in MELAS: analysis of neurovascular cellular mechanisms. Curr Neurovasc Res. 2005;2:29–45.
24. Mancuso M, Orsucci D, Angelini C, Bertini E, Carelli V, Comi GP, Donati A, Minetti C, Moggio M, Mongini T, Servidei S, Tonin P, Toscano A, Uziel G, Bruno C, Ienco EC, Filosto M, Lamperti C, Catteruccia M, Moroni I, Musumeci O, Pegoraro E, Ronchi D, Santorelli FM, Sauchelli D, Scarpelli M, Sciacco M, Valentino ML, Vercelli L, Zeviani M, Siciliano G. The m.3243A>G mitochondrial DNA mutation and related phenotypes. A matter of gender? J Neurol. 2014;261(3):504–10.
25. Pickett SJ, Grady JP, Ng YS, Gorman GS, Schaefer AM, Wilson IJ, Cordell HJ, Turnbull DM, Taylor RW, McFarland R. Phenotypic heterogeneity in m.3243A>G mitochondrial disease: the role of nuclear factors. Ann Clin Transl Neurol. 2018;5(3):333–45.
26. Tzoulis C, Neckelmann G, Mørk SJ, Engelsen BE, Viscomi C, Moen G, Ersland L, Zeviani M, Bindoff LA. Localized cerebral energy failure in DNA polymerase gamma-associated encephalopathy syndromes. Brain. 2010;133(Pt 5):1428–37.
27. Demarest ST, Whitehead MT, Turnacioglu S, Pearl PL, Gropman AL. Phenotypic analysis of epilepsy in the mitochondrial encephalomyopathy, lactic acidosis, and strokelike episodes-associated mitochondrial DNA A3243G mutation. J Child Neurol. 2014;29(9):1249–56.
28. Lee HN, Eom S, Kim SH, Kang HC, Lee JS, Kim HD, Lee YM. Epilepsy characteristics and clinical outcome in patients with mitochondrial encephalomyopathy, lactic acidosis, and stroke-like episodes (MELAS). Pediatr Neurol. 2016;64:59–65.
29. Nesbitt V, Pitceathly RD, Turnbull DM, Taylor RW, Sweeney MG, Mudanohwo EE, Rahman S, Hanna MG, McFarland R. The UK MRC mitochondrial disease patient cohort study: clinical phenotypes associated with the m.3243A>G mutation-implications for diagnosis and management. J Neurol Neurosurg Psychiatry. 2013;84(8):936–8.
30. Vollono C, Primiano G, Della Marca G, Losurdo A, Servidei S. Migraine in mitochondrial disorders: prevalence and characteristics. Cephalalgia. 2018;38(6):1093–106.

31. Kärppä M, Herva R, Moslemi AR, Oldfors A, Kakko S, Majamaa K. Spectrum of myopathic findings in 50 patients with the 3243A>G mutation in mitochondrial DNA. Brain. 2005;128(Pt 8):1861–9.
32. Chinnery PF, Howell N, Lightowlers RN. Turnbull DM molecular pathology of MELAS and MERRF. The relationship between mutation load and clinical phenotypes. Brain. 1997;120(Pt 10):1713–21.
33. El-Hattab AW, Adesina AM, Jones J, Scaglia F. MELAS syndrome: clinical manifestations, pathogenesis, and treatment options. Mol Genet Metab. 2015;116(1–2):4–12.
34. Luigetti M, Sauchelli D, Primiano G, Cuccagna C, Bernardo D, Monaco L, Servidei S. Eur J Neurol. 2016;23(6):1020–7.
35. García-Velasco A, Gómez-Escalonilla C, Guerra-Vales JM, Cabello A, Campos Y, Arenas J. Intestinal pseudo-obstruction and urinary retention: cardinal features of a mitochondrial DNA-related disease. J Intern Med. 2003;253(3):381–5.
36. Chang TM, Chi CS, Tsai CR, Lee HF, Li MC. Paralytic ileus in MELAS with phenotypic features of MNGIE. Pediatr Neurol. 2004;31(5):374–7.
37. Primiano G, Plantone D, Forte F, Sauchelli D, Scaldaferri F, Gasbarrini A, Servidei S. Acute refractory intestinal pseudo-obstruction in MELAS: efficacy of prucalopride. Neurology. 2014;82(21):1932–4.
38. Ng YS, Feeney C, Schaefer AM, Holmes CE, Hynd P, Alston CL, Grady JP, Roberts M, Maguire M, Bright A, Taylor RW, Yiannakou Y, McFarland R, Turnbull DM, Gorman GS. Pseudo-obstruction, stroke, and mitochondrial dysfunction: a lethal combination. Ann Neurol. 2016;80(5):686–92.
39. Ng YS, Grady JP, Lax NZ, Bourke JP, Alston CL, Hardy SA, Falkous G, Schaefer AG, Radunovic A, Mohiddin SA, Ralph M, Alhakim A, Taylor RW, McFarland R, Turnbull DM, Gorman GS. Sudden adult death syndrome in m.3243A>G-related mitochondrial disease: an unrecognized clinical entity in young, asymptomatic adults. Eur Heart J. 2016;37(32):2552–9.
40. Betts J, Barron MJ, Needham SJ, Schaefer AM, Taylor RW, Turnbull DM. Gastrointestinal tract involvement associated with the 3243A>G mitochondrial DNA mutation. Neurology. 2008;70(15):1290–2.
41. Al-Gadi IS, Haas RH, Falk MJ, Goldstein A, McCormack SE. Endocrine disorders in primary mitochondrial disease. J Endocr Soc. 2018;2(4):361–73.
42. Menotti F, Brega A, Diegoli M, Grasso M, Modena MG, Arbustini E. A novel mtDNA point mutation in tRNA(Val) is associated with hypertrophic cardiomyopathy and MELAS. Ital Heart J. 2004;5(6): 460–5.
43. Wortmann SB, Rodenburg RJ, Backx AP, Schmitt E, Smeitink JA, Morava E. Early cardiac involvement in children carrying the A3243G mtDNA mutation. Acta Paediatr. 2007;96(3):450–1.
44. Hollingsworth KG, Gorman GS, Trenell MI, McFarland R, Taylor RW, Turnbull DM, MacGowan GA, Blamire AM, Chinnery PF. Cardiomyopathy is common in patients with the mitochondrial DNA m.3243A>G mutation and correlates with mutation load. Neuromuscul Disord. 2012;22(7):592–6.
45. Bates MG, Bourke JP, Giordano C, d'Amati G, Turnbull DM, Taylor RW. Cardiac involvement in mitochondrial DNA disease: clinical spectrum, diagnosis, and management. Eur Heart J. 2012;33(24):3023–33.
46. Wahbi K, Bougouin W, Béhin A, Stojkovic T, Bécane HM, Jardel C, Berber N, Mochel F, Lombès A, Eymard B, Duboc D, Laforêt P. Long-term cardiac prognosis and risk stratification in 260 adults presenting with mitochondrial diseases. Eur Heart J. 2015;36(42):2886–93.
47. Hotta O, Inoue CN, Miyabayashi S, Furuta T, Takeuchi A, Taguma Y. Clinical and pathologic features of focal segmental glomerulosclerosis with mitochondrial tRNALeu(UUR) gene mutation. Kidney Int. 2001;59:1236–43.
48. Kaufmann P, Shungu DC, Sano MC, Jhung S, Engelstad K, Mitsis E, Mao X, Shanske S, Hirano M, DiMauro S, De Vivo DC. Cerebral lactic acidosis correlates with neurological impairment in MELAS. Neurology. 2004;62(8):1297–302.
49. DiMauro S, Bonilla E. Mitochondrial encephalomyopathies. In: Rosenberg RN, Prusiner SB, DiMauro S, Barchi RL, editors. The molecular and genetic basis of neurological disease. Boston, MA: Butterworth-Heinemann; 1997. p. 201–35.
50. Filosto M, Tomelleri G, Tonin P, Scarpelli M, Vattemi G, Rizzuto N, Padovani A, Simonati A. Neuropathology of mitochondrial diseases. Biosci Rep. 2007;27:23–30.
51. Silvestri G, Rana M, Odoardi F, Modoni A, Paris E, Papacci M, Tonali P, Servidei S. Single-fiber PCR in MELAS(3243) patients: correlations between intratissue distribution and phenotypic expression of the mtDNA(A3243G) genotype. Am J Med Genet. 2000;94(3):201–6.
52. Hasegawa H, Matsuoka T, Goto Y, Nonaka I. Strongly succinate dehydrogenase-reactive blood vessels in muscles from patients with mitochondrial myopathy, encephalopathy, lactic acidosis, and stroke-like episodes. Ann Neurol. 1991;29:601–5.
53. Kaufmann P, Pascual JM, Anziska Y, Gooch CL, Engelstad K, Jhung S, DiMauro S, De Vivo DC. Nerve conduction abnormalities in patients with MELAS and the A3243G mutation. Arch Neurol. 2006;63:746–8.
54. Whitehead MT, Wien M, Lee B, Bass N, Gropman A. Black. Toenail sign in MELAS syndrome. Pediatr Neurol. 2017;75:61–5.
55. Finsterer J. Laminar cortical necrosis in mitochondrial disorders. Clin Neurol Neurosurg. 2009;111(8):655–8.
56. Tschampa HJ, Urbach H, Greschus S, Kunz WS, Kornblum C. Neuroimaging characteristics in

mitochondrial encephalopathies associated with them.3243A>G MTTL1 mutation. J Neurol. 2013;260(4):1071–80.
57. Primiano G, Servidei S. Intestinal pseudo-obstruction in mitochondrial diseases. Ann Neurol. 2017;81(1):158–9.
58. Tsujikawa K, Senda J, Yasui K, Hasegawa Y, Hoshiyama M, Katsuno M, Sobue G. Distinctive distribution of brain volume reductions in MELAS and mitochondrial DNA A3243G mutation carriers: a voxel-based morphometric study. Mitochondrion. 2016;30:229–35.
59. Alston CL, Rocha MC, Lax NZ, Turnbull DM, Taylor RW. The genetics and pathology of mitochondrial disease. J Pathol. 2017;241(2):236–50.
60. Abe K, Yoshimura H, Tanaka H, Fujita N, Hikita T, Sakoda S. Comparison of conventional and diffusion-weighted MRI and proton MR spectroscopy in patients with mitochondrial encephalomyopathy, lactic acidosis, and stroke-like events. Neuroradiology. 2004;46(2):113–7.
61. Weiduschat N, Kaufmann P, Mao X, Engelstad KM, Hinton V, DiMauro S, De Vivo D, Shungu D. Cerebral metabolic abnormalities in A3243G mitochondrial DNA mutation carriers. Neurology. 2014;82(9):798–805.
62. McDonnell MT, Schaefer AM, Blakely EL, McFarland R, Chinnery PF, Turnbull DM, Taylor RW. Noninvasive diagnosis of the 3243A > G mitochondrial DNA mutation using urinary epithelial cells. Eur J Hum Genet. 2004;12:778–81.
63. Shanske S, Pancrudo J, Kaufmann P, Engelstad K, Jhung S, Lu J, Naini A, DiMauro S, De Vivo DC. Varying loads of the mitochondrial DNA A3243G mutation in different tissues: implications for diagnosis. Am J Med Genet A. 2004;130A:134–7.
64. Rahman S, Poulton J, Marchington D, Suomalainen A. Decrease of 3243 A->G mtDNA mutation from blood in MELAS syndrome: a longitudinal study. Am J Hum Genet. 2001;68(1):238–40.
65. Goto Y, Nonaka I, Horai S. A new mtDNA mutation associated with mitochondrial myopathy, encephalopathy, lactic acidosis and stroke-like episodes (MELAS). Biochim Biophys Acta. 1991;1097:238–40.
66. Morten KJ, Cooper JM, Brown GK, Lake BD, Pike D. Poulton J. a new point mutation associated with mitochondrial encephalomyopathy. Hum Mol Genet. 1993;2:2081–7.
67. Goto Y, Tsugane K, Tanabe Y, Nonaka I, Horai S. A new point mutation at nucleotide pair 3291 of the mitochondrial tRNA(Leu(UUR)) gene in a patient with mitochondrial myopathy, encephalopathy, lactic acidosis, and stroke-like episodes (MELAS). Biochem Biophys Res Commun. 1994;202:1624–30.
68. Sato W, Hayasaka K, Shoji Y, Takahashi T, Takada G, Saito M, Fukawa O, Wachi E. A mitochondrial tRNA(Leu)(UUR) mutation at 3,256 associated with mitochondrial myopathy, encephalopathy, lactic acidosis, and stroke-like episodes (MELAS). Biochem Mol Biol Int. 1994;33:1055–61.
69. Nishino I, Komatsu M, Kodama S, Horai S, Nonaka I, Goto Y. The 3260 mutation in mitochondrial DNA can cause mitochondrial myopathy, encephalopathy, lactic acidosis, and strokelike episodes (MELAS). Muscle Nerve. 1996;19:1603–4.
70. Hanna MG, Nelson IP, Morgan-Hughes JA, Wood NW. MELAS: a new disease associated mitochondrial DNA mutation and evidence for further genetic heterogeneity. J Neurol Neurosurg Psychiatry. 1998;65:512–7.
71. Taylor RW, Chinnery PF, Haldane F, Morris AA, Bindoff LA, Wilson J, Turnbull DM. MELAS associated with a mutation in the valine transfer RNA gene of mitochondrial DNA. Ann Neurol. 1996;40:459–62.
72. Tanji K, Kaufmann P, Naini AB, Lu J, Parsons TC, Wang D, Willey JZ, Shanske S, Hirano M, Bonilla E, Khandji A, DiMauro S, Rowland LP. A novel tRNA(Val) mitochondrial DNA mutation causing MELAS. J Neurol Sci. 2008;270:23–7.
73. Bataillard M, Chatzoglou E, Rumbach L, Sternberg D, Tournade A, Laforet P, Jardel C, Maisonobe T, Lombes A. Atypical MELAS syndrome associated with a new mitochondrial tRNA glutamine point mutation. Neurology. 2001;56:405–7.
74. Herrero-Martín MD, Ayuso T, Tuñón MT, Martín MA, Ruiz-Pesini E, Montoya JA. MELAS/MERRF phenotype associated with the mitochondrial DNA 5521G>A mutation. J Neurol Neurosurg Psychiatry. 2010;81:471–2.
75. Manfredi G, Schon EA, Bonilla E, Moraes CT, Shanske S, DiMauro S. Identification of a mutation in the mitochondrial tRNA(Cys) gene associated with mitochondrial encephalopathy. Hum Mutat. 1996;7:158–63.
76. Lindberg C, Moslemi AR, Oldfors A. MELAS syndrome in a patient with a point mutation in MTTS1. Acta Neurol Scand. 2008;117:128–32.
77. Calvaruso MA, Willemsen MA, Rodenburg RJ, van den Brand M, Smeitink JA, Nijtmans L. New mitochondrial tRNA HIS mutation in a family with lactic acidosis and stroke-like episodes (MELAS). Mitochondrion. 2011;11:778–82.
78. Abu-Amero KK, Al-Dhalaan H, Bohlega S, Hellani A, Taylor RW. A patient with typical clinical features of mitochondrial encephalopathy, lactic acidosis and stroke-like episodes (MELAS) but without an obvious genetic cause: a case report. J Med Case Rep. 2009;3:77.
79. Campos Y, Lorenzo G, Martin MA, Torregrosa A, del Hoyo P, Rubio JC, Garcia A, Arenas J. A mitochondrial tRNA(Lys) gene mutation (T8316C) in a patient with mitochondrial myopathy, lactic acidosis, and stroke-like episodes. Neuromuscul Disord. 2000;10:493–6.
80. Sakuta R, Honzawa S, Murakami N, Goto Y, Nagai T. Atypical MELAS associated with mitochondrial tRNA(Lys) gene A8296G mutation. Pediatr Neurol. 2002;27:397–400.
81. Malfatti E, Bugiani M, Invernizzi F, de Souza CF, Farina L, Carrara F, Lamantea E, Antozzi C,

Confalonieri P, Sanseverino MT, Giugliani R, Uziel G, Zeviani M. Novel mutations of ND genes in complex I deficiency associated with mitochondrial encephalopathy. Brain. 2007;130:1894–904.
82. Kirby DM, McFarland R, Ohtake A, Dunning C, Ryan MT, Wilson C, Ketteridge D, Turnbull DM, Thorburn DR, Taylor RW. Mutations of the mitochondrial ND1 gene as a cause of MELAS. J Med Genet. 2004;41:784–9.
83. Tam EW, Feigenbaum A, Addis JB, Blaser S, Mackay N, Al-Dosary M, Taylor RW, Ackerley C, Cameron JM. Robinson BH. A novel mitochondrial DNA mutation in COX1 leads to strokes, seizures, and lactic acidosis. Neuropediatrics. 2008;39:328–34.
84. Manfredi G, Schon EA, Moraes CT, Bonilla E, Berry GT, Sladky JT, DiMauro S. A new mutation associated with MELAS is located in a mitochondrial DNA polypeptide-coding gene. Neuromuscul Disord. 1995;5:391–8.
85. Santorelli FM, Tanji K, Kulikova R, Shanske S, Vilarinho L, Hays AP, DiMauro S. Identification of a novel mutation in the mtDNA ND5 gene associated with MELAS. Biochem Biophys Res Commun. 1997;238:326–8.
86. Liolitsa D, Rahman S, Benton S, Carr LJ, Hanna MG. Is the mitochondrial complex I ND5 gene a hotspot for MELAS causing mutations? Ann Neurol. 2003;53:128–32.
87. Naini AB, Lu J, Kaufmann P, Bernstein RA, Mancuso M, Bonilla E, Hirano M, DiMauro S. Novel mitochondrial DNA ND5 mutation in a patient with clinical features of MELAS and MERRF. Arch Neurol. 2005;62:473–6.
88. Crimi M, Galbiati S, Moroni I, Bordoni A, Perini MP, Lamantea E, Sciacco M, Zeviani M, Biunno I, Moggio M, Scarlato G, Comi GP. A missense mutation in the mitochondrial ND5 gene associated with a Leigh-MELAS overlap syndrome. Neurology. 2003;60:1857–61.
89. Corona P, Antozzi C, Carrara F, D'Incerti L, Lamantea E, Tiranti V, Zeviani M. A novel mtDNA mutation in the ND5 subunit of complex I in two MELAS patients. Ann Neurol. 2001;49:106–10.
90. McKenzie M, Liolitsa D, Akinshina N, Campanella M, Sisodiya S, Hargreaves I, Nirmalananthan N, Sweeney MG, Abou-Sleiman PM, Wood NW, Hanna MG, Duchen MR. Mitochondrial ND5 gene variation associated with encephalomyopathy and mitochondrial ATP consumption. J Biol Chem. 2007;282:36845–52.
91. Ravn K, Wibrand F, Hansen FJ, Horn N, Rosenberg T, Schwartz M. An mtDNA mutation, 14453G>A, in the NADH dehydrogenase subunit 6 associated with severe MELAS syndrome. Eur J Hum Genet. 2001;9:805–9.
92. De Coo IF, Renier WO, Ruitenbeek W, Ter Laak HJ, Bakker M, Schagger H, Van Oost BA, Smeets HJ. A 4-base pair deletion in the mitochondrial cytochrome b gene associated with parkinsonism/MELAS overlap syndrome. Ann Neurol. 1999;1999(45):130–3.
93. Emmanuele V, Sotiriou E, Rios PG, Ganesh J, Ichord R, Foley AR, Akman HO, DiMauro S. A novel mutation in the mitochondrial DNA cytochrome b gene (MTCYB) in a patient with mitochondrial encephalomyopathy, lactic acidosis, and strokelike episodes syndrome. J Child Neurol. 2013;28:236–42.
94. Manwaring N, Jones MM, Wang JJ, Rochtchina E, Howard C, Mitchell P, Sue CM. Population prevalence of the MELAS A3243G mutation. Mitochondrion. 2007;7(3):230–3.
95. Grady JP, Pickett SJ, Ng YS, Alston CL, Blakely EL, Hardy SA, Feeney CL, Bright AA, Schaefer AM, Gorman GS, McNally RJ, Taylor RW, Turnbull DM, McFarland R. mtDNA heteroplasmy level and copy number indicate disease burden in m.3243A>G mitochondrial disease. EMBO Mol Med. 2018;
96. Majamaa-Voltti KA, Winqvist S, Remes AM, Tolonen U, Pyhtinen J, Uimonen S, Kärppä M, Sorri M, Peuhkurinen K, Majamaa K. A 3-year clinical follow-up of adult patients with 3243A>G in mitochondrial DNA. Neurology. 2006;66:1470–5.
97. Malfatti E, Laforet P, Jardel C, Stojkovic T, Behin A, Eymard B, Lombes A, Benmalek A, Becane H-M, Berber N, Meune C, Duboc D, Wahbi K. High risk of severe cardiac adverse events in patients with mitochondrial m.3243A-G mutation. Neurology. 2013;80:100–5.
98. Barends M, Verschuren L, Morava E, Nesbitt V, Turnbull D, McFarland R. Causes of death in adults with mitochondrial disease. JIMD Rep. 2016;26:103–13.
99. Glover EI, Martin J, Maher A, Thornhill RE, Moran GR, Tarnopolsky MA. A randomized trial of coenzyme Q10 in mitochondrial disorders. Muscle Nerve. 2010;42:739–48.
100. Rodriguez MC, MacDonald JR, Mahoney DJ, Parise G, Beal MF, Tarnopolsky MA. Beneficial effects of creatine, CoQ10, and lipoic acid in mitochondrial disorders. Muscle Nerve. 2007;35:235–42.
101. Napolitano A, Salvetti S, Vista M, Lombardi V, Siciliano G, Giraldi C. Long-term treatment with idebenone and riboflavin in a patient with MELAS. Neurol Sci. 2000;21:S981–2.
102. Kaufmann P, Engelstad K, Wei Y, Jhung S, Sano MC, Shungu DC, Millar WS, Hong X, Gooch CL, Mao X, Pascual JM, Hirano M, Stacpoole PW, DiMauro S, De Vivo DC. Dichloroacetate causes toxic neuropathy in MELAS: a randomized, controlled clinical trial. Neurology. 2006;66(3):324–30.
103. Pfeffer G, Majamaa K, Turnbull DM, Thorburn D. Chinnery PFTreatment for mitochondrial disorders. Cochrane Database Syst Rev. 2012;4:CD004426.
104. Camp KM, Krotoski D, Parisi MA, Gwinn KA, Cohen BH, Cox CS, Enns GM, Falk MJ, Goldstein AC, Gopal-Srivastava R, Gorman GS, Hersh SP, Hirano M, Hoffman FA, Karaa A, MacLeod EL, McFarland R, Mohan C, Mulberg AE, Odenkirchen JC, Parikh S, Rutherford PJ, Suggs-Anderson SK, Tang WH, Vockley J, Wolfe LA, Yannicelli S, Yeske PE, Coates PM. Nutritional interventions in primary

mitochondrial disorders: developing an evidence base. Mol Genet Metab. 2016;119(3):187–206.
105. Koga Y, Akita Y, Nishioka J, Yatsuga S, Povalko N, Tanabe Y, Fujimoto S, Matsuishi T. L-arginine improves the symptoms of strokelike episodes in MELAS. Neurology. 2005;64(4):710–2.
106. Koga Y, Akita Y, Junko N, Yatsuga S, Povalko N, Fukiyama R, Ishii M, Matsuishi T. Endothelial dysfunction in MELAS improved by L-arginine supplementation. Neurology. 2006;66(11):1766–9.
107. El-Hattab AW, Hsu JW, Emrick LT, Wong LJ, Craigen WJ, Jahoor F, Scaglia F. Restoration of impaired nitric oxide production in MELAS syndrome with citrulline and arginine supplementation. Mol Genet Metab. 2012;105(4):607–14.
108. El-Hattab AW, Emrick LT, Hsu JW, Chanprasert S, Almannai M, Craigen WJ, Jahoor F, Scaglia F. Impaired nitric oxide production in children with MELAS syndrome and the effect of arginine and citrulline supplementation. Mol Genet Metab. 2016;117(4):407–12.
109. Ohsawa Y, Hagiwara H, Nishimatsu SI, Hirakawa A, Kamimura N, Ohtsubo H, Fukai Y, Murakami T, Koga Y, Goto YI, Ohta S, Sunada Y, KN01 Study Group. Taurine supplementation for prevention of stroke-like episodes in MELAS: a multicentre, open-label, 52-week phase III trial. J Neurol Neurosurg Psychiatry. 2018;
110. Koenig MK, Emrick L, Karaa A, Korson M, Scaglia F, Parikh S, Goldstein A. Recommendations for the management of strokelike episodes in patients with mitochondrial encephalomyopathy, lactic acidosis, and strokelike episodes. JAMA Neurol. 2016;73(5):591–4.
111. Rodan LH, Wells GD, Banks L, Thompson S, Schneiderman JE, Tein I. Cerebral hyperperfusion and decreased cerebrovascular reactivity correlate with neurologic disease severity in MELAS. Mitochondrion. 2015;22:66–74.
112. Fryer RH, Bain JM, De Vivo DC. Mitochondrial encephalomyopathy lactic acidosis and stroke-like episodes (MELAS): a case report and critical reappraisal of treatment options. Pediatr Neurol. 2016;56:59–61.
113. Primiano G, Vollono C, Dono F, Servidei S. Drug-resistant epilepsy in MELAS: safety and potential efficacy of lacosamide. Epilepsy Res. 2018;139:135–6.
114. Karaa A, Goldstein A. The spectrum of clinical presentation, diagnosis, and management of mitochondrial forms of diabetes. Pediatr Diabetes. 2015;16(1):1–9.
115. Scarpelli M, Zappini F, Filosto M, Russignan A, Tonin P, Tomelleri G. Mitochondrial sensorineural hearing loss: a retrospective study and a description of cochlear implantation in a MELAS patient. Genet Res Int. 2012;2012:287432.
116. Karaa A, Elsharkawi I, Clapp MA, Balcells C. Effects of mitochondrial disease/dysfunction on pregnancy: a retrospective study. Mitochondrion. 2018; https://doi.org/10.1016/j.mito.2018.06.007.
117. Kang E, Wu J, Gutierrez NM, Koski A, Tippner-Hedges R, Agaronyan K, Platero-Luengo A, Martinez-Redondo P, Ma H, Lee Y, Hayama T, Van Dyken C, Wang X, Luo S, Ahmed R, Li Y, Ji D, Kayali R, Cinnioglu C, Olson S, Jensen J, Battaglia D, Lee D, Wu D, Huang T, Wolf DP, Temiakov D, Belmonte JC, Amato P, Mitalipov S. Mitochondrial replacement in human oocytes carrying pathogenic mitochondrial DNA mutations. Nature. 2016;540(7632):270–5.

Myoclonus Epilepsy with Ragged-Red Fibers (MERRF)

Costanza Lamperti and Michelangelo Mancuso

Introduction

In 1921 Ramsay Hunt described six patients with a disorder resembling Friedreich ataxia characterized by ataxia, myoclonus, and epilepsy, which he called "dyssynergia cerebellaris myoclonica" [1]. Fifty years later, a family with mitochondrial myopathy, hallmarked by the presence of ragged-red fibers associated with familial myoclonic epilepsy, was first described [2].

The acronym MERRF (myoclonus epilepsy with ragged-red fibers) was coined later to describe two patients with a syndrome whose clinical and histological features became diagnostic criteria for the disease: myoclonus, generalized epilepsy, cerebellar ataxia, and myopathy with ragged-red fibers on muscle biopsy [3]. MERRF has two historical distinctions: it was the first human disease in which a maternal inheritance pattern was clearly demonstrated, thus suggesting a defect in mt-DNA, and it was also the first mitochondrial encephalomyopathy in which a molecular defect of mt-DNA was identified [4].

Finally the mt-DNA $tRNA^{Lys}$ mutation was reported as genetic cause of MERRF [5, 6].

MERRF syndrome (OMIM number #545000) was one of the three major, multisystem syndromes first classified as "mitochondrial encephalomyopathy" together with MELAS and Kearns-Sayre syndrome [7]. It is a worldwide disorder with no known ethnic predilection.

Three epidemiological studies in Northern European countries have estimated the prevalence of the m.8344A>G mutation, the variant primary cause for MERRF, in affected adulthood to be 0.2 (0.1–0.5) $\times 10^{-5}$ [8–11] and 0.5 $\times 10^{-5}$ in adults and at risk kids. Onset of clinical manifestations is in infancy, childhood, or adolescence [12]; being a degenerating disorder, its course gradually progresses over years: it is usually slow in affected adults, whereas in juveniles it may be rapid with a fatal outcome [13]. Symptoms and physical findings vary greatly between affected individuals in the same family and between different families. About 80% of patients have a family history of mitochondrial encephalomyopathy, although not always full-blown MERRF [14].

Maternal family members may be symptomatic, oligosymptomatic, or asymptomatic. The age of death has ranged from 7 to 79 years of age [14].

C. Lamperti
Division of Medical Genetics and Neurogenetics, IRCCS Foundation National Neurological Institute "C. Besta", Milan, Italy
e-mail: costanza.lamperti@istituto-besta.it

M. Mancuso (✉)
Department of Clinical and Experimental Medicine, Neurological Institute, University of Pisa, Pisa, Italy
e-mail: michelangelo.mancuso@unipi.it

M. Mancuso, T. Klopstock (eds.), *Diagnosis and Management of Mitochondrial Disorders*,
https://doi.org/10.1007/978-3-030-05517-2_6

Clinical Features

The disease is multisystem, involving different organs. Although the hallmark symptom is myoclonus epilepsy, frequent manifestations of the disease include sensorineural hearing loss, myopathy, muscle wasting, myalgia (exercise-induced or at rest), intellectual disability, psychiatric disorder or dementia, short stature, exercise intolerance, and optic atrophy. Peripheral neuropathy is not uncommon, being usually sensory-motor and contributing to the onset and progression of gait ataxia. Moreover, at least one case was reported with predominant motor symptoms, thus phenocopying Charcot-Marie-Tooth and Leigh disease [15].

Less common clinical signs (seen in <50% of the patients) include pigmentary retinopathy, pyramidal signs, ophthalmoplegia, and the appearance of multiple lipomas, particularly in the neck and upper trunk Fig. 1b.

In 2013, Mancuso and the Italian Network of the mitochondrial diseases studied 42 patients carrying the m.8344A>G mutation. The great majority did not have full-blown MERRF syndrome. Myoclonus was present in one of five patients, whereas myopathic signs and symptoms, generalized seizures, hearing loss, eyelid ptosis, and multiple lipomatosis represented the most common clinical features. Interestingly, myoclonus was more strictly associated with ataxia than generalized seizures in adult m.8344A>G subjects.

A German study from the multicentric registry of the German network for mitochondrial disorders mitoNET [16] studied the clinical phenotype of 34 patients with the m.8344A>G mutation. Mean age at symptom onset was 24.5 years ±10.9 (6–48 years) with adult onset in 75% of the patients. In this cohort, the canonical features seizures, myoclonus, cerebellar ataxia, and ragged-red fibers that are traditionally associated with MERRF occurred in only 61, 59, 70, and 63% of the patients, respectively. In contrast, other features such as hearing impairment were even more frequently present (72%). Other common features in the cohort were migraine (52%), psychiatric disorders (54%), respiratory dysfunction (45%), gastrointestinal symptoms (38%), dysarthria (36%), and dysphagia (35%).

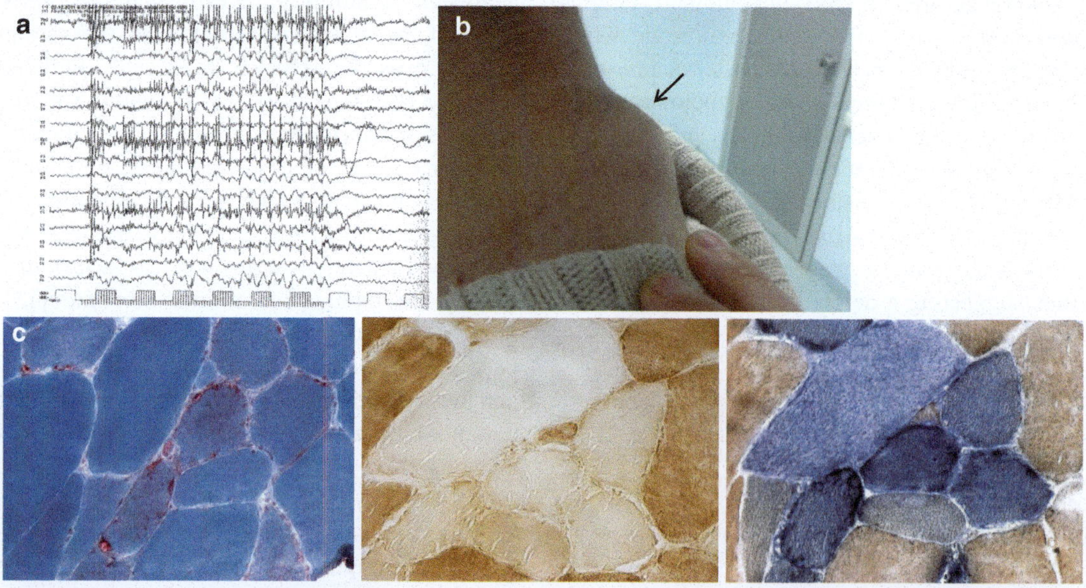

Fig. 1 (**a**) EEG of patient showing sharp/waives activity. (**b**) An example of lipoma positioned on the neck in a MERRF patient. (**c**) Histochemical images of a group of altered muscular fibers in a MERRF patient obtained with modified Gomori Trichrome stain (left), cytochrome oxydase (COX) staining (middle) and double COX-SDH reaction (right). Note the presence of ragged-red fibers, one big white fiber and some COX-deficient fibers

Cardiac involvement as cardiomyopathy and arrhythmias has been reported to be frequent in individuals with the m.8344A>G. In a study of 18 patients with this mutation, several had cardiac involvement (dilated cardiopathy, Wolff-Parkinson-White syndrome, incomplete left bundle branch block, left ventricular dysfunction and premature ventricular beats), and two died of heart failure [17].

An Italian study showed that cardiac involvement was observed in 53% of fifteen m.8344A>G MERRF patients, and a restrictive respiratory insufficiency requiring ventilatory support was observed in about half of the patients [13].

A few unusual clinical presentations, characterized by overlap symptoms between MERRF and MELAS, have been reported. One patient presented with parkinsonism without myoclonus, epilepsy, or ataxia [18], and a child presented with acute demyelination in the central and peripheral nervous system [19].

Other possible symptoms associated to MERRF are migraine, gastrointestinal dysmotility, vomiting, dysphagia, diabetes, and hypothyroidism [20]. Although respiratory failure is not so common, it should always been investigated because it could be the cause of death in this patients.

Finally, rare clinical features are of uncertain relationship to MERRF: dystonia, dyskinesia, spasmodic dysphonia (focal dystonia), cataract, arterial hypertension, pulmonary hypertension, chronic pancreatitis, aseptic pancreatitis, anemia, clubfeet, and psoriasis [20].

Laboratory Tests

The diagnosis is based on "canonical" clinical features (myoclonus, generalized epilepsy, ataxia), muscle biopsy finding of ragged-red fibers, and/or identification of an mtDNA pathogenic variant. Among serum screening patients with typical MERRF have elevated blood lactate and pyruvate at rest, both (abnormally) increasing excessively after moderate activity.

Blood leukocyte and urine sediment DNA should be screened for an mt-DNA point mutation to obviate the need for a costly and invasive muscle biopsy.

Electrocardiogram (ECG) often reveals preexcitation or partial cardiac conduction block demonstrating cardiomyopathy.

Electromyography (EMG) and nerve conduction velocity (NCV) studies are usually compatible with a predominantly myopathic pattern, except when motor peripheral neuropathy is clearly present. Typically, there are decreased amplitudes of compound muscle or nerve action potentials indicating axonal degeneration [21].

Electroencephalography (EEG) may show atypical generalized spike and wave discharges, with abnormal background slowing; focal epileptiform discharges may also be seen [22] (Fig. 1a). Somatosensory evoked responses may show giant cortical evoked responses [22].

Brain imaging with CT or MRI may be normal or may show basal ganglia calcification as well as cerebral and/or cerebellar atrophy [23, 24], cortical/subcortical atrophy, white matter abnormalities, periaqueductal lesions, cysts or vacuolated lesions, brainstem atrophy, and stroke-like lesions [24]. Neuronal loss and gliosis in the brain involve preferentially the dentate nucleus in the cerebellum, the inferior olivary nucleus, the red nucleus and the substantia nigra in the brain stem, and the thoracic nucleus of Clarke, the anterior and the posterior horns in the spinal cord. Demyelinization affects preferentially the superior cerebellar peduncles and the posterior columns and lateral spinocerebellar tracts of the spinal cord, whereas the pyramidal system is usually spared or mildly affected.

Phosphorus magnetic resonance spectroscopy may evidence a mitochondrial dysfunction by increased relative intracellular inorganic phosphate (Pi) concentration and decreased phosphocreatine to Pi ratio in gastrocnemius muscle [25] but not in the brain.

Mitochondrial enzyme activities can be measured in whole muscle homogenate or in isolated mitochondria and usually demonstrate multiple respiratory chain defects, particularly in complex IV [26]. Complex II is always preserved.

Histological examination of cytochrome c oxidase (COX) activity in skeletal muscle biopsies seems to be consistently decreased in individual muscle fibers. Ragged-red fibers on modified Gomori trichrome stain are the hallmark histological feature present in over 90% of MERRF patients [14] (Fig. 1c). Occasionally, RRFs may not be observed [27].

The succinate dehydrogenase stain (SDH) reveals hyperactive fibers darker than normal reaction and represents a more sensitive indicator of mitochondrial proliferation.

Ultrastructural studies may confirm the increased number of mitochondria, as well as morphologically abnormal mitochondria, which sometimes contain paracrystalline inclusions.

Differential Diagnosis

The clinical differential diagnosis of syndromes characterized by myoclonus epilepsy and ataxia includes Unverricht-Lundborg disease, Lafora body disease, neuronal ceroid lipofuscinosis, and sialidosis [28, 29] and degenerative cerebellar ataxia syndromes. Although genetic differential diagnosis may be reached with next-generation sequencing testing such as mt-DNA sequencing, phenotype-driven gene panel testing, whole exome sequencing, and whole genome sequencing, the identification of variants of uncertain significance may complicate diagnosis requiring biochemical and histologic approaches [20].

Genotype

MERRF syndrome is caused by pathogenic variants in mt-DNA and is transmitted by maternal inheritance. For all mutations, clinical expression depends on three factors: heteroplasmy, tissue distribution of mutant mitochondria, and the dependence of that tissue of mitochondrial activity (respiration, ATP production, oxidative stress). There is no clear correlation between the percentage of the prevalent mutation m.8344A>G in muscle and clinical severity [30]. In addition, it was observed that regional pathology in brain areas and in skeletal muscle is due to an increase of mt-DNA copy number and a high mutation percentage in these tissues [31].

The principal MERRF mutations affect highly conserved nucleotides in the MT-TK gene, coding for mt-tRNA^{Lys}, since it is clearly a hot spot for mutations causing MERRF [32].

The most frequent mutation, present in more than 80% of affected individuals with typical findings, is an A-to-G transition at nucleotide 8344 (m.8344A>G) in the T-Ψ-C loop of mt-tRNA^{Lys} [14, 30]. It is virtually always heteroplasmic, and its phenotypic threshold for determining typical MERRF is usually high or very high (i.e., about 60–90% of total mt-DNA), which suggests that this mutation is relatively benign [6].

In 1975 Karl Ekbom [33] described multiple lipomas in association with hereditary ataxia, photomyoclonus, and skeletal deformities in a family in which the 8344A>G mutation was later documented [34, 35]. These tumors varying in size from small subcutaneous nodules to disfiguring masses are usually located in the nape of the neck and in the shoulder area in MERRF patients [36, 37].

In an Italian retrospective analysis of over 42 carriers of the m.8344A>G, the large majority had not the four canonical features of MERRF, e.g., had not myoclonus or displayed myoclonus associated with cerebellar ataxia instead of epilepsy, and showed marked heterogeneity, reaching from asymptomatic to lethal multisystem diseases [38]. The authors suggested that the acronym MERRF could better be read as "myoclonic encephalomyopathy with ragged-red fibers." In 34 adult subjects with m.8344A>G in the German mitoNET registry, the association between myoclonus and ataxia was not significant, but a trend was observed ($p = 0.0699$) [16].

If the m.8344A>G variant is the most common variant causing the MERRF phenotype, three other MT-TK variants (m.8356T>C, m.8363G>A, and m.8361G>A) account for another approximately 10% of the pathogenic variants in individuals with MERRF [12]. Thus, 90% of the MERRF variants are located in the MT-TK gene.

The point mutation m.8356T>C, located in the T-Ψ-C loop in the MT-TK gene, was discovered simultaneously in an American family with typical MERRF [39] and in an Italian family with a MERRF/MELAS overlap syndrome [40]. Both families presented with hyperthyroidism, which is rather unusual in mitochondrial diseases. A third family was later reported from Japan: the proband had typical MERRF, but a maternal aunt had stroke-like episodes, another example of MERRF/MELAS overlap [41].

Mutation m.8363G>A is located in the aminoacyl acceptor stem of the putative cloverleaf (secondary) structure of mt-tRNA^{Lys} transcript. It was first identified in two unrelated American families with maternally inherited cardiomyopathy [32]. Additional signs included encephalomyopathy, neurosensory hearing loss, progressive external ophthalmoparesis, mental retardation, limb weakness, and peripheral neuropathy, variably affecting members of both families. Cerebellar symptoms were frequent, including ataxia, dysmetria, slurred speech, and gait instability. One proband had "horse collar" lipomas. The same mutation was later identified in two unrelated Japanese patients with typical MERRF, one of whom also had cardiomyopathy [42] (Fig. 2).

In a case of childhood-onset MERRF, a substitution m.8361G>A within the mt-tRNA^{Lys} gene

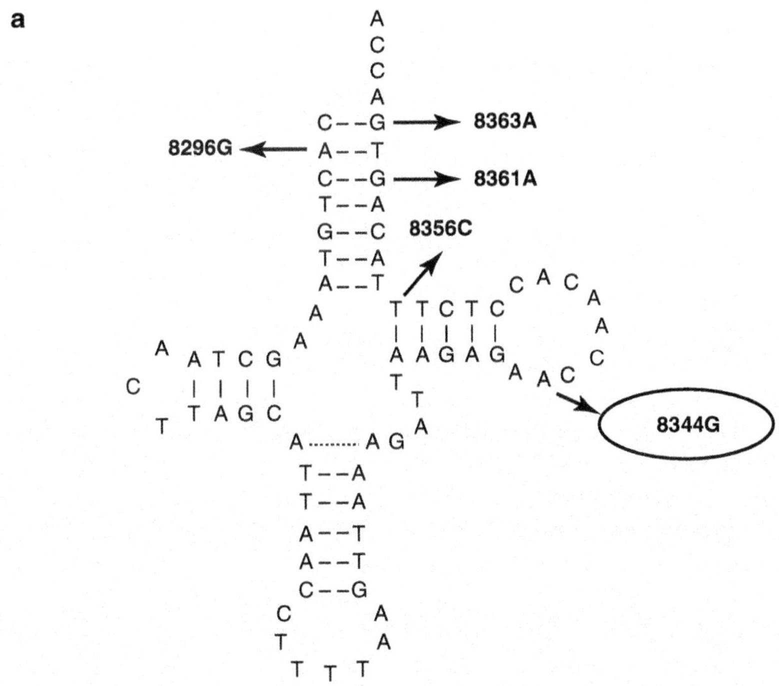

Fig. 2 (**a**) Cloverleaf structures of the human mt-tRNA^{Lys}. The arrows indicate the positions and the nucleotide changes associated to MERRF syndrome. In the circle the most common MERRF mutation m.8344A>G. (**b**) PCR-RFLP (restriction fragment length polymorphism) strategy. The MERRF mutation does not alter recognition sequences for commercially available restriction enzymes; hence the fragment of mtDNA containing the MERRF mutation m.8344A>G is amplified using a forward primer from position 8186 and a reverse mismatched primer (from 8386 to 8345) where two nucleotides close to the position 8344 are changed. The fragment amplified by PCR consists of 201 nucleotides (wt). If the m.8344A>G mutation is present, a *Bgl*I site is generated from nt 8344 to 8354 (GCCNNNNNGGC), and digestion with enzyme produces two fragments of 165 and 36 nucleotides, respectively (mut). In the black box, the guanosine in position 8344; asterisks show the modified nucleotides; triangle indicates the cut site of *Bgl*I enzyme. (**c**) Quantification of m.8344A>G mutation by PCR-RFLP analysis. The gel electrophoresis of DNA fragments amplified and digested by *Bgl*I enzyme performed in samples obtained from subjects belonging to a family with m.8344A>G mutation shows two different bands: the uncut fragment (201 bp) representing the wt molecules, and a shorter fragment (165 bp) resulting by *Bgl*I cut; the 36 bp fragment is not shown. The panel shows the PCR-RFLP analysis performed on DNA extracted from tissues of two MERRF patients and their unaffected mother. The proportion of mutant molecules versus wt (heteroplasmy) is calculated by densitometry and is reported. *M* muscle, *U* urinary sediment, *L* lymphocytes

Fig. 2 (continued)

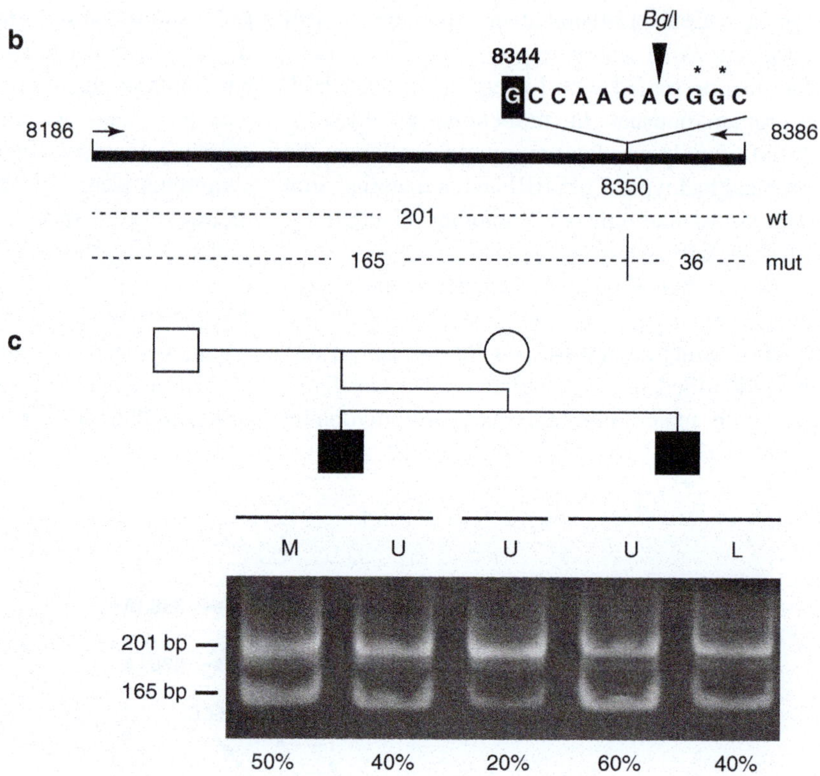

was identified as the cause of the disease. It was maternally inherited, heteroplasmic in all tissues tested, and correlated with mitochondrial dysfunction in individual muscle fibers. He developed seizures and myoclonus, followed by ataxia, cognitive impairment, and sensorineural hearing loss. Maternal relatives were oligosymptomatic [43].

Pathogenic variants in other genes have also been described in a subset of individuals affected by MERRF, listed in Table 1. Moreover, an overlap phenotype between MERRF and progressive external ophthalmoplegia [55] and MERRF and Leigh syndrome [15, 73] has been described.

A single patient with canonical MERRF symptoms and, in addition, peripheral neuropathy, dementia, and mild cerebral and severe cerebellar atrophy had no mutation in the $tRNA^{Lys}$ gene but multiple mtDNA deletions in the muscle, suggesting impairment in a nuclear gene product controlling mtDNA integrity, for instance, POLG1 [74]. Numerous variants in POLG1 can be associated with MERRF-like presentation. POLG1 syndromes have highly variable phenotypes, but myoclonic epilepsy is a prominent clinical feature in patients with mitochondrial recessive ataxia syndrome. This class of POLG1 patients has various designations in the literature: sensory ataxic neuropathy with mtDNA deletions; spinocerebellar ataxia with epilepsy; epilepsy, progressive myoclonic, with sensory ataxic neuropathy; epilepsy, progressive myoclonic; sensory ataxic neuropathy, dysarthria, and ophthalmoparesis; and myoclonic epilepsy, myopathy, and sensory ataxia [20].

Pathological Mechanism

It is unclear how the mitochondrial DNA point mutations cause the MERRF clinical phenotype. Studies on cybrids harboring the m.8344A>G or the m.8356T>C showed that high proportions of the mutation correlated with decreased protein synthesis and oxygen consumption and COX deficiency [75, 76].

The m.8344A>G-induced protein synthesis defects not only reduce oxygen consumption and

Table 1 List of variants reported in the literature or databases as "definitely pathogenic", "possibly/probably pathogenic" or "neutral" for MERRF phenotype

Gene	Mutation	Comments	References
List of variants reported in the literature or databases as "definitely pathogenic" for MERRF phenotype according to the modified Yarham Criteria [44, 45] *and to the 2017 Smith Gene-Disease Relationship criteria* [46]			
MT-TF	611G>A	MERRF	[47, 48]
MT-TH	12147G>A	MERRF/MELAS	[49, 50]
MT-TI	4279A>G	MERRF	[51]
	4284G>A	MERRF	[52, 53]
MT-TK	8344A>G	MERFF, MERRF/PEO, Pigmentary retinopathy	[54, 55]
	8356T>C	MERRF, MERRF/MELAS	[56]
	8361G>A	MERRF	[43]
	8363G>A	MERRF	[32, 42]
MT-TL1	3243A>G	MERRF, MERRF/KSS, MERRF/PEO, MERRF/MELAS	[56, 57]
	3255G>A	MERRF/KSS	[58]
	3271T>C	MERRF	[59]
	3291T>C	MERRF/KSS, MERRF/MELAS/KSS	[60, 61]
MT-TL2	12300G>A	MERRF/NARP. Variant also reported as a suppressor for the m.3243A>G variant when present at low levels	[62]
MT-TP	15967G>A	MERRF	[63, 64]
MT-TS1	7471_7472insC	MERRF. Variant commonly reported as 7472insC	[65]
	7512A>G	MERRF, MERRF/MELAS	[66]
MT-TS2	12207G>A	Incorrectly characterized as MERRF/MELAS in original publication but phenotype is consistent with Leigh disease	[67]
MT-TW	5521G>A	MERRF/MELAS	[68]
MT-ND3	10191T>C	Atypical MERRF lacking ragged-red and COX deficient fibers	[55]
POLG1		Numerous variants associated with MERRF-like presentation	http://polg.bmb.msu.edu/index.php

Gene	Mutation	Comments	References	Pathogenic/ Neutral
List of variants reported in the literature or in the databases as "possibly/probably pathogenic" or "neutral" for MERRF phenotype according to the modified Yarham Criteria [44, 45] *and to the 2017 Smith Gene-Disease Relationship criteria* [46]				
MT-TD	7543A>G	Myoclonic epilepsy, developmental delay without ragged-red fibers	[69]	Neutral
MT-TI	8296A>G	Multiple reports but normal cybrid studies	[20]	Neutral
MT-TT	15923A>G	MERRF	[70, 71]	Possibly pathogenic
MT-RNN2	2294A>G	MERRF	[55]	Neutral
	3145A>G	MERRF	[55]	Neutral
MT-ND5	13042G>A	MERRF/MELAS	[72]	Probably pathogenic

ATP synthesis but may also increase oxidative stress [77].

Both in cybrids and cultured myotubules [78] carrying high percentage of mutant mt-DNA the polypeptides containing more lysine residues were severely affected by the mutations, suggesting that the $tRNA^{Lys}$ mutation directly inhibits protein synthesis. Presence of aberrant mitochondrial protein was probably due to ribosomal frame-shifting. Decreased levels of $tRNA^{Lys}$ and aminoacylated $tRNA^{Lys}$ have been observed in cells harboring the m.8344A>G mutation [79]. The lack of modification in $tRNA^{Lys}$ leads to impaired protein synthesis [80]. Studies of in vitro transcribed $tRNA^{Lys}$ mutants showed that the mutations associated with MERRF had no effect on lysylation efficiency [81].

The mutation appeared to be functionally recessive, because only about 15% wild-type mt-DNA was needed to restore translation and COX activities to near normal levels.

Human cybrid cells harboring the classical MERRF mutation are more prone to undergo apoptosis then their wild-type counterpart when challenged with various apoptotic inducers, such as staurosporine. This may be mediated by perturbed calcium homeostasis induced by mitochondrial dysfunction [82].

Treatment and Management

As with other mitochondrial encephalomyopathies, there is no specific therapy for MERRF. Therefore patients are empirically treated with "cocktails" of vitamins and cofactors. Symptomatic management includes conventional therapy for all the organs involved in the disease.

Epilepsy is one of the hallmarks of the disease. There are no controlled studies to compare efficacy of different antiepileptic regimens: as with all mitochondrial diseases, valproate has to be used with caution [83].

The conventional anticonvulsant therapy may be used to treat the seizures of MERRF.

Myoclonus can be controlled with clonazepam (0.5–1 mg three times a day) or zonisamide although Levetiracetam is the first choice in MERRF [84].

The muscle weakness is another important symptom of the disease. Thus, there are no effective drugs for weakness; aerobic exercise is helpful in MERRF to improve any impaired motor function [85]. Lactic acidosis can be controlled by bicarbonate, which, however, has only a transient buffering effect and may exacerbate the cerebral symptoms. It is important to monitor the ventilator activity and the saturation. As others patients with muscle impairment, MERRF patients can present an important weakness in respiratory muscles, leading to respiratory failure. Moreover, the low level of O_2 and the high level of CO_2 could improve the epileptic status and the myoclonus. For these reasons, a saturimetry and the CPAP support have to be proposed to MERRF patients if the initial respiratory failure is present.

Heart involvements are not so frequent; nevertheless, standard pharmacologic therapy is allowed for cardiac symptoms.

In general anesthesia, drugs that lower seizure threshold should be avoided; anesthetic drugs such as succinylcholine and non-depolarizing muscle relaxants should also be avoided. Preparatory fasting could be risky in mitochondrial patients, and increment of lactic acid should be prevented avoiding hypoglycemia, hypoxia, and hypotension.

Actually no treatment for the genetic defect is available; therefore patients are empirically treated with "cocktails" of vitamins and cofactors, including idebenone at high dosage (150 mg × 3 daily), L-carnitine (1 g daily), and coenzyme Q10 (100–400 mg three times a day) [86]. Recently it has been shown that the C-terminal domain of human mt-$tRNA^{Leu}$ synthetase rescues the pathologic phenotype associated either with the m.3243A>G mutation in mt-$tRNA^{Leu}$ or with mutations in the mt-$tRNA^{Ile}$. Moreover, by using the human transmitochondrial cybrid model, it has been shown that the C-terminal was also able to improve the phenotype caused by the m.8344A>G mutation in mt-$tRNA^{Lys}$. The same rescuing ability was retained by two C term-derived short peptides, β30_31 and β32_33, which were effective toward both the m.8344A>G and the m.3243A>G mutations. In vitro these peptides bound with high affinity, wild-type, and mutant human mt-$tRNA^{Leu}$ and mt-$tRNA^{Lys}$ and stabilized mutant mt-$tRNA^{Leu}$ [87]. An important part of MERRF management is genetic counseling. Women with mt-DNA mutations associated with MERRF can give birth to children, but they are at risk of passing the mutation to their progeny. It is difficult to know the percentage of mutation present in fetus, and as a consequence it is difficult to predict if the baby will be affected or not. Nevertheless prenatal testing of the fetus may be useful; however, there are no significant published data about how confident the prediction of pathology is. Right now it is possible to do a preimplantation diagnosis of MERRF.

References

1. Hunt JR. Dyssynergia cerebellaris myoclonica-primary atrophy of the dentate system: a contribution to the pathology and symptomatology of the cerebellum. Brain. 1921;44:490–538.
2. Tsairis P, Engel W, Park P. Familial myoclonic epilepsy syndrome associated with skeletal muscle abnormalities. Neurology. 1973;23:408.
3. Fukuhara N, Tokigushi S, Shirakawa K, Tsubaki T. Myoclonus epilepsy associated with ragged-red fibers (mitochondrial abnormalities): disease entity or syndrome. Light and electron microscopic studies of two cases and review of the literature. J Neurol Sci. 1980;47:117–33.
4. Rosing HS, Hopkins LC, Wallace DC, Epstein CM, Weidenheim K. Maternally inherited mitochondrial myopathy and myoclonic epilepsy. Ann Neurol. 1985;17(3):228–37.
5. Yoneda M, Tanno Y, Horai S, Ozawa T, Miyatake T, Tsuji S. A common mitochondrial DNA mutation in the tRNA-lys of patients with myoclonus epilepsy associated with ragged-red fibers. Biochem Int. 1990;21:789–96.
6. Shoffner JM, Lott MT, Lezza A, Seigel P, Ballinger S, Wallace DC. Myoclonic epilepsy and ragged-red fiber disease (MERRF) is associated with a mitochondrial DNA tRNALys mutation. Cell. 1990;61:931–7.
7. DiMauro S, Bonilla E, Zeviani M, Nakagawa M, DeVivo DC. Mitochondrial myopathies. Ann Neurol. 1985;17:521–38.
8. Chinnery PF, Johnson MA, Wardell TM, et al. The epidemiology of pathogenic mitochondrial DNA mutations. Ann Neurol. 2000;48:188–93.
9. Darin N, Oldfors A, Moslemi AR, Holme E, Tulinius M. The incidence of mitochondrial encephalomyopathies in childhood: clinical features and morphological, biochemical, and DNA abnormalities. Ann Neurol. 2001;49:377–83.
10. Gorman GS, Schaefer AM, Ng Y, Gomez N, Blakely EL, Alston CL, Feeney C, Horvath R, Yu-Wai-Man P, Chinnery PF, Taylor RW, Turnbull DM, McFarland R. Prevalence of nuclear and mitochondrial DNA mutations related to adult mitochondrial disease. Ann Neurol. 2015;77:753–9.
11. Remes AM, Karppa M, Moilanen JS, et al. Epidemiology of the mitochondrial DNA 8344A>G mutation for the myoclonus epilepsy and ragged red fibres (MERRF) syndrome. J Neurol Neurosurg Psychiatry. 2003;74:1158–9.
12. DiMauro S, Hirano M. MERRF. In: Adam MP, Ardinger HH, Pagon RA, et al., eds. GeneReviews® [Internet]. Seattle, WA: University of Washington, Seattle; 2003:1993–2017. https://www.ncbi.nlm.nih.gov/books/NBK1520/. Jun 3 Updated 2015 Jan 29.
13. Catteruccia M, Sauchelli D, Della Marca G, Primiano G, Cuccagna C, Bernardo D, Leo M, Camporeale A, Sanna T, Cianfoni A, Servidei S. "Myo-cardiomyopathy" is commonly associated with the A8344G "MERRF" mutation. J Neurol. 2015;262:701–10.
14. Hirano M, DiMauro S. Clinical features of mitochondrial myopathies and encephalomyopathies. In: Lane RJ, editor. Handbook of muscle disease. New York: Marcel Dekker; 1996. p. 479–504.
15. Howell N, Kubacka I, Smith R, Frerman F, Parks JK, Parker WD Jr. Association of the mitochondrial 8344 MERRF mutation with maternally inherited spinocerebellar degeneration and Leigh disease. Neurology. 1996;46:219–22.
16. Altmann J, Büchner B, Nadaj-Pakleza A, Schäfer J, Jackson S, Lehmann D, Deschauer M, Kopajtich R, Lautenschläger R, Kuhn KA, Karle K, Schöls L, Schulz JB, Weis J, Prokisch H, Kornblum C, Claeys KG, Klopstock T. Expanded phenotypic spectrum of the m.8344A>G "MERRF" mutation: data from the German mitoNET registry. J Neurol. 2016;263(5):961–72.
17. Wahbi K, Larue S, Jardel C, et al. Cardiac involvement is frequent in patients with the m.8344A>G mutation of mitochondrial DNA. Neurology. 2010;74:674–7.
18. Horvath R, Kley RA, Lochmuller H, Vorgerd M. Parkinson syndrome, neuropathy, and myopathy caused by the mutation A8344G (MERRF) in tRNALys. Neurology. 2007;68:56–8.
19. Erol I, Alehan F, Horvath R, Schneiderat P, Talim B. Demyelinating disease of central and peripheral nervous systems associated with a A8344G mutation in tRNALys. Neuromuscul Disord. 2009;19:275–8.
20. Finsterer J, Zarrouk-Mahjoub S, Shoffner JM. MERRF classification: implications for diagnosis and clinical trials. Pediatr Neurol. 2018;80:8–23.
21. Chu CC, Huang CC, Fang W, Chu NS, Pang CY, Wei YH. Peripheral neuropathy in mitochondrial encephalomyopathies. Eur Neurol. 1997;37:110–5.
22. So N, Berkovic S, Andermann F, Kuziecky R, Gendron D, Quesney L. Myoclonus epilepsy and ragged-red fibres (MERRF) 2. Electrophysiological studies and comparison with other progressive myoclonus epilepsies. Brain. 1989;112:1261–76.
23. Berkovic SF, Carpenter S, Evans A, et al. Myoclonus epilepsy and ragged-red fibers (MERRF): a clinical,

pathological biochemical magnetic resonance spectrographic and positron emission tomographic study. Brain. 1989;112:1231–60.

24. Mancuso M, Orsucci D, Angelini C, Bertini E, Carelli V, Comi GP, Minetti C, Moggio M, Mongini T, Servidei S, Tonin P, Toscano A, Uziel G, Bruno C, Caldarazzo Ienco E, Filosto M, Lamperti C, Martinelli D, Moroni I, Musumeci O, Pegoraro E, Ronchi D, Santorelli FM, Sauchelli D, Scarpelli M, Sciacco M, Spinazzi M, Valentino ML, Vercelli L, Zeviani M, Siciliano G. Phenotypic heterogeneity of the 8344A>G mtDNA "MERRF" mutation. Neurology. 2013;80(22):2049–54.
25. Rahman S. Mitochondrial disease and epilepsy. Dev Med Child Neurol. 2012;54(5):397–406.
26. Lombes A, Mendell JR, Nakase H, et al. Myoclonic epilepsy and ragged-red fibers with cytochrome c oxidase deficiency: neuropathology, biochemistry, and molecular genetics. Ann Neurol. 1989;26:20–33.
27. Mancuso M, Petrozzi L, Filosto M, et al. MERRF syndrome without ragged-red fibers: the need for molecular diagnosis. Biochem Biophys Res Commun. 2007;354:1058–60.
28. Andermann F, Berkovic S, Carpenter S, Andermann E. The Ramsay Hunt syndrome is no longer a useful diagnostic category. Mov Disord. 1989;4:13–7.
29. Marsden C, Obeso J. Viewpoints on the Ramsay Hunt syndrome. The Ramsay Hunt syndrome is a useful clinical entity. Mov Disord. 1989;4:6–12.
30. Silvestri G, Ciafaloni E, Santorelli F, et al. Clinical features associated with the A->G transition at nucleotide 8344 of mtDNA ("MERRF" mutation). Neurology. 1993;43:1200–6.
31. Brinckmann A, Weiss C, Wilbert F, et al. Regionalized pathology correlates with augmentation of mtDNA copy numbers in a patient with myoclonic epilepsy with ragged-red fibers (MERRF-syndrome). PLoS One. 2010;5(10):e13513.
32. Santorelli FM, Mak S-C, El-Schahawi M, et al. Maternally inherited cardiomyopathy and hearing loss associated with a novel mutation in the mitochondrial DNA tRNALys gene (G8363A). Am J Hum Genet. 1996;58:933–9.
33. Ekbom K. Hereditary ataxia, photomyoclonus, skeletal deformities and lipoma. Acta Neurol Scand. 1975;51:393–404.
34. Berkovic S, Shoubridge E, Andermann F, Carpenter S. Clinical spectrum of mitochondrial DNA mutations at base pair 8344. Lancet. 1991;338:457.
35. Traff J, Holme E, Nilsson BY. Ekbom's syndrome of photomyoclonus, cerebellar ataxia and cervical lipoma is associated with tRNALys A8344G mutation in mitochondrial DNA. Acta Neurol Scand. 1995;92:394–7.
36. Austin SA, Vriesendorp FJ, Thandroyen FT, Hecht JT, Jones OT, Johns DR. Expanding phenotype of the 8334 transfer tRNA lysine mitochondrial DNA mutation. Neurology. 1998;51:1447–50.
37. Larsson NG, Tulinius MH, Holme E, et al. Segregation and manifestations of the mtDNA tRNALys A->G(8344) mutation of myoclonus epilepsy and ragged-red fibers (MERRF) syndrome. Am J Hum Genet. 1992;51:1201–12.
38. Mancuso M, Orsucci D, Angelini C, et al. Myoclonus in mitochondrial disorders. Mov Disord. 2014;29(6):722–8.
39. Silvestri G, Moraes CT, Shanske S, Oh S, DiMauro S. A new mtDNA mutation in the tRNALys gene associated with myoclonic epilepsy and ragged-red fibers (MERRF). Am J Hum Genet. 1992;51:1213–7.
40. Zeviani M, Muntoni F, Savarese N, et al. A MERRF/MELAS overlap syndrome associated with a new point mutation in the mitochondrial DNA tRNALys gene. Eur J Hum Genet. 1992;1:80–7.
41. Sano M, Ozawa M, Shiota S, Momose Y, Uchigata M, Goto Y. The T-C (8356) mitochondrial DNA mutation in a Japanese family. J Neurol. 1996;243:441–4.
42. Ozawa M, Nishino I, Horai S, Nonaka I, Goto YI. Myoclonus epilepsy associated with ragged-red fibers: a G-to-A mutation at nucleotide pair 8363 in mitochondrial tRNA(lys) in two families. Muscle Nerve. 1997;20:271–8.
43. Rossmanith W, Raffelsberger T, Roka J, et al. The expanding mutational spectrum of MERRF substitution G8361 in the mitochondrial tRNALys gene. Ann Neurol. 2003;54:820–3.
44. Gonzalez-Vioque E, Bornstein B, Gallardo ME, Fernandez-Moreno MA, Garesse R. The pathogenicity scoring system for mitochondrial tRNA mutations revisited. Mol Genet Genomic Med. 2014;2:107–14.
45. Yarham JW, Al-Dosary M, Blakely EL, et al. A comparative analysis approach to determining the pathogenicity of mitochondrial tRNA mutations. Hum Mutat. 2011;32:1319–25.
46. Smith ED, Radtke K, Rossi M, et al. Classification of genes: standardized clinical validity assessment of gene-disease associations aids diagnostic exome analysis and reclassifications. Hum Mutat. 2017;38:600–8.
47. Mancuso M, Filosto M, Mootha VK, et al. A novel mitochondrial tRNAPhe mutation causes MERRF syndrome. Neurology. 2004;62(11):2119–21.
48. Ling J, Roy H, Qin D, et al. Pathogenic mechanism of a human mitochondrial tRNAPhe mutation associated with myoclonic epilepsy with ragged red fibers syndrome. Proc Natl Acad Sci U S A. 2007;104:15299–304.
49. Melone MA, Tessa A, Petrini S, et al. Revelation of a new mitochondrial DNA mutation (G12147A) in a MELAS/MERRF phenotype. Arch Neurol. 2004;61(2):269–72.
50. Taylor RW, Schaefer AM, McDonnell MT, et al. Catastrophic presentation of mitochondrial disease due to a mutation in the tRNA(His) gene. Neurology. 2004;62:1420–3.
51. Zsurka G, Becker F, Heinen M, et al. Mutation in the mitochondrial tRNA(Ile) gene causes progressive myoclonus epilepsy. Seizure. 2013;22:483–6.
52. Hahn A, Schänzer A, Neubauer BA, Gizewski E, Ahting U, Rolinski B. MERRF-like phenotype asso-

ciated with a rare mitochondrial tRNA-Ile mutation (m.4284 G>A). Neuropediatrics. 2011;42(4):148–51.
53. Corona P, Lamantea E, Greco M, et al. Novel heteroplasmic mtDNA mutation in a family with heterogeneous clinical presentations. Ann Neurol. 2002;51:118–22.
54. Isashiki Y, Nakagawa M, Ohba N, et al. Retinal manifestations in mitochondrial diseases associated with mitochondrial DNA mutation. Acta Ophthalmol Scand. 1998;76:6–13.
55. Choi BO, Hwang JH, Cho EM, et al. Mutational analysis of whole mitochondrial DNA in patients with MELAS and MERRF diseases. Exp Mol Med. 2010;42:446–55.
56. Nakamura M, Yabe I, Sudo A, et al. MERRF/MELAS overlap syndrome: a double pathogenic mutation in mitochondrial tRNA genes. J Med Genet. 2010;47(10):659–64.
57. Brackmann F, Abicht A, Ahting U, Schroder R, Trollmann R. Classical MERRF phenotype associated with mitochondrial tRNA(Leu) (m.3243A>G) mutation. Eur J Pediatr. 2012;171(5):859–62.
58. Nishigaki Y, Tadesse S, Bonilla E, et al. A novel mitochondrial tRNALeu(UUR) mutation in a patient with features of MERRF and Kearns-Sayre syndrome. Neuromuscul Disord. 2003;13:334–40.
59. Tokunaga M, Mita S, Sakuta R, Nonaka I, Araki S. Increased mitochondrial DNA in blood vessels and ragged-red fibers in mitochondrial myopathy, encephalopathy, lactic acidosis, and stroke-like episodes (MELAS). Ann Neurol. 1993;33:275–80.
60. Emmanuele V, Silvers DS, Sotiriou E, Tanji K, DiMauro S, Hirano M. MERRF and Kearns-Sayre overlap syndrome due to the mitochondrial DNA m.3291T>C mutation. Muscle Nerve. 2011;44(3):448–51.
61. Liu K, Zhao H, Ji K, Yan C. MERRF/MELAS overlap syndrome due to the m.3291T>C mutation. Metab Brain Dis. 2014;29(1):139–44.
62. Martín-Jiménez R, Martín-Hernández E, Cabello A, et al. Clinical and cellular consequences of the mutation m.12300G>A in the mitochondrial tRNA(Leu(CUN)) gene. Mitochondrion. 2012;12(2):288–93.
63. Murphy JL, Ratnaike TE, Shang E, et al. Cytochrome c oxidase intermediate fibres: importance in understanding the pathogenesis and treatment of mitochondrial myopathy. Neuromuscul Disord. 2012;22:690–8.
64. Blakely EL, Trip SA, Swalwell H, et al. A new mitochondrial transfer RNAPro gene mutation associated with myoclonic epilepsy with ragged-red fibers and other neurological features. Arch Neurol. 2009;66:399–402.
65. Tiranti V, Chariot P, Carella F, et al. Maternally inherited hearing loss ataxia and myoclonus associated with a novel point mutation in mitochondrial tRNASer(UCN) gene. Hum Mol Genet. 1995;4:1421–7.
66. Nakamura M, Nakano S, Goto Y, et al. A novel point mutation in the mitochondrial tRNA(Ser(UCN)) gene detected in a family with MERRF/MELAS overlap syndrome. Biochem Biophys Res Commun. 1995;214(1):86–93.
67. Wong LJ, Yim D, Bai RK, et al. A novel mutation in the mitochondrial tRNA(Ser(AGY)) gene associated with mitochondrial myopathy, encephalopathy, and complex I deficiency. J Med Genet. 2006;43:e46.
68. Herrero-Martin MD, Ayuso T, Tunon MT, Martin MA, Ruiz-Pesini E, Montoya J. A MELAS/MERRF phenotype associated with the mitochondrial DNA 5521G>A mutation. J Neurol Neurosurg Psychiatry. 2010;81:471–2.
69. Shtilbans A, El-Schahawi M, Malkin E, Shanske S, Musumeci O, DiMauro S. A novel mutation in the mitochondrial DNA transfer ribonucleic acid Asp gene in a child with myoclonic epilepsy and psychomotor regression. J Child Neurol. 1999;14:610–3.
70. Del Mar O'CM, Emperador S, et al. New mitochondrial DNA mutations in tRNA associated with three severe encephalopamyopathic phenotypes: neonatal, infantile, and childhood onset. Neurogenetics. 2012;13:245–50.
71. Yoon KL, Ernst SG, Rasmussen C, Dooling EC, Aprille JR. Mitochondrial disorder associated with newborn cardiopulmonary arrest. Pediatr Res. 1993;33:433–40.
72. Naini AB, Lu J, Kaufmann P, et al. Novel mitochondrial DNA ND5 mutation in a patient with clinical features of MELAS and MERRF. Arch Neurol. 2005;62(3):473–6.
73. Shtilbans A, Shanske S, Goodman S, et al. G8363A mutation in the mitochondrial DNA transfer ribonucleic acidLys gene: another cause of Leigh syndrome. J Child Neurol. 2000;15:759–61.
74. Blumenthal DT, Shanske S, Schochet SS, et al. Myoclonus epilepsy with ragged red fibers and multiple mtDNA deletions. Neurology. 1998;50(2):524–5.
75. Chomyn A, Meola G, Bresolin N, Lai ST, Scarlato G, Attardi G. In vitro genetic transfer of protein synthesis and respiration defects to mitochondrial DNA-less cells with myopathy-patient mitochondria. Mol Cell Biol. 1991;11:2236–44.
76. Masucci JP, Davidson M, Koga Y, Schon EA, King MP. In vitro analysis of mutations causing myoclonus epilepsy with ragged-red fibers in the mitochondrial tRNALys gene: two genotypes produce similar phenotypes. Mol Cell Biol. 1995;15:2872–81.
77. Wu SB, Ma YS, Wu YT, Chen YC, Wei YH. Mitochondrial DNA mutation-elicited oxidative stress, oxidative damage, and altered gene expression in cultured cells of patients with MERRF syndrome. Mol Neurobiol. 2010;41:256–66.
78. Boulet L, Karpati G, Shoubridge EA. Distribution and threshold expression of the tRNA mutation in skeletal muscle of patients with myoclonic epilepsy and ragged-red fibers (MERRF). Am J Hum Genet. 1992;51:1187–200.
79. Enriquez JA, Chomyn A, Attardi G. MtDNA mutation in MERRF syndrome causes defective aminoacyla-

tion of tRNA(Lys) and premature translation termination. Nat Genet. 1995;10(1):47–55.
80. Yasukawa T, Suzuki T, Ishii N, Ohta S, Watanabe K. Wobble modification defect in tRNA disturbs codon-anticodon interaction in a mitochondrial disease. EMBO J. 2001;20(17):4794–802.
81. Sissler M, Helm M, Frugier M, Giege R, Florentz C. Aminoacylation properties of pathology-related human mitochondrial tRNA(Lys) variants. RNA. 2004;10(5):841–53.
82. Rommelaere G, Michel S, Malaisse J, Charlier S, Arnould T, Renard P. Hypersensitivity of A8344G MERRF mutated cybrid cells to staurosporine-induced cell death is mediated by calcium-dependent activation of calpains. Int J Biochem Cell Biol. 2012;44(1):139–49.
83. DiMauro S, Hirano M, Schon EA. Mitochondrial encephalomyopathies: therapeutic approaches. Neurol Sci. 2000;21:S901–8.
84. Crest C, Dupont S, Leguern E, Adam C, Baulac M. Levetiracetam in progressive myoclonic epilepsy: an exploratory study in 9 patients. Neurology. 2004;62(4):640–3.
85. Taivassalo T, Haller RG. Implications of exercise training in mtDNA defects--use it or lose it. Biochim Biophys Acta. 2004;1659(2–3):221–31.
86. Farge G, Pham XH, Holmlund T, et al. The accessory subunit B of DNA polymerase gamma is required required for mitochondrial replisome function. NucleicAcids Res. 2007;35:902–11.
87. Perli E, Fiorillo A, Giordano C, Pisano A, Montanari A, Grazioli P, Campese AF, Di Micco P, Tuppen HA, Genovese I, Poser E, Preziuso C, Taylor RW, Morea V, Colotti G, d'Amati G. Short peptides from leucyl-tRNA synthetase rescue disease-causing mitochondrial tRNA point mutations. Hum Mol Genet. 2016;25(5):903–15.

Diseases of DNA Polymerase Gamma

Omar Hikmat, Pirjo Isohanni, Anu Suomalainen, and Laurence A. Bindoff

Introduction

Polymerase gamma (Polγ) is the DNA-dependent DNA polymerase responsible for replicating mitochondrial DNA. The enzyme is a trimer and comprises one catalytic subunit (POLG), which contains the polymerase activity together with proofreading exonuclease activity, and two accessory subunits (POLG2) that promote DNA binding and processivity. Replication of mtDNA requires several additional proteins: in vitro studies have shown that the minimal replication machinery consists of the helicase Twinkle, mitochondrial RNA polymerase and single-stranded binding protein [1], but others may be required in vivo [2]. Mutations in *POLG* are one of the most common causes of mitochondrial disease and responsible for a wide range of phenotypes. Mutations in *POLG2* are rare. Disease caused by mutations in Twinkle gives a similar spectrum of disease to those caused by POLG and we will discuss them together where this is appropriate.

At the molecular level, mutations in *POLG* cause damage to mtDNA, but the type of damage appears to depend on the tissue involved: for example in neurons, studies have shown that there is depletion of mtDNA and that damage, in the form of point mutations and deletions, accumulates over time [3]. In liver, mtDNA depletion occurs, while in skeletal muscle mtDNA deletions are the major genetic defect [4].

The Clinical Picture

POLG-related disease can affect multiple-organ systems, including the central and peripheral nervous systems, skeletal muscle, liver, endocrine glands and gut [5, 6], or apparently arise in a

O. Hikmat
Department of Pediatrics, Haukeland University Hospital, Bergen, Norway

Department of Clinical Medicine (K1), University of Bergen, Bergen, Norway

P. Isohanni
Department of Child Neurology, Children's Hospital, University of Helsinki and Helsinki University Hospital, Helsinki, Finland

Research Programs Unit, Molecular Neurology, Biomedicum Helsinki, University of Helsinki, Helsinki, Finland

A. Suomalainen
Research Programs Unit, Molecular Neurology, Biomedicum Helsinki, University of Helsinki, Helsinki, Finland

Neuroscience Center, University of Helsinki, Helsinki, Finland

L. A. Bindoff (✉)
Department of Clinical Medicine (K1), University of Bergen, Bergen, Norway

Department of Neurology, Haukeland University Hospital, Bergen, Norway
e-mail: laurence.bindoff@nevro.uib.no

M. Mancuso, T. Klopstock (eds.), *Diagnosis and Management of Mitochondrial Disorders*,
https://doi.org/10.1007/978-3-030-05517-2_7

single tissue, e.g. skeletal muscle (progressive external ophthalmoplegia) [7]. Describing the range of phenotypes is an ongoing process and we believe that the clinical manifestations form a continuum rather than well-defined and distinct syndromes. Onset of disease ranges from infancy to late adulthood and it is clear that the age at which the disease starts plays a major role in both the type of clinical manifestation and outcome of POLG-related disease [8–10]. To facilitate discussion and recognition of POLG-related disease, we will describe the spectrum of phenotypes according to the age of onset highlighting the earlier nomenclature as appropriate. We would reiterate that the plethora of terminologies in current usage does more to confuse the field than it helps clarify disease aetiology.

Early-Onset Disease

The early-onset phenotypes, i.e. those presenting from birth to adolescence, are among the most severe and dramatic in the POLG-related disease spectrum. These diseases often affect brain and liver, but can affect multiple other tissues, and are associated with a high morbidity and mortality [11]. The phenotypes have been named myocerebrohepatopathy spectrum disorder (MCHS) and Alpers-Huttenlocher syndrome (AHS). The former is less common and the essential difference between them is the lack of epilepsy in MCHS.

The earliest form of POLG-related disease frequently manifests between the neonatal period and 3 years of age, and the disease is characterised by the triad of myopathy (or hypotonia), developmental delay and/or encephalopathy and liver dysfunction. Other clinical features include cataract, optic atrophy, faltering growth and renal tubular acidosis [11, 12]. Seizures are not a recognised feature of this early phenotype. It is necessary to perform a full sequence analysis of the entire *POLG* gene because the common founder mutations (c.1399G>A, p.Ala467Thr and c.2243G>C, p.Trp748Ser) are rarely associated with this phenotype.

The other major early-onset phenotype is characterised by progressive encephalopathy with psychomotor regression, refractory epilepsy and characteristic liver disease [6, 13, 14]. This disease was first recognised in 1931 before its genetic basis was clarified and named Alpers syndrome, based on the typical brain pathology. Subsequently, when the association with liver involvement was recognised it was called Alpers-Huttenlocher syndrome (AHS) (OMIM # 203700) [15].

The link to polymerase gamma was made in 1999 [16] and pathogenic *POLG* mutations were first reported in 2004 [17]. AHS is the most frequently reported phenotype in infants and early childhood [12] and one of the most severe forms in the *POLG*-related disease spectrum. AHS presents most frequently during infancy, typically around 1 year of age, thus overlapping with MCHS [11], although adolescent and early adult onset has also been reported [18]. Patients with later onset are usually asymptomatic at birth and the majority develop normally prior to disease onset. A prodromal phase with mild development delay, hypotonia and flattening growth may occur and an infectious illness may precede the disease onset.

Refractory epilepsy is a major clinical feature of AHS and is present in the vast majority of the patients early in the disease [11]. Focal seizures, commonly evolving into bilateral convulsive seizures, are the most common seizure types with epileptiform discharges predominantly occurring over the occipital regions, at least initially [11, 19, 20]. The characteristic manifestation of occipital lobe involvement with visual hallucination, vomiting and headache is less clearly delineated in young children than older children and adults. The majority of the patients develop myoclonic seizures and episodes of epilepsia partialis continua (EPC) and/or generalised status epilepticus (SE). Patients with AHS may also present with refractory SE from which they might never recover [6, 11, 19, 21]. Other major predominant clinical features are faltering growth, progressive regression of psychomotor skills and hypotonia [11, 22].

Patients with AHS have epileptic encephalopathy and may develop episodes of acute exacerbation previously called stroke-like episodes

(SLEs). These episodes are characterised by acute or subacute neurological dysfunction and may be associated with EPC. The aetiology of these episodes is neuronal dysfunction leading to damage, not vascular occlusion. In the older age group, prodromal symptoms such as migraine-like headaches, visual disturbance and mental changes may occur. Clinically, such episodes are less often reported in children compared with adults, but radiological evidence of cortical lesions is common in both [3, 11].

Hepatic involvement is a major feature of the early-onset POLG disease and may progress rapidly to end-stage liver failure; however, affected children with normal, mild and transient abnormalities of liver function are well recognised [11, 23, 24]. Liver failure can be triggered by sodium valproate, and can occur spontaneously without the exposure to this drug [9, 25]. Recovery after transient liver failure and after the discontinuation of sodium valproate has been documented [20]. Nevertheless, sodium valproate clearly accelerates the development of liver failure in patients with *POLG* mutations and its use is absolutely contraindicated.

In addition to the above, patients in this age group may present with other phenotypes including a syndrome resembling mitochondrial neurogastrointestinal encephalopathy (MNGIE-like phenotype). These children have predominantly gastrointestinal symptoms including severe dysmotility, failure to thrive, vomiting, abdominal pain, cachexia and neurological symptoms including encephalopathy [11]. A Leigh-like phenotype has also been described [26] and some present with ataxia without epilepsy or evidence of hepatic involvement (author's personal unpublished data) similar to the adolescent/adult form.

Early-onset disease is in general associated with high mortality with the main causes of death being liver failure, sepsis and status epilepticus. A recent study of 27 patients with bi-allelic *POLG* mutations and age of onset <12 years showed that the median survival time of patients with disease onset ≤12 months was 3.6 months (range 0.5–181) compared to 10 months (range 1.4–82) for those with disease onset >12 months [11].

Adolescent and Young Adult Onset Disease

Mitochondrial recessive ataxia syndrome (MIRAS) and mitochondrial spinocerebellar ataxia with epilepsy (MSCAE) describe similar conditions differing only in the presence of epilepsy. They are the same as myoclonic epilepsy myopathy sensory ataxia (MEMSA) and overlap with sensory ataxic neuropathy, dysarthria, and ophthalmoparesis (SANDO), also called ataxia neuropathy spectrum syndrome (ANS).

This form of POLG-related disease manifests a combination of central and peripheral nervous system involvement and while the balance between these can vary the crucial element appears to be the presence or absence of epilepsy. Almost all of the patients develop ataxia that is usually a combination of central, i.e. cerebellar dysfunction, and sensory involvement particularly posterior column involvement and a peripheral neuropathy. Patients in this age group will also develop hepatic necrosis if exposed to sodium valproate or spontaneously particularly in the terminal phases of the disease. Many develop epilepsy and encephalopathic episodes that mimic stroke (see above). There is therefore much overlap with the disease presenting earlier.

The phenotype comprising epilepsy and ataxia is one of the major forms of adolescent POLG-related disease. Seizures can be the first manifestation and presentation in status epilepticus is not uncommon. Ataxia, which is combined central and sensory and an axonal/demyelinating peripheral neuropathy, either is present at onset or develops thereafter. Myopathy and, depending on age, ophthalmoplegia develop if the patient survives [8, 13, 19]. Seizure semiology in this and the early-onset disease is similar; focal seizures, commonly evolving into bilateral convulsive seizures, are the most common seizure types; however myoclonic seizures, epilepsia partialis continua and generalised SE are frequently reported [27]. Occipital lobe features are common and may include simple flickering, coloured light, visual hallucinations, scotomata, hemianopia, amaurosis, nystagmus and ocular clonus [8, 9, 28]. Episodes of encephalopathy leading to cerebral damage, previously called SLEs, are more readily detected in these patients compared with early-onset disease [3]. Headache and vomiting, resembling migraine with aura, occur and may precede the episodes. Hepatic involvement including liver failure is also a feature and can be triggered by usage of sodium valproate [9, 29].

A later presentation (i.e. adult) with predominant ataxia and neuropathy is associated with prolonged survival. In this group, patients also develop cognitive decline and psychiatric symptoms; ophthalmoplegia is more often a late feature and predominant myopathy rare [10, 24, 30]. This phenotype is the most common form (MIRAS) in Finland. That seizures and hepatic involvement also occur reinforces the point that these conditions are part of a continuum rather than distinct syndromes [6, 13].

Interestingly, epilepsy occurs more frequently in some populations [31] than others [8]. In the Norwegian population, epilepsy is the presenting symptom in about 65% of patients [19]. In Finland, the most common manifestation is with peripheral neuropathy and ataxia that are initially sensory but later also cerebellar in origin.

Both MELAS-like [32] and MNGIE-like phenotypes have been reported [33] in adolescent and adult-onset disease. Again, it is worth reiterating that the SLEs are not vascular [3] but encephalopathic in origin.

Late-Onset Disease

The major clinical features in this age group are progressive external ophthalmoplegia (PEO), myopathy, peripheral neuropathy and ataxia.

Mutations in *POLG* can give PEO that shows either autosomal dominant or recessive inheritance [7]. Affected individuals suffer from progressive weakness of the extraocular muscles leading to unilateral or bilateral ptosis and loss of eye movement both in the vertical and horizontal directions. Systemic involvement such as ataxia, peripheral neuropathy and generalised myopathy occurs more frequently in autosomal recessive progressive external ophthalmoplegia (arPEO) than the autosomal dominant form (adPEO) [7, 13, 34–37]. Other features may include sensorineural hearing loss [24], parkinsonism [30, 38], premature menopause [30, 34], male infertility [39], cataract [30] and depression [30]. Although reported, diabetes mellitus [24] and cardiomyopathy [40] are not typical features.

Diseases Caused by Mutations in Twinkle

The clinical phenotypes caused by mutations in the gene encoding Twinkle, the replicative mtDNA helicase, mimic those caused by *POLG*. An adult-onset, pure mitochondrial myopathy with progressive external ophthalmoplegia is a typical manifestation of dominant Twinkle mutations [41–43], but ataxia and peripheral neuropathy can also occur [44]. The recessive form of Twinkle disease manifests as infantile-onset spinocerebellar ataxia, IOSCA, a severe, progressive neurodegenerative disorder characterised by infantile-onset ataxia and athetosis. Subsequently, ophthalmoplegia and sensorineural hearing impairment develop in childhood, together with loss of ambulation and deafness: In adolescence, the syndrome is characterised by sensory axonal neuropathy, optic atrophy and female hypogonadotropic hypogonadism. Most IOSCA patients develop epilepsy: this is similar to that seen in POLG-related disease and it is often refractory and may lead to fatal encephalopathy with epilepsia partialis continua and status epilepticus [45–47]. More severe [48, 49] and milder phenotypes have been reported including Perrault syndrome (sensorineural hearing impairment and ovarian dysfunction) accompanied by neurological involvement [50].

Diagnosis

Clinical Awareness

The confirmation or exclusion of *POLG* disease is a major clinical challenge particularly in infants. A single clinical feature or diagnostic criterion is rarely sufficient to establish the diagnosis. The current approach is to incorporate clinical, biochemical, neuroradiological, pathological and molecular information in order to reach the diagnosis.

Age of onset may provide a clue to the diagnosis; onset soon after birth with hypotonia, faltering growth and liver failure, but no seizures, would suggest early-onset POLG-related disease. Intractable epilepsy with mild-to-moderate developmental delay after an uneventful neonatal period would suggest Alpers-Huttenlocher syndrome in both infants and early adolescents particularly if the liver enzymes were also raised. Presentation with acute-onset status epilepticus preceded by headache and visual disturbances and MRI changes suggestive of ischaemia in an adolescent or adults may raise the suspicion for POLG-related disease. This is true whether the individual has signs of liver dysfunction or not. These patients may have a history of migraine, psychiatric symptoms or poor motor performance in childhood, but the history may also be unremarkable. EEG findings and seizure semiology may give clue to the diagnosis; focal and focal evolving to bilateral tonic–clonic seizures with epileptiform discharge predominantly over the occipital lobes should raise the suspicion of POLG-related disease. MRI changes can provide early clues, e.g. with the finding of thalamic high T2 signal and/or occipital changes in someone with epilepsy. POLG-related disease should also be considered in any patients with intractable epilepsy and encephalopathy.

Biochemical Analysis

There are no specific blood biochemical markers for POLG-related disease. Elevated blood lactate is a marker for mitochondrial disease generally; however, in POLG-related disease elevation can be mild, transient or even absent. Further, inappropriate collection, particularly in infants/children, may result in falsely high levels. Pyruvate is used, often as a ratio with lactate, to indicate OXPHOS impairment [11, 51]. Both can be measured in the CSF that is less prone to false positivity. Again, lack of specificity limits the diagnostic value and elevated CSF lactate occurs in other conditions, e.g. seizures, stroke, CNS inflammation and infection [52], and CSF lactate can be normal in POLG-related disease.

Fibroblast growth factor 21 (FGF21) [53] and growth differentiation factor 15 (GDF15) [54] are both potential biomarkers for mitochondrial myopathy. FGF21 appears more consistently elevated in those with a predominantly muscle phenotype and both can be used as additional biomarkers in the initial screening process when POLG-related disease is suspected [53]. Negative results should not exclude the diagnosis and, typically, FGF21 and GDF15 are lower in patients with POLG than with Twinkle disease.

Routine investigations including full blood count, glucose, creatine kinase (CK), transaminases, liver and renal function tests are indicated to evaluate the systemic involvement of the disease. Metabolic screening with measurement of plasma amino acid and acylcarnitine profiles and urinary organic acids is helpful to exclude other metabolic disorders. Raised CSF protein is a common finding in patients with POLG-related disease and this can be used as a biomarker both to facilitate early diagnosis and to identify those with high risk to develop epilepsy [55].

Neurophysiological Findings

EEG findings may give a clue to the diagnosis of POLG-related disease: predominant ictal and interictal occipital epileptic activity, in both adults and children with *POLG* disease, is highly suggestive (Fig. 1) particularly in the early phase. Focal epileptic discharges may also occur in the temporal and frontal regions, and multifocal or generalised epileptic activity may occur during seizure evolution and SE [11, 19, 27]. Other EEG changes as rhythmic high amplitude with delta (RHADs) and focal slowing are frequently observed [20, 27].

Nerve conduction studies will confirm the presence and nature of the peripheral neuropathy that is often present [9]. While this is mostly axonal, with major sensory and some motor components, demyelinating motor neuropathy has also been reported [56, 57].

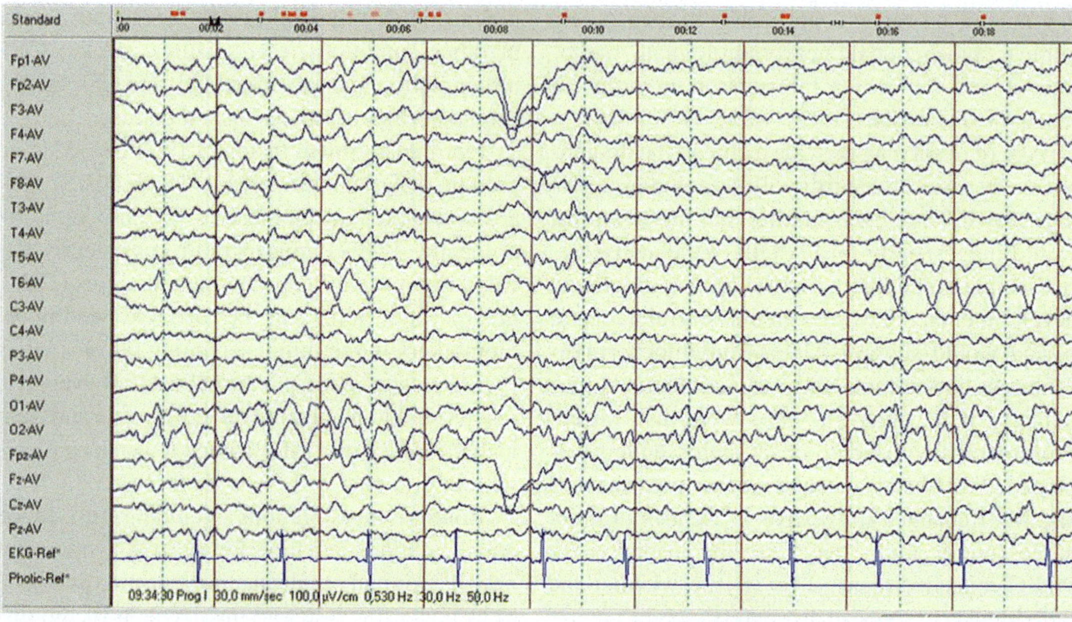

Fig. 1 Interictal EEG from patient 10 (4/0128) taken in 2004. Prior to this EEG, she had had three secondary generalised tonic–clonic seizures on different occasions. The EEG shows focal slow wave activity with sharp components in T6, O1 and O2 with suppression by eye opening. During seizures, epileptic activity was seen in O1 and O2 (data not shown) (Published in Brain 2008 Mar;131 (Pt 3):818–28; Figure 2. Used with permission.)

Neuroimaging

Magnetic resonance imaging (MRI) is the modality of choice, and the most sensitive sequences are T2 fluid-attenuated inversion recovery (FLAIR-T2) and diffusion-weighted imaging (DWI). The most frequently seen changes are T2/T2-FLAIR hyperintensities in the cerebral cortex, also known as cortical focal lesions (CFLs), which occur in patients with epilepsy and mainly affect the occipital lobes although they may also involve parietal, temporal and frontal lobes (Fig. 2). Cortical focal lesions have an acute/subacute onset, occur during episodes of encephalopathic exacerbation and may evolve over days or weeks. Subsequent partial or complete regression may occur [3, 9, 11, 27]. Notably, early neuroimaging study may be normal.

Involvement of other regions includes the thalamus, olivary nucleus and cerebellar white matter in which lesions usually remain stable throughout the disease. Generalised brain atrophy develops later during the disease course and is progressive reflecting the clinical progression of the disease [3, 27, 29].

Magnetic resonance spectroscopy (MRS) of CFLs typically show a prominent lactate peak due to impaired aerobic respiration and decreased N-acetyl aspartate concentration which reflects neuronal loss [3]. Ictal cerebral ^{18}F-fluoro-deoxy-glucose-positron emission tomography (FDG-PET) imaging shows increased glucose uptake in acute phase [29].

Histopathology and Respiratory Chain Enzyme Assay

Classical mitochondrial muscle pathology findings such as ragged-red and cytochrome oxidase-negative fibres are seen in patients with POLG-related disease; however, normal findings are also seen especially in the early-onset disease [11, 58]. Adolescent patients may have less than 1% of COX-negative fibres, emphasising the major manifestations to be in CNS. In addition to morphological examinations, mitochondrial respiratory chain enzyme (RC) analysis of biopsied muscle is helpful to confirm RC complex defects and provide a clue

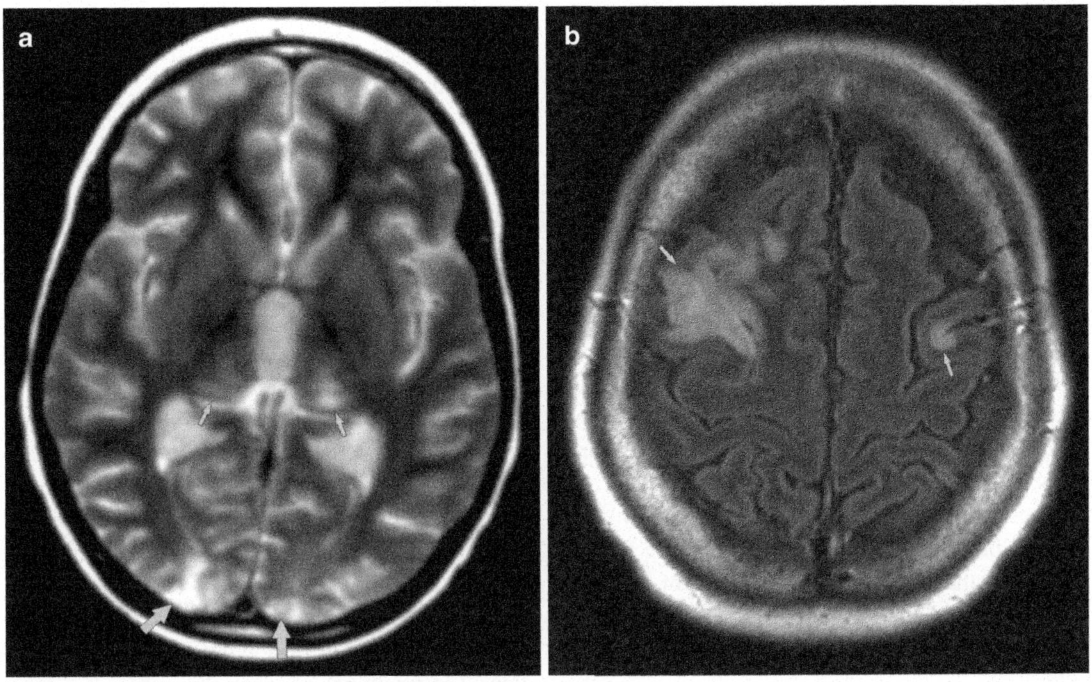

Fig. 2 (**a**) Axial T2-weighted MRI showing high signal lesions in the thalami (small arrows) and occipital cortices (large arrows). (**b**) Axial FLAIR MRI showing high signal intensity changes in the frontal cortex bilaterally (arrows) in a patient with focal motor status epilepticus (Published in Brain 2008 Mar;131(Pt 3):818–28; Figure 9. Used with permission.)

for the diagnosis. RC enzyme analysis may show isolated enzyme deficiency or combined deficiencies of multiple enzymes, especially in patients with primary muscle involvement, but may also be normal [11]. *POLG* mutations demonstrate tissue predilections and thus RC enzyme deficiencies may only be identified in clinically affected tissues such as liver or brain.

Molecular Genetics

The finding of pathological variants in *POLG* establishes the diagnosis: in recessive diseases, these are bi-allelic and in dominantly inherited disorders heterozygous. The most common inherited dominant variant is the p.Tyr955Cys, which is typically associated with mitochondrial myopathy, sensory neuropathy, parkinsonism and female premature menopause [7, 30]. A single patient with mutation of the same site (Tyr955His) had early-onset disease with bilateral sensorineural hearing loss, cataract, myopathy and liver failure [59].

Screening for the common founder mutations p.Ala467Thr, p.Trp784Ser, p.Gly848Ser and p. Tyr955Cys is an appropriate initial genetic investigation when population frequencies are known. If not, direct sequence analysis of *POLG* gene is the most appropriate first-line investigation and inclusion of *POLG* in next-generation sequencing gene panels for epilepsy, ataxia and mitochondrial disease will probably facilitate early diagnosis. This is particularly important in early-onset disease [11].

There are a large number of neutral and pathogenic *POLG* variants making interpretation difficult in some cases. It is also important to remember that some pathogenic POLG alleles comprise multiple nucleotide changes that change amino acids; for example, a common, recessively inherited allele may carry changes that cause Gln497His, Trp748Ser and Glu1443Gln in one POLG polypeptide. It is, therefore, crucial to evaluate segregation of the alleles since an individual carrying all these heterozygous changes can be a carrier and unaffected. A useful resource in judging pathogenicity is the Human DNA Polymerase Gamma Mutation Database (https://tools.niehs.nih.gov/polg/).

Management

Currently, there are no cures for POLG-related disease. Clinical management depends largely on symptomatic and supportive measures based usually on conventional approaches to treat the clinical manifestations and associated complications. This disease is often fatal, particularly in the young and those that develop epilepsy, and despite heroic efforts. It is vital therefore to consider the ethical aspects of management carefully to ensure that the treatment provided is in the best interest of the patient.

Management of Epilepsy

Epilepsy is the single most important prognostic factor for survival and the presence of seizures is associated with increased morbidity in patients with POLG-related disease. Early recognition and immediate, aggressive seizure treatment are crucial in improving patient survival. Many patients, regardless of age of onset, develop therapy-resistant seizures [9, 11] and this is particularly true for infants and children. Treatment with a single antiepileptic drug (AED) is rarely effective and high-dose polytherapy is often required [27]. There are currently no consensus recommendations for epilepsy management in POLG-related disease, and several AEDs have been used in various dosages and combinations.

Sodium valproate is absolutely contraindicated due to the risk of acute, progressive hepatic necrosis [9]. Transient liver failure with recovery after discontinuation of sodium valproate has been documented [20]. We suggest sequencing of the *POLG* gene be performed before prescribing sodium valproate to a patient with status epilepticus of unknown aetiology, especially an infant, if the clinical features raise any suspicion of POLG-related disease [25].

Since the most common seizure type is focal and focal evolving to bilateral convulsive, AEDs such as oxcarbazepine, carbamazepine, lacosamide and perampanel are appropriate, and can be used in combination with a benzodiazepine such as clobazam or clonazepam. Lamotrigine, topiramate and levetiracetam have also been used, but lamotrigine can worsen myoclonic seizures and should be used with caution.

Patients with POLG-related disease may present with or develop status epilepticus (SE) at any time. Management of SE is challenging: benzodiazepines, phenytoin and levetiracetam can be used as first-line treatment, but should not be pursued if initially ineffective. In this case, generalised anaesthesia using propofol or a barbiturate (pentothal) should be instituted, following the general guidelines for treatment of convulsive SE. Ketamine [60], magnesium infusion [61] and corticosteroids [20] have been effective in terminating SE in single cases, but lack of sufficient data (and our own experience) means that the use of these drugs cannot be recommended. Functional hemispherectomy as a palliative procedure can be considered when the short-term benefits outweigh the risk [62].

Epilepsia partialis continua is generally resistant to pharmacotherapy. Transcranial direct current stimulation gave promising results in one case [63], but requires further evaluation. Other non-pharmacological alternatives include ketogenic diet and vagus nerve stimulation, and these can be tried in therapy-resistant epilepsy [64]. There are, however, no clinical trials confirming the benefit of either in patients with POLG-related disease.

Some POLG patients show low CSF folate, and in these cases folinate supplementation has improved clinical functionality. For muscle weakness, our experience indicates improvement in muscle strength with niacin, a precursor of NAD+ (personal communication, A Suomalainen).

Nutritional supplements, referred to as 'mitochondrial cocktails' which include coenzyme

Q10, carnitine, L-arginine, EPI-734 and multiple vitamins, have been widely used; however, there is no clear evidence showing any significant clinical effect [65].

Supportive Management

Gastrointestinal and Nutritional

Faltering growth, feeding difficulties, gastric dysmotility and vomiting are common features of POLG-related disease in the very young, and dysmotility and vomiting can be seen regardless of the age of onset [11, 33]. The involvement of a gastroenterologist and dietician is recommended and use of a gastric tube/gastrostomy should be considered early, especially in early-onset disease to provide adequate nutrition, but also on older patients to facilitate management and nutrition.

Hepatic Involvement

Hepatic involvement is a common feature whatever the age and mild and/or transiently elevated liver enzymes are common. Patients can develop liver failure spontaneously, even without previous exposure to sodium valproate. Spontaneous resolution of liver failure after exposure to sodium valproate has been reported [66]. Measurement of liver enzymes (AST, ALT, GGT) and functional parameters (ammonia, albumin, bilirubin, prothrombin time, INR) should be performed frequently and at least every 3–4 months, especially in early- and adolescent-onset disease.

There is some controversy around the use of liver transplantation in this disease [67–69]. It has, however, been performed in patients with acute liver failure prior to the diagnosis of POLG disease with encouraging results. Further, experience with transplantation is growing and in some centres it is a preferred form of treatment. In all cases, careful evaluation of the ethical aspects and an individualised risk-benefit analysis are needed before proceeding to transplantation [70–72]. Survival after liver transplantation in adult-onset disease is better than with early-onset disease [9, 35, 71].

Movement Disorders and POLG

Parkinsonism is a feature of late-onset disease [30] and usually occurs together with peripheral neuropathy and PEO, and premature amenorrhea/menopause in women. Early-onset parkinsonism was reported in two sisters who also had neuropathy, but not PEO [38]. Treatment with L-DOPA [73] appears more successful in the late-onset disease.

The use of benzodiazepines can reduce the severity of other non-epileptic movement disorders including myoclonus, tremor and palatal myoclonus. Dystonia must be treated using established treatments such as botulinum toxin.

Ophthalmological Manifestations

Ophthalmological manifestations including cortical blindness, nystagmus, ptosis and ophthalmoplegia are features of POLG-related disease and may need intervention. Referral to ophthalmologist should be considered. Surgery for ptosis may provide some symptomatic relieve; however relapse may frequently occur.

Multidisciplinary Team

Due to the complexity and severity of these diseases, we would recommend that a multidisciplinary team manage individuals with POLG-related disease. The team should include neurologist/paediatric neurologist, gastroenterologist, dietician, occupational therapist, physiotherapist and ophthalmologist. Local health services should actively be involved to coordinate and provide services at community level. Screening for cognitive impairment and psychiatric symptoms will necessitate the involvement of psychiatrist, neuropsychologist and/or psychologist as appropriate and genetic counselling should be offered as soon as the diagnosis is established. Information about the nature of the disease, prognosis, mode of inheritance, carrier status, recurrence risk and implications for future decisions concerning choice of education, career and family planning, including the possibility for pre-implantation testing, should be discussed together with members of the team.

References

1. Korhonen JA, Pham XH, Pellegrini M, Falkenberg M. Reconstitution of a minimal mtDNA replisome in vitro. EMBO J. 2004;23(12):2423–9.
2. Wanrooij S, Falkenberg M. The human mitochondrial replication fork in health and disease. Biochim Biophys Acta. 2010;1797(8):1378–88.
3. Tzoulis C, Neckelmann G, Mork SJ, Engelsen BE, Viscomi C, Moen G, et al. Localized cerebral energy failure in DNA polymerase gamma-associated encephalopathy syndromes. Brain J Neurol. 2010;133(Pt 5):1428–37.
4. Muller-Hocker J, Horvath R, Schafer S, Hessel H, Muller-Felber W, Kuhr J, et al. Mitochondrial DNA depletion and fatal infantile hepatic failure due to mutations in the mitochondrial polymerase gamma (POLG) gene: a combined morphological/enzyme histochemical and immunocytochemical/biochemical and molecular genetic study. J Cell Mol Med. 2011;15(2):445–56.
5. Hudson G, Chinnery PF. Mitochondrial DNA polymerase-gamma and human disease. Hum Mol Genet. 2006;15(2):R244–52.
6. Saneto RP, Naviaux RK. Polymerase gamma disease through the ages. Dev Disabil Res Rev. 2010;16(2):163–74.
7. Van Goethem G, Dermaut B, Lofgren A, Martin JJ, Van Broeckhoven C. Mutation of POLG is associated with progressive external ophthalmoplegia characterized by mtDNA deletions. Nat Genet. 2001;28(3):211–2.
8. Winterthun S, Ferrari G, He L, Taylor RW, Zeviani M, Turnbull DM, et al. Autosomal recessive mitochondrial ataxic syndrome due to mitochondrial polymerase gamma mutations. Neurology. 2005;64(7):1204–8.
9. Tzoulis C, Engelsen BA, Telstad W, Aasly J, Zeviani M, Winterthun S, et al. The spectrum of clinical disease caused by the A467T and W748S POLG mutations: a study of 26 cases. Brain J Neurol. 2006;129(Pt 7):1685–92.
10. Hakonen AH, Heiskanen S, Juvonen V, Lappalainen I, Luoma PT, Rantamaki M, et al. Mitochondrial DNA polymerase W748S mutation: a common cause of autosomal recessive ataxia with ancient European origin. Am J Hum Genet. 2005;77(3):430–41.
11. Hikmat O, Tzoulis C, Chong WK, Chentouf L, Klingenberg C, Fratter C, et al. The clinical spectrum and natural history of early-onset diseases due to DNA polymerase gamma mutations. Genet Med. 2017;19(11):1217–25.
12. Nguyen KV, Sharief FS, Chan SS, Copeland WC, Naviaux RK. Molecular diagnosis of Alpers syndrome. J Hepatol. 2006;45(1):108–16.
13. Cohen BH, Chinnery PF, Copeland WC. POLG-related disorders. In: Pagon RA, Adam MP, Ardinger HH, Wallace SE, Amemiya A, LJH B, et al., editors. GeneReviews(R). Seattle (WA): University of Washington; 1993.
14. Harding BN. Progressive neuronal degeneration of childhood with liver disease (Alpers-Huttenlocher syndrome): a personal review. J Child Neurol. 1990;5(4):273–87.
15. Alpers BJ. DIffuse progressive degeneration of the gray matter of the cerebrum. Arch Neurol Psychiatr. 1931;25(3):469–505.
16. Naviaux RK, Nyhan WL, Barshop BA, Poulton J, Markusic D, Karpinski NC, et al. Mitochondrial DNA polymerase gamma deficiency and mtDNA depletion in a child with Alpers' syndrome. Ann Neurol. 1999;45(1):54–8.
17. Naviaux RK, Nguyen KV. POLG mutations associated with Alpers' syndrome and mitochondrial DNA depletion. Ann Neurol. 2004;55(5):706–12.
18. Uusimaa J, Hinttala R, Rantala H, Paivarinta M, Herva R, Roytta M, et al. Homozygous W748S mutation in the POLG1 gene in patients with juvenile-onset Alpers syndrome and status epilepticus. Epilepsia. 2008;49(6):1038–45.
19. Engelsen BA, Tzoulis C, Karlsen B, Lillebo A, Laegreid LM, Aasly J, et al. POLG1 mutations cause a syndromic epilepsy with occipital lobe predilection. Brain J Neurol. 2008;131(Pt 3):818–28.
20. Wolf NI, Rahman S, Schmitt B, Taanman JW, Duncan AJ, Harting I, et al. Status epilepticus in children with Alpers' disease caused by POLG1 mutations: EEG and MRI features. Epilepsia. 2009;50(6):1596–607.
21. Bindoff LA, Engelsen BA. Mitochondrial diseases and epilepsy. Epilepsia. 2012;53(Suppl 4):92–7.
22. Saneto RP, Cohen BH, Copeland WC, Naviaux RK. Alpers-Huttenlocher syndrome. Pediatr Neurol. 2013;48(3):167–78.
23. de Vries MC, Rodenburg RJ, Morava E, van Kaauwen EP, ter Laak H, Mullaart RA, et al. Multiple oxidative phosphorylation deficiencies in severe childhood multi-system disorders due to polymerase gamma (POLG1) mutations. Eur J Pediatr. 2007;166(3):229–34.
24. Horvath R, Hudson G, Ferrari G, Futterer N, Ahola S, Lamantea E, et al. Phenotypic spectrum associated with mutations of the mitochondrial polymerase gamma gene. Brain J Neurol. 2006;129(Pt 7):1674–84.
25. Saneto RP, Lee IC, Koenig MK, Bao X, Weng SW, Naviaux RK, et al. POLG DNA testing as an emerging standard of care before instituting valproic acid therapy for pediatric seizure disorders. Seizure. 2010;19(3):140–6.
26. Taanman JW, Rahman S, Pagnamenta AT, Morris AA, Bitner-Glindzicz M, Wolf NI, et al. Analysis of mutant DNA polymerase gamma in patients with mitochondrial DNA depletion. Hum Mutat. 2009;30(2):248–54.
27. Anagnostou ME, Ng YS, Taylor RW, McFarland R. Epilepsy due to mutations in the mitochondrial polymerase gamma (POLG) gene: a clinical and molecular genetic review. Epilepsia. 2016;57(10):1531–45.

28. Hikmat O, Eichele T, Tzoulis C, Bindoff LA. Understanding the epilepsy in POLG related disease. Int J Mol Sci. 2017;18(9):E1845.
29. Janssen W, Quaegebeur A, Van Goethem G, Ann L, Smets K, Vandenberghe R, et al. The spectrum of epilepsy caused by POLG mutations. Acta Neurol Belg. 2016;116(1):17–25.
30. Luoma P, Melberg A, Rinne JO, Kaukonen JA, Nupponen NN, Chalmers RM, et al. Parkinsonism, premature menopause, and mitochondrial DNA polymerase gamma mutations: clinical and molecular genetic study. Lancet (London, England). 2004;364(9437):875–82.
31. Hakonen AH, Davidzon G, Salemi R, Bindoff LA, Van Goethem G, Dimauro S, et al. Abundance of the POLG disease mutations in Europe, Australia, New Zealand, and the United States explained by single ancient European founders. Eur J Hum Genet. 2007;15(7):779–83.
32. Deschauer M, Tennant S, Rokicka A, He L, Kraya T, Turnbull DM, et al. MELAS associated with mutations in the POLG1 gene. Neurology. 2007;68(20):1741–2.
33. Van Goethem G, Schwartz M, Lofgren A, Dermaut B, Van Broeckhoven C, Vissing J. Novel POLG mutations in progressive external ophthalmoplegia mimicking mitochondrial neurogastrointestinal encephalomyopathy. Eur J Hum Genet. 2003;11(7):547–9.
34. Pagnamenta AT, Taanman JW, Wilson CJ, Anderson NE, Marotta R, Duncan AJ, et al. Dominant inheritance of premature ovarian failure associated with mutant mitochondrial DNA polymerase gamma. Hum Reprod. 2006;21(10):2467–73.
35. Wong LJ, Naviaux RK, Brunetti-Pierri N, Zhang Q, Schmitt ES, Truong C, et al. Molecular and clinical genetics of mitochondrial diseases due to POLG mutations. Hum Mutat. 2008;29(9):E150–72.
36. Milone M, Brunetti-Pierri N, Tang LY, Kumar N, Mezei MM, Josephs K, et al. Sensory ataxic neuropathy with ophthalmoparesis caused by POLG mutations. Neuromuscul Disord. 2008;18(8):626–32.
37. Pitceathly RD, Tomlinson SE, Hargreaves I, Bhardwaj N, Holton JL, Morrow JM, et al. Distal myopathy with cachexia: an unrecognised phenotype caused by dominantly-inherited mitochondrial polymerase gamma mutations. J Neurol Neurosurg Psychiatry. 2013;84(1):107–10.
38. Davidzon G, Greene P, Mancuso M, Klos KJ, Ahlskog JE, Hirano M, et al. Early-onset familial parkinsonism due to POLG mutations. Ann Neurol. 2006;59(5):859–62.
39. Nowak R, Zub R, Skoneczna I, Sikora K, Ligaj M. CAG repeat polymorphism in the DNA polymerase gamma gene in a Polish population: an association with testicular cancer risk. Ann Oncol. 2005;16(7):1211–2.
40. Van Goethem G, Luoma P, Rantamaki M, Al Memar A, Kaakkola S, Hackman P, et al. POLG mutations in neurodegenerative disorders with ataxia but no muscle involvement. Neurology. 2004;63(7):1251–7.
41. Suomalainen A, Majander A, Haltia M, Somer H, Lonnqvist J, Savontaus ML, et al. Multiple deletions of mitochondrial DNA in several tissues of a patient with severe retarded depression and familial progressive external ophthalmoplegia. J Clin Invest. 1992;90(1):61–6.
42. Suomalainen A, Majander A, Wallin M, Setala K, Kontula K, Leinonen H, et al. Autosomal dominant progressive external ophthalmoplegia with multiple deletions of mtDNA: clinical, biochemical, and molecular genetic features of the 10q-linked disease. Neurology. 1997;48(5):1244–53.
43. Spelbrink JN, Li FY, Tiranti V, Nikali K, Yuan QP, Tariq M, et al. Human mitochondrial DNA deletions associated with mutations in the gene encoding Twinkle, a phage T7 gene 4-like protein localized in mitochondria. Nat Genet. 2001;28(3):223–31.
44. Hudson G, Deschauer M, Busse K, Zierz S, Chinnery PF. Sensory ataxic neuropathy due to a novel C10Orf2 mutation with probable germline mosaicism. Neurology. 2005;64(2):371–3.
45. Koskinen T, Santavuori P, Sainio K, Lappi M, Kallio AK, Pihko H. Infantile onset spinocerebellar ataxia with sensory neuropathy: a new inherited disease. J Neurol Sci. 1994;121(1):50–6.
46. Nikali K, Suomalainen A, Saharinen J, Kuokkanen M, Spelbrink JN, Lonnqvist T, et al. Infantile onset spinocerebellar ataxia is caused by recessive mutations in mitochondrial proteins Twinkle and Twinky. Hum Mol Genet. 2005;14(20):2981–90.
47. Lonnqvist T, Paetau A, Valanne L, Pihko H. Recessive twinkle mutations cause severe epileptic encephalopathy. Brain J Neurol. 2009;132(Pt 6):1553–62.
48. Hakonen AH, Isohanni P, Paetau A, Herva R, Suomalainen A, Lonnqvist T. Recessive Twinkle mutations in early onset encephalopathy with mtDNA depletion. Brain J Neurol. 2007;130(Pt 11):3032–40.
49. Sarzi E, Goffart S, Serre V, Chretien D, Slama A, Munnich A, et al. Twinkle helicase (PEO1) gene mutation causes mitochondrial DNA depletion. Ann Neurol. 2007;62(6):579–87.
50. Morino H, Pierce SB, Matsuda Y, Walsh T, Ohsawa R, Newby M, et al. Mutations in Twinkle primase-helicase cause Perrault syndrome with neurologic features. Neurology. 2014;83(22):2054–61.
51. Debray FG, Mitchell GA, Allard P, Robinson BH, Hanley JA, Lambert M. Diagnostic accuracy of blood lactate-to-pyruvate molar ratio in the differential diagnosis of congenital lactic acidosis. Clin Chem. 2007;53(5):916–21.
52. Chow SL, Rooney ZJ, Cleary MA, Clayton PT, Leonard JV. The significance of elevated CSF lactate. Arch Dis Child. 2005;90(11):1188–9.
53. Suomalainen A, Elo JM, Pietilainen KH, Hakonen AH, Sevastianova K, Korpela M, et al. FGF-21 as a biomarker for muscle-manifesting mitochondrial respiratory chain deficiencies: a diagnostic study. Lancet Neurol. 2011;10(9):806–18.

54. Yatsuga S, Fujita Y, Ishii A, Fukumoto Y, Arahata H, Kakuma T, et al. Growth differentiation factor 15 as a useful biomarker for mitochondrial disorders. Ann Neurol. 2015;78(5):814–23.
55. Hikmat O, Naess K, Engvall M, Klingenberg C, Rasmussen M, Tallaksen CME, et al. Elevated cerebrospinal fluid protein in POLG-related epilepsy: diagnostic and prognostic implications. Epilepsia. 2018;59(8):1595–602.
56. Menezes MP, Rahman S, Bhattacharya K, Clark D, Christodoulou J, Ellaway C, et al. Neurophysiological profile of peripheral neuropathy associated with childhood mitochondrial disease. Mitochondrion. 2016;30:162–7.
57. Horga A, Pitceathly RD, Blake JC, Woodward CE, Zapater P, Fratter C, et al. Peripheral neuropathy predicts nuclear gene defect in patients with mitochondrial ophthalmoplegia. Brain J Neurol. 2014;137(Pt 12):3200–12.
58. Isohanni P, Hakonen AH, Euro L, Paetau I, Linnankivi T, Liukkonen E, et al. POLG1 manifestations in childhood. Neurology. 2011;76(9):811–5.
59. Siibak T, Clemente P, Bratic A, Bruhn H, Kauppila TES, Macao B, et al. A multi-systemic mitochondrial disorder due to a dominant p.Y955H disease variant in DNA polymerase gamma. Hum Mol Genet. 2017;26(13):2515–25.
60. Pruss H, Holtkamp M. Ketamine successfully terminates malignant status epilepticus. Epilepsy Res. 2008;82(2–3):219–22.
61. Visser NA, Braun KPJ, Leijten FSS, van Nieuwenhuizen O, Wokke JHJ, van den Bergh WM. Magnesium treatment for patients with refractory status epilepticus due to POLG1-mutations. J Neurol. 2011;258(2):218–22.
62. Lupashko S, Malik S, Donahue D, Hernandez A, Perry MS. Palliative functional hemispherectomy for treatment of refractory status epilepticus associated with Alpers' disease. Childs Nerv Syst. 2011;27(8):1321–3.
63. Ng YS, van Ruiten H, Lai HM, Scott R, Ramesh V, Horridge K, et al. The adjunctive application of transcranial direct current stimulation in the management of de novo refractory epilepsia partialis continua in adolescent-onset POLG-related mitochondrial disease. Epilepsia Open. 2018;3(1):103–8.
64. Martikainen MH, Paivarinta M, Jaaskelainen S, Majamaa K. Successful treatment of POLG-related mitochondrial epilepsy with antiepileptic drugs and low glycaemic index diet. Epileptic Disord. 2012;14(4):438–41.
65. Pfeffer G, Horvath R, Klopstock T, Mootha VK, Suomalainen A, Koene S, et al. New treatments for mitochondrial disease-no time to drop our standards. Nat Rev Neurol. 2013;9(8):474–81.
66. McFarland R, Hudson G, Taylor RW, Green SH, Hodges S, McKiernan PJ, et al. Reversible valproate hepatotoxicity due to mutations in mitochondrial DNA polymerase gamma (POLG1). Arch Dis Child. 2008;93(2):151–3.
67. Thomson MA, Lynch S, Strong R, Shepherd RW, Marsh W. Orthotopic liver transplantation with poor neurologic outcome in valproate-associated liver failure: a need for critical risk-benefit appraisal in the use of valproate. Transplant Proc. 2000;32(1):200–3.
68. Mindikoglu AL, King D, Magder LS, Ozolek JA, Mazariegos GV, Shneider BL. Valproic acid-associated acute liver failure in children: case report and analysis of liver transplantation outcomes in the United States. J Pediatr. 2011;158(5):802–7.
69. Kelly DA. Liver transplantation: to do or not to do? Pediatr Transplant. 2000;4(3):170–2.
70. Parikh S, Karaa A, Goldstein A, Ng YS, Gorman G, Feigenbaum A, et al. Solid organ transplantation in primary mitochondrial disease: proceed with caution. Mol Genet Metab. 2016;118(3):178–84.
71. Hynynen J, Komulainen T, Tukiainen E, Nordin A, Arola J, Kalviainen R, et al. Acute liver failure after valproate exposure in patients with POLG1 mutations and the prognosis after liver transplantation. Liver Transpl. 2014;20(11):1402–12.
72. Park S, Kang HC, Lee JS, Park YN, Kim S, Koh H. Alpers-Huttenlocher syndrome first presented with hepatic failure: can liver transplantation be considered as treatment option? Pediatr Gastroenterol Hepatol Nutr. 2017;20(4):259–62.
73. Martikainen MH, Ng YS, Gorman GS, Alston CL, Blakely EL, Schaefer AM, et al. Clinical, genetic, and radiological features of extrapyramidal movement disorders in mitochondrial disease. JAMA Neurol. 2016;73(6):668–74.

Mitochondrial Optic Neuropathies

Valerio Carelli, Chiara La Morgia,
and Thomas Klopstock

Introduction

In 1988, the first point mutation affecting the gene encoding subunit ND4 of complex I in mitochondrial DNA (mtDNA) was associated by Doug Wallace with Leber's hereditary optic neuropathy (LHON) [1], contributing to start the field of "mitochondrial medicine" [2]. It took time before the second most frequent inherited optic neuropathy, dominant optic atrophy (DOA), was recognized to be the nuclear counterpart of LHON, when in 2000 it was associated with heterozygous mutations in the OPA1 gene encoding for a major factor regulating mitochondrial dynamics [3, 4]. It is not surprising that almost all inherited forms of optic neuropathy are now recognized as mitochondrial diseases [5, 6]. Mitochondrial dysfunction affects critically specialized tissues with high metabolic requirements, and the retina sits on the top of the hierarchy, as a highly sophisticated organ of sense, which is also the only component of the central nervous system being exposed out of the skull [7].

Leber's Hereditary Optic Neuropathy

This inherited optic neuropathy, described initially by the German ophthalmologists von Graefe [8] and Theodor Leber [9], is now recognized as the most frequent mitochondrial disease [10]. LHON has a very distinctive clinical course characterized by a rapid neurodegenerative loss of retinal ganglion cells (RGCs), starting from the macula, thus affecting first the small axons of the papillomacular bundle [11, 12]. From the clinical standpoint, this translates into a subacute loss of central vision with central scotoma at visual fields, defective color vision, and contrast sensitivity loss, which evolves over weeks to months into a profound vision defect, frequently qualifying as legal blindness [13, 14]. The rapid neurodegenerative process characterizing LHON is in most cases defined by specific funduscopic appearance [15, 16], which is now quantified by optical coherence tomography (OCT) measurements. The initial 6 months after disease onset, now defined as the "subacute phase" [17], are characterized by loss of nerve fibers on the

V. Carelli (✉) · C. La Morgia
IRCCS Istituto di Scienze Neurologiche di Bologna, Bologna, Italy

Dipartimento di Scienze Biomediche e Neuromotorie, Universita' di Bologna, Bologna, Italy
e-mail: valerio.carelli@unibo.it

T. Klopstock
Department of Neurology, Friedrich-Baur-Institute, Ludwig-Maximilians-University of Munich, Munich, Germany

German Center for Neurodegenerative Diseases (DZNE), Munich, Germany

Munich Cluster for Systems Neurology (SyNergy), Munich, Germany

M. Mancuso, T. Klopstock (eds.), *Diagnosis and Management of Mitochondrial Disorders*,
https://doi.org/10.1007/978-3-030-05517-2_8

temporal side of the optic nerve disc leading to temporal atrophy, whereas the remaining quadrants are characterized by nerve fibers swelling, defined as "pseudoedema," and microangiopathy with vessel tortuosity [13, 14] (Fig. 1a–c). In the second 6 months, now defined as the "dynamic phase," this fundus picture evolves toward a resolution of the swelling, which leads to generalized loss of retinal nerve fibers and complete optic atrophy, with normalization of the vascular abnormalities. By about 1 year after disease onset, the patient enters the "chronic phase" with stabilization of the funduscopic picture, demonstrating variable degrees of optic atrophy with pale optic discs [13, 14] (Fig. 1d–f). Yet, in the first years of chronicity, a subset of LHON patients may experience some degree of spontaneous recovery of visual function, with rates that might differ depending on the mtDNA mutation type [13, 14]. The recent introduction of OCT redefined in a quantitative way the seminal but accurate descriptions based just on fundus oculi appearance of the pre-OCT era. Thus, the natural history of subsequent stages of retinal nerve fiber

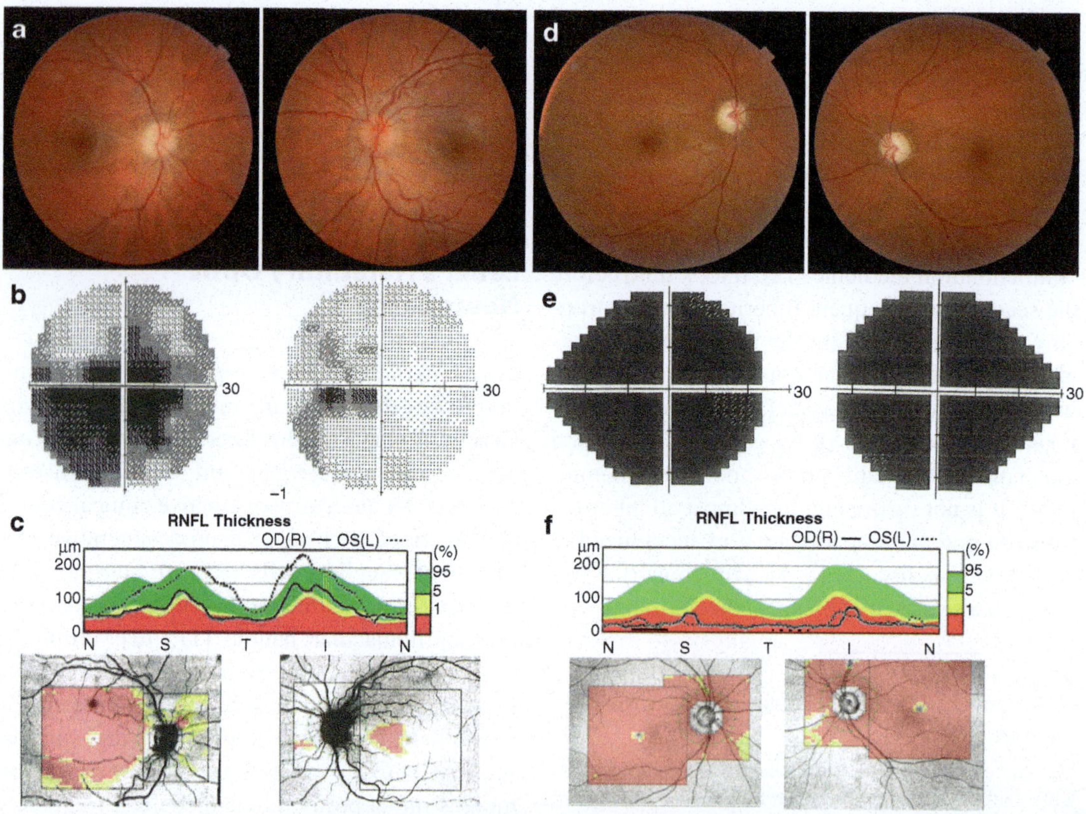

Fig. 1 LHON. (**a**) Fundus appearance of a LHON patient during the subacute phase. Note the asymmetry between eyes, with OD (left panel) displaying optic disc pallor more evident on the temporal sector, whereas OS (right panel) still has a hyperemic disc with nerve fiber swelling on the superior and inferior sectors. (**b**) The asymmetry noticeable at fundus is also reflected in the dimension of the central scotoma at visual fields, much larger in OD (left panel) than in OS (right panel). (**c**) The OCT assessments of RNFL thickness and of GCC, compatible with the fundus appearance and visual fields, reveal a substantial loss of GCC (lower left panel) and reduction of RNFL thickness (upper panel, continuous line) in OD, whereas OS has only minimal loss of GCC (lower right panel) and substantial increased RNFL thickness (upper panel, dotted line) due to fiber swelling. (**d**) Fundus appearance of a LHON patient during the chronic stage, displaying diffusely pale optic discs of both eyes. (**e**) Visual fields of both eyes show a profound and generalized loss of sensitivity. (**f**) The OCT assessment of RNFL thickness and GCC shows in both eyes profound loss of GCC and reduction in thickness of RNFL, confirming the profound bilateral optic atrophy

layer (RNFL) swelling and atrophy, quadrant by quadrant, has been quantified [18], as well as the macular ganglion cell complex (GCC) early loss is now defined [19]. Similarly, after the introduction of the angio-OCT module, the dynamic changes of choroid and retinal vasculature have been assessed, revealing that choroidal changes follow the loss of RGCs and the development of optic atrophy [20], whereas the microangiopathic features increase preceding the subacute phase of RNFL thickening and GCC loss [21]. These OCT and angio-OCT measurements, defining in a quantitative fashion the staging of natural history, not only represent a formidable tool to understand the disease but will also be incrementally instrumental as disease biomarkers to assessing the therapeutic efficacy of any drug being tested in LHON. Similarly to affected individuals, fundus changes [22] and OCT measurements [23, 24] define the amount of sub- or preclinical abnormalities that may characterize the unaffected mutation carriers, allowing again for an informative follow-up of the patients, possibly predicting, in the future, the conversion to affected [25].

LHON is essentially a clinical diagnosis of bilateral or sequential subacute visual loss and optic neuropathy with absence of inflammatory features [26, 27], as also reinforced by the lack of efficacy of corticosteroids during the subacute/dynamic phase [17] and supported by the frequent maternal inheritance in the family history [28]. Currently, the clinical suspicion can be rapidly confirmed by genetic testing. After the seminal discovery of the first LHON primary mutation m.11778G>A in the *MT-ND4* subunit gene of complex I [1], two other mutations m.3460G>A/*MT-ND1* and m.14484T>C/*MT-ND6* are now considered as frequent, overall covering about 90% of worldwide patients [29–32]. There is also an increasing number of "rare" primary mutations, with enough evidence fulfilling the criteria of pathogenicity [33]. Recently, LHON has also been linked to peculiar combinations of individually nonpathogenic missense mtDNA variants [34], broadening the defining criteria for pathogenicity of an mtDNA mutation and blurring the border between pathogenic and polymorphic variants. Thus, the most accurate diagnostic paradigm currently suggested is the sequence analysis of the entire mtDNA.

LHON remains peculiar for three remarkable features, considering that this is an mtDNA-related disease. These are:

1. The three common primary mtDNA mutations (m.11778G>A/*MT-ND4*, m.3460G>A/*MT-ND1*, and m.14484T>C/*MT-ND6*) are in the large majority of cases homoplasmic (100% mutant mtDNAs in all cells of all tissues) in every maternally related individual of a family; however, disease penetrance is incomplete in mutation carriers with most of them remaining unaffected lifelong.
2. Penetrance is strikingly higher in males than females, accounting for roughly about 50% of males and 10% of females.
3. Notwithstanding the mutation is homoplasmic in all cells of all tissues of the human body, only RGCs are affected in the retina.

The LHON conundrum has now some partial answers. Historically, the initial hypothesis postulated to explain male prevalence was the possible existence of a modifying gene on the X chromosome [35, 36], but, despite different loci having been reported by different studies, no relevant variant could be identified in any gene so far [37–39]. Furthermore, one assumption for the X-linked modifying effect predicted a skewed inactivation of the X chromosome in affected female patients, which has never been found in multiple studies, even assessing multiple tissues including the retina [40–42]. More recently, in vitro cell studies suggested that estrogens are partially protective in females by optimizing a compensatory response mainly based on increased mitochondrial biogenesis [43]. Expanding from this observation, it has been shown [44], and independently replicated [45], that mitochondrial biogenesis is efficiently activated as a successful compensatory strategy driving incomplete penetrance in both genders. The simplest biomarker of mitochondrial biogenesis is the assessment of mtDNA copy number in circulating blood cells, which distinguishes affected individuals from unaffected mutation carriers [44, 45]. Remarkably, as environmental factors such as tobacco and alcohol consumption have been confirmed to trigger LHON [46, 47], a recent study demonstrated in vitro that tobacco extracts lower mtDNA copy number, potentially hampering the compensatory response [48]. Thus, taking into account the exposure to triggering factors, it has been proposed that LHON patients could be broadly distinguished in two categories, those affected at young-adult age and mostly due to the genetic background (type I) and those with later onset (older than 40) triggered mostly by the prolonged toxic exposure (long-lasting tobacco smokers) (type II) [49]. This possible subcategorization of LHON patients by age of onset, as related to prevalent genetic predisposition opposed to the prevalent exposure to environmental triggers, remains debated [50], as a different study on late-onset LHON failed to observe such association with environmental factors [51]. Overall, it remains still unclear what is the possible contribution of nuclear genome variants as modulators of the compensatory activation of mitochondrial biogenesis, ultimately impinging on penetrance [52]. Scattered reports on the association of a few putative modifying variants in nuclear genes (*PARL* and *YARS2*) with LHON [53–55] were not reproduced in different patient cohorts ([44, 56] and Valerio Carelli, Pio D'Adamo, Patrick Chinnery unpublished data), possibly pointing to a substantial heterogeneity of genetic modifiers in LHON in different population-specific combinations. At difference with the still uncertain role of nuclear modifying variants, the role attributed to the mtDNA haplogroup J background in LHON is well established [57, 58], and evidence has been presented for coincidental association of primary mutations with private variants as modulatory factors for penetrance [59, 60].

Besides the incomplete penetrance and male prevalence, we must consider the third peculiarity of LHON, the cell specificity of the pathological mechanism driven by defective complex I, which leads to selective neurodegeneration of RGCs. Three decades of cell studies, mainly exploiting the cybrid cell model [61] and patient-derived cell lines (lymphoblasts and fibroblasts), substantiated that the biochemical defect affecting complex I leads to reduced bioenergetic efficiency, increased oxidative stress, and propensity to activate apoptotic cell death [5–7, 13, 14]. These functional alterations somehow relate to RGC architecture. These retinal neurons generate a long intraretinal unmyelinated axonal segment, allowing for retinal transparency to light but representing a metabolic choke point. Myelination is then acquired by RGC axons as they pass the lamina cribrosa and form the retrobulbar optic nerve. As a consequence there is an asymmetric distribution of axonal mitochondria, which must be very abundant in the unmyelinated axonal segment, reflecting on the compensatory mitochondrial biogenesis activated by LHON mutations, so that the smallest axons are the most vulnerable for their unfavorable metabolic requirements [13, 14]. Ultimately, RGCs may undergo a catastrophic crisis precipitated by many possible mechanisms, and axonal loss then follows the documented pattern affecting first the smaller axons [11, 12], which has also been reproduced in a genetic mouse model of LHON [62]. Despite our understanding of LHON has substantially increased in the last three decades, there are many areas that still remain to be fully explored and defined. These include the roles played by vascular changes, myelin maintenance and remodeling, and astrocytes, and, ultimately, we still need to understand how the key mechanisms regulating mitochondrial homeostasis, including mitochondrial dynamics, biogenesis, and mitophagic removal, are at work in the pathophysiology of LHON [7].

Nowadays, LHON represents a major paradigm for development of therapeutic strategies that might be of relevance for other mitochondrial and neurodegenerative disorders. The natural history of LHON is now fairly well characterized and efficiently measured by various technical approaches, including the innovative OCT [18–21]. Thus, the combination of a relatively predictable disease course, with good technical assessment of visual function biomarkers, elected LHON as the ideal disease for clinical trials ranging from idebenone [63, 64], approved in Europe in 2015, to gene therapy with the allotopic expression strategy [65], with trials ongoing in 2018. This latter approach exploits nuclear expression of a recoded wild-type version of the mutant ND subunit, targeted to mitochondrial import by a mitochondrial import sequence inserted in the construct packaged in the AAV vector. The imported wild-type ND subunit is assumed to compete with the mutant one within mitochondria and ultimately to assemble in complex I, complementing the biochemical dysfunction [65].

Dominant Optic Atrophy

In 1959 the Danish ophthalmologist Poul Kjer described a series of families with dominant inheritance of a slowly progressive form of optic atrophy with onset in childhood [66], now defined as DOA [67]. DOA is reported to have a prevalence of 1:50,000–1:10,000 in Denmark [68]. Typically, a roughly bilateral and symmetrical visual loss is recognized since childhood, accompanied by central scotoma, impairment of color vision (tritanopia), and temporal pallor of the optic discs (Fig. 2a–c). Frequently the patient is unaware of a vision defect, and the disease is recognized by chance during routine vision testing (school eye screenings). The disease progression may be quite variable in different individuals even in the same family, ranging from mild cases with essentially stable visual acuity, to slowly progressing cases, to cases with steplike decreases of visual acuity [13, 14]. This variable expressivity includes severe cases with legal blindness as final outcome, as well as

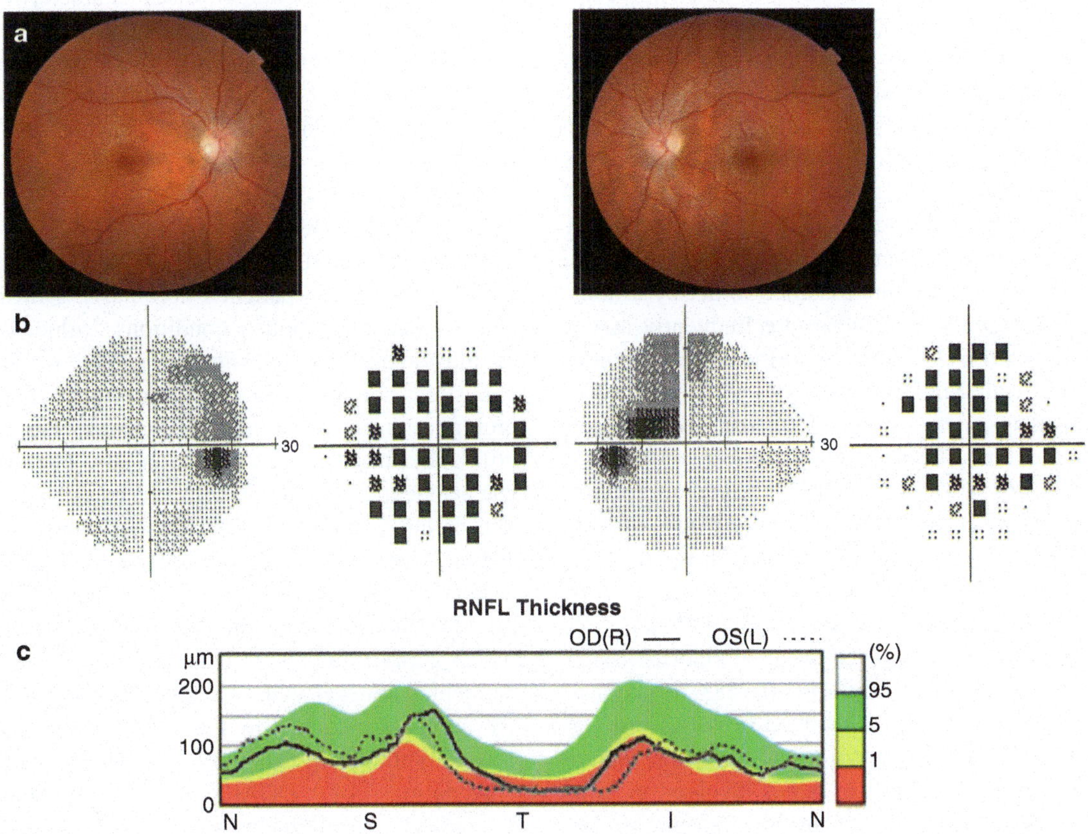

Fig. 2 DOA. (**a**) Fundus appearance is characterized by selective atrophy of the temporal side of optic discs. (**b**) Visual fields reveal a bilateral central scotoma. (**c**) OCT assessment of RNFL thickness confirms a selective loss of fibers limited to the temporal sector (T)

asymptomatic, non-penetrant cases [69, 70]. It must be emphasized that despite the obvious difference in age of onset and natural history, the central pattern of visual loss and preference for the papillomacular bundle in DOA overlaps substantially with LHON [13, 14], suggesting that there might be common final pathways leading to neurodegeneration of RGCs [5, 6]. Since the preclinical era, there were also reports of families with DOA combined with deafness, as well as more complex syndromes including chronic progressive external ophthalmoplegia (CPEO) and myopathy, peripheral neuropathy, and central nervous system involvement [71, 72], now denominated as "DOA plus" [73].

The first genetic defect associated with DOA was discovered in the year 2000, as heterozygous mutations were found in the optic atrophy type 1 (*OPA1*) gene [3, 4], whose major function, among many, is to carry out fusion of inner mitochondrial membranes [74, 75]. OPA1 is a dynamin-related GTPase also involved in regulating cristae morphology [76] and apoptosis [77, 78], in sensing oxidative phosphorylation and ensuring its efficiency [79, 80], as well as in mtDNA maintenance [81, 82]. Interestingly, while most *OPA1* mutations associated with DOA result in haploinsufficiency, missense mutations affecting the GTPase domain and assumed to act by a dominant negative mechanism are frequently associated with DOA "plus," with the hallmark feature of affecting mtDNA stability [73, 81]. However, DOA is genetically heterogeneous, and dominant mutations affecting *OPA1* cover only about 60–70% of DOA cases [67]. Mutations in other genes are currently reported as causative of DOA or "DOA plus," such as those affecting the *MFN2* gene [83] involved in fusion of external mitochondrial membranes, the *DRP1* [84] and *OPA3* [85, 86] genes involved in mitochondrial fission, and the *SPG7* [87] and *AFG3L2* [88, 89] cognate proteases, somehow involved in OPA1 processing of long to short isoforms [90]. Thus, there is a clear convergence of genes involved in mitochondrial dynamics as causative for optic atrophy with the classical pattern of mitochondrial optic neuropathies [5–7, 91]. Furthermore, it is remarkable that these same genes may also lead to CPEO with mitochondrial myopathy and mtDNA multiple deletions, frequently within the frame of a complex syndrome with further recurrent features such as sensorineural deafness and peripheral neuropathy [5–7, 91].

As in LHON, many areas of DOA remain blurry, in particular concerning the variability in expressivity and penetrance [52]. The possible modifying role of mtDNA haplogroups in OPA1-DOA, for example, has been downplayed by two studies, but doubts remain about the study design [92, 93]. One interesting finding in OPA1-DOA, as observed by OCT measurements assessing the dimension of optic discs, is the significantly smaller disc area characterizing these patients compared with controls, which lead to the suggestion that DOA is a congenital condition with various degrees of hypoplasia of the optic nerve head [94]. The size of the optic disc is also influential in LHON, as larger discs characterize unaffected mutation carriers and patients with better prognosis, introducing in LHON the well-known concept of "disc at risk" that applies to non-arteritic ischemic optic neuropathy (NAION) [95].

The pathogenic mechanism of OPA1-DOA has been studied both in cell and in animal models (*Drosophila* and mouse). The initial studies have been run using patient's fibroblasts, grown under basal metabolic conditions (glucose medium) as well as challenged by classic metabolic stress conditions (galactose medium), thus forcing cells to use oxidative phosphorylation [96]. Under basal conditions, the in vitro phenotype is essentially well compensated by the presence of the wild-type allele, whereas galactose medium leads to the emergence of a pathological phenotype characterized by impaired respiration and ATP synthesis through complex I substrates and impaired mitochondrial fusion with hyperfragmented network with loss of cristae morphology at ultrastructure and ultimately with cell propensity to undergo apoptosis [97–99].

Modeling of DOA in OPA1-mutant *Drosophila* highlighted the relevance of increased ROS production in the disease pathogenesis as the phenotype was partially neutralized by antioxidant therapy [100]. This result, in conjunction with the decreased efficiency of complex I evidenced in patient-derived fibroblasts, prompted to test the first therapeutic approaches with the antioxidant idebenone in human patients with DOA [101]. DOA has also been studied in two mouse models carrying heterozygous *OPA1* mutations recapitulating haploinsufficiency, both characterized by about 50% reduction of OPA1 expression (embryonically lethal in the homozygous condition), inducing a mild, age-dependent ocular phenotype with evidence of RGC dysfunction, but limited loss of RGCs [102, 103]. Interestingly, increased autophagy in RGCs was reported in one of the mouse models [104], a feature that has also been seen in fibroblasts from patients with specific *OPA1* mutations leading to unusual neurodegenerative phenotypes such as Parkinsonism and dementia [105], as well as cases with biallelic *OPA1* mutations and severe multisystemic phenotype [106]. Another finding of interest was obtained by studying the RGC's synaptic connectivity in the same mouse showing that the earliest pathological changes occur in the form of dendritic pruning and marked reduction in synaptic connectivity, qualifying this as a dendropathy [107, 108]. Thus, counterintuitively, the neurodegeneration of RGCs induced by OPA1 does not seem to affect first the axons but the maintenance of the dendritic tree, for which OPA1 seems to play a crucial role [109]. A third knock-in mouse model carrying the human common *OPA1* microdeletion c.2708_2711delTTAG was phenotypically characterized by a multisystemic poly-degenerative phenotype, with visual failure, deafness, encephalomyelopathy, peripheral neuropathy, ataxia, and cardiomyopathy [110]. Furthermore, there were age-related axonal and myelin degeneration, increased autophagy and mitophagy, and mitochondrial supercomplex instability preceding degeneration and cell death [110]. Thus, this mouse model displayed most of the features typical of DOA "plus," despite the purported pathogenic mechanism of haploinsufficiency, similar to the other two OPA1 mouse models.

Overall, we now consider OPA1 to be a multifunctional protein, ruling many processes within mitochondria, as a crossroad among mitochondrial dynamics, sensing of oxidative phosphorylation, mtDNA maintenance, apoptosis regulation, autophagic removal of mitochondria by mitophagy, and mitochondrial cristae architecture [75]. The *OPA1* gene is expressed in eight isoforms by alternative splicing, which may be further processed from long to short isoforms [75]. To clarify the possible role of this very complex OPA1 expression profile, each isoform was recently reexpressed in OPA1-null mouse embryonic fibroblasts, or silenced in different combinations in HeLa cells, reaching the interesting conclusion that each of the isoforms may ensure the recovery of bioenergetics, cristae shape, and mtDNA maintenance, but only a specific balance between long and short isoforms in the presence of an adequate amount of OPA1 can actually recover mitochondrial dynamics (fusion) [111]. This knowledge is a prerequisite for setting gene therapy in humans [111, 112], as this therapeutic approach is being tested in mice [113]. This is a very active research area, as slight overexpression of OPA1 seems to be therapeutic in many different pathologic scenarios variously characterized by mitochondrial dysfunction [114, 115]. The use of reprogrammed stem cells from patient-derived fibroblasts to generate target tissues, such as dopaminergic neurons in the case of the OPA1 mutations associated with Parkinsonism and dementia, has been recently undertaken to model the pathogenic mechanisms (necroptosis) and test therapies [116].

Recessive and X-linked Optic Neuropathies

Recessively or X-linked inherited, nonsyndromic optic neuropathies are rare entities, which only recently started to be better defined, thanks to the identification of a few genetic causes (Table 1). As predictable, most of the genes identified to date affect mitochondrial proteins, obeying the general rule that RGCs and their optic nerve-forming axons are primary targets of mitochondrial dysfunction [5–7]. In 2003, Barbet and colleagues mapped

Table 1 Nuclear genes associated with isolated or dominant optic atrophy

Disease	OMIM	Inheritance	*Gene* (or locus)	References
OPA1	125250	AD	*OPA1*	[3, 4]
OPA2	311050	XR	(chr.Xp11.4–p11.21)	[129]
OPA3	165300	AR, AD	*OPA3*	[85, 128]
OPA4	605293	AD	(chr.18q12.2–q12.3)	[5, 6]
OPA5	610708	AD	(chr.22q12.1–q13.1), DNM1L	[5, 6, 84]
OPA6	258500	AR	(chr. 8q21–q22)	[117]
OPA7	612989	AR	*TMEM126A*	[118]
OPA8	616648	AD	(chr.16q21–q22)	[5, 6]
OPA9	616289	AR	*ACO2*	[119]
OPA10	616732	AR	*RTN4IP1*	[120]
OPA11	617302	AR	*YME1L1*	[121]

the first locus for a recessive optic neuropathy at 8q21–q22 defined as OPA6 (OPA6), which still lacks the identification of the causative gene [117]. Instead, identified genes now include *TMEM126A* (OPA7) [118], *ACO2* (OPA9) [119], *RTN4IP1* (OPA10) [120], and *YME1L1* (OPA11) [121]. TMEM126A protein is located in the inner mitochondrial membrane and its function remains unknown [122], whereas ACO2 is a matrix enzyme implicated in tricarboxylic acid cycle, catalyzing interconversion of citrate into isocitrate [119]. RTN4IP1 is another mitochondrial protein associated with the outer mitochondrial membrane and a quinone oxidoreductase activity, predicted to interact with the partner protein RTN4 localized to the endoplasmic reticulum [120, 123]. YME1L1 is a mitochondrial protease, which together with OMA1 is implicated in the Proteolytic cleavage of OPA1 long forms to short [74]. It is not infrequent that allelic mutations may underlie both isolated optic atrophy or more complex diseases, being optic atrophy very frequently described in many neurodegenerative recessive disorders, such as Behr and Costeff syndromes [124, 125]. Interestingly, recessive mutations in OPA1 were recently associated with Behr syndrome [126, 127], whereas Costeff syndrome is due to recessive mutations in OPA3 [128], being in both cases implicated disturbed mitochondrial dynamics.

Finally, concerning the X-linked optic neuropathy, there is a locus for which no gene has been identified yet [129, 130]. It must be mentioned that syndromic optic atrophy, typically associated with deafness and dystonia, clinically characterizes the X-linked Mohr-Tranebjaerg syndrome, which is due to mutations in the TIMM8a gene [131].

Conclusions and Future Directions

Mitochondrial optic neuropathies remain a major paradigm of mitochondrial mono-organ disease, for which we actively entered the era of therapy. This paradigm will be probably valuable for a larger landscape of rare mitochondrial disorders, as the understanding of pathogenic mechanisms leading to neurodegeneration of RGCs may be generalized to other neuronal systems [7]. The paucity of mouse models of mitochondrial diseases, in particular of those related to mtDNA mutations, has hampered the development of the field. However, new powerful tools are now available, in particular the reprogramming of stem cells from patient-derived primary cell lines (iPSCs) and the generation of organoids that will possibly fill the gap of animal modeling in mitochondrial disorders [7]. The continuous refinement of these techniques leading to better differentiated mini-eyes and mini-brains may truly become a new avenue to test therapies, screening drug libraries and applying gene editing, as now possible with many different tailored nucleases including CRISPR/Cas9, mitoTalen [132], and mitoZFN [133]. The mtDNA genome remains more problematic than the nuclear in this respect, because, despite the many efforts, we do not have yet clear-cut tools to introduce DNA within the mitochondria [134]. The times to come will be interesting for the field and most importantly will hopefully provide solutions to the patients, which will finally be offered a cure.

References

1. Wallace DC, Singh G, Lott MT, Hodge JA, Schurr TG, Lezza AM, Elsas LJ 2nd, Nikoskelainen EK. Mitochondrial DNA mutation associated with Leber's hereditary optic neuropathy. Science. 1988;242:1427–30.
2. Luft R. The development of mitochondrial medicine. Proc Natl Acad Sci U S A. 1994;91:8731–8.
3. Alexander C, Votruba M, Pesch UEA, Thiselton DL, Mayer S, Moore A, Rodriguez M, Kellner U, Leo-Kottler B, Auburger G, Bhattacharya SS, Wissinger B. OPA1, encoding a dynamin-related GTPase, is mutated in autosomal dominant optic atrophy linked to chromosome 3q28. Nat Genet. 2000;26:211–5.
4. Delettre C, Lenaers G, Griffoin J-M, Gigarel N, Lorenzo C, Belenguer P, Pelloquin L, Grosgeorge J, Turc-Carel C, Perret E, Astarie-Dequeker C, Lasquellec L, Arnaud B, Ducommun B, Kaplan J, Hamel CP. Nuclear gene OPA1, encoding a mitochondrial dynamin-related protein, is mutated in dominant optic atrophy. Nat Genet. 2000;26:207–10.
5. Maresca A, la Morgia C, Caporali L, Valentino ML, Carelli V. The optic nerve: a "mito-window" on mitochondrial neurodegeneration. Mol Cell Neurosci. 2013;55:62–76.
6. Yu-Wai-Man P, Votruba M, Burté F, La Morgia C, Barboni P, Carelli V. A neurodegenerative perspective on mitochondrial optic neuropathies. Acta Neuropathol. 2016;132:789–806.
7. Carelli V, La Morgia C, Ross-Cisneros FN, Sadun AA. Optic neuropathies: the tip of the neurodegeneration iceberg. Hum Mol Genet. 2017;26(R2):R139–50.
8. Von Graefe A. Ein ungewőhnlicher Fall von hereditärer Amaurose. Arch Ophthalmol. 1858;4:266–8.
9. Leber T. Uber hereditare und congenital-angelegte Sehnervenleiden. Arch Ophthalmol. 1871;17:249–91.
10. Gorman GS, Schaefer AM, Ng Y, Gomez N, Blakely EL, Alston CL, Feeney C, Horvath R, Yu-Wai-Man P, Chinnery PF, Taylor RW, Turnbull DM, McFarland R. Prevalence of nuclear and mitochondrial DNA mutations related to adult mitochondrial disease. Ann Neurol. 2015;77:753–9.
11. Sadun AA, Win PH, Ross-Cisneros FN, Walker SO, Carelli V. Leber's hereditary optic neuropathy differentially affects smaller axons in the optic nerve. Trans Am Ophthalmol Soc. 2000;98:223–32; discussion 232–5
12. Pan BX, Ross-Cisneros FN, Carelli V, Rue KS, Salomao SR, Moraes-Filho MN, Moraes MN, Berezovsky A, Belfort R Jr, Sadun AA. Mathematically modeling the involvement of axons in Leber's hereditary optic neuropathy. Invest Ophthalmol Vis Sci. 2012;53:7608–17.
13. Carelli V, Ross-Cisneros FN, Sadun AA. Mitochondrial dysfunction as a cause of optic neuropathies. Prog Retin Eye Res. 2004;23:53–89.
14. Yu-Wai-Man P, Griffiths PG, Chinnery PF. Mitochondrial optic neuropathies -disease mechanisms and therapeutic strategies. Prog Retin Eye Res. 2011;30:81–114.
15. Smith JL, Hoyt WF, Susac JO. Ocular fundus in acute Leber optic neuropathy. Arch Ophthalmol. 1973;90:349–54.
16. Nikoskelainen E, Hoyt WF, Nummelin K. Ophthalmoscopic findings in Leber's hereditary optic neuropathy. II. The fundus findings in the affected family members. Arch Ophthalmol. 1983;101:1059–68.
17. Carelli V, Carbonelli M, de Coo IF, Kawasaki A, Klopstock T, Lagrèze WA, La Morgia C, Newman NJ, Orssaud C, Pott JWR, Sadun AA, van Everdingen J, Vignal-Clermont C, Votruba M, Yu-Wai-Man P, Barboni P. International consensus statement on the clinical and therapeutic management of Leber hereditary optic neuropathy. J Neuroophthalmol. 2017;37:371–81.
18. Barboni P, Carbonelli M, Savini G, Ramos Cdo V, Carta A, Berezovsky A, Salomao SR, Carelli V, Sadun AA. Natural history of Leber's hereditary optic neuropathy: longitudinal analysis of the retinal nerve fiber layer by optical coherence tomography. Ophthalmology. 2010;117:623–7.
19. Balducci N, Savini G, Cascavilla ML, La Morgia C, Triolo G, Giglio R, Carbonelli M, Parisi V, Sadun AA, Bandello F, Carelli V, Barboni P. Macular nerve fibre and ganglion cell layer changes in acute Leber's hereditary optic neuropathy. Br J Ophthalmol. 2016;100:1232–7.
20. Borrelli E, Triolo G, Cascavilla ML, La Morgia C, Rizzo G, Savini G, Balducci N, Nucci P, Giglio R, Darvizeh F, Parisi V, Bandello F, Sadun AA, Carelli V, Barboni P. Changes in choroidal thickness follow the RNFL changes in Leber's hereditary optic neuropathy. Sci Rep. 2016;6:37332.
21. Balducci N, Cascavilla ML, Ciardella A, La Morgia C, Triolo G, Parisi V, Bandello F, Sadun AA, Carelli V, Barboni P. Peripapillary vessel density changes in Leber's hereditary optic neuropathy: a new biomarker. Clin Experiment Ophthalmol. 2018;46(9):1055–62.
22. Nikoskelainen E, Hoyt WF, Nummelin K. Ophthalmoscopic findings in Leber's hereditary optic neuropathy. I. Fundus findings in asymptomatic family members. Arch Ophthalmol. 1982;100:1597–602.
23. Savini G, Barboni P, Valentino ML, Montagna P, Cortelli P, De Negri AM, Sadun F, Bianchi S, Longanesi L, Zanini M, Carelli V. Retinal nerve fiber layer evaluation by optical coherence tomography in unaffected

carriers with Leber's hereditary optic neuropathy mutations. Ophthalmology. 2005;112:127–31.
24. Barboni P, Savini G, Feuer WJ, Budenz DL, Carbonelli M, Chicani F, Ramos Cdo V, Salomao SR, Negri AD, Parisi V, Carelli V, Sadun AA. Retinal nerve fiber layer thickness variability in Leber hereditary optic neuropathy carriers. Eur J Ophthalmol. 2012;22:985–91.
25. Hwang TJ, Karanjia R, Moraes-Filho MN, Gale J, Tran JS, Chu ER, Salomao SR, Berezovsky A, Belfort R Jr, Moraes MN, Sadun F, DeNegri AM, La Morgia C, Barboni P, Ramos CDVF, Chicani CF, Quiros PA, Carelli V, Sadun AA. Natural history of conversion of Leber's hereditary optic neuropathy: a prospective case series. Ophthalmology. 2017;124:843–50.
26. Nikoskelainen E, Hoyt WF, Nummelin K, Schatz H. Fundus findings in Leber's hereditary optic neuroretinopathy. III. Fluorescein angiographic studies. Arch Ophthalmol. 1984;102:981–9.
27. La Morgia C, Carbonelli M, Barboni P, Sadun AA, Carelli V. Medical management of hereditary optic neuropathies. Front Neurol. 2014;5:141.
28. Erickson RP. Leber's optic atrophy, a possible example of maternal inheritance. Am J Hum Genet. 1972;24:348–9.
29. Howell N, Bindoff LA, McCullough DA, Kubacka I, Poulton J, Mackey D, Taylor L, Turnbull DM. Leber hereditary optic neuropathy: identification of the same mitochondrial ND1 mutation in six pedigrees. Am J Hum Genet. 1991;49:939–50.
30. Huoponen K, Vilkki J, Aula P, Nikoskelainen EK, Savontaus ML. A new mtDNA mutation associated with Leber hereditary optic neuroretinopathy. Am J Hum Genet. 1991;48:1147–53.
31. Mackey D, Howell N. A variant of Leber hereditary optic neuropathy characterized by recovery of vision and by an unusual mitochondrial genetic etiology. Am J Hum Genet. 1992;51:1218–28.
32. Johns DR, Neufeld MJ, Park RD. An ND-6 mitochondrial DNA mutation associated with Leber hereditary optic neuropathy. Biochem Biophys Res Commun. 1992;187:1551–7.
33. Achilli A, Iommarini L, Olivieri A, Pala M, Hooshiar Kashani B, Reynier P, La Morgia C, Valentino ML, Liguori R, Pizza F, Barboni P, Sadun F, De Negri AM, Zeviani M, Dollfus H, Moulignier A, Ducos G, Orssaud C, Bonneau D, Procaccio V, Leo-Kottler B, Fauser S, Wissinger B, Amati-Bonneau P, Torroni A, Carelli V. Rare primary mitochondrial DNA mutations and probable synergistic variants in Leber's hereditary optic neuropathy. PLoS One. 2012;7:e42242.
34. Caporali L, Iommarini L, La Morgia C, Olivieri A, Achilli A, Maresca A, Valentino ML, Capristo M, Tagliavini F, Del Dotto V, Zanna C, Liguori R, Barboni P, Carbonelli M, Cocetta V, Montopoli M, Martinuzzi A, Cenacchi G, De Michele G, Testa F, Nesti A, Simonelli F, Porcelli AM, Torroni A, Carelli V. Peculiar combinations of individually non-pathogenic missense mitochondrial DNA variants cause low penetrance Leber's hereditary optic neuropathy. PLoS Genet. 2018;14:e1007210.
35. Bu XD, Rotter JI. X chromosome-linked and mitochondrial gene control of Leber hereditary optic neuropathy: evidence from segregation analysis for dependence on X chromosome inactivation. Proc Natl Acad Sci U S A. 1991;88:8198–202.
36. Bu X, Rotter JI. Leber hereditary optic neuropathy: estimation of number of embryonic precursor cells and disease threshold in heterozygous affected females at the X-linked locus. Clin Genet. 1992;42:143–8.
37. Hudson G, Keers S, Yu-Wai-Man P, Griffiths P, Huoponen K, Savontaus ML, Nikoskelainen E, Zeviani M, Carrara F, Horvath R, Karcagi V, Spruijt L, de Coo IF, Smeets HJ, Chinnery PF. Identification of an X-chromosomal locus and haplotype modulating the phenotype of a mitochondrial DNA disorder. Am J Hum Genet. 2005;77:1086–91.
38. Shankar SP, Fingert JH, Carelli V, Valentino ML, King TM, Daiger SP, Salomao SR, Berezovsky A, Belfort R Jr, Braun TA, Sheffield VC, Sadun AA, Stone EM. Evidence for a novel x-linked modifier locus for leber hereditary optic neuropathy. Ophthalmic Genet. 2008;29:17–24.
39. Ji Y, Jia X, Li S, Xiao X, Guo X, Zhang Q. Evaluation of the X-linked modifier loci for Leber hereditary optic neuropathy with the G11778A mutation in Chinese. Mol Vis. 2010;16:416–24.
40. Pegoraro E, Carelli V, Zeviani M, Cortelli P, Montagna P, Barboni P, Angelini C, Hoffman EP. X-inactivation patterns in female Leber's hereditary optic neuropathy patients do not support a strong X-linked determinant. Am J Med Genet. 1996;61:356–62.
41. Pegoraro E, Vettori A, Valentino ML, Molon A, Mostacciuolo ML, Howell N, Carelli V. X-inactivation pattern in multiple tissues from two Leber's hereditary optic neuropathy (LHON) patients. Am J Med Genet A. 2003;119A:37–40.
42. Hudson G, Carelli V, Horvath R, Zeviani M, Smeets HJ, Chinnery PF. X-inactivation patterns in females harboring mtDNA mutations that cause Leber hereditary optic neuropathy. Mol Vis. 2007;13:2339–43.
43. Giordano C, Montopoli M, Perli E, Orlandi M, Fantin M, Ross-Cisneros FN, Caparrotta L, Martinuzzi A, Ragazzi E, Ghelli A, Sadun AA, d'Amati G, Carelli V. Oestrogens ameliorate mitochondrial dysfunction in Leber's hereditary optic neuropathy. Brain. 2011;134:220–34.
44. Giordano C, Iommarini L, Giordano L, Maresca A, Pisano A, Valentino ML, Caporali L, Liguori R, Deceglie S, Roberti M, Fanelli F, Fracasso F, Ross-Cisneros FN, D'Adamo P, Hudson G, Pyle A, Yu-Wai-Man P, Chinnery PF, Zeviani M, Salomao SR, Berezovsky A, Belfort R Jr, Ventura DF, Moraes M, Moraes Filho M, Barboni P, Sadun F, De Negri A, Sadun AA, Tancredi A, Mancini M, d'Amati G, Loguercio Polosa P, Cantatore P, Carelli V. Efficient mitochondrial biogenesis drives incomplete penetrance in Leber's hereditary optic neuropathy. Brain. 2014;137:335–53.

45. Bianco A, Martínez-Romero I, Bisceglia L, D'Agruma L, Favia P, Ruiz-Pesini E, Guerriero S, Montoya J, Petruzzella V. Mitochondrial DNA copy number differentiates the Leber's hereditary optic neuropathy affected individuals from the unaffected mutation carriers. Brain. 2016;139:e1.
46. Sadun AA, Carelli V, Salomao SR, Berezovsky A, Quiros PA, Sadun F, DeNegri AM, Andrade R, Moraes M, Passos A, Kjaer P, Pereira J, Valentino ML, Schein S, Belfort R. Extensive investigation of a large Brazilian pedigree of 11778/haplogroup J Leber hereditary optic neuropathy. Am J Ophthalmol. 2003;136:231–8.
47. Kirkman MA, Yu-Wai-Man P, Korsten A, Leonhardt M, Dimitriadis K, De Coo IF, Klopstock T, Chinnery PF. Gene-environment interactions in Leber hereditary optic neuropathy. Brain. 2009;132:2317–26.
48. Giordano L, Deceglie S, d'Adamo P, Valentino ML, La Morgia C, Fracasso F, Roberti M, Cappellari M, Petrosillo G, Ciaravolo S, Parente D, Giordano C, Maresca A, Iommarini L, Del Dotto V, Ghelli AM, Salomao SR, Berezovsky A, Belfort R Jr, Sadun AA, Carelli V, Loguercio Polosa P, Cantatore P. Cigarette toxicity triggers Leber's hereditary optic neuropathy by affecting mtDNA copy number, oxidative phosphorylation and ROS detoxification pathways. Cell Death Dis. 2015;6:e2021.
49. Carelli V, d'Adamo P, Valentino ML, La Morgia C, Ross-Cisneros FN, Caporali L, Maresca A, Loguercio Polosa P, Barboni P, De Negri A, Sadun F, Karanjia R, Salomao SR, Berezovsky A, Chicani F, Moraes M, Moraes Filho M, Belfort R Jr, Sadun AA. Parsing the differences in affected with LHON: genetic versus environmental triggers of disease conversion. Brain. 2016;139:e17.
50. Yu-Wai-Man P, Hudson G, Klopstock T, Chinnery PF. Reply: parsing the differences in affected with LHON: genetic versus environmental triggers of disease conversion. Brain. 2016;139:e18.
51. Dimitriadis K, Leonhardt M, Yu-Wai-Man P, Kirkman MA, Korsten A, De Coo IF, Chinnery PF, Klopstock T. Leber's hereditary optic neuropathy with late disease onset: clinical and molecular characteristics of 20 patients. Orphanet J Rare Dis. 2014;9:158.
52. Caporali L, Maresca A, Capristo M, Del Dotto V, Tagliavini F, Valentino ML, La Morgia C, Carelli V. Incomplete penetrance in mitochondrial optic neuropathies. Mitochondrion. 2017;36:130–7.
53. Phasukkijwatana N, Kunhapan B, Stankovich J, Chuenkongkaew WL, Thomson R, Thornton T, Bahlo M, Mushiroda T, Nakamura Y, Mahasirimongkol S, Tun AW, Srisawat C, Limwongse C, Peerapittayamongkol C, Sura T, Suthammarak W, Lertrit P. Genome-wide linkage scan and association study of PARL to the expression of LHON families in Thailand. Hum Genet. 2010;128:39–49.
54. Istikharah R, Tun AW, Kaewsutthi S, Aryal P, Kunhapan B, Katanyoo W, Chuenkongkaew W, Lertrit P. Identification of the variants in PARL, the nuclear modifier gene, responsible for the expression of LHON patients in Thailand. Exp Eye Res. 2013;116:55–7.
55. Jiang P, Jin X, Peng Y, Wang M, Liu H, Liu X, Zhang Z, Ji Y, Zhang J, Liang M, Zhao F, Sun YH, Zhang M, Zhou X, Chen Y, Mo JQ, Huang T, Qu J, Guan MX. The exome sequencing identified the mutation in YARS2 encoding the mitochondrial tyrosyl-tRNA synthetase as a nuclear modifier for the phenotypic manifestation of Leber's hereditary optic neuropathy-associated mitochondrial DNA mutation. Hum Mol Genet. 2016;25:584–96.
56. Zhang AM, Jia X, Zhang Q, Yao YG. No association between the SNPs (rs3749446 and rs1402000) in the PARL gene and LHON in Chinese patients with m.11778G>A. Hum Genet. 2010;128:465–8.
57. Carelli V, Achilli A, Valentino ML, Rengo C, Semino O, Pala M, Olivieri A, Mattiazzi M, Pallotti F, Carrara F, Zeviani M, Leuzzi V, Carducci C, Valle G, Simionati B, Mendieta L, Salomao S, Belfort R Jr, Sadun AA, Torroni A. Haplogroup effects and recombination of mitochondrial DNA: novel clues from the analysis of Leber hereditary optic neuropathy pedigrees. Am J Hum Genet. 2006;78:564–74.
58. Hudson G, Carelli V, Spruijt L, Gerards M, Mowbray C, Achilli A, Pyle A, Elson J, Howell N, La Morgia C, Valentino ML, Huoponen K, Savontaus ML, Nikoskelainen E, Sadun AA, Salomao SR, Belfort R Jr, Griffiths P, Yu-Wai-Man P, de Coo RF, Horvath R, Zeviani M, Smeets HJ, Torroni A, Chinnery PF. Clinical expression of Leber hereditary optic neuropathy is affected by the mitochondrial DNA-haplogroup background. Am J Hum Genet. 2007;81:228–33.
59. Yang J, Zhu Y, Chen L, Zhang H, Tong Y, Huang D, Zhang Z, Chen S, Han X, Ma X. Novel A14841G mutation is associated with high penetrance of LHON/C4171A family. Biochem Biophys Res Commun. 2009;386:693–6.
60. Yang J, Zhu Y, Tong Y, Zhang Z, Chen L, Chen S, Cao Z, Liu C, Xu J, Ma X. The novel G10680A mutation is associated with complete penetrance of the LHON/T14484C family. Mitochondrion. 2009;9:273–8.
61. King MP, Attardi G. Human cells lacking mtDNA: repopulation with exogenous mitochondria by complementation. Science. 1989;246:500–3.
62. Lin CS, Sharpley MS, Fan W, Waymire KG, Sadun AA, Carelli V, Ross-Cisneros FN, Baciu P, Sung E, McManus MJ, Pan BX, Gil DW, Macgregor GR, Wallace DC. Mouse mtDNA mutant model of Leber hereditary optic neuropathy. Proc Natl Acad Sci U S A. 2012;109:20065–70.
63. Klopstock T, Yu-Wai-Man P, Dimitriadis K, Rouleau J, Heck S, Bailie M, Atawan A, Chattopadhyay S, Schubert M, Garip A, Kernt M, Petraki D, Rummey C, Leinonen M, Metz G, Griffiths PG, Meier T, Chinnery PF. A randomized placebo-controlled trial of idebenone in Leber's hereditary optic neuropathy. Brain. 2011;134:2677–86.

64. Carelli V, La Morgia C, Valentino ML, Rizzo G, Carbonelli M, De Negri AM, Sadun F, Carta A, Guerriero S, Simonelli F, Sadun AA, Aggarwal D, Liguori R, Avoni P, Baruzzi A, Zeviani M, Montagna P, Barboni P. Idebenone treatment in Leber's hereditary optic neuropathy. Brain. 2011;134:e188.
65. Guy J, Qi X, Pallotti F, Schon EA, Manfredi G, Carelli V, Martinuzzi A, Hauswirth WW, Lewin AS. Rescue of a mitochondrial deficiency causing Leber hereditary optic neuropathy. Ann Neurol. 2002;52:534–42.
66. Kjer P. Infantile optic atrophy with dominant mode of inheritance: a clinical and genetic study of 19 Danish families. Acta Ophthalmol Scand. 1959;37:1–146.
67. Lenaers G, Hamel C, Delettre C, Amati-Bonneau P, Procaccio V, Bonneau D, Reynier P, Milea D. Dominant optic atrophy. Orphanet J Rare Dis. 2012;7:46.
68. Newman NJ. Dominant optic atrophy. In: Miller NR, Newman NJ, editors. Walsh and Hoyt's clinical neuro-ophthalmology. Baltimore, MD: Williams & Wilkins; 1998. p. 753–6.
69. Toomes C, Marchbank NJ, Mackey DA, Craig JE, Newbury-Ecob RA, Bennett CP, Vize CJ, Desai SP, Black GC, Patel N, Teimory M, Markham AF, Inglehearn CF, Churchill AJ. Spectrum, frequency and penetrance of OPA1 mutations in dominant optic atrophy. Hum Mol Genet. 2001;10:1369–78.
70. Cohn AC, Toomes C, Potter C, Towns KV, Hewitt AW, Inglehearn CF, Craig JE, Mackey DA. Autosomal dominant optic atrophy: penetrance and expressivity in patients with OPA1 mutations. Am J Ophthalmol. 2007;143:656–62.
71. Treft RL, Sanborn GE, Carey J, Swartz M, Crisp D, Wester DC, Creel D. Dominant optic atrophy, deafness, ptosis, ophthalmoplegia, dystaxia, and myopathy. A new syndrome. Ophthalmology. 1984;91:908–15.
72. Meire F, De Laey JJ, de Bie S, van Staey M, Matton MT. Dominant optic nerve atrophy with progressive hearing loss and chronic progressive external ophthalmoplegia (CPEO). Ophthalmic Paediatr Genet. 1985;5:91–7.
73. Yu-Wai-Man P, Griffiths PG, Gorman GS, Lourenco CM, Wright AF, Auer-Grumbach M, Toscano A, Musumeci O, Valentino ML, Caporali L, Lamperti C, Tallaksen CM, Duffey P, Miller J, Whittaker RG, Baker MR, Jackson MJ, Clarke MP, Dhillon B, Czermin B, Stewart JD, Hudson G, Reynier P, Bonneau D, Marques W Jr, Lenaers G, McFarland R, Taylor RW, Turnbull DM, Votruba M, Zeviani M, Carelli V, Bindoff LA, Horvath R, Amati-Bonneau P, Chinnery PF. Multi-system neurological disease is common in patients with OPA1 mutations. Brain. 2010;133:771–86.
74. MacVicar T, Langer T. OPA1 processing in cell death and disease - the long and short of it. J Cell Sci. 2016;129:2297–306.
75. Del Dotto V, Fogazza M, Carelli V, Rugolo M, Zanna C. Eight human OPA1 isoforms, long and short: what are they for? Biochim Biophys Acta Bioenerg. 1859;2018:263–9.
76. Frezza C, Cipolat S, Martins de Brito O, Micaroni M, Beznoussenko GV, Rudka T, Bartoli D, Polishuck RS, Danial NN, De Strooper B, Scorrano L. OPA1 controls apoptotic cristae remodeling independently from mitochondrial fusion. Cell. 2006;126:177–89.
77. Cipolat S, Rudka T, Hartmann D, Costa V, Serneels L, Craessaerts K, Metzger K, Frezza C, Annaert W, D'Adamio L, Derks C, Dejaegere T, Pellegrini L, D'Hooge R, Scorrano L, De Strooper B. Mitochondrial rhomboid PARL regulates cytochrome c release during apoptosis via OPA1-dependent cristae remodeling. Cell. 2006;126:163–75.
78. Olichon A, Elachouri G, Baricault L, Delettre C, Belenguer P, Lenaers G. OPA1 alternate splicing uncouples an evolutionary conserved function in mitochondrial fusion from a vertebrate restricted function in apoptosis. Cell Death Differ. 2007;14:682–92.
79. Mishra P, Carelli V, Manfredi G, Chan DC. Proteolytic cleavage of Opa1 stimulates mitochondrial inner membrane fusion and couples fusion to oxidative phosphorylation. Cell Metab. 2014;19:630–41.
80. Cogliati S, Frezza C, Soriano ME, Varanita T, Quintana-Cabrera R, Corrado M, Cipolat S, Costa V, Casarin A, Gomes LC, Perales-Clemente E, Salviati L, Fernandez-Silva P, Enriquez JA, Scorrano L. Mitochondrial cristae shape determines respiratory chain supercomplexes assembly and respiratory efficiency. Cell. 2013;155:160–71.
81. Amati-Bonneau P, Valentino ML, Reynier P, Gallardo ME, Bornstein B, Boissière A, Campos Y, Rivera H, de la Aleja JG, Carroccia R, Iommarini L, Labauge P, Figarella-Branger D, Marcorelles P, Furby A, Beauvais K, Letournel F, Liguori R, La Morgia C, Montagna P, Liguori M, Zanna C, Rugolo M, Cossarizza A, Wissinger B, Verny C, Schwarzenbacher R, Martín MA, Arenas J, Ayuso C, Garesse R, Lenaers G, Bonneau D, Carelli V. OPA1 mutations induce mitochondrial DNA instability and optic atrophy 'plus' phenotypes. Brain. 2008;131:338–51.
82. Elachouri G, Vidoni S, Zanna C, Pattyn A, Boukhaddaoui H, Gaget K, Yu-Wai-Man P, Gasparre G, Sarzi E, Delettre C, Olichon A, Loiseau D, Reynier P, Chinnery PF, Rotig A, Carelli V, Hamel CP, Rugolo M, Lenaers G. OPA1 links human mitochondrial genome maintenance to mtDNA replication and distribution. Genome Res. 2011;21:12–20.
83. Rouzier C, Bannwarth S, Chaussenot A, Chevrollier A, Verschueren A, Bonello-Palot N, Fragaki K, Cano A, Pouget J, Pellissier JF, Procaccio V, Chabrol B, Paquis-Flucklinger V. The MFN2 gene is responsible for mitochondrial DNA instability and optic atrophy 'plus' phenotype. Brain. 2012;135:23–34.
84. Gerber S, Charif M, Chevrollier A, Chaumette T, Angebault C, Kane MS, Paris A, Alban J, Quiles M, Delettre C, Bonneau D, Procaccio V, Amati-Bonneau P, Reynier P, Leruez S, Calmon R, Boddaert N, Funalot B, Rio M, Bouccara D, Meunier I, Sesaki H, Kaplan J, Hamel CP, Rozet JM, Lenaers G. Mutations in DNM1L, as in OPA1, result in dominant optic atrophy despite opposite effects on mitochondrial fusion and fission. Brain. 2017;140:2586–96.

85. Reynier P, Amati-Bonneau P, Verny C, Olichon A, Simard G, Guichet A, Bonnemains C, Malecaze F, Malinge MC, Pelletier JB, Calvas P, Dollfus H, Belenguer P, Malthièry Y, Lenaers G, Bonneau D. OPA3 gene mutations responsible for autosomal dominant optic atrophy and cataract. J Med Genet. 2004;41:e110.
86. Ryu SW, Jeong HJ, Choi M, Karbowski M, Choi C. Optic atrophy 3 as a protein of the mitochondrial outer membrane induces mitochondrial fragmentation. Cell Mol Life Sci. 2010;67:2839–50.
87. Klebe S, Depienne C, Gerber S, Challe G, Anheim M, Charles P, Fedirko E, Lejeune E, Cottineau J, Brusco A, Dollfus H, Chinnery PF, Mancini C, Ferrer X, Sole G, Destée A, Mayer JM, Fontaine B, de Seze J, Clanet M, Ollagnon E, Busson P, Cazeneuve C, Stevanin G, Kaplan J, Rozet JM, Brice A, Durr A. Spastic paraplegia gene 7 in patients with spasticity and/or optic neuropathy. Brain. 2012;135:2980–93.
88. Charif M, Roubertie A, Salime S, Mamouni S, Goizet C, Hamel CP, Lenaers G. A novel mutation of AFG3L2 might cause dominant optic atrophy in patients with mild intellectual disability. Front Genet. 2015;6:311.
89. Colavito D, Maritan V, Suppiej A, Del Giudice E, Mazzarolo M, Miotto S, Farina S, Dalle Carbonare M, Piermarocchi S, Leon A. Non-syndromic isolated dominant optic atrophy caused by the p.R468C mutation in the AFG3 like matrix AAA peptidase subunit 2 gene. Biomed Rep. 2017;7:451–4.
90. Martinelli P, Rugarli EI. Emerging roles of mitochondrial proteases in neurodegeneration. Biochim Biophys Acta. 1797;2010:1–10.
91. Burté F, Carelli V, Chinnery PF, Yu-Wai-Man P. Disturbed mitochondrial dynamics and neurodegenerative disorders. Nat Rev Neurol. 2015;11:11–24.
92. Han J, Thompson-Lowrey AJ, Reiss A, Mayorov V, Jia H, Biousse V, Newman NJ, Brown MD. OPA1 mutations and mitochondrial DNA haplotypes in autosomal dominant optic atrophy. Genet Med. 2006;8:217–25.
93. Pierron D, Ferré M, Rocher C, Chevrollier A, Murail P, Thoraval D, Amati-Bonneau P, Reynier P, Letellier T. OPA1-related dominant optic atrophy is not strongly influenced by mitochondrial DNA background. BMC Med Genet. 2009;10:70.
94. Barboni P, Carbonelli M, Savini G, Foscarini B, Parisi V, Valentino ML, Carta A, De Negri A, Sadun F, Zeviani M, Sadun AA, Schimpf S, Wissinger B, Carelli V. OPA1 mutations associated with dominant optic atrophy influence optic nerve head size. Ophthalmology. 2010;117:1547–53.
95. Ramos Cdo V, Bellusci C, Savini G, Carbonelli M, Berezovsky A, Tamaki C, Cinoto R, Sacai PY, Moraes-Filho MN, Miura HM, Valentino ML, Iommarini L, De Negri AM, Sadun F, Cortelli P, Montagna P, Salomao SR, Sadun AA, Carelli V, Barboni P. Association of optic disc size with development and prognosis of Leber's hereditary optic neuropathy. Invest Ophthalmol Vis Sci. 2009;50:1666–74.
96. Robinson BH, Petrova-Benedict R, Buncic JR, Wallace DC. Nonviability of cells with oxidative defects in galactose medium: a screening test for affected patient fibroblasts. Biochem Med Metab Biol. 1992;48:122–6.
97. Chevrollier A, Guillet V, Loiseau D, Gueguen N, de Crescenzo MA, Verny C, Ferre M, Dollfus H, Odent S, Milea D, Goizet C, Amati-Bonneau P, Procaccio V, Bonneau D, Reynier P. Hereditary optic neuropathies share a common mitochondrial coupling defect. Ann Neurol. 2008;63:794–8.
98. Zanna C, Ghelli A, Porcelli AM, Karbowski M, Youle RJ, Schimpf S, Wissinger B, Pinti M, Cossarizza A, Vidoni S, Valentino ML, Rugolo M, Carelli V. OPA1 mutations associated with dominant optic atrophy impair oxidative phosphorylation and mitochondrial fusion. Brain. 2008;131:352–67.
99. Agier V, Oliviero P, Lainé J, L'Hermitte-Stead C, Girard S, Fillaut S, Jardel C, Bouillaud F, Bulteau AL, Lombès A. Defective mitochondrial fusion, altered respiratory function, and distorted cristae structure in skin fibroblasts with heterozygous OPA1 mutations. Biochim Biophys Acta. 1822;2012:1570–80.
100. Yarosh W, Monserrate J, Tong JJ, Tse S, Le PK, Nguyen K, Brachmann CB, Wallace DC, Huang T. The molecular mechanisms of OPA1-mediated optic atrophy in Drosophila model and prospects for antioxidant treatment. PLoS Genet. 2008;4:e6.
101. Barboni P, Valentino ML, La Morgia C, Carbonelli M, Savini G, De Negri A, Simonelli F, Sadun F, Caporali L, Maresca A, Liguori R, Baruzzi A, Zeviani M, Carelli V. Idebenone treatment in patients with OPA1-mutant dominant optic atrophy. Brain. 2013;136:e231.
102. Alavi MV, Bette S, Schimpf S, Schuettauf F, Schraermeyer U, Wehrl HF, Ruttiger L, Beck SC, Tonagel F, Pichler BJ, Knipper M, Peters T, Laufs J, Wissinger B. A splice site mutation in the murine Opa1 gene features pathology of autosomal dominant optic atrophy. Brain. 2007;130:1029–42.
103. Davies VJ, Hollins AJ, Piechota MJ, Yip W, Davies JR, White KE, Nicols PP, Boulton ME, Votruba M. Opa1 deficiency in a mouse model of autosomal dominant optic atrophy impairs mitochondrial morphology, optic nerve structure and visual function. Hum Mol Genet. 2007;16:1307–18.
104. White KE, Davies VJ, Hogan VE, Piechota MJ, Nichols PP, Turnbull DM, Votruba M. OPA1 deficiency associated with increased autophagy in retinal ganglion cells in a murine model of dominant optic atrophy. Invest Ophthalmol Vis Sci. 2009;50:2567–71.
105. Carelli V, Musumeci O, Caporali L, Zanna C, La Morgia C, Del Dotto V, Porcelli AM, Rugolo M, Valentino ML, Iommarini L, Maresca A, Barboni P, Carbonelli M, Trombetta C, Valente EM, Patergnani S, Giorgi C, Pinton P, Rizzo G, Tonon C, Lodi R, Avoni P, Liguori R, Baruzzi A, Toscano A, Zeviani M. Syndromic parkinsonism and dementia

associated with OPA1 missense mutations. Ann Neurol. 2015;78:21–38.
106. Liao C, Ashley N, Diot A, Morten K, Phadwal K, Williams A, Fearnley I, Rosser L, Lowndes J, Fratter C, Ferguson DJ, Vay L, Quaghebeur G, Moroni I, Bianchi S, Lamperti C, Downes SM, Sitarz KS, Flannery PJ, Carver J, Dombi E, East D, Laura M, Reilly MM, Mortiboys H, Prevo R, Campanella M, Daniels MJ, Zeviani M, Yu-Wai-Man P, Simon AK, Votruba M, Poulton J. Dysregulated mitophagy and mitochondrial organization in optic atrophy due to OPA1 mutations. Neurology. 2017;88:131–42.
107. Williams PA, Morgan JE, Votruba M. Opa1 deficiency in a mouse model of dominant optic atrophy leads to retinal ganglion cell dendropathy. Brain. 2010;133:2942–51.
108. Williams PA, Piechota M, von Ruhland C, Taylor E, Morgan JE, Votruba M. Opa1 is essential for retinal ganglion cell synaptic architecture and connectivity. Brain. 2012;135:493–505.
109. Li Z, Okamoto K, Hayashi Y, Sheng M. The importance of dendritic mitochondria in the morphogenesis and plasticity of spines and synapses. Cell. 2004;119:873–87.
110. Sarzi E, Angebault C, Seveno M, Gueguen N, Chaix B, Bielicki G, Boddaert N, Mausset-Bonnefont AL, Cazevieille C, Rigau V, Renou JP, Wang J, Delettre C, Brabet P, Puel JL, Hamel CP, Reynier P, Lenaers G. The human OPA1delTTAG mutation induces premature age-related systemic neurodegeneration in mouse. Brain. 2012;135:3599–613.
111. Del Dotto V, Mishra P, Vidoni S, Fogazza M, Maresca A, Caporali L, McCaffery JM, Cappelletti M, Baruffini E, Lenaers G, Chan D, Rugolo M, Carelli V, Zanna C. OPA1 isoforms in the hierarchical organization of mitochondrial functions. Cell Rep. 2017;19:2557–71.
112. Del Dotto V, Fogazza M, Lenaers G, Rugolo M, Carelli V, Zanna C. OPA1: how much do we know to approach therapy? Pharmacol Res. 2018;131:199–210.
113. Sarzi E, Seveno M, Piro-Mégy C, Elzière L, Quilès M, Péquignot M, Müller A, Hamel CP, Lenaers G, Delettre C. OPA1 gene therapy prevents retinal ganglion cell loss in a dominant optic atrophy mouse model. Sci Rep. 2018;8:2468.
114. Civiletto G, Varanita T, Cerutti R, Gorletta T, Barbaro S, Marchet S, Lamperti C, Viscomi C, Scorrano L, Zeviani M. Opa1 overexpression ameliorates the phenotype of two mitochondrial disease mouse models. Cell Metab. 2015;21:845–54.
115. Varanita T, Soriano ME, Romanello V, Zaglia T, Quintana-Cabrera R, Semenzato M, Menabò R, Costa V, Civiletto G, Pesce P, Viscomi C, Zeviani M, Di Lisa F, Mongillo M, Sandri M, Scorrano L. The OPA1-dependent mitochondrial cristae remodeling pathway controls atrophic, apoptotic, and ischemic tissue damage. Cell Metab. 2015;21:834–44.
116. Iannielli A, Bido S, Folladori L, Segnali A, Cancellieri C, Maresca A, Massimino L, Rubio A, Morabito G, Caporali L, Tagliavini F, Musumeci O, Gregato G, Bezard E, Carelli V, Tiranti V, Broccoli V. Pharmacological inhibition of necroptosis protects from dopaminergic neuronal cell death in Parkinson's disease models. Cell Rep. 2018;22:2066–79.
117. Barbet F, Gerber S, Hakiki S, Perrault I, Hanein S, Ducroq D, Tanguy G, Dufier JL, Munnich A, Rozet JM, et al. A first locus for isolated autosomal recessive optic atrophy (ROA1) maps to chromosome 8q. Eur J Hum Genet. 2003;11:966–71.
118. Hanein S, Perrault I, Roche O, Gerber S, Khadom N, Rio M, Boddaert N, Jean-Pierre M, Brahimi N, Serre V, Chretien D, Delphin N, Fares-Taie L, Lachheb S, Rotig A, Meire F, Munnich A, Dufier JL, Kaplan J, Rozet JM. TMEM126A, encoding a mitochondrial protein, is mutated in autosomal-recessive nonsyndromic optic atrophy. Am J Hum Genet. 2009;84:493–8.
119. Metodiev MD, Gerber S, Hubert L, Delahodde A, Chretien D, Gérard X, Amati-Bonneau P, Giacomotto MC, Boddaert N, Kaminska A, Desguerre I, Amiel J, Rio M, Kaplan J, Munnich A, Rötig A, Rozet JM, Besmond C. Mutations in the tricarboxylic acid cycle enzyme, aconitase 2, cause either isolated or syndromic optic neuropathy with encephalopathy and cerebellar atrophy. J Med Genet. 2014;51:834–8.
120. Angebault C, Guichet PO, Talmat-Amar Y, Charif M, Gerber S, Fares-Taie L, Gueguen N, Halloy F, Moore D, Amati-Bonneau P, Manes G, Hebrard M, Bocquet B, Quiles M, Piro-Mégy C, Teigell M, Delettre C, Rossel M, Meunier I, Preising M, Lorenz B, Carelli V, Chinnery PF, Yu-Wai-Man P, Kaplan J, Roubertie A, Barakat A, Bonneau D, Reynier P, Rozet JM, Bomont P, Hamel CP, Lenaers G. Recessive mutations in RTN4IP1 cause isolated and syndromic optic neuropathies. Am J Hum Genet. 2015;97:754–60.
121. Hartmann B, Wai T, Hu H, MacVicar T, Musante L, Fischer-Zirnsak B, Stenzel W, Gräf R, van den Heuvel L, Ropers HH, Wienker TF, Hübner C, Langer T, Kaindl AM. Homozygous YME1L1 mutation causes mitochondriopathy with optic atrophy and mitochondrial network fragmentation. Elife. 2016;5. pii: e16078
122. Hanein S, Garcia M, Fares-Taie L, Serre V, De Keyzer Y, Delaveau T, Perrault I, Delphin N, Gerber S, Schmitt A, Masse JM, Munnich A, Kaplan J, Devaux F, Rozet JM. TMEM126A is a mitochondrial located mRNA (MLR) protein of the mitochondrial inner membrane. Biochim Biophys Acta. 1830;2013:3719–33.
123. Hu WH, Hausmann ON, Yan MS, Walters WM, Wong PK, Bethea JR. Identification and characterization of a novel Nogo-interacting mitochondrial protein (NIMP). J Neurochem. 2002;81:36–45.
124. Behr C. Die komplizierte, hereditaer familiaere Optikusatrophie des Kindesalters. Ein bisher nicht beschriebener Symptomcomplex Klin Monatsbl Augenheilkd. 1909;47:138.

125. Costeff H, Gadoth N, Apter N, Prialnic M, Savir H. A familial syndrome of infantile optic atrophy, movement disorder, and spastic paraplegia. Neurology. 1989;39:595–7.
126. Bonneau D, Colin E, Oca F, Ferré M, Chevrollier A, Guéguen N, Desquiret-Dumas V, N'Guyen S, Barth M, Zanlonghi X, Rio M, Desguerre I, Barnerias C, Momtchilova M, Rodriguez D, Slama A, Lenaers G, Procaccio V, Amati-Bonneau P, Reynier P. Early-onset Behr syndrome due to compound heterozygous mutations in OPA1. Brain. 2014;137:e301.
127. Carelli V, Sabatelli M, Carrozzo R, Rizza T, Schimpf S, Wissinger B, Zanna C, Rugolo M, La Morgia C, Caporali L, Carbonelli M, Barboni P, Tonon C, Lodi R, Bertini E. 'Behr syndrome' with OPA1 compound heterozygote mutations. Brain. 2015;138:e321.
128. Anikster Y, Kleta R, Shaag A, Gahl WA, Elpeleg O. Type III 3-methylglutaconic aciduria (optic atrophy plus syndrome, or Costeff optic atrophy syndrome): identification of the OPA3 gene and its founder mutation in Iraqi Jews. Am J Hum Genet. 2001;69:1218–24.
129. Assink JJ, Tijmes NT, ten Brink JB, Oostra RJ, Riemslag FC, de Jong PT, Bergen AA. A gene for X-linked optic atrophy is closely linked to the Xp11.4-Xp11.2 region of the X chromosome. Am J Hum Genet. 1997;61:934–9.
130. Katz BJ, Zhao Y, Warner JE, Tong Z, Yang Z, Zhang K. A family with X-linked optic atrophy linked to the OPA2 locus Xp11.4-Xp11.2. Am J Med Genet A. 2006;140:2207–11.
131. Ha AD, Parratt KL, Rendtorff ND, Lodahl M, Ng K, Rowe DB, Sue CM, Hayes MW, Tranebjaerg L, Fung VS. The phenotypic spectrum of dystonia in Mohr-Tranebjaerg syndrome. Mov Disord. 2012 Jul;27(8):1034–40.
132. Hashimoto M, Bacman SR, Peralta S, Falk MJ, Chomyn A, Chan DC, Williams SL, Moraes CT. MitoTALEN: a general approach to reduce mutant mtDNA loads and restore oxidative phosphorylation function in mitochondrial diseases. Mol Ther. 2015;23:1592–9.
133. Gammage PA, Van Haute L, Minczuk M. Engineered mtZFNs for manipulation of human mitochondrial DNA heteroplasmy. Methods Mol Biol. 2016;1351:145–62.
134. Gammage PA, Moraes CT, Minczuk M. Mitochondrial genome engineering: the revolution may not be CRISPR-Ized. Trends Genet. 2018;34:101–10.

Mitochondrial Myopathies, Chronic Progressive External Ophthalmoparesis, and Kearns-Sayre Syndrome

Thomas Klopstock and Michelangelo Mancuso

Introduction

Myopathy manifesting as exercise intolerance or as overt muscle weakness is a common symptom in mitochondrial diseases. It can be the only or the most prominent clinical feature, or be associated with additional "mitochondrial red flag" manifestations [1]. In 2017, a consortium of international experts defined primary mitochondrial myopathies (PMM) as genetically determined disorders leading to defects of oxidative phosphorylation affecting predominantly, but not exclusively, skeletal muscle [2].

The most common presentation of PMM is chronic progressive external ophthalmoparesis (CPEO or PEO) characterized by a predominant affection of external eye muscles. If PEO is accompanied by extramuscular mitochondrial signs, it is often designated PEO plus. A particularly severe form of PEO plus is Kearns-Sayre syndrome (KSS), which was historically defined by the early onset of PEO before age 20 years, pigmentary retinopathy, and at least one of the following: cerebellar ataxia, cardiac conduction block, or cerebrospinal fluid protein levels >0.1 g/L [3]. Isolated mitochondrial myopathy (MiMy), without affection of extraocular muscles, is much rarer than PEO, and—for the lack of red flags—more difficult to diagnose.

Here we provide a comprehensive overview on historical aspects, clinical features, genetic background, and therapeutic options in MiMy, PEO, and KSS.

T. Klopstock (✉)
Department of Neurology, Friedrich-Baur-Institute, Ludwig-Maximilians-University of Munich, Munich, Germany

German Center for Neurodegenerative Diseases (DZNE), Munich, Germany

Munich Cluster for Systems Neurology (SyNergy), Munich, Germany
e-mail: Thomas.Klopstock@med.LMU.de

M. Mancuso
Department of Clinical and Experimental Medicine, Neurological Institute, University of Pisa, Pisa, Italy

Historical Aspects

A syndrome of progressive weakness of the external eye muscles with ptosis was first described in 1856 by Albrecht von Graefe (1828–1870), a renowned German ophthalmologist [4] who—by the way—also provided the first description of Leber's hereditary optic neuropathy [5] (LHON, cf. chapter "Mitochondrial Optic Neuropathies"). The first report on this syndrome in the Anglo-Saxon literature followed more than 20 years later under the name "ophthalmoplegia externa" [6]. In the following decades, a scholarly dispute developed over the question of whether the ophthalmoplegia was a primary myopathy of the eye muscles or a primary neuropathy of the oculomotor nerves. In 1951, Kiloh

M. Mancuso, T. Klopstock (eds.), *Diagnosis and Management of Mitochondrial Disorders*,
https://doi.org/10.1007/978-3-030-05517-2_9

and Nevin summarized the previously published cases in a much-noticed essay and judged that the neuronal changes found were too small to explain pronounced ophthalmoplegia [7]. On the basis of biopsies of eye and limb muscles, they favored the myopathy hypothesis and introduced the term "ocular myopathy." From a today's perspective, it is likely that these early descriptions comprise not only cases of mitochondrial CPEO but also cases of oculopharyngeal muscular dystrophy (OPMD), two disorders of rather similar phenotype which can only be discriminated by twentieth-century methods of muscle morphology and genetics [8].

In 1958, Kearns and Sayre described two patients with the clinical triad of "retinitis pigmentosa, external ophthalmoplegia, and complete AV block," thus the title of their famous publication [3]. Berenberg et al. suggested in 1977 to name the syndrome Kearns-Sayre syndrome (KSS) and proposed the following diagnostic criteria: external ophthalmoplegia, "atypical" retinitis pigmentosa, and onset before the age of 20 plus one of the following symptoms: cardiac conduction disorder, CSF protein >1 g/L, or ataxia [9].

Many patients have symptoms beyond CPEO without meeting the definition of KSS. This was already recognized by Drachman in 1968 who coined the term "ophthalmoplegia plus" for these cases [10]. Later, Bastiaensen refined the use of this term to designate a disease with external ophthalmoplegia, muscle weakness, retinal pigment disorder, and other neurological and non-neurological manifestations caused by mitochondrial dysfunction [11]. Today, such cases are referred to as ophthalmoplegia plus or (C)PEO plus.

The term "mitochondrial myopathy" was formerly often used for the entirety of mitochondrial diseases. In view of the often multisystemic nature of mitochondrial diseases, this is obviously misleading. Today, the term "primary mitochondrial myopathies" (PMM) should be reserved for genetically determined disorders leading to defects of oxidative phosphorylation affecting predominantly, but not exclusively, skeletal muscle [2].

Clinical Features

CPEO is characterized by slowly progressive eyelid drooping (ptosis) and limitation of eye movements in all directions of gaze (ophthalmoparesis, ophthalmoplegia), cf. Fig. 1. Both ptosis and ophthalmoparesis are usually symmetric but there are exceptions to the point of unilateral involvement. Sometimes, ptosis may precede ophthalmoparesis for years [12], while ophthalmoparesis without ptosis is extremely rare. Internal eye muscles are always spared; that is, pupillary reactions are normal. To compensate for the impaired vision by the drooping eyelids, patients tend to innervate their frontalis muscle and recline their head. Previously, diplopia has been considered to be rare but numerous studies of PEO patients have found high rates of transient or constant diplopia [13], corresponding to

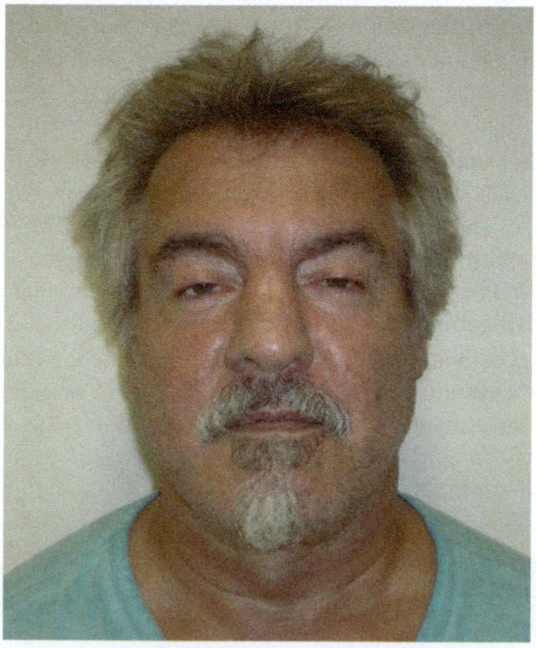

Fig. 1 56-Year-old patient with progressive ptosis, ophthalmoparesis, and diplopia from age 44 years. There was no family history of mitochondrial disease. Beyond eye muscle involvement, there was moderate exercise intolerance but no extramuscular symptoms. Muscle biopsy revealed multiple ragged red and COX-negative fibers as well as a single deletion of mtDNA, thus confirming the diagnosis of chronic progressive external ophthalmoparesis (CPEO)

asymmetric involvement of eyes. Many patients are able to avoid diplopia by facultative suppression, most probably because they have learned to do so over the long time course of ocular misalignment [13]. Interestingly, patients without diplopia are often not aware of their ophthalmoparesis, even if severe. One study found that only 8/45 (17.8%) patients with ophthalmoplegia on examination were aware of limited extraocular motility [14]. Obviously, these patients perfect their compensatory head movements during the long habituation process.

CPEO may be accompanied by other muscular symptoms like muscle weakness (42.9%), exercise intolerance (23.1%), and muscle wasting (17.5%) [15]. Myopathy predominantly affects the proximal hip and shoulder girdle muscles as well as the axial neck flexor muscles. Muscle weakness may also cause dysphagia and dysarthria due to oropharyngeal weakness, as well as respiratory failure.

If there are additional nonmuscular symptoms as part of the syndromic presentation of the patient, this is commonly designated as **CPEO plus**. The most common of these nonmuscular symptoms are ataxia (19.8%), hearing loss (15.3%), cognitive impairment (13.5%), seizures (7.5%), pyramidal signs (7.3%), and less frequently (<5%) tremor, stroke-like episodes, impaired consciousness, dystonia, microcephaly, nystagmus, myoclonus, and parkinsonism [15].

KSS has been defined historically (see above) but can ultimately be regarded as a particularly severe manifestation of CPEO plus by both etiology and phenomenology. The classical KSS definition comprises a triad of CPEO, pigmentary retinopathy, and onset before age 20 years plus at least one of the following symptoms: heart block, cerebellar syndrome, or cerebrospinal fluid protein above 100 mg/dl. Obviously, this historic definition brings along many inconsistencies and limitations: (1) age limit and protein levels are arbitrary; (2) multisystem clinical features strongly associated with KSS (for example hearing loss, failure to thrive, short stature, cognitive involvement, tremor, and cardiomyopathy) are excluded from the current criteria; and (3) there is a continuum from CPEO via CPEO plus to KSS. To overcome some of these limitations, the Italian Network of mitochondrial diseases in a large cohort of 228 patients tested simplified criteria for a newly defined category "KSS spectrum" (ptosis and/or ophthalmoparesis due to an mtDNA single large-scale deletion and at least one of the following: retinopathy, ataxia, cardiac conduction defects, hearing loss, failure to thrive/short stature, cognitive involvement, tremor, cardiomyopathy), as opposed to PEO (ptosis and/or ophthalmoparesis due to an mtDNA single large-scale deletion not fulfilling the new "KSS spectrum" criteria). In this view, "classic" KSS represents the most severe extreme of the KSS spectrum. With these new criteria, it was possible to classify nearly all single-deletion patients: 64.5% PEO, 31.6% KSS spectrum (including classic KSS 6.6%), and 2.6% Pearson syndrome [16].

While CPEO is the most frequent type of primary mitochondrial myopathies (PMM), there are also patients who manifest with myopathy without affection of extraocular muscles. This phenotype may be designated as isolated or pure mitochondrial myopathy (**MiMy**). Muscle involvement may manifest as permanent muscle weakness or as exercise-related symptoms, or both. If there is permanent muscle weakness, it shows the same characteristics as the axial and proximal limb myopathy in CPEO (see above). Exercise-related symptoms may include exercise intolerance, myalgia, fatigue, muscle cramps, and recurrent rhabdomyolysis with myoglobinuria. Again, there is a continuum between MiMy and CPEO (e.g., slowed saccades without overt limitation of eye movements) and also a continuum to multisystemic mitochondrial disease as MiMy may be accompanied by nonmuscular symptoms (MiMy plus).

PMM including MiMy, CPEO, and their plus forms may manifest at any age with a clear correlation of younger age of onset with the severity of the disorder. In early-onset forms, the phenotype is often dominated by hypotonia, floppy infant syndrome, failure to thrive, and respiratory insufficiency [17].

Prominent ophthalmoplegia is also found in other multisystemic mitochondrial diseases, some of them being discussed in separate chapters of this book, e.g., MELAS, MERRF, POLGopathies, OPA1-associated autosomal dominant optic atrophy, mitochondrial depletion syndromes, and MNGIE.

While we discussed mitochondrial CPEO so far in the context of genetic diseases, the same syndrome may rarely occur as a consequence of mitochondrial drug toxicity. This has been found in nucleoside reverse transcriptase inhibitor use for human immunodeficiency virus infection [18, 19], and a change in medications may halt progression or even reverse PEO [18]. HMG-CoA reductase inhibitors (statins) for hyperlipidemia have well-known systemic muscle toxicity. An investigation of 256 reports of ptosis, diplopia, and/or ophthalmoplegia associated with statin use found 62 cases of symptom resolution with drug cessation and 14 cases of symptom recurrence with drug reinitiation [20]. This led to a World Health Organization criteria-based conclusion that statin drugs can possibly cause ophthalmoparesis.

Differential Diagnosis of CPEO: Non-mitochondrial Look-Alikes

In the presence of ophthalmoparesis and ptosis, CPEO is one of the most likely and most frequent underlying disorders. The most important differential diagnosis is certainly ocular **myasthenia gravis** or generalized myasthenia with prominent ocular involvement, both because it is relatively frequent and amenable to treatment. The distinction of CPEO and myasthenia is rather straightforward, however. While both disorders show a predilection of extraocular muscles, the weakness is permanent in CPEO but marked by prominent diurnal and exercise-related fluctuations in myasthenia. Accordingly, reported diplopia and eye motility are stereotypical in CPEO but markedly variable in myasthenia. In addition, autoimmune myasthenia gravis is usually confirmed by the presence of acetylcholine receptor or other antibodies, a decrement in repetitive nerve stimulation, and a treatment response to acetylcholine esterase inhibitors, e.g., pyridostigmine, and/or corticosteroids. Of note, single-fiber EMG has no major role in the differential diagnosis, since both disorders show abnormal jitter [21]. There are two important exceptions to the strict and easy distinction of CPEO and myasthenia: (1) there may be a slight fatigue-induced deterioration of ptosis and eye motility in CPEO on top of the fixed muscle weakness, e.g., eyelid drooping or diplopia getting worse in the evening; this component may benefit from treatment with low-dose pyridostigmine; (2) hereditary, congenital forms of myasthenia often manifest with fixed weakness of extraocular muscles without diurnal fluctuations; this renders the phenotype virtually indistinguishable from CPEO, and if not by age of onset (congenital or early infantile in **congenital myasthenia**, mostly later in CPEO) the discrimination will require a muscle biopsy or genetic testing.

Another important differential diagnosis of therapeutic relevance is **thyroid-associated ophthalmopathy** (TAO, Graves' disease) which may also present with restricted extraocular motility and diplopia. Unlike CPEO, however, there is no ptosis but eyelid retraction in most cases. Moreover, TAO shows acute or subacute onset and progression, and is associated with orbital inflammatory signs including conjunctival swelling and redness, periocular edema, and proptosis [13]. On orbital MRI imaging, extraocular muscles are usually thickened in TAO as opposed to atrophic muscles in CPEO [22]. Laboratory tests and treatment response to corticosteroids are of further relevance in the differential diagnosis.

Ocular myositis can cause diffuse motility abnormalities but, unlike PEO, is associated with orbital inflammatory signs, pain, and acute onset [13]. Again, orbital MRI imaging, laboratory tests, and treatment responses may support differential diagnosis.

Congenital fibrosis of the extraocular muscles (CFEOM), a form of congenital cranial dysinnervation, is a heterogeneous group of disorders marked by congenital maldevelopment of ocular motor cranial nerves with secondary fibrosis of the corresponding extraocular muscles [23]. Unlike CPEO, this phenotype of severe ptosis and paretic strabismus is fully penetrant from birth and not progressing afterwards.

Oculopharyngeal muscular dystrophy (OPMD) is a late-onset muscle disorder characterized by progressive ptosis, dysphagia, and limb muscle weakness. Most cases are transmitted in an autosomal dominant fashion, although some occur in a recessive or sporadic pattern [24]. Dominant OPMD is caused by triplet-repeat expansions in the polyadenylation binding protein 2 (PABP2) gene, which leads to mutated PABP2 oligomers accumulating as filamentous inclusions in nuclei. The phenotype of OPMD can be very similar to late-onset CPEO but, as a rule of thumb, there is much more dysphagia in OPMD. Diagnosis is confirmed by typical muscle biopsy findings and ultimately by genetic testing.

Ophthalmoplegia is also common in **congenital myopathies** [25] but can be discriminated from CPEO by age of onset, distribution of weakness, muscle morphology, and ultimately genetic testing.

Miller Fisher syndrome (MFS) is a variant of Guillain-Barre syndrome characterized by ataxia, areflexia, and ophthalmoparesis [13]. The acute onset and parainfectious nature of this disorder distinguish it rather easily from PEO. MFS benefits from treatment with plasmapheresis or intravenous immunoglobulins.

Another differential diagnosis of therapeutic relevance is **Wernicke's encephalopathy** due to thiamine deficiency, usually in patients with severe alcohol abuse. It is characterized by a triad of ophthalmoplegia, ataxia, and confusion. The latter is usually not found in CPEO. Thiamine supplementation is of utmost importance in this syndrome and often leads to improvement or even complete resolution of the symptoms.

Progressive supranuclear palsy (PSP) causes vertical, later also horizontal, gaze palsy. Such conjugated gaze palsies of central nervous origin can easily be differentiated from the omnidirectional ophthalmoparesis of muscular origin in CPEO, e.g., by oculocephalic reflex maneuvers. In addition, PSP is characterized by parkinsonism.

An interesting differential diagnosis to CPEO is **age-related dehiscence of the levator palpebrae muscle** causing ptosis in conjunction with age-related sagging eye syndrome (SES) causing strabismus. While this constellation can mimic CPEO, SES cases can be distinguished by normal saccadic velocity and full adduction and depression on motility testing [26].

Etiology and Pathogenesis

CPEO and KSS are **sporadic** in approximately 50% of cases, the most common underlying cause being a single large de novo deletion of the mtDNA. Size and location of the single deletion seem to predict the clinical phenotype with larger deletions leading to more severe disease [16, 27]. Of note, even in so far sporadic cases, the transmission risk of single mtDNA deletions is not zero but approximately 4% [28], an important point for genetic counselling.

The remaining 50% of cases are inherited through autosomal dominant (AD), autosomal recessive (AR), or maternal transmission. **AD-PEO** has been associated with mutations in at least eight genes encoded by nuclear DNA, including POLG1 [29], POLG2, ANT1 [30], Twinkle [31, 32], RRM2B [33], DNA2 [34], SPG7 [35], and OPA1 [36], with POLG1 being the most common. The consequences of these nuclear DNA mutations are impaired mtDNA maintenance and replication resulting in multiple deletions or depletion of mtDNA, as discussed in detail in chapter "Diseases of DNA Polymerase Gamma" of this book. AD-PEO may manifest as pure CPEO or more frequently as CPEO plus, featuring nonmuscular symptoms such as parkinsonism, dementia, ataxia, myoclonus, and seizures. Peripheral neuropathy is the clinical feature with the highest predictive value for a nuclear DNA mutation [37].

AR-PEO is less common and may be caused by mutations in TYMP, POLG1, DGUOK, TK2, MGM1, RRM2B, RNASEH1, and SPG7 genes, leading to either multiple mtDNA deletions or mtDNA depletion. These disorders are almost always multisystemic syndromes, and some of them including MNGIE due to TYMP mutations are discussed in detail in chapters "Mitochondrial Depletion Syndromes" and "Mitochondrial Neurogastrointestinal Encephalomyopathy Disease (MNGIE)."

Of note, mutations in three genes (POLG1, RRM2B, and SPG7) can lead either to AD-PEO (heterozygous mutations) or to AR-PEO (homozygous or compound heterozygous mutations).

Maternally inherited CPEO is caused by point mutations of the mtDNA, most frequently the m.3243A>G mutation, which is usually associated with MELAS syndrome (cf. chapter "Mitochondrial Encephalomyopathy, Lactic Acidosis, and Stroke-Like Episodes (MELAS)") but can rarely lead to CPEO or CPEO plus [38]. Other mtDNA point mutations leading to maternal CPEO have been identified in several mt-tRNA genes [13]. Ophthalmoplegia is less often associated with the m.8344A>G "MERRF" mutation of the mtDNA (cf. chapter "Myoclonus Epilepsy with Ragged Red Fibers (MERRF)"), being present in about 5% of patients in an Italian cohort, whereas eyelid ptosis occurred in 25% of cases [39].

In view of these manifold genetic causes leading to CPEO, it is important to keep in mind that sporadic cases (i.e., without any other affected family members) are mostly due to single mtDNA deletions with low transmission risk to offspring but that all other genetic causes can lead to "pseudo-sporadic" occurrence. This is particularly true in recessive gene defects but can also happen in dominant or maternal inheritance, e.g., due to reduced penetrance of the respective mutations. As a consequence, it is not sufficient to confirm the diagnosis of CPEO by detecting RRF in muscle but identification of the genetic cause is indispensable for proper genetic counselling.

Diagnostic Workup

Today, diagnosis of many mitochondrial disorders can be confirmed by doing molecular genetics from blood or urine. This is obviously the case in all Mendelian disorders (including AD-PEO and AR-PEO) where the respective mutations are found in any tissue. It is also true for mtDNA point mutations in multisystemic diseases (cf. chapters "Mitochondrial Disease Genetics," "Mitochondrial Encephalomyopathy, Lactic Acidosis, and Stroke-Like Episodes (MELAS)," and "Myoclonus Epilepsy with Ragged Red Fibers (MERRF)"). An important exception is the disorders discussed here where a **muscle biopsy** is still the diagnostic gold standard. In CPEO and KSS, mtDNA deletions are preferentially found in postmitotic tissues like muscle and often absent from blood. When CPEO or KSS is clinically suspected, the finding of RRF and COX-negative fibers in muscle confirms the diagnosis (cf. chapter "Mitochondria: Muscle Morphology"). In addition, the subsequent detection of a single mtDNA deletion points at sporadic occurrence (with the limitations discussed above) while the detection of multiple mtDNA deletions entails further genetic testing for one of the nuclear gene defects discussed above. Moreover, morphological analysis of muscle biopsies is also extremely helpful to distinguish CPEO from other disorders of similar phenotype, e.g., OPMD.

Muscle biopsy is also necessary in suspected MiMy because it helps in the broad differential diagnosis to other myopathies and because MiMy can be due to muscle-specific mtDNA mutations.

Further measures of diagnostic workup are discussed in chapters "Diagnostic Approach to Mitochondrial Diseases" and "Neuroimaging Findings of Mitochondrial Cytopathies."

Treatment

Until now, all treatment for PMM is symptom-oriented and no disease-modifying therapies are available. It should be stressed, however, that the benefit from proper symptomatic management must not be underestimated in mitochondrial disorders: it can much improve activities of daily living and quality of life. Here we will first describe current symptomatic management regimes, and then give an outlook on more causally oriented treatment options in development.

Treatment of Ophthalmic Manifestations of CPEO and KSS

The key questions in **ptosis** treatment are whether, when, and how. A clear medical indication is given when ptosis causes visual obstruction, like a curtain falling from above. This entails compensatory frontalis muscle contraction and chin-up position which in turn may evoke headache and neck pain. Before visual obstruction occurs, any measure against ptosis is just for aesthetic reasons, which is only rarely demanded by patients. Neurologists and ophthalmologists also mostly advise to postpone ptosis surgery as long as possible, both for possible adverse effects and limited effect duration of the operation. Eyelid crutches are a nonsurgical solution to mechanically elevate the eyelids [40] but are often not tolerated well. The mainstay of ptosis treatment is surgery. The surgical technique depends on the function of the levator palpebrae superioris (LPS) muscle. If it is only mildly impaired, resection and/or advancement of the levator tendon along the superior tarsus is preferred. With more advanced LPS impairment, frontalis suspension procedures tethering the superior eyelid to the frontalis muscle using a silicone or fascia lata sling are preferred [13]. Of note, CPEO patients are at high risk for corneal exposure and severe dryness following frontalis suspension procedures, and postoperative lubrication is often required [41].

Ophthalmoparesis is often asymptomatic in CPEO and does not require treatment. If bothersome diplopia occurs, however, smaller angle ocular misalignments may be corrected with prismatic glasses. A more invasive option is strabismus surgery which may lead to marked improvement in alignment. It is, however, important to set realistic expectations before surgery since the progressive nature of CPEO along with poor fusional amplitudes contributes to a high rate of strabismus recurrence and persistent postoperative diplopia in this patient population [42].

As mentioned above in the differential diagnosis to myasthenia gravis, low doses of pyridostigmine may improve a possible fatigue-induced component of ptosis and eye motility impairment in CPEO.

Treatment of Non-ophthalmic Myopathy Manifestations of PMM

Dysphagia occurs in approximately half of PMM patients, and is often due to cricopharyngeal achalasia. These patients should be seen by gastroenterologists, ENT specialists, and speech/swallowing therapists. Therapeutic options include physical swallowing therapy, cricopharyngeal myotomy, and percutaneous external gastrostomy [43].

Physical therapy, exercise, and training are a mainstay of treatment in mitochondrial myopathy manifestations. They are discussed in detail in chapter "The Pathophysiology of Exercise and Effect of Training in Mitochondrial Myopathies."

Treatment of Nonmuscular Multisystem Manifestations of PMM

Since all forms of PMM may be accompanied by nonmuscular multisystem manifestations, this should be thoroughly evaluated. Most important is the detection of **cardiac conduction abnormalities and cardiomyopathy** which are found in not only KSS but also CPEO plus and MiMy plus. Both arrhythmias and cardiomyopathy can lead to life-threatening episodes, disability, and even sudden cardiac death. For this reason, all patients with a new diagnosis of PMM should undergo a 12-lead ECG and a transthoracic echocardiogram [44]. We also recommend 24-h Holter monitoring. These investigations should be regularly repeated even in cardiologically asymptomatic patients. Serious cardiac conduction abnormalities will benefit from pacemaker/defibrillator placement. Cardiac transplantation may be an option in selected patients where cardiomyopathy dominates the clinical picture.

Sensorineural hearing loss is a common manifestation of mitochondrial dysfunction in patients with PMM. One study in patients with KSS or CPEO plus [45] found manifest hearing loss in 5/17 patients (29.4%) and pathological audiometry in 10/17 (58.8%). Hearing loss may be compensated by hearing aids or cochlear implantation [46].

Endocrinopathies including diabetes mellitus, hypothyroidism, hypoparathyroidism, and adrenal failure are common in mitochondrial patients. As these are treatable manifestations, they should be regularly screened for.

Dietary Supplements

Numerous **dietary supplements or "nutraceuticals"** have been tested in mitochondrial disorders under the hypothesis that they may improve respiratory chain function, reduce oxidative stress, or augment cellular energy pools. Unfortunately, these compounds have mostly been tested in single cases or very small patient series, precluding clear conclusions.

An open-label study of **coenzyme Q** (CoQ, 2 mg/kg/day) in 44 patients with CPEO or KSS resulted in a lower lactate level after exercise in 16 patients after 6 months of treatment. However, a subsequent double-blind study in these 16 patients showed no significant advantage of CoQ over placebo [47]. An indisputable indication for CoQ supplementation, however, is diseases with primary or secondary CoQ deficiency. This applies in particular to **CoQ deficiency myopathy with ETFDH mutations**, a form of PMM. All patients in the literature and in our own experience improved significantly with administration of CoQ (up to 500 mg/day), mostly in combination with riboflavin 100 mg/day [48].

Creatine supplementation showed no significant effects on physical performance, eye movements, activities of daily living, and MR-spectroscopic parameters in two small randomized, placebo-controlled crossover studies in 16 and 15 patients, respectively, with CPEO, KSS, or mitochondrial myopathy [49, 50].

These and other symptomatic treatment approaches are discussed in detail in chapter "Mitochondrial Symptomatic Treatments."

Disease-Modifying Treatment Options in Development or in Clinical Studies

In a cell model, the "common deletion" of mtDNA which is the most frequent cause of CPEO and KSS could be partially eliminated by the use of mitochondrially targeted zinc finger nucleases. Subsequent repopulation of wild-type mtDNA partially restored mitochondrial respiratory function. This study provided proof of principle that, through heteroplasmy manipulation, delivery of site-specific nuclease activity to mitochondria can alleviate a severe biochemical phenotype in primary mitochondrial disease arising from deleted mtDNA species [51].

More advanced is the development of elamipretide, an aromatic-cationic tetrapeptide that readily penetrates cell membranes and transiently localizes to the inner mitochondrial membrane where it associates with cardiolipin. In preclinical studies, elamipretide increased the synthesis of ATP and reduced reactive oxygen species production [52]. A phase I/II multicenter, randomized, double-blind, placebo-controlled trial in 36 participants with genetically confirmed PMM showed increased exercise performance after 5 days of treatment [53]. As of March 2019, this drug is investigated in a large international phase 3 trial.

Other experimental therapies are discussed in chapters "Experimental Therapies" and "Reproductive Options for Women with Mitochondrial Disease."

References

1. Gorman GS, Chinnery PF, DiMauro S, Hirano M, Koga Y, McFarland R, et al. Mitochondrial diseases. Nat Rev Dis Primers. 2016;2:16080.
2. Mancuso M, McFarland R, Klopstock T, Hirano M, consortium on Trial Readiness in Mitochondrial Myopathies. International Workshop: outcome measures and clinical trial readiness in primary

mitochondrial myopathies in children and adults. Consensus recommendations. Neuromuscul Disord. 2017;27(12):1126–37.
3. Kearns TP, Sayre GP. Retinitis pigmentosa, external ophthalmoplegia, and complete heart block: unusual syndrome with histologic study in one of two cases. AMA Arch Ophthalmol. 1958;60:280–9.
4. von Graefe A. Verhandlungen ärztlicher Gesellschaften. Berlin Klin Wochenschr. 1856;5:125–7.
5. von Graefe A. Ein ungewoehnlicher Fall von hereditaerer Amaurose [An unusual case of hereditary amaurosis]. Arch f Ophthalmol. 1858;4:266–8.
6. Hutchinson J. On ophthalmoplegia externa or symmetrical immobility (partial) of the eyes, with ptosis. Trans R Med Clin Soc. 1879;62:307–29.
7. Kiloh LG, Nevin S. Progressive dystrophy of the external ocular muscles (ocular myopathy). Brain. 1951;74:115–43.
8. Klopstock T. Albrecht von Graefe (1828–1870). Nervenarzt. 2004;75:831.
9. Berenberg RA, Pellock JM, DiMauro S, et al. Lumping or splitting? "Ophthalmoplegia-plus" or Kearns-Sayre syndrome? Ann Neurol. 1977;1(1):37–54.
10. Drachman DA. Ophthalmoplegia plus. The neurodegenerative disorders associated with progressive external ophthalmoplegia. Arch Neurol. 1968;18(6):654–74.
11. Bastiaensen LA, Joosten EM, de Rooij JA, et al. Ophthalmoplegia-plus, a real nosological entity. Acta Neurol Scand. 1978;58(1):9–34.
12. Siciliano G, Viacava P, Rossi B, Andreani D, Muratorio A, Bevilacqua G. Ocular myopathy without ophthalmoplegia can be a form of mitochondrial myopathy. Clin Neurol Neurosurg. 1992;94(2):133–41.
13. McClelland C, Manousakis G, Lee MS. Progressive external ophthalmoplegia. Curr Neurol Neurosci Rep. 2016;16(6):53.
14. Petty RK, Harding AE, Morgan-Hughes JA. The clinical features of mitochondrial myopathy. Brain. 1986;109(Pt 5):915–38.
15. Orsucci D, Angelini C, Bertini E, Carelli V, Comi GP, Federico A, Minetti C, Moggio M, Mongini T, Santorelli FM, Servidei S, Tonin P, Ardissone A, Bello L, Bruno C, Ienco EC, Diodato D, Filosto M, Lamperti C, Moroni I, Musumeci O, Pegoraro E, Primiano G, Ronchi D, Rubegni A, Salvatore S, Sciacco M, Valentino ML, Vercelli L, Toscano A, Zeviani M, Siciliano G, Mancuso M. Revisiting mitochondrial ocular myopathies: a study from the Italian Network. J Neurol. 2017;264:1777–84.
16. Mancuso M, Orsucci D, Angelini C, et al. Redefining phenotypes associated with mitochondrial DNA single deletion. J Neurol. 2015;262(5):1301–9.
17. Pitceathly RD, McFarland R. Mitochondrial myopathies in adults and children: management and therapy development. Curr Opin Neurol. 2014;27(5):576–82.
18. Pfeffer G, Cote HC, Montaner JS, Li CC, Jitratkosol M, Mezei MM. Ophthalmoplegia and ptosis: mitochondrial toxicity in patients receiving HIV therapy. Neurology. 2009;73(1):71–2.
19. Pineles SL, Demer JL, Holland GN, Ransome SS, Bonelli L, Velez FG. External ophthalmoplegia in human immunodeficiency virus-infected patients receiving antiretroviral therapy. J AAPOS. 2012;16:529–33.
20. Fraunfelder FW, Richards AB. Diplopia, blepharoptosis, and ophthalmoplegia and 3-hydroxy-3-methylglutaryl-CoA reductase inhibitor use. Ophthalmology. 2008;115(12):2282–5.
21. Krendel DA, Sanders DB, Massey JM. Single fiber electromyography in chronic progressive external ophthalmoplegia. Muscle Nerve. 1987;10(4):299–302.
22. Strianese D. Update on Graves disease: advances in treatment of mild, moderate and severe thyroid eye disease. Curr Opin Ophthalmol. 2017;28:505–13.
23. Assaf AA. Congenital innervation dysgenesis syndrome (CID)/congenital cranial dysinnervation disorders (CCDDs). Eye (Lond). 2011;25:1251–61.
24. Luigetti M, Lo Monaco M, Mirabella M, Primiano G, Lucchini M, Monforte M, Servidei S. Oculopharyngeal muscular dystrophy: clinical and neurophysiological features. Clin Neurophysiol. 2015;126(12):2406–8.
25. Jones KJ, North KN. External ophthalmoplegia in neuromuscular disorders; case report and review of the literature. Neuromuscul Disord. 1997;7:143–51.
26. Chaudhuri Z, Demer JL. Sagging eye syndrome: connective tissue involution as a cause of horizontal and vertical strabismus in older patients. JAMA Ophthalmol. 2013;131(5):619–25.
27. Grady JP, Campbell G, Ratnaike T, Blakely EL, Falkous G, Nesbitt V, Schaefer AM, McNally RJ, Gorman GS, Taylor RW, Turnbull DM, McFarland R. Disease progression in patients with single, large-scale mitochondrial DNA deletions. Brain. 2014;137:323–34.
28. Chinnery PF, DiMauro S, Shanske S, Schon EA, Zeviani M, Mariotti C, Carrara F, Lombes A, Laforet P, Ogier H, Jaksch M, Lochmüller H, Horvath R, Deschauer M, Thorburn DR, Bindoff LA, Poulton J, Taylor RW, Matthews JN, Turnbull DM. Risk of developing a mitochondrial DNA deletion disorder. Lancet. 2004;364:592–6.
29. Lamantea E, Tiranti V, Bordoni A, et al. Mutations of mitochondrial DNA polymerase gammaA are a frequent cause of autosomal dominant or recessive progressive external ophthalmoplegia. Ann Neurol. 2002;52(2):211–9.
30. Kaukonen J, Juselius JK, Tiranti V, et al. Role of adenine nucleotide translocator 1 in mtDNA maintenance. Science. 2000;289(5480):782–5.
31. Spelbrink JN, Li FY, Tiranti V, et al. Human mitochondrial DNA deletions associated with mutations in the gene encoding Twinkle, a phage T7 gene 4-like protein localized in mitochondria. Nat Genet. 2001;28(3):223–31.

32. Suomalainen A, Kaukonen J, Amati P, et al. An autosomal locus predisposing to deletions of mitochondrial DNA. Nat Genet. 1995;9(2):146–51.
33. Tyynismaa H, Ylikallio E, Patel M, Molnar MJ, Haller RG, Suomalainen A. A heterozygous truncating mutation in RRM2B causes autosomal-dominant progressive external ophthalmoplegia with multiple mtDNA deletions. Am J Hum Genet. 2009;85(2):290–5.
34. Ronchi D, Di Fonzo A, Lin W, et al. Mutations in DNA2 link progressive myopathy to mitochondrial DNA instability. Am J Hum Genet. 2013;92:293–300.
35. Pfeffer G, Gorman GS, Griffin H, et al. Mutations in the SPG7 gene cause chronic progressive external ophthalmoplegia through disordered mitochondrial DNA maintenance. Brain. 2014;137:1323–36.
36. Hudson G, Amati-Bonneau P, Blakely EL, et al. Mutation of OPA1 causes dominant optic atrophy with external ophthalmoplegia, ataxia, deafness and multiple mitochondrial DNA deletions: a novel disorder of mtDNA maintenance. Brain. 2008;131:329–37.
37. Horga A, Pitceathly RD, Blake JC, et al. Peripheral neuropathy predicts nuclear gene defect in patients with mitochondrial ophthalmoplegia. Brain. 2014;137(Pt 12):3200–12.
38. Mariotti C, Savarese N, Suomalainen A, et al. Genotype to phenotype correlations in mitochondrial encephalomyopathies associated with the A3234G mutation of mitochondrial DNA. J Neurol. 1995;242:304–12.
39. Mancuso M, Orsucci D, Angelini C, Bertini E, Carelli V, Comi GP, Minetti C, Moggio M, Mongini T, Servidei S, Tonin P, Toscano A, Uziel G, Bruno C, Caldarazzo Ienco E, Filosto M, Lamperti C, Martinelli D, Moroni I, Musumeci O, Pegoraro E, Ronchi D, Santorelli FM, Sauchelli D, Scarpelli M, Sciacco M, Spinazzi M, Valentino ML, Vercelli L, Zeviani M, Siciliano G. Phenotypic heterogeneity of the 8344A>G mtDNA "MERRF" mutation. Neurology. 2013;80:2049–54.
40. Lapid O, Lapid-Gortzak R, Barr J, Rosenberg L. Eyelid crutches for ptosis: a forgotten solution. Plast Reconstr Surg. 2000;106:1213–4.
41. Ahn J, Kim NJ, Choung HK, et al. Frontalis sling operation using silicone rod for the correction of ptosis in chronic progressive external ophthalmoplegia. Br J Ophthalmol. 2008;92:1685–8.
42. Tinley C, Dawson E, Lee J. The management of strabismus in patients with chronic progressive external ophthalmoplegia. Strabismus. 2010;18(2):41–7.
43. St Guily JL, Perie S, Willig TN, Chaussade S, Eymard B, Angelard B. Swallowing disorders in muscular diseases: functional assessment and indications of cricopharyngeal myotomy. Ear Nose Throat J. 1994;73(1):34–40.
44. Pfeffer G, Chinnery PF. Diagnosis and treatment of mitochondrial myopathies. Ann Med. 2013;45(1):4–16.
45. Kornblum C, Broicher R, Walther E, et al. Sensorineural hearing loss in patients with chronic progressive external ophthalmoplegia or Kearns-Sayre syndrome. J Neurol. 2005;252(9):1101–7.
46. Sinnathuray AR, Raut V, Awa A, Magee A, Toner JG. A review of cochlear implantation in mitochondrial sensorineural hearing loss. Otol Neurotol. 2003;24(3):418–26.
47. Bresolin N, Doriguzzi C, Ponzetto C, et al. Ubidecarenone in the treatment of mitochondrial myopathies: a multi-center double-blind trial. J Neurol Sci. 1990;100:70–8.
48. Gempel K, Topaloglu H, Talim B, et al. The myopathic form of coenzyme Q10 deficiency is caused by mutations in the electron-transferring-flavoprotein dehydrogenase (ETFDH) gene. Brain. 2007;130:2037–44.
49. Klopstock T, Querner V, Schmidt F, et al. A placebo-controlled crossover trial of creatine in mitochondrial diseases. Neurology. 2000;55:1748–51.
50. Kornblum C, Schroder R, Muller K, et al. Creatine has no beneficial effect on skeletal muscle energy metabolism in patients with single mitochondrial DNA deletions: a placebo-controlled, double-blind 31P-MRS crossover study. Eur J Neurol. 2005;12:300–9.
51. Gammage PA, Rorbach JF, Vincent AI, Rebar EJ, Minczuk M. Mitochondrially targeted ZFNs for selective degradation of pathogenic mitochondrial genomes bearing large-scale deletions or point mutations. EMBO Mol Med. 2014;6(4):458–66.
52. Siegel M, Kruse S, Percival J, et al. Mitochondrial-targeted peptide rapidly improves mitochondrial energetic and skeletal muscle performance in aged mice. Aging Cell. 2013;12:763–71.
53. Karaa A, Haas R, Goldstein A, Vockley J, Weaver WD, Cohen BH. Randomized dose-escalation trial of elamipretide in adults with primary mitochondrial myopathy. Neurology. 2018;90:e1212–21.

Leigh Syndrome

Albert Zishen Lim and Robert McFarland

Introduction

Leigh syndrome is the most common paediatric presentation of mitochondrial disease. Also known as subacute necrotising encephalomyelopathy, this early-onset neurodegenerative disorder is caused by more than 80 pathogenic gene mutations, encoded in two genomes (mitochondrial and nuclear) [1, 2].

History

This eponymous condition was first reported by Dr. Denis Archibald Leigh in 1951 while he was working at the Maudsley Hospital, London [3]. He described a 7-month-old male infant who presented to King's College Hospital in 1947 and died within 6 weeks from a central nervous system disorder. This infant had a normal birth and satisfactory development until 6 weeks of age, but from that point developed a range of neurological features including somnolence, blindness, deafness and spasticity of the limbs. Bilateral focal symmetrical subacute necrotic lesions extending from thalamus to the pons, inferior olives and posterior columns of the spinal cord were noted in post-mortem autopsy [3]. Dr. Leigh used the term "subacute necrotising encephalomyelopathy" to encapsulate the features of this condition.

It was initially postulated that the underlying mechanism in subacute necrotising encephalomyelopathy, or later known as "Leigh syndrome", was a biochemical defect in thiamine metabolism [4]. The brain tissue from a patient with subacute necrotising encephalomyelopathy contained essentially no thiamine triphosphate, although thiamine and its other phosphate esters were present. These findings suggested a relationship between this disease and thiamine triphosphate [4]. A defect in energy metabolism was first linked to Leigh syndrome in 1968 [5]. High serum lactate and pyruvate were noted in a 1-year-old boy with clinical features of Leigh encephalomyelopathy and a family history of deaths in three siblings. One of his siblings had a brain autopsy that showed lesions consistent with Leigh syndrome. In this boy's liver biopsy, there was an almost complete absence of the enzyme pyruvate carboxylase, which converts pyruvic acid to oxaloacetic acid in the process of gluconeogenesis. It was concluded that Leigh syndrome in this family may be a consequence of the lack of pyruvate carboxylase [5].

Although Hommes' description had provided the first association of Leigh syndrome with defective energy metabolism, it was not until

A. Z. Lim · R. McFarland (✉)
Wellcome Centre for Mitochondrial Research, Institute of Neuroscience, The Medical School, Newcastle University, Newcastle Upon Tyne, UK
e-mail: robert.mcfarland@ncl.ac.uk

M. Mancuso, T. Klopstock (eds.), *Diagnosis and Management of Mitochondrial Disorders*,
https://doi.org/10.1007/978-3-030-05517-2_10

1977 that Leigh syndrome was first related to mitochondrial respiratory chain dysfunction. A 6-year-old girl, with autopsy-confirmed subacute necrotising encephalomyelopathy, had previously been shown to have raised blood lactate:pyruvate and beta-hydroxybutyrate:acetoacetate ratios, suggesting a defect in mitochondrial oxidation [6]. Cytochrome *c* oxidase deficiency was subsequently demonstrated in post-mortem skeletal muscle tissue [6]. The first genetic diagnoses of Leigh syndrome were made in 12 patients with typical clinical features and a T > G mutation at position 8993 in mitochondrial DNA (mtDNA) [7] in 1993. Initially this mutation had been linked with another form of mitochondrial disease presenting with neurogenic weakness, ataxia and retinitis pigmentosa (NARP) but there have been many subsequent reports of it causing Leigh syndrome at higher levels of heteroplasmy.

Diagnosis

Since Dr. Leigh's original report, Leigh syndrome has moved on from a post-mortem neuro-histopathological diagnosis to one that can be made in life. There is heterogeneity between patients with respect to age of onset, duration of illness and symptomatology, but despite this variation Leigh syndrome is typically characterised by stepwise developmental regression or developmental delay, specific neuroradiological features and abnormal mitochondrial energy metabolism. Stringent diagnostic criteria was first proposed in 1996 to define Leigh syndrome [8], followed by two revisions in 2014 [9] and 2016 [1]. Three main criteria are generally agreed (see Table 1). "Leigh-like syndrome" terminology is frequently used if patients have clinical features strongly suggestive of Leigh syndrome, but do not satisfy all of these stringent criteria. This "Leigh-like" designation is often a result of atypical (or normal) neuroimaging, normal blood and/or CSF lactate levels or unusual neuropathology.

Table 1 Diagnostic criteria for Leigh syndrome

1. Stepwise clinical deterioration	Progressive neurological disease characterised by *stepwise* decompensation during intercurrent illness. Motor and intellectual developmental delay or regression is often followed by a period of stabilisation or recovery before another decline. Seizures and peripheral neuropathy are often associated
2. Bilateral neuroradiological features	Signs and symptoms of brain stem and/or basal ganglia disease (dystonia spasticity, movement disorder, ataxia and nystagmus). These correspond with bilateral symmetric hyper-intense signal changes in the brain stem and/or basal ganglia on T2-weighted magnetic resonance imaging (MRI) of the brain. Proton magnetic resonance spectroscopy could pick up areas of raised lactate levels
3. Abnormal mitochondrial energy metabolism	Elevation of blood and/or CSF lactate levels. Increased lactate is more consistent in CSF than blood. Plasma amino acid might show raised alanine level. These result from defective oxidative phosphorylation (OXPHOS) or pyruvate dehydrogenase complex (PDHc) activities

"Leigh-like syndrome" terminology is frequently used if patients have features strongly suggestive of Leigh syndrome but do not satisfy all these criteria. These may be due to atypical/normal neuroimaging, normal blood/CSF lactate levels or unusual neuropathology

Prevalence

The birth prevalence of Leigh syndrome and Leigh-like syndrome is generally estimated to be 1:40,000 [8]. In western Swedish preschool children, the estimated prevalence was up to 1:34,000 [10], but there are significant founder effects influencing the prevalence of Leigh syndrome in some populations. For example, a form of Leigh syndrome due to a specific homozygous mutation in the *LRPPRC* gene, occurs in the French-Canadian population living in the Saguenay-Lac-Saint-Jean region, where the incidence reaches

1 in 2000 live births [11]. Until recently, mutations in *LRPPRC* were not described outside of this small insular population. This form of Leigh syndrome was thought to be unique to the region, but subsequent descriptions of Leigh and Leigh-like syndromes due to mutations in *LRPPRC* have now been reported in a diverse range of ethnicities [12]. Another example is that of a Leigh-like syndrome, more specifically encephalomyopathy and methylmalonic acidaemia, caused by mutations in *SUCLA2*, where the incidence in the Faroe Islands, a community of approximately 49,000 people, approaches 1 in 1700 [13].

Clinical Manifestations

The onset of Leigh syndrome is typically between 3 and 12 months [8] although symptoms can occur in the early neonatal period or infrequently, later in adult life [14]. The median age of onset is estimated to be around 7 months, with more than 80% of patients presenting before 2 years old [15, 16]. Late presentation (later than the first year of life) and slow progression have been observed in some patients, with occasional long-term survival. The underlying genetic defect appears to predict the life expectancy and extraneurological features [17]. A multicentre study on Leigh syndrome in Europe revealed that the median time from disease onset to death was 1.8 years with a median age at death of 2.4 years [16].

The initial clinical features during the early infantile period may be non-specific. Feeding difficulties (dysphagia), persistent vomiting and failure to thrive are reported to be frequent presentations but these are often difficult to distinguish from gastro-oesophageal reflux or from other non-mitochondrial-related causes. The onset of Leigh syndrome is often triggered by metabolic challenges, such as respiratory or gastrointestinal viral infections, and are accompanied, or quickly followed, by a loss of acquired developmental skills [9]. Central nervous system features such as encephalopathy, hypotonia, dystonia, spasticity and seizures predominate early in the course of the disease, though as the condition progresses the involvement of the neuromuscular system can become increasingly obvious such as peripheral neuropathy, ptosis and muscle wasting. This combined central nervous and neuromuscular system involvement has a profound impact on motor function in a developing brain and children with Leigh syndrome can exhibit a wide range of abnormal motor findings [16, 18].

A prominent feature of Leigh syndrome is impaired control of eye movement; with nystagmus, strabismus, ptosis and ophthalmoplegia being common clinical findings [18–20]. Visual impairment and optic atrophy may also be present depending on the precise genetic aetiology of the Leigh syndrome [19, 20]. Epileptic seizures are common, with both generalised and focal convulsions witnessed in many patients. The basal ganglia and/or brainstem lesions can cause an extrapyramidal movement disorder, respiratory difficulties (apnoea/hypopnoea), bulbar palsy and abnormal thermoregulation [16]. Sensorineural hearing impairment occurs in approximately 20% of patients with Leigh syndrome [16]. Extraneurological manifestation of Leigh syndrome is not uncommon with dilated or hypertrophic cardiomyopathy, hepatic failure, renal tubulopathy and diffuse glomerulocystic kidney disease previously reported [15, 21–24]. A summary of extraneurological features that are associated with Leigh or Leigh-like syndrome can be found in Table 2.

The clinical indicators of poor survival for Leigh syndrome as reported in a multicentre European study were a history of epileptic seizures, failure to thrive, brainstem lesions and intensive care admissions [16]. Age of onset before 6 months also signifies a poor prognosis though that is true more generally for mitochondrial diseases with the exception of reversible infantile-onset respiratory chain deficiency [25, 26]. Elevated CSF lactate has been linked to early onset of disease, hypotonia, frequent exacerbations and brainstem lesions, although no correlation had been found between high CSF lactate and survival outcome [16]. The presence of cardiomyopathy in children with any form of mitochondrial disease usually denotes an unfavourable survival outcome [27] and cardiac assessment should therefore form part of the clinical assessments of children with Leigh syndrome.

Table 2 Summary of extraneurological features that are associated with Leigh or Leigh-like syndrome

Distinguishing extraneurological features	Mitochondrial pathology	Genes
Cardiac		
Hypertrophic cardiomyopathy	Complex I deficiencies	*NDUFS2, NDUFS4, NDUFS8, NDUFA2, NDUFV2, NDUFA10*
	Complex IV deficiencies	*COX10, COX15, SCO2*
	Lipoic acid synthesis defect	*LIAS*
	Mitochondrial translation defect	*TSFM*
	mt-tRNA modification	*GTPBP3, MTO1*
	Short-chain enoyl-CoA hydratase deficiency	*ECHS1*
Liver		
Hepatic dysfunction	Mitochondrial DNA depletion	*SUCLG2*
	mt-tRNA modification	*TRMU (*reversible)*
	Glutamyl aminoacyl tRNA synthetase deficiency	*EARS2*
	Lipoic acid synthesis defect	*LIPT1*
Renal		
Nephrotic syndrome	Coenzyme Q10 deficiency	*PDSS2*
Proximal renal tubulopathy	Complex III deficiency	*BCS1L*
Endocrine		
Hypoglycaemia	Disrupted mitochondrial modelling	*SERAC1*
Visual		
Cataracts	Isoleucyl aminoacyl tRNA synthetase deficiency	*IARS2*
	Mitochondrial chaperone deficiency	*CLPB*
Facial dysmorphism	Complex IV deficiency	*LRPPRC*
	Mitochondrial DNA depletion	*FBXL4*
Other		
Acrocyanosis	Ethylmalonic aciduria	*ETHE1*
Hypertrichosis	Complex I deficiency	*NDUFA12*
	Complex IV deficiency	*SURF1*

Clinical Investigations

A high index of clinical suspicion is key in assessing infants or children who present with stepwise regression of their developmental milestones. In order to establish the clinical diagnosis of Leigh syndrome, a series of assessments and investigations should be considered (see Table 3).

Table 3 Suggested investigations and evaluations of Leigh syndrome

1. Detailed developmental assessment, especially serial assessments
2. Neuroimaging (MRI and MRS of brain stem/basal ganglia)
3. Electrophysiology studies (EEG if epileptic seizures and nerve conduction studies if peripheral neuropathy is suspected)
4. Ophthalmic examination to assess ocular abnormalities
5. Cardiac assessment including echocardiography and ECG
6. Metabolic biochemical studies including serum and CSF lactate and pyruvate levels; urinary organic acids; pH studies
7. Respiratory chain enzyme studies
8. Referral to experts in genetics/mitochondrial service for the consideration of genetics studies (panels, exome- or whole-genome sequencing)

Differential Diagnoses

A number of disorders share similarities to Leigh syndrome especially those presenting with bilateral brainstem and/or basal ganglia involvement. In clinical practice, viral related causes of encephalopathy should be clinically obvious and have to be sought early in the diagnostic process. Postinfectious encephalopathy secondary to influenzae A and adenovirus can present with bilateral symmetrical lesions in brainstem and thalami, which respond to high-dose steroid therapy [28]. Another infection-related condition that mimics Leigh syndrome is the acute necrotising encephalopathy (ANE), a disorder where previously healthy young children develop a rapidly progressive encephalopathy within days of the onset of a viral infection [29]. In the acute phase, the cerebral MR imaging typically shows symmetric lesions affecting the basal ganglia [29]. Although this condition is sporadic, a familial (incompletely penetrant) autosomal dominant ANE (ADANE), due to mutations in the *RANBP2* gene, has been reported [30]. Other metabolic disorders, especially organic acidurias (methylmalonic aciduria [31] and propionic acidaemia [32]) or pantothenate kinase-associated neurodegeneration [33] (PKAN), can lead to symmetrical basal ganglia involvement. The analysis of blood and urine samples could distinguish these from Leigh syndrome.

Dietary thiamine deficiency secondary to malnutrition or systemic illness could lead to Wernicke's encephalopathy (WE) in children of which the typical neuroradiological features include mammillary body degeneration, as well as bilateral basal ganglia and putaminal MR changes [34]. This underdiagnosed condition is immediately responsive to thiamine. Thiamine can also be used, in combination with biotin, to treat another Leigh syndrome mimic, the biotin-responsive basal ganglia disease (BRBGD). This disorder is caused by mutations in the *SLC19A3* gene, which encodes a thiamine transporter, and can be difficult to distinguish from mitochondrial disease without genetic testing. The brain imaging usually shows symmetric bilateral lesions in the caudate nucleus, putamen and brainstem [35]. This thiamine transporter-2 deficiency can be treated at an early stage with thiamine and high-dose biotin with significant clinical improvement [36]. One other "treatable" condition which can be phenotypically similar to Leigh syndrome is biotinidase deficiency due to mutations in the *BTD* gene [37, 38]. Children with this condition have deafness, ataxia, optic atrophy, seizures and characteristic organic aciduria [37]. The treatment for this condition is with high dose of biotin supplementation and, newborn screening programmes are available in some countries [39].

Leigh-like presentations can overlap with other mitochondrial encephalopathies. *MTND5* and *MTND3* mutations can have features of both Leigh syndrome and mitochondrial encephalomyopathy, lactic acidosis and stroke-like episodes (MELAS) syndrome [40, 41]. Large-scale mitochondrial DNA deletions that usually cause Pearson's or Kearns-Sayre syndromes might have some Leigh-like pathology [42]. *POLG* mutations, usually associated with Alpers-Huttenlocher syndrome, in Leigh-like patients can have characteristics of both syndromes [43].

Biochemical Basis

A major aspect of the process of energy transfer in mitochondria is the system of oxidative phosphorylation (OXPHOS), which is performed sequentially within the mitochondrial inner membrane by five complexes, four of which (complexes I–IV) comprise the mitochondrial respiratory chain with the fifth complex being an ATPase (complex V) [42]. The serial transfer of electrons between these mitochondrial respiratory chain complexes is facilitated by co-substrates, namely the lipophilic ubiquinone, also known as coenzyme-Q, and the hydrophilic heme protein cytochrome *c* [44, 45]. Defective energy metabolism within mitochondria is believed to underline the biochemical basis of Leigh syndrome [44].

Biochemical analysis of respiratory chain enzyme activity in a patient with Leigh syndrome may reveal decreased activity of any of these complexes, but this is not always in isolation and more than one complex may be deficient. Respiratory chain enzyme activity deficiencies of complex I or IV are the most frequent abnormality though multiple respiratory chain deficiencies also occur with mt-tRNA mutations and defects of mtDNA maintenance or synthesis (e.g. *SUCLA2*, *RRM2B*). Histological and histochemical analysis of the muscle biopsy remains one of the most important diagnostic screens for detecting mitochondrial abnormalities [46]. The skeletal muscle tissue is often affected and is fairly accessible. About 10–20% of patients with normal respiratory chain enzyme activity in skeletal muscle may have defects in liver or cardiac muscle [47].

A "hypocapnic hypothesis" has been proposed that questions energy deprivation as the mechanism causing the typical features of Leigh syndrome [48]. The hypocapnic hypothesis assumes that, for OXPHOS-deficient brain cells, the primary harmful factor in triggering Leigh syndrome is a decrease in pCO_2 (hypocapnia) associated with increase in pH (alkalisation) occurring during hyperventilation and not energy deprivation. Evidence supporting this hypothesis remains rather circumstantial.

Genetic Mutations

Our understanding of the genetic aetiology of Leigh syndrome has improved enormously over the last 20 years (see Fig. 1) with more than 80 genes that have now been identified in affected patients [1]. Nevertheless, a substantial proportion of patients with Leigh sydrome remain without a genetic diagnosis indicating that there are aspects of mitochondrial metabolism that have not yet been elucidated but are important in maintaining normal mitochondrial function. The genetic basis of Leigh syndrome can be divided into two broad categories—the nuclear DNA and the mitochondrial DNA-associated Leigh syndrome. These genes and their possible functions are summarised in a schematic diagram (see Fig. 2).

Nuclear DNA-Associated Leigh Syndrome

Complex I Deficiency

The most common biochemical defect in Leigh syndrome is complex I deficiency and mutations affecting the *NDUFS4* (NADH dehydrogenase) subunit appear to be the most frequent cause of this deficiency, although this may reflect some degree

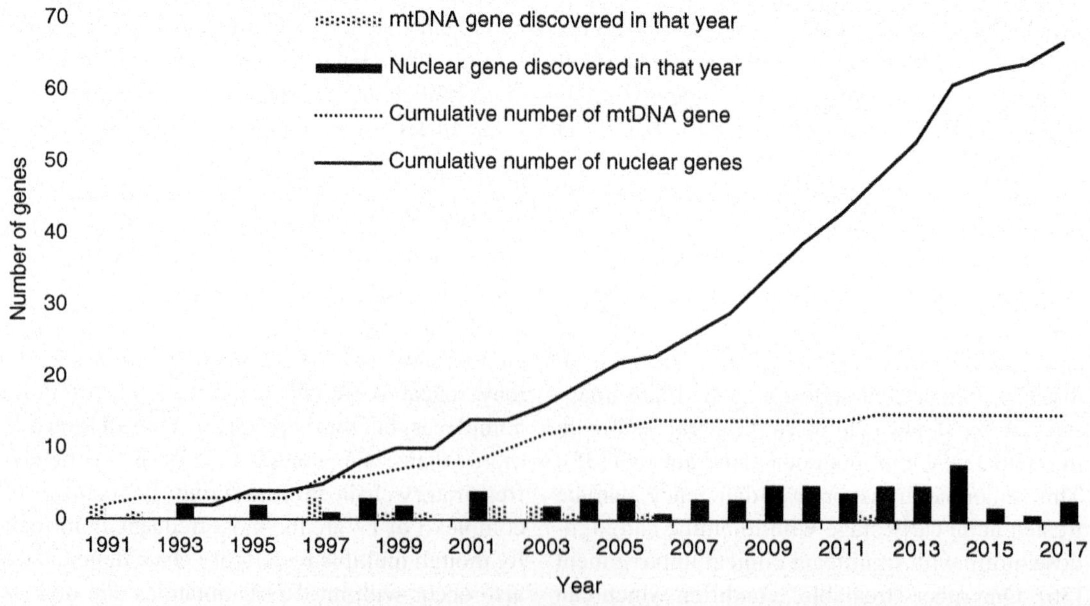

Fig. 1 Timeline demonstrates the number of nuclear and mitochondrial genes associated with Leigh syndrome discovered in each year. Line shows cumulative number of genes over the years (full line—nuclear genes; dotted line—mitochondrial genes). Courtesy of Prof. David Thorburn

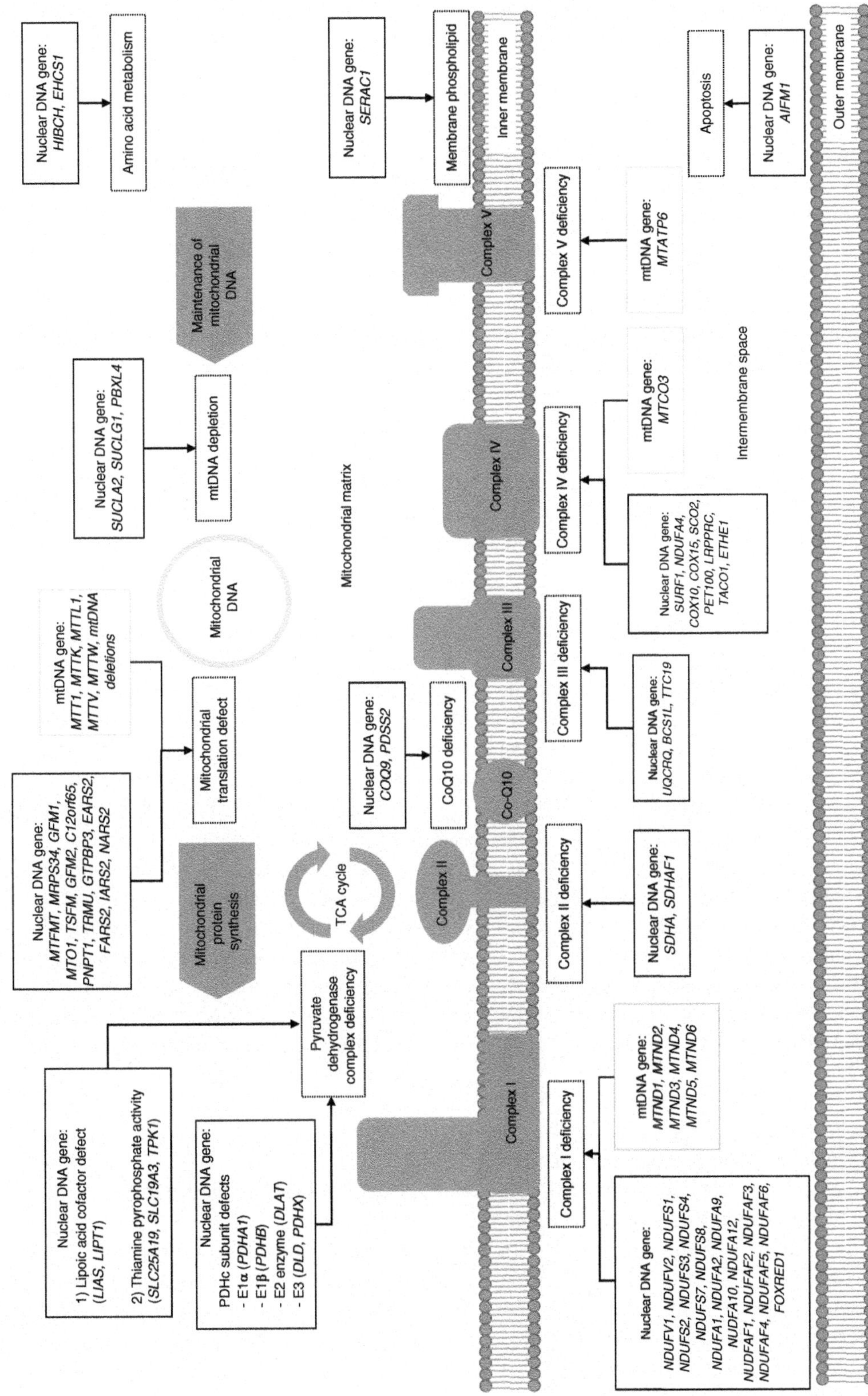

Fig. 2 Schematic diagram showing pathogenic mechanism of genes that are associated with Leigh syndrome

of reporting bias [49]. Almost all patients with *NDUFS4* mutations have Leigh syndrome with a characteristic initial presentation at 8 months old and, a rapidly progressive course with death occurring by 30 months [49, 50]. The neuroradiological findings in these infants showed bilateral symmetrical basal ganglia lesions and approximately one-third of cases have hypertrophic cardiomyopathy [50]. Several other nuclear genetic mutations associated with Leigh syndrome or Leigh-like syndrome can affect complex I activity. Leigh syndrome mediated by *NDUFS4*, *NDUFV1* and *NDUFS1* seems to have the more severe forms of the disease [1]. *NDUFV1* and *NDUFS1* are both core subunits of complex I [51] and the complete loss of these proteins is probably incompatible with life. The children with these mutations also have lower median age of death compared to other forms of Leigh syndrome [1, 16].

Complex IV Deficiency

Patients with complex IV deficiency constitute approximately 15% of Leigh syndrome [8, 16]. The most common cause of complex IV-deficient Leigh syndrome is mutations in *SURF1*, which encodes a complex IV assembly factor [17]. *SURF1* patients tend to survive longer than those with Leigh syndrome due to other genetic aetiologies, with a median age of death at 5.4 years [17]. Another important genetic variant that affects the function of complex IV is the *ETHE1 gene* which impairs the sulphide detoxification; sulphide is a powerful inhibitor of complex IV and its accumulation causes a functional cytochrome oxidase deficiency and leads to an encephalopathy resembling Leigh syndrome [52]. This fatal condition has been shown to be "treatable" by reducing sulphide accumulation with metronidazole and N-acetylcysteine [53]. As noted above, the inherited homozygous *LRPPRC* mutations are a cause of Leigh syndrome with severely low complex IV activities in brain and liver tissue within the population at Saguenay-Lac-Saint-Jean region of Quebec [54]. Leigh syndrome associated with this population has typical mild facial dysmorphism and liver dysfunction [55]. Although the gene product of LPPPRC has a role in the stability and translation of the mRNA for mitochondrially encoded complex IV subunits [56], *LRPPRC* is increasingly recognised to have a broader effect on mitochondrial energy processes including ATP synthase [57].

Complex II, III and Ubiquinone Deficiencies

The nuclear gene mutations affecting complex II, complex III and ubiquinone deficiencies are rare causes of Leigh syndrome. Leigh syndrome that has been reported with these biochemical deficiencies include mutations in *SDHA* and *SDHAF1* (complex II); *UQCRQ*, *BCS1L* and *TTC19* (complex III); and *COQ9* and *PDSS2* (ubiquinone). From a clinical perspective, the early identification of ubiquinone (CoQ10)-deficient Leigh syndrome could facilitate initiation of replacement therapy with large doses of CoQ10, with a good survival outcome into adulthood being reported [58]. The *PDSS2* mutations are known to be associated with refractory seizures and nephrotic syndrome [59]. Mutation in *the SDHA* gene (complex II) was one of the earliest reported nuclear mutations described in Leigh syndrome [60]. This early-onset disease was associated with a rapid demise, but some patients might experience a milder course with survival into late childhood and preservation of cognitive abilities [61, 62]. Mutation in the *TTC19* gene which codes for a complex III assembly factor causes a form of Leigh syndrome with characteristic neuroimaging changes that include lesions in the putamen and caudate nuclei, cerebellar atrophy and the unusual finding of hypertrophic olivary nuclei degeneration [63].

Mitochondrial DNA Depletion

Nuclear genes that cause mitochondrial DNA depletion can affect the availability of mitochondrial DNA to synthesise key components for complex I, III, IV and V. One of the most common causes of mitochondrial-DNA-depleted Leigh syndrome is mutation in *SUCLA2* which encodes subunits of succinyl-coA synthetase within the citric acid cycle [64]. The accumulation of succinyl-CoA due to a failure in the conversion to succinate leads to methylmalonic aciduria. The *SUCLA2* mutations can cause hypotonia, muscle atrophy, hearing loss and growth retardation [13]. Manifestation of *SUCLG2* is similar but primarily recurrent hepatic failure [65]. These two mutations, *SUCLA2* and *SUCLG2*, are thought to impact the interaction of succinyl-CoA synthetase and nucleoside diphosphate kinase which is responsible for mitochondrial nucleotide supply [13]. Another gene mutation that results in mitochondrial DNA depletion is *FBXL4*. Patients with this mutation present with Leigh-like syndrome along with facial dysmorphism, gastrointestinal dysmotility and renal tubular acidosis [66, 67].

Mitochondrial Translation Defects Caused by Nuclear Genes

The more recently characterised forms of Leigh syndrome are those caused by mutations in genes encoding the mitochondrial tRNA-modifying enzymes (*MTFMT*, *MTO1*, *TRMU* and *GTPBP3*). These enzymes are responsible for the post-transcriptional modification of mitochondrial tRNAs essential for successful mitochondrial DNA translation. Consequently, Leigh syndrome resulting from such mutations typically has combined mitochondrial respiratory chain deficiencies. Other genes involved in the mitochondrial DNA translation machinery that typically lead to a combined mitochondrial respiratory chain deficiency include *MRPS34* [68], *GFM1* [69], *TSFM* [70], *GFM2* [71], *C12orf65* [72] and *PNPT1* [73], while those encoding mitochondrial tRNA synthetases (*EARS2* [74], *FARS2* [67], *IARS2* [75] and *NARS2* [76]) often have a more variable impact on the mitochondrial respiratory chain activities [77]. In 2011 mitochondrial methionyl-tRNA formyltransferase (*MTFMT*) mutations were discovered in two unrelated children with Leigh syndrome with, microcephaly and a combined oxidative phosphorylation pathway deficiency [78]. Almost all subsequently identified cases are compound heterozygotes carrying one copy of the c.626C>T mutation identified in the original cases. Since its discovery, mutations in *MTFMT* have become one of the most common nuclear genetic causes of Leigh syndrome in the European population, with a carrier frequency of approximately 1 in 1000 [79].

Pyruvate Dehydrogenase Complex (PDHc) Deficiency

The pyruvate dehydrogenase complex is a multi-enzyme platform located on the inner mitochondrial membrane that catalyses the conversion of pyruvate to acetyl CoA and carbon dioxide. The acetyl CoA generated enters the tricarboxylic acid cycle and thus PDHc is a crucial step in the energy transduction process. PDHc-deficient Leigh syndrome presents with many of the typical features of the condition and the presence of corpus callosum dysgenesis, epilepsy and an elevated serum lactate:pyruvate ratio of more than 20 may be diagnostic clues to the genetic aetiology [80]. Autosomal recessive PDHc deficiencies can be subdivided into several main categories: (1) lipoic acid synthesis defects (*LIAS and LIPT1*) [81, 82]; (2) PDHc subunit E3 defects (*DLD* and *PDHX*) [83, 84]; and (3) absence of thiamine pyrophosphate (TPP) activity (*PDHA1*, *SLC25A19*, *SLC19A3* and *TPK1*) [85]. Of particular note are mutations in *PDHA1* an X-linked gene encoding the E1 alpha subunit of the complex and where unfavourable X-inactivation frequently results in symptomatic females. The gene also has a high de novo mutation rate and *PDHA1* mutations are thought to be the leading cause of PDHc-deficient Leigh syndrome [80, 86].

Mitochondrial DNA-Associated Leigh Syndrome

Mitochondrial DNA (mtDNA) is inherited maternally in multiple copies and is considerably more prone to mutation than the nuclear DNA (nDNA) because it lacks many of the repair and protective mechanisms present for the nDNA. While not completely determining disease expression, the proportion of mutated mtDNA present (the level of heteroplasmy) is nevertheless a key factor in the clinical severity of disease, with tissue-specific thresholds for each individual and each mutation. This concept of a heteroplasmy threshold determining the expression of a biochemical abnormality (and therefore clinical disease) is important in explaining why some family members with subthreshold heteroplasmy levels remain asymptomatic. Numerous mitochondrial genes have been associated with Leigh syndrome including six that encode for complex I subunits (*MTND1, MTND2, MTND3, MTND4, MTND5* and *MTND6*), one for complex IV subunits (*MTCO3*) and one for complex V subunits (*MTATP6*). Among all these, *MTND3*, *MTND5* and *MTATP6* are the leading causes of mitochondrial DNA-associated Leigh syndrome. *MTATP6* (m.8993T>G or m.8993T>C) is believed to be the basis of about 1 in 10 cases in this category of Leigh syndrome [8, 61]. Mitochondrial DNA-associated Leigh syndrome usually has heteroplasmy level above 90%, though several different mutations in the *MTND5* gene have been linked with Leigh syndrome at mutant load below 50% [87]. Another group of mitochondrial DNA mutations that are associated with Leigh syndrome are those that caused translational defects (*MTT1, MTTK, MTTL1, MTTV and MTTW*). Although m.3243A>G in *MTTL1* is typically associated with mitochondrial encephalomyopathy, lactic acidosis and stroke-like episodes (MELAS) or maternally inherited diabetes and deafness (MIDD) phenotypes and m.8344A>G in *MTTK* is associated with MERRF, Leigh syndrome has been observed in carriers of these two common mitochondrial tRNA translation defects [88].

Diagnostic Strategy

After taking a comprehensive medical history with family pedigree and bedside examination, a series of investigation should be undertaken to define the neuroradiological and biochemical characteristics. Some patients have a constellation of findings that is suggestive of a specific mutation, which, if identified, might avoid the need for expensive and invasive muscle or skin biopsies for measurement of defective oxidative phosphorylation (OXPHOS) or pyruvate dehydrogenase complex (PDHc) activities. The Multigene panel testing has become a popular mean of investigating a wide range of clinical disorders including mitochondrial disease, but panel is quickly become obsolete with new gene discoveries and with whole-exome or whole-genome sequencing now being employed in the diagnostic algorithm in a number of specialist laboratories [89, 90]. These powerful next-generation sequencing techniques can detect both nuclear and mitochondrial DNA defects [89, 91].

Management

Specific Treatments

There are possibly six Leigh or Leigh-like syndromes that could be treated with varying degrees of response expected depending on the underlying genetic mutations. These conditions should be sought at an early stage in the diagnostic process to avoid a delay in instigating disease-modifying treatment. All of these conditions have been discussed in other sections of this chapter and are summarised in Table 4. Where there is high clinical index of suspicion of a particular form of Leigh syndrome, it would be reasonable to commence a trial of the relevant supplements while waiting for genetic confirmation.

General Supportive Care

There are currently no specific curative treatments for other causes of Leigh syndrome. However, the management of symptoms (e.g. spasticity and dystonia) is important, as is prevention, recognition and prompt treatment of exacerbating factors such as fever, dehydration and poor nutrition. Epileptic seizures should be managed by a paediatric neurologist with appropriate use of anticonvulsant medication, keto-

Table 4 Six Leigh or Leigh-like syndromes that had specific treatment with varying degrees of success

Gene	Biochemical defect	Distinguishing features	Treatment (response)
SLC19A3	Thiamine transporter 2 deficiency	Episodic encephalopathy, paraparesis, dystonia, bilateral necrosis of caudate/putamen	Biotin 5–10 mg/kg/ day and thiamine 300–900 mg daily (fairly good) [92]
BTD	Biotinidase deficiency	Deafness, optic atrophy, seizures, ataxia, organic aciduria	Biotin 5–10 mg daily (fairly good) [93]
PDSS2	Coenzyme Q10 deficiency	Refractory seizures, nephrotic syndrome	Coenzyme Q10 10–30 mg/kg/day (variable [93, 94]
ETHE1	Ethylmalonic encephalopathy	Developmental regression, pyramidal and extrapyramidal signs, acrocyanosis, ethylmalonic aciduria	Metronidazole and N-acetylcysteine (variable) [53] (variable); liver transplant (single patient) [95]
PDHA1	Pyruvate dehydrogenase complex deficiency	Seizures, dystonia, microcephaly, cerebral atrophy, dysgenesis of corpus callosum, low serum lactate:pyruvate ratio	Thiamine 30–40 mg/kg/day (variable) [96] Ketogenic diet [118]
TPK1	Thiamine pyrophosphokinase deficiency	Episodic encephalopathy, dystonia, spasticity	Thiamine 20 mg/kg/day (variable) [97]

genic diet and on occasion epilepsy surgery (vagal nerve stimulator). It is probably advisable to avoid sodium valproate due to its inhibitory effect on mitochondrial function, though its adverse effects in this respect have not been ubiquitously demonstrated in all types of mitochondrial disease and it has proved to be an effective anticonvulsant in some patients [92, 93]. Dystonia is a common feature in Leigh syndrome of which baclofen, benzhexol, tetrabenazine and gabapentin are useful treatments. Cardiomyopathy could be one of the manifestations of Leigh syndrome [94] and anti-congestive therapy should be led by specialist cardiologists. General health surveillance at regular intervals (6–12 months) to monitor progression is generally recommended.

During acute acidotic crises, sodium bicarbonate or sodium citrate can be considered with close monitoring. Dichloroacetate (DCA) reduces blood lactate by activating pyruvate dehydrogenase complex. DCA is well tolerated by young children with congenital lactic acidosis [95]. However, correcting lactic acidosis using DCA might be complicated by peripheral nerve toxicity [96]. Therefore, the focus of management should be in optimising general supportive care rather than correcting lactate values which might not have clear benefits [95, 96].

Experimental Treatment

Supplementation

A variety of vitamin supplementations, such as riboflavin, thiamine and CoQ10, have been used in Leigh syndrome generally with the hope of improving mitochondrial function [97]. However, the clinical efficacy of each of these vitamin supplements in Leigh syndrome remains unproven. In a double-blind randomised controlled trial EPI-743, a modified form of CoQ10, reportedly has a 1000-fold increased antioxidant activity compared to native Co-Q10 [98]. Open-label trials using EPI-743 appeared to slow disease progression, but a phase 2b randomised placebo-controlled clinical trial failed to meet its primary endpoint. Nevertheless, studies with EPI-743 and other drugs (KH167, elamipretide, idebenone and acipimox) are ongoing in mitochondrial disease though with the exception of EPI-743, not specifically Leigh syndrome.

Ketogenic Diet

Ketogenic diet is a high-fat, low-carbohydrate-content diet which is used typically to treat severe epilepsy. This diet encourages hepatic conversion of fat into ketone bodies which then replace glucose as the main energy source for the brain. The evidence of its clinical efficacy in patients with mitochondrial disease is currently limited. Ketones have been reported to reduce mitochondrial DNA deletion load in cybrid models [99] but this effect was not reproducible in an experimental mouse model of mitochondrial disease. Instead, the ketogenic diet appeared to slow the rate of progression of myopathy and hepatopathy in some mouse models [100, 101]. Another possible therapeutic avenue is the use of an active component in the ketogenic diet known as decanoic acid. Decanoic acid has been shown to stimulate mitochondrial biogenesis in fibroblast cell cultures from patients with complex I-deficient Leigh syndrome [102]. However, with the notable exception of pyruvate dehydrogenase deficiency, where the ketogenic diet is offered more routinely, the clinical application of ketogenic diet (or its derivatives) has yet to be fully explored in Leigh syndrome.

Mitochondrial Biogenesis

Another promising area of research is using nicotinamide analogues such as nicotinamide riboside or nicotinamide mononucleotide to increase nicotinamide adenine dinucleotide (NAD) levels and to induce mitochondrial biogenesis via the PGC1α (peroxisome proliferator-activated receptor gamma coactivator-1-alpha) pathway [103]. Nicotinamide riboside in myopathic mitochondrial mouse models has been shown to delay disease progression [104, 105]. It has also demonstrated modest results in fibroblast of patient with *NDUFS1* Leigh syndrome [103]. In the mouse model of Alzheimer's disease, nicotinamide mononucleotide was able to enhance mitochondrial respiratory chain function [106]. Although all these are promising avenues for research purposes, these techniques are still far from clinical application in children with Leigh syndrome.

Gene Therapy

Presently, there are no clinical trials using gene therapy in Leigh syndrome, but in laboratory and in animal models of mitochondrial disease, gene therapy has been shown to reduce mtDNA heteroplasmy below threshold levels. Pathogenic variant m.8993T>G in *MTATP6* underlies one of the most common maternally inherited causes of Leigh syndrome [107]. The ATP synthesis defect caused by this pathogenic variant can be rescued by allotopic expression of an *MTATP6* construct transfected to the nucleus [108]. An alternative approach is to recognise and degrade the m.8993T>G pathogenic variant using a mitochondrially targeted restriction endonuclease (mtRE) [109–111]. At present this technique is limited to a small number of disease-causing restriction sites within mtDNA. Another reagent to selective degrade mutant mtDNA, which can be modified to overcome targeting limitations of mtRE, is the mitochondrially targeted zinc-finger nuclease (mtZFN) [112, 113]. More recently, mtZFN has selectively eliminated NARP-causing variant of m.8993T>G by cleaving site-specific DNA [114]. The mtDNA heteroplasmy could also be reduced by using mitochondrially targeted transcription activator-like effector nucleases (mito-TALENs). MitoTALENs have been shown to eliminate mutant mitochondrial DNA from cytoplasmic hybrids that harbour m.14459G>A [115], a variant within the *MTND6* gene which had been previously reported to have Leigh syndrome manifestation [116].

Family Counselling

An extensive, multigenerational family pedigree should be defined during the history-taking process. Most of the nuclear DNA gene mutations of Leigh syndrome will be inherited in an autosomal recessive manner though some, such as *PDHA1*, *NDUFA1* and *AIFM1*, showed X-linked inheritance. Mitochondrial DNA mutations, on the other hand, are often maternally inherited though some occur de novo in the patient. Patients and family members of those with known or suspected to have mitochondrial DNA pathogenic variant should have up-to-date genetic counselling at specialised centres to explore all potential outcomes ranging from prenatal diagnosis to reproductive options [117]. Given that the understanding of genotype, phenotype and potential treatment options of Leigh syndrome will improve in future, DNA banking should be considered for affected individuals. Following the identification of a pathogenic variant in an affected member, there are several options available to prevent the transmission of mitochondrial disease including prenatal diagnosis, preimplantation genetic diagnosis and mitochondrial donation. These preventative strategies are discussed elsewhere and while relevant are beyond the scope of this chapter.

References

1. Lake NJ, Compton AG, Rahman S, Thorburn DR. Leigh syndrome: one disorder, more than 75 monogenic causes. Ann Neurol. 2016;79(2):190–203.
2. Rahman J, Noronha A, Thiele I, Rahman S. Leigh map: a novel computational diagnostic resource for mitochondrial disease. Ann Neurol. 2017;81(1):9–16.
3. Leigh D. Subacute necrotizing encephalomyelopathy in an infant. J Neurol Neurosurg Psychiatry. 1951;14(3):216–21.
4. Cooper JR, Itokawa Y, Pincus JH. Thiamine triphosphate deficiency in subacute necrotizing encephalomyelopathy. Science. 1969;164(3875):74–5.
5. Hommes FA, Polman HA, Reerink JD. Leigh's encephalomyelopathy: an inborn error of gluconeogenesis. Arch Dis Child. 1968;43(230):423–6.
6. Willems JL, Monnens LA, Trijbels JM, et al. Leigh's encephalomyelopathy in a patient with cytochrome c oxidase deficiency in muscle tissue. Pediatrics. 1977;60(6):850–7.
7. Santorelli FM, Shanske S, Macaya A, DeVivo DC, DiMauro S. The mutation at nt 8993 of mitochondrial DNA is a common cause of Leigh's syndrome. Ann Neurol. 1993;34(6):827–34.
8. Rahman S, Blok RB, Dahl HH, et al. Leigh syndrome: clinical features and biochemical and DNA abnormalities. Ann Neurol. 1996;39(3):343–51.
9. Baertling F, Rodenburg RJ, Schaper J, et al. A guide to diagnosis and treatment of Leigh syndrome. J Neurol Neurosurg Psychiatry. 2014;85(3):257–65.
10. Darin N, Oldfors A, Moslemi AR, Holme E, Tulinius M. The incidence of mitochondrial encephalomyopathies in childhood: clinical features and morphological, biochemical, and DNA abnormalities. Ann Neurol. 2001;49(3):377–83.
11. Morin C, Mitchell G, Larochelle J, et al. Clinical, metabolic, and genetic aspects of cytochrome C oxidase deficiency in Saguenay-Lac-Saint-Jean. Am J Hum Genet. 1993;53(2):488–96.
12. Olahova M, Hardy SA, Hall J, et al. LRPPRC mutations cause early-onset multisystem mitochondrial disease outside of the French-Canadian population. Brain. 2015;138(Pt 12):3503–19.
13. Ostergaard E, Hansen FJ, Sorensen N, et al. Mitochondrial encephalomyopathy with elevated methylmalonic acid is caused by SUCLA2 mutations. Brain. 2007;130(Pt 3):853–61.
14. McKelvie P, Infeld B, Marotta R, Chin J, Thorburn D, Collins S. Late-adult onset Leigh syndrome. J Clin Neurosci. 2012;19(2):195–202.
15. Naess K, Freyer C, Bruhn H, et al. MtDNA mutations are a common cause of severe disease phenotypes in children with Leigh syndrome. Biochim Biophys Acta. 2009;1787(5):484–90.
16. Sofou K, De Coo IF, Isohanni P, et al. A multicenter study on Leigh syndrome: disease course and predictors of survival. Orphanet J Rare Dis. 2014;9:52.
17. Wedatilake Y, Brown RM, McFarland R, et al. SURF1 deficiency: a multi-centre natural history study. Orphanet J Rare Dis. 2013;8:96.
18. Ruhoy IS, Saneto RP. The genetics of Leigh syndrome and its implications for clinical practice and risk management. Appl Clin Genet. 2014;7:221–34.
19. Han J, Lee Y-M, Kim SM, Han SY, Lee JB, Han S-H. Ophthalmological manifestations in patients with Leigh syndrome. Br J Ophthalmol. 2015;99(4):528–35.
20. Åkebrand R, Andersson S, Seyedi Honarvar AK, et al. Ophthalmological characteristics in children with Leigh syndrome–A long-term follow-up. Acta Ophthalmol. 2016;94(6):609–17.
21. Wang SB, Weng WC, Lee NC, Hwu WL, Fan PC, Lee WT. Mutation of mitochondrial DNA G13513A presenting with Leigh syndrome, Wolff-Parkinson-White syndrome and cardiomyopathy. Pediatr Neonatol. 2008;49(4):145–9.
22. Hadzsiev K, Maasz A, Kisfali P, et al. Mitochondrial DNA 11777C>A mutation associated Leigh syndrome: case report with a review of the previously described pedigrees. NeuroMolecular Med. 2010;12(3):277–84.
23. Van Hove JL, Saenz MS, Thomas JA, et al. Succinyl-CoA ligase deficiency: a mitochondrial hepatoencephalomyopathy. Pediatr Res. 2010;68(2):159–64.
24. Duff RM, Shearwood AM, Ermer J, et al. A mutation in MT-TW causes a tRNA processing defect and reduced mitochondrial function in a family with Leigh syndrome. Mitochondrion. 2015;25:113–9.
25. Zeharia A, Shaag A, Pappo O, et al. Acute infantile liver failure due to mutations in the TRMU gene. Am J Hum Genet. 2009;85(3):401–7.
26. Uusimaa J, Jungbluth H, Fratter C, et al. Reversible infantile respiratory chain deficiency is a unique, genetically heterogenous mitochondrial disease. J Med Genet. 2011;48(10):660–8.
27. Holmgren D, Wahlander H, Eriksson BO, Oldfors A, Holme E, Tulinius M. Cardiomyopathy in children with mitochondrial disease; clinical course and cardiological findings. Eur Heart J. 2003;24(3):280–8.
28. Suwa K, Yamagata T, Momoi MY, et al. Acute relapsing encephalopathy mimicking acute necrotizing encephalopathy in a 4-year-old boy. Brain Dev. 1999;21(8):554–8.

29. Mizuguchi M, Abe J, Mikkaichi K, et al. Acute necrotising encephalopathy of childhood: a new syndrome presenting with multifocal, symmetric brain lesions. J Neurol Neurosurg Psychiatry. 1995;58(5):555–61.
30. Neilson DE, Eiben RM, Waniewski S, et al. Autosomal dominant acute necrotizing encephalopathy. Neurology. 2003;61(2):226–30.
31. Zwickler T, Haege G, Riderer A, et al. Metabolic decompensation in methylmalonic aciduria: which biochemical parameters are discriminative? J Inherit Metab Dis. 2012;35(5):797–806.
32. North KN, Korson MS, Gopal YR, et al. Neonatal-onset propionic acidemia: neurologic and developmental profiles, and implications for management. J Pediatr. 1995;126(6):916–22.
33. Egan RA, Weleber RG, Hogarth P, et al. Neuro-ophthalmologic and electroretinographic findings in pantothenate kinase-associated neurodegeneration (formerly Hallervorden-Spatz syndrome). Am J Ophthalmol. 2005;140(2):267–74.
34. Zuccoli G, Siddiqui N, Bailey A, Bartoletti SC. Neuroimaging findings in pediatric Wernicke encephalopathy: a review. Neuroradiology. 2010;52(6):523–9.
35. Tabarki B, Al-Shafi S, Al-Shahwan S, et al. Biotin-responsive basal ganglia disease revisited: Clinical, radiologic, and genetic findings. Neurology. 2013;80(3):261–7.
36. Fassone E, Wedatilake Y, DeVile CJ, Chong WK, Carr LJ, Rahman S. Treatable Leigh-like encephalopathy presenting in adolescence. BMJ Case Rep. 2013;2013:200838.
37. Mitchell G, Ogier H, Munnich A, et al. Neurological deterioration and lactic acidemia in biotinidase deficiency. A treatable condition mimicking Leigh's disease. Neuropediatrics. 1986;17(3):129–31.
38. Wolf B. First microdeletion involving only the biotinidase gene that can cause biotinidase deficiency: a lesson for clinical practice. Mol Genet Metab Rep. 2016;6:74–6.
39. Weber P, Scholl S, Baumgartner ER. Outcome in patients with profound biotinidase deficiency: relevance of newborn screening. Dev Med Child Neurol. 2004;46(7):481–4.
40. Chol M, Lebon S, Benit P, et al. The mitochondrial DNA G13513A MELAS mutation in the NADH dehydrogenase 5 gene is a frequent cause of Leigh-like syndrome with isolated complex I deficiency. J Med Genet. 2003;40(3):188–91.
41. Wang Z, Qi XK, Yao S, et al. Phenotypic patterns of MELAS/LS overlap syndrome associated with m.13513G>A mutation, and neuropathological findings in one autopsy case. Neuropathology. 2010;30(6):606–14.
42. Santorelli FM, Barmada MA, Pons R, Zhang LL, DiMauro S. Leigh-type neuropathology in Pearson syndrome associated with impaired ATP production and a novel mtDNA deletion. Neurology. 1996;47(5):1320–3.
43. Scalais E, Francois B, Schlesser P, et al. Polymerase gamma deficiency (POLG): clinical course in a child with a two stage evolution from infantile myocerebrohepatopathy spectrum to an Alpers syndrome and neuropathological findings of Leigh's encephalopathy. Eur J Paediatr Neurol. 2012;16(5):542–8.
44. DiMauro S, Schon EA. Mitochondrial respiratory-chain diseases. N Engl J Med. 2003;348(26):2656–68.
45. Kroger A, Klingenberg M. The kinetics of the redox reactions of ubiquinone related to the electron-transport activity in the respiratory chain. Eur J Biochem. 1973;34(2):358–68.
46. Old SL, Johnson MA. Methods of microphotometric assay of succinate dehydrogenase and cytochrome c oxidase activities for use on human skeletal muscle. Histochem J. 1989;21(9-10):545–55.
47. Thorburn DR, Chow CW, Kirby DM. Respiratory chain enzyme analysis in muscle and liver. Mitochondrion. 2004;4(5-6):363–75.
48. Pronicka E. Hypocapnic hypothesis of Leigh disease. Med Hypotheses. 2017;101:23–7.
49. Fassone E, Rahman S. Complex I deficiency: clinical features, biochemistry and molecular genetics. J Med Genet. 2012;49(9):578–90.
50. Assouline Z, Jambou M, Rio M, et al. A constant and similar assembly defect of mitochondrial respiratory chain complex I allows rapid identification of NDUFS4 mutations in patients with Leigh syndrome. Biochim Biophys Acta. 2012;1822(6):1062–9.
51. Mimaki M, Wang X, McKenzie M, Thorburn DR, Ryan MT. Understanding mitochondrial complex I assembly in health and disease. Biochim Biophys Acta. 2012;1817(6):851–62.
52. Tiranti V, Viscomi C, Hildebrandt T, et al. Loss of ETHE1, a mitochondrial dioxygenase, causes fatal sulfide toxicity in ethylmalonic encephalopathy. Nat Med. 2009;15(2):200–5.
53. Viscomi C, Burlina AB, Dweikat I, et al. Combined treatment with oral metronidazole and N-acetylcysteine is effective in ethylmalonic encephalopathy. Nat Med. 2010;16(8):869–71.
54. Merante F, Petrova-Benedict R, MacKay N, et al. A biochemically distinct form of cytochrome oxidase (COX) deficiency in the Saguenay-Lac-Saint-Jean region of Quebec. Am J Hum Genet. 1993;53(2):481–7.
55. Debray FG, Morin C, Janvier A, et al. LRPPRC mutations cause a phenotypically distinct form of Leigh syndrome with cytochrome c oxidase deficiency. J Med Genet. 2011;48(3):183–9.
56. Xu F, Morin C, Mitchell G, Ackerley C, Robinson BH. The role of the LRPPRC (leucine-rich pentatricopeptide repeat cassette) gene in cytochrome oxidase assembly: mutation causes lowered levels of COX (cytochrome c oxidase) I and COX III mRNA. Biochem J. 2004;382(Pt 1):331–6.
57. Mourier A, Ruzzenente B, Brandt T, Kuhlbrandt W, Larsson NG. Loss of LRPPRC causes ATP synthase deficiency. Hum Mol Genet. 2014;23(10):2580–92.

58. Van Maldergem L, Trijbels F, DiMauro S, et al. Coenzyme Q-responsive Leigh's encephalopathy in two sisters. Ann Neurol. 2002;52(6):750–4.
59. Lopez LC, Schuelke M, Quinzii CM, et al. Leigh syndrome with nephropathy and CoQ10 deficiency due to decaprenyl diphosphate synthase subunit 2 (PDSS2) mutations. Am J Hum Genet. 2006;79(6):1125–9.
60. Bourgeron T, Rustin P, Chretien D, et al. Mutation of a nuclear succinate dehydrogenase gene results in mitochondrial respiratory chain deficiency. Nat Genet. 1995;11(2):144–9.
61. Ma YY, Wu TF, Liu YP, et al. Genetic and biochemical findings in Chinese children with Leigh syndrome. J Clin Neurosci. 2013;20(11):1591–4.
62. Pagnamenta AT, Hargreaves IP, Duncan AJ, et al. Phenotypic variability of mitochondrial disease caused by a nuclear mutation in complex II. Mol Genet Metab. 2006;89(3):214–21.
63. Koch J, Freisinger P, Feichtinger RG, et al. Mutations in TTC19: expanding the molecular, clinical and biochemical phenotype. Orphanet J Rare Dis. 2015;10:40.
64. Elpeleg O, Miller C, Hershkovitz E, et al. Deficiency of the ADP-forming succinyl-CoA synthase activity is associated with encephalomyopathy and mitochondrial DNA depletion. Am J Hum Genet. 2005;76(6):1081–6.
65. Valayannopoulos V, Haudry C, Serre V, et al. New SUCLG1 patients expanding the phenotypic spectrum of this rare cause of mild methylmalonic aciduria. Mitochondrion. 2010;10(4):335–41.
66. Huemer M, Karall D, Schossig A, et al. Clinical, morphological, biochemical, imaging and outcome parameters in 21 individuals with mitochondrial maintenance defect related to FBXL4 mutations. J Inherit Metab Dis. 2015;38(5):905–14.
67. Shamseldin HE, Alshammari M, Al-Sheddi T, et al. Genomic analysis of mitochondrial diseases in a consanguineous population reveals novel candidate disease genes. J Med Genet. 2012;49(4):234–41.
68. Lake NJ, Webb BD, Stroud DA, et al. Biallelic mutations in MRPS34 lead to instability of the small mitoribosomal subunit and leigh syndrome. Am J Hum Genet. 2017;101(2):239–54.
69. Valente L, Tiranti V, Marsano RM, et al. Infantile encephalopathy and defective mitochondrial DNA translation in patients with mutations of mitochondrial elongation factors EFG1 and EFTu. Am J Hum Genet. 2007;80(1):44–58.
70. Ahola S, Isohanni P, Euro L, et al. Mitochondrial EFTs defects in juvenile-onset Leigh disease, ataxia, neuropathy, and optic atrophy. Neurology. 2014;83(8):743–51.
71. Glasgow RIC, Thompson K, Barbosa IA, et al. Novel GFM2 variants associated with early-onset neurological presentations of mitochondrial disease and impaired expression of OXPHOS subunits. Neurogenetics. 2017;18(4):227–35.
72. Antonicka H, Ostergaard E, Sasarman F, et al. Mutations in C12orf65 in patients with encephalomyopathy and a mitochondrial translation defect. Am J Hum Genet. 2010;87(1):115–22.
73. Vedrenne V, Gowher A, De Lonlay P, et al. Mutation in PNPT1, which encodes a polyribonucleotide nucleotidyltransferase, impairs RNA import into mitochondria and causes respiratory-chain deficiency. Am J Hum Genet. 2012;91(5):912–8.
74. Martinelli D, Catteruccia M, Piemonte F, et al. EPI-743 reverses the progression of the pediatric mitochondrial disease--genetically defined Leigh Syndrome. Mol Genet Metab. 2012;107(3):383–8.
75. Schwartzentruber J, Buhas D, Majewski J, et al. Mutation in the nuclear-encoded mitochondrial isoleucyl-tRNA synthetase IARS2 in patients with cataracts, growth hormone deficiency with short stature, partial sensorineural deafness, and peripheral neuropathy or with Leigh syndrome. Hum Mutat. 2014;35(11):1285–9.
76. Simon M, Richard EM, Wang X, et al. Mutations of human NARS2, encoding the mitochondrial asparaginyl-tRNA synthetase, cause nonsyndromic deafness and Leigh syndrome. PLoS Genet. 2015;11(3):e1005097.
77. Boczonadi V, Horvath R. Mitochondria: Impaired mitochondrial translation in human disease. Int J Biochem Cell Biol. 2014;48(100):77–84.
78. Tucker EJ, Hershman SG, Kohrer C, et al. Mutations in MTFMT underlie a human disorder of formylation causing impaired mitochondrial translation. Cell Metab. 2011;14(3):428–34.
79. Haack TB, Gorza M, Danhauser K, et al. Phenotypic spectrum of eleven patients and five novel MTFMT mutations identified by exome sequencing and candidate gene screening. Mol Genet Metab. 2014;111(3):342–52.
80. Patel KP, O'Brien TW, Subramony SH, Shuster J, Stacpoole PW. The spectrum of pyruvate dehydrogenase complex deficiency: clinical, biochemical and genetic features in 371 patients. Mol Genet Metab. 2012;106(3):385–94.
81. Soreze Y, Boutron A, Habarou F, et al. Mutations in human lipoyltransferase gene LIPT1 cause a Leigh disease with secondary deficiency for pyruvate and alpha-ketoglutarate dehydrogenase. Orphanet J Rare Dis. 2013;8:192.
82. Baker PR 2nd, Friederich MW, Swanson MA, et al. Variant non ketotic hyperglycinemia is caused by mutations in LIAS, BOLA3 and the novel gene GLRX5. Brain. 2014;137(Pt 2):366–79.
83. Schiff M, Mine M, Brivet M, et al. Leigh's disease due to a new mutation in the PDHX gene. Ann Neurol. 2006;59(4):709–14.
84. Quinonez SC, Leber SM, Martin DM, Thoene JG, Bedoyan JK. Leigh syndrome in a girl with a novel DLD mutation causing E3 deficiency. Pediatr Neurol. 2013;48(1):67–72.
85. Mayr JA, Freisinger P, Schlachter K, et al. Thiamine pyrophosphokinase deficiency in encephalopathic

children with defects in the pyruvate oxidation pathway. Am J Hum Genet. 2011;89(6):806–12.
86. DeBrosse SD, Okajima K, Zhang S, et al. Spectrum of neurological and survival outcomes in pyruvate dehydrogenase complex (PDC) deficiency: lack of correlation with genotype. Mol Genet Metab. 2012;107(3):394–402.
87. Kirby DM, Boneh A, Chow CW, et al. Low mutant load of mitochondrial DNA G13513A mutation can cause Leigh's disease. Ann Neurol. 2003;54(4):473–8.
88. Hammans SR, Sweeney MG, Brockington M, et al. The mitochondrial DNA transfer RNA(Lys) A-->G(8344) mutation and the syndrome of myoclonic epilepsy with ragged red fibres (MERRF). Relationship of clinical phenotype to proportion of mutant mitochondrial DNA. Brain. 1993;116(Pt 3):617–32.
89. Carroll CJ, Brilhante V, Suomalainen A. Next-generation sequencing for mitochondrial disorders. Br J Pharmacol. 2014;171(8):1837–53.
90. DePristo MA, Banks E, Poplin R, et al. A framework for variation discovery and genotyping using next-generation DNA sequencing data. Nat Genet. 2011;43(5):491–8.
91. Calvo SE, Compton AG, Hershman SG, et al. Molecular diagnosis of infantile mitochondrial disease with targeted next-generation sequencing. Sci Transl Med. 2012;4(118):118ra110.
92. Anderson CM, Norquist BA, Vesce S, et al. Barbiturates induce mitochondrial depolarization and potentiate excitotoxic neuronal death. J Neurosci. 2002;22(21):9203–9.
93. Melegh B, Trombitas K. Valproate treatment induces lipid globule accumulation with ultrastructural abnormalities of mitochondria in skeletal muscle. Neuropediatrics. 1997;28(5):257–61.
94. Ruiter EM, Siers MH, van den Elzen C, et al. The mitochondrial 13513G>A mutation is most frequent in Leigh syndrome combined with reduced complex I activity, optic atrophy and/or Wolff-Parkinson-White. Eur J Hum Genet. 2007;15(2):155–61.
95. Stacpoole PW, Kurtz TL, Han Z, Langaee T. Role of dichloroacetate in the treatment of genetic mitochondrial diseases. Adv Drug Deliv Rev. 2008;60(13-14):1478–87.
96. Kaufmann P, Engelstad K, Wei Y, et al. Dichloroacetate causes toxic neuropathy in MELAS: a randomized, controlled clinical trial. Neurology. 2006;66(3):324–30.
97. Kanabus M, Heales SJ, Rahman S. Development of pharmacological strategies for mitochondrial disorders. Br J Pharmacol. 2014;171(8):1798–817.
98. Enns GM, Kinsman SL, Perlman SL, et al. Initial experience in the treatment of inherited mitochondrial disease with EPI-743. Mol Genet Metab. 2012;105(1):91–102.
99. Santra S, Gilkerson RW, Davidson M, Schon EA. Ketogenic treatment reduces deleted mitochondrial DNAs in cultured human cells. Ann Neurol. 2004;56(5):662–9.
100. Ahola-Erkkila S, Carroll CJ, Peltola-Mjosund K, et al. Ketogenic diet slows down mitochondrial myopathy progression in mice. Hum Mol Genet. 2010;19(10):1974–84.
101. Purhonen J, Rajendran J. Ketogenic diet attenuates hepatopathy in mouse model of respiratory chain complex III deficiency caused by a Bcs1l mutation. Sci Rep. 2017;7(1):957.
102. Kanabus M, Fassone E, Hughes SD, et al. The pleiotropic effects of decanoic acid treatment on mitochondrial function in fibroblasts from patients with complex I deficient Leigh syndrome. J Inherit Metab Dis. 2016;39(3):415–26.
103. Felici R, Lapucci A, Cavone L, Pratesi S, Berlinguer-Palmini R, Chiarugi A. Pharmacological NAD-boosting strategies improve mitochondrial homeostasis in human complex I-mutant fibroblasts. Mol Pharmacol. 2015;87(6):965–71.
104. Cerutti R, Pirinen E, Lamperti C, et al. NAD(+)-dependent activation of Sirt1 corrects the phenotype in a mouse model of mitochondrial disease. Cell Metab. 2014;19(6):1042–9.
105. Khan NA, Auranen M, Paetau I, et al. Effective treatment of mitochondrial myopathy by nicotinamide riboside, a vitamin B3. EMBO Mol Med. 2014;6(6):721–31.
106. Long AN, Owens K, Schlappal AE, Kristian T, Fishman PS, Schuh RA. Effect of nicotinamide mononucleotide on brain mitochondrial respiratory deficits in an Alzheimer's disease-relevant murine model. BMC Neurol. 2015;15:19.
107. White SL, Shanske S, McGill JJ, et al. Mitochondrial DNA mutations at nucleotide 8993 show a lack of tissue- or age-related variation. J Inherit Metab Dis. 1999;22(8):899–914.
108. Manfredi G, Fu J, Ojaimi J, et al. Rescue of a deficiency in ATP synthesis by transfer of MTATP6, a mitochondrial DNA-encoded gene, to the nucleus. Nat Genet. 2002;30(4):394–9.
109. Bacman SR, Williams SL, Hernandez D, Moraes CT. Modulating mtDNA heteroplasmy by mitochondria-targeted restriction endonucleases in a 'differential multiple cleavage-site' model. Gene Ther. 2007;14(18):1309–18.
110. Tanaka M, Borgeld HJ, Zhang J, et al. Gene therapy for mitochondrial disease by delivering restriction endonuclease SmaI into mitochondria. J Biomed Sci. 2002;9(6 Pt 1):534–41.
111. Alexeyev MF, Venediktova N, Pastukh V, Shokolenko I, Bonilla G, Wilson GL. Selective elimination of mutant mitochondrial genomes as therapeutic strategy for the treatment of NARP and MILS syndromes. Gene Ther. 2008;15(7):516–23.
112. Kim YG, Cha J, Chandrasegaran S. Hybrid restriction enzymes: zinc finger fusions to Fok I cleavage domain. Proc Natl Acad Sci U S A. 1996;93(3):1156–60.

113. Minczuk M, Papworth MA, Kolasinska P, Murphy MP, Klug A. Sequence-specific modification of mitochondrial DNA using a chimeric zinc finger methylase. Proc Natl Acad Sci U S A. 2006;103(52):19689–94.
114. Gammage PA, Gaude E, Van Haute L, et al. Near-complete elimination of mutant mtDNA by iterative or dynamic dose-controlled treatment with mtZFNs. Nucleic Acids Res. 2016;44(16):7804–16.
115. Bacman SR, Williams SL, Pinto M, Peralta S, Moraes CT. Specific elimination of mutant mitochondrial genomes in patient-derived cells by mitoTALENs. Nat Med. 2013;19(9):1111–3.
116. Kirby DM, Kahler SG, Freckmann M-L, Reddihough D, Thorburn DR. Leigh disease caused by the mitochondrial DNA G14459A mutation in unrelated families. Ann Neurol. 2000;48(1):102–4.
117. Poulton J, Turnbull DM. 74th ENMC international workshop: mitochondrial diseases 19-20 November 1999, Naarden, The Netherlands. Neuromusc Dis. 2000;10(6):460–2.
118. Sofou K, Dahlin M, Hallböök T, Lindefeldt M, Viggedal G, Darin N. Ketogenic diet in pyruvate dehydrogenase complex deficiency: short- and long-term outcomes. J Inherit Metab Dis. 2017;40(2):237–45.

Coenzyme Q_{10} Deficiency

Catarina M. Quinzii and Luis Carlos Lopez

Functions and Biosynthesis of Coenzyme Q_{10}

Coenzyme Q_{10} (CoQ_{10}) is a lipophilic molecule with redox capacity localized in cell membranes [1]. In the mitochondrial inner membrane, CoQ_{10} plays a central role in the electron transport chain (mtETC), where it is required for the transfer of electrons between NADH:ubiquinone oxidoreductase (complex I) and coenzyme Q:cytochrome c—oxidoreductase (complex III). CoQ_{10} and its oxidation by the mtETC is also required for the function of several enzymes that link the mtETC to other metabolic pathways, as tricarboxylic acid (TCA) cycle, through succinate dehydrogenase (SDH or complex II); β-oxidation, through electron-transfer flavoprotein-ubiquinone oxidoreductase (ETFDH); shuttle of reduction equivalents from the cytoplasm, through glycerol-3-phosphate dehydrogenase (G3PDH); pyrimidine biosynthesis, through dihydroorotate dehydrogenase (DODH); glycine metabolism, through choline dehydrogenase (CHDH); arginine and proline metabolism, through proline dehydrogenase (PDH); and seleno-amino acid metabolism and sulfur assimilation, through sulfide:quinone oxidoreductase (SQOR) [1] (Fig. 1). Moreover, CoQ_{10} is an important endogenous antioxidant in the cell membranes [1].

The biosynthesis of CoQ occurs in a complex biosynthetic pathway, in which the initial substrates are the decaprenyl diphosphate, produced by the decaprenyl diphosphate synthase, and the 4-hydroxybenzoic acid (4-HB) (Fig. 2). The first step is the prenylation of the benzoquinone ring, precursor of CoQ, followed by seven reactions (one decarboxylation, three hydroxylation, and three methylation) that produce the fully substituted benzoquinone ring of CoQ. This process involves at least 12 genes that encode catalytic enzymes or regulatory proteins. Moreover, most of these proteins form a CoQ multiprotein complex for CoQ biosynthesis. The most represented CoQ in human has ten isoprenyl groups and thus is called CoQ_{10} [1].

Clinical Presentations and Molecular Mechanisms of CoQ_{10} Deficiency

Encephalomyopathy

Although encephalopathy was the first phenotype associated with CoQ_{10} deficiency, few patients with this presentation have been described so far,

C. M. Quinzii (✉)
Department of Neurology, Columbia University Medical Center, New York, NY, USA
e-mail: cmq2101@cumc.columbia.edu

L. C. Lopez
Department of Physiology, Centro de Investigación Biomédica, Universidad de Granada, Granada, Spain
e-mail: luisca@ugr.es

M. Mancuso, T. Klopstock (eds.), *Diagnosis and Management of Mitochondrial Disorders*,
https://doi.org/10.1007/978-3-030-05517-2_11

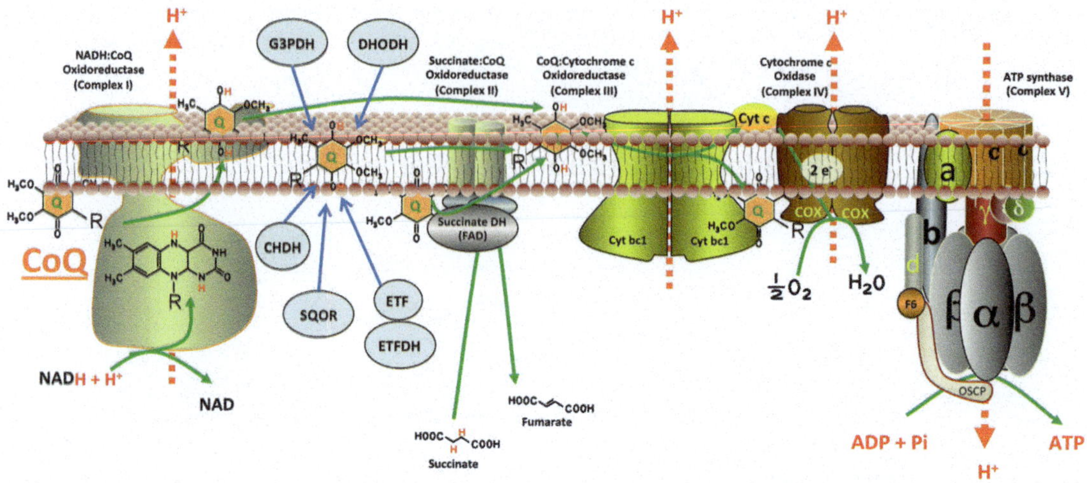

Fig. 1 CoQ functions in the mitochondria, indicating all protein complexes and enzymes that provide electrons to CoQ

and most lack molecular diagnosis. In 1989, Ogasahara and colleagues described two sisters who, after normal early development, presented with exercise intolerance and slowly progressive weakness of axial and proximal limb muscles. After 5 years of age, brain involvement manifested with learning disability in both sisters, seizures in one, and cerebellar syndrome in the other. In addition, both had episodes of myoglobinuria following seizures or intercurrent infections. Laboratory abnormalities included lactic acidosis and increased serum creatine kinase (CK). EMG showed myopathic features. Muscle biopsies showed ragged red fibers (RRF) and excessive accumulation of lipid droplets in type I fibers, decreased activities of mitochondrial respiratory chain complexes I + III and II + III, and markedly decreased concentration of CoQ_{10} in muscle, but normal in serum and cultured fibroblasts [2]. Since then, four patients with the same clinical triad of mitochondrial myopathy, recurrent myoglobinuria, and encephalopathy have been reported [3–6]. Mutations in *ADCK3* (now renamed *COQ8A*) have been found in one patient [7].

Interestingly, Salviati and colleagues reported a patient with severe hypotonia, congenital myopathy, moderate mental retardation, and dysmorphic features, associated with haploinsufficiency of *COQ4* caused by a 3.9 Mb deletion of chromosome 9q34 [8].

Infantile Multisystemic Disease

The infantile, multisystemic presentation is usually caused by mutations in genes directly involved in CoQ_{10} biosynthesis [9]. To date, mutations in *COQ1* (*PDSS1* and *PDSS2*), *COQ2*, *COQ4*, *COQ6*, *COQ7*, and *COQ9* genes have been identified in patients with this phenotype. Due to its early onset and frequent lethality, this manifestation of CoQ_{10} deficiency is probably underdiagnosed. However, in the last decade, next-generation sequencing techniques, where available, have increased the diagnostic rate [10]. Low levels of CoQ_{10} in cultured fibroblasts and early renal involvement seem to be hallmarks of primary infantile multisystemic syndromes [11–16]. Intriguingly, whereas kidney involvement is a prevalent manifestation in patients with multisystemic disease caused by mutations in *COQ1* (PDSS2 subunit), *COQ2*, *COQ6*, and *COQ9* genes, to date, it has never been associated with mutations in *COQ4* gene [17]. On the contrary, cardiomyopathy has been described in patients with mutations in *COQ4* [18–20], *PDSS1* [14], *PDSS2* [11], *COQ2* [16], and *COQ9* [21].

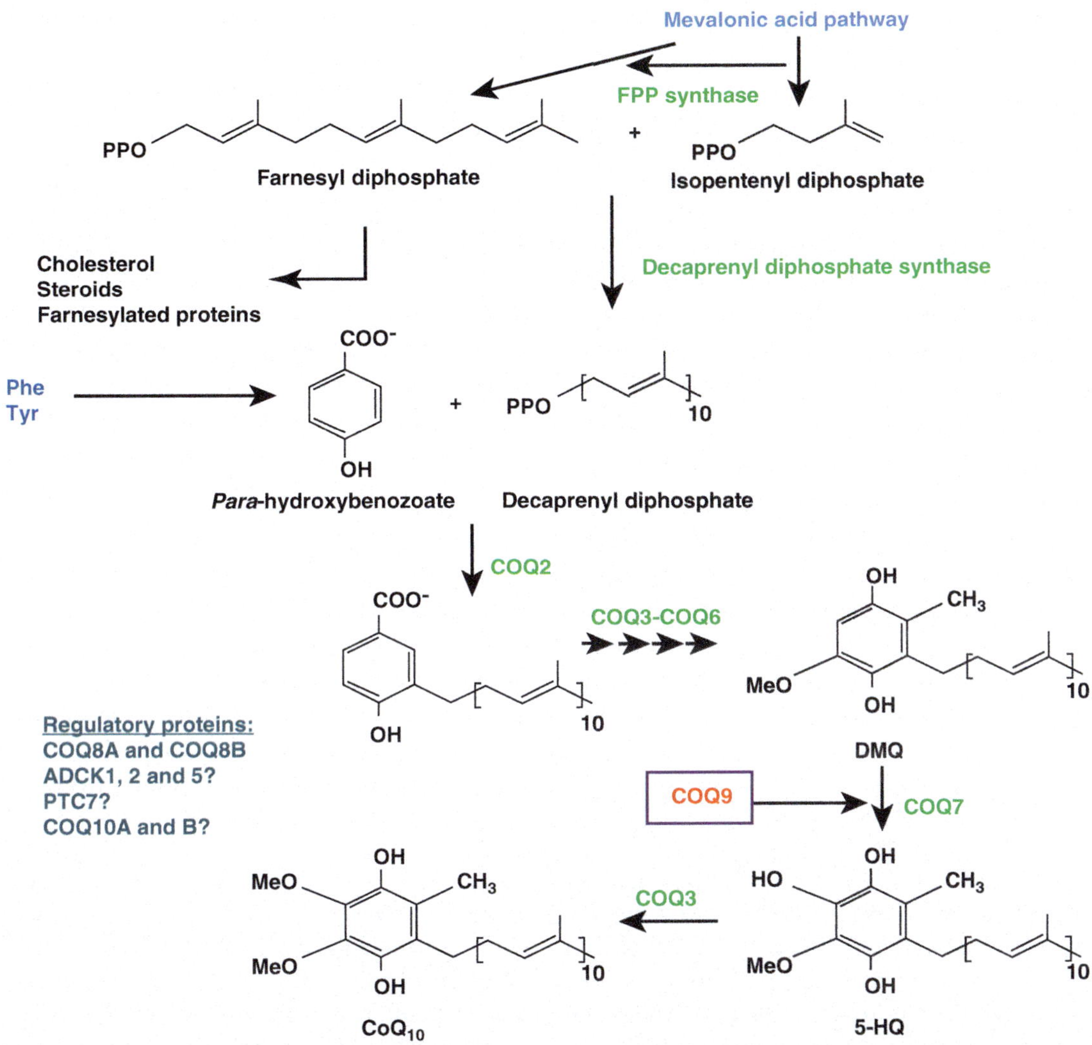

Fig. 2 Biochemical pathway of CoQ biosynthesis. The quinone ring is derived from tyrosine or phenylalanine, and the isoprenoid side chain is produced by addition of isopentenyl diphosphate molecules to farnesyl diphosphate in multiple steps catalyzed by decaprenyl diphosphate synthase. Decaprenyl diphosphate and para-hydroxybenzoate (PHB) are condensed in a reaction catalyzed by PHB-polyprenyl transferase or COQ2, and the benzoate ring is then modified by at least six enzymes, which catalyze methylation, decarboxylation, and hydroxylation reactions to synthesize CoQ

Hearing loss, encephalopathy (as Leigh syndrome and stroke-like episodes), lactic acidosis, and hepatopathy are other frequent manifestations. The combination of sensory hearing loss and nephropathy is typical of *COQ6* mutations [22], which will be further described in the nephropathy section of this chapter.

The first reported patients with multisystemic manifestation of CoQ_{10} deficiency were three siblings who presented soon after birth with neurological symptoms, including nystagmus, optic atrophy, sensorineural hearing loss, ataxia, dystonia, weakness, rapidly progressive nephropathy, and widespread CoQ_{10} deficiency [23], associated with mutations in *PDSS2* (Rötig, personal communication). Later, we reported a male infant with nephrotic syndrome and Leigh syndrome due to mutations in *PDSS2* [11]. The boy presented with neonatal pneumonia and hypotonia. At 3 months of age, he developed seizures; subsequently became progressively floppy; had difficulty feeding, severe episodic vomiting, and lactic acidosis; and died at 8 months of age due to status epilepticus [11]. Similar phenotypes with severe Leigh syndrome, glomerular nephropathy, and CoQ_{10} deficiency in muscle were described in another infant with compound heterozygous mutations in the *PDSS2* gene [24]. Interestingly, Leigh syndrome was previously reported in two sisters with CoQ_{10} deficiency, encephalopathy, growth retardation, infantilism, ataxia, deafness, lactic acidosis, and unknown molecular defect [25].

In a consanguineous family, two siblings had CoQ_{10} deficiency due to a homozygous *PDSS1* mutation manifesting as a multisystem disease with early-onset deafness, encephaloneuropathy, obesity, livedo reticularis, and cardiac valvulopathy [14].

In 2005, we reported two siblings, who shared a homozygous missense mutation in the *COQ2* gene [12, 26]. The proband was a 33-month-old boy who developed nystagmus at 2 months. At 12 months of age, he was hospitalized because of a severe nephrotic syndrome and neurological examination showed hypotonia and mild psychomotor delay. At 18 months of age, he developed frequent vomiting, psychomotor regression, tremor, weakness, and status epilepticus. Brain MRI showed cerebral and cerebellar atrophy and stroke-like lesions. He received a successful renal transplant at 3 years of age. The sister developed nephrotic syndrome at 12 months of age without any clinical signs of neurological involvement [13, 26]. Both siblings improved with CoQ_{10} supplementation [13, 27]. Rötig's group subsequently reported two siblings harboring a homozygous base-pair deletion in exon 7 of the *COQ2* gene. The girl had neonatal neurologic distress, nephrotic syndrome, hepatopathy, pancytopenia, diabetes mellitus, seizures, and lactic acidosis progressing to fatal multiorgan failure at age 12 days [14]. The older brother also had anemia, liver failure, and renal insufficiency, and died at the age of 1 day.

In the last year, other five patients with multisystemic disease and novel mutations in *COQ2* have been reported [13, 28–30]. Interestingly, there was no evidence for renal involvement in a dizygotic twin from consanguineous Turkish parents carrying a novel homozygous mutation in *COQ2*, reported by Jakobs [29]. The children were born prematurely and died at the age of 5 and 6 months, respectively, after an undulating disease course involving apneas, seizures, feeding problems, and generalized edema, alternating with relatively stable periods without the need of artificial ventilation [29]. One patient had the interesting combination of retinitis pigmentosa and multiple system atrophy (MSA) [30]. The association between *COQ2* variants and MSA will be further addressed in the cerebellar ataxia section of this chapter.

Desbats et al. reported a patient with mutations in *COQ2* who presented at birth with severe lactic acidosis, proteinuria, dicarboxylic aciduria, and hepatic insufficiency. She also had dilation of left ventricle on echocardiography. Her neurological condition rapidly worsened and despite aggressive care she died at 23 h of life [31].

To date, 12 recessive mutations in *COQ4* have been reported in patients presenting neonatal encephalopathy and severe CoQ_{10} deficiency. Chung reported five recessive missense *COQ4* mutations in five patients with severe, early-onset mitochondrial disease presenting encephalopathy and/or cardiomyopathy and lactic acidosis [19]. A very similar phenotype was observed in an infant with profound mitochondrial disease presenting with perinatal seizures, hypertrophic cardiomyopathy, and severe muscle CoQ_{10} deficiency, associated with gastroesophageal reflux requiring fundoplication, delayed visual maturation without structural abnormality of the eyes, bilateral hearing loss, profound hypotonia, and absence of development [20]. Brea-Calvo reported six pathogenic, autosomal recessive, variants in five patients with early-onset mitochondrial disease and CoQ_{10} deficiency. The clinical phenotypes of the five subjects varied widely, but four had a prenatal or perinatal onset with early fatal outcome.

Two unrelated individuals presented with severe hypotonia, bradycardia, respiratory insufficiency, and heart failure; two sisters showed antenatal cerebellar hypoplasia, neonatal respiratory-distress syndrome, and epileptic encephalopathy. The fifth subject had an early onset but slowly progressive clinical course dominated by neurological deterioration with hardly any involvement of other organs [18]. In Chung et al., five out of five patients had hypotonia and five out of six patients presented with cardiomyopathy, yet the prevalence of hypotonia and cardiomyopathy in the cohort reported by Brea-Calvo was one in five and two in five, respectively [18, 19]. Nevertheless, as mentioned before, among all reported patients harboring *COQ4* mutations, cardiomyopathy is the most prominent feature.

Although mutations in *COQ6* have been associated typically with nephropathy and hearing loss, a 10-month-old boy was described with nephrotic syndrome associated with extrarenal manifestations including hearing loss, cardiovascular abnormality, motor and mental retardation, and unilateral ptosis. Importantly, CoQ_{10} supplementation improved renal function and growth, but not hearing loss [32], confirming previous results of supplementation in another patient [22].

Only two patients have been reported with mutations in *COQ7*; although they both present hearing loss, one was a 6-year-old girl with spasticity and bilateral sensorineural hearing loss [33], while the other one had earlier onset with a complex clinical picture and multiple organ involvement including neonatal lung hypoplasia, contractures, early infantile hypertension, and cardiac hypertrophy, hypothesized to be secondary to his prenatal kidney dysplasia with renal dysfunction which surprisingly resolved during his first year, mild psychomotor delay with hearing, and visual impairment [34].

Also mutations in *COQ9* have been reported only in two patients. In 2001, Rahman and colleagues reported a newborn with generalized limb hypertonia, reduced truncal tone, lactic acidosis, renal tubulopathy, and left ventricular hypertrophy with global hypokinesia. Brain MRI revealed cerebral and cerebellar atrophy. He developed severe seizures and dystonia, and died at 2 years of age [21]. The second patient was a boy born premature, small for gestational age, with poor respiratory efforts, muscular hypotonia, bradycardia, and generalized cyanosis. Laboratory investigations revealed lactic acidosis. Cranial ultrasound results were suggestive of neonatal Leigh-like syndrome. After seizures and recurrent episodes of apnea and bradycardia, the boy died due to cardiorespiratory failure at 18 days of age [35].

A single patient with cardiofaciocutaneous syndrome due to a *BRAF* gene mutation also had muscle CoQ_{10} deficiency (2.7 nmol/gr; normal = 24–39.5 nmol/gr) [36].

In 2003, Leshinsky-Silver and colleagues reported a patient who presented with neonatal liver disease, pancreatic insufficiency, tyrosinemia, hyperammonemia, subsequent sensorineural hearing loss, and Leigh syndrome. Although CoQ_{10} level and molecular defect in this patient are unknown, liver biopsy revealed markedly reduced complex I + III and II + III activity that was restored by addition of CoQ_{10} to the liver homogenate indicating CoQ_{10} deficiency [37].

Nephropathy

Steroid-resistant nephrotic syndrome is one of the most common manifestations of CoQ_{10} deficiency, with mutations in *COQ6* and *COQ8B* (previously named *ADCK4*) as the most frequent responsible molecular defects [17].

As mentioned above, of the first two siblings described carrying *COQ2* mutations, the sister developed nephrotic syndrome at 12 months of age without any clinical signs of neurological involvement [26]. In 2007, other two patients with early-onset glomerulopathy due to mutations in the *COQ2* gene were described [13]. The first patient presented with steroid-resistant nephrotic syndrome at age 18 months as a result of collapsing glomerulopathy, without extrarenal manifestations. The second patient presented at 5 days of life with oliguria, had severe extracapillary proliferation on renal biopsy, rapidly developed end-stage renal disease, and died at the age of 6 months after a course complicated by progressive epileptic encephalopathy. Combined complex II + III activity and CoQ_{10} level were decreased in renal cortex as well as in skeletal muscle [13].

An extensive screening of *COQ2* and *PDSS2* mutations performed in 117 European non-Finnish patients with congenital nephrotic syndrome was negative, suggesting that mutations in those genes are rare causes of early-onset nephrotic syndrome [38]. At the contrary, a patient with *COQ2* mutations was identified by a recent screening performed in UK in 36 pediatric patients with NS, identified a patient with *COQ2* mutations [39]. Although the onset of nephropathy associated with *COQ2* mutations is usually in infancy, a patient with adolescence onset was described [40].

Mutations in *COQ6* were initially reported in 13 individuals (7 families) with steroid-resistant nephrotic syndrome, neurosensory deafness, and encephalomyopathy [22]. In the two patients treated, CoQ_{10} supplementation improved proteinuria but not hearing function [22]. Park reported seven patients with nephrotic syndrome and hearing loss [41], and Gigante reported a patient with isolated nephrotic syndrome [40].

Mutations in *COQ8B* have been identified in 76 individuals with steroid-resistant nephrotic syndrome, and therefore are the first cause of CoQ_{10} deficiency [41–45]. In patients with *COQ8B* mutations, compared to other cases of coenzyme Q_{10} biosynthesis defects, extrarenal involvement appears less frequent and renal disease develops on average at older age (adolescence) and responds to CoQ_{10} supplementation [41–45]. Four children with onset in the first decade of life were described [41, 44]. Extrarenal manifestations include seizures, mental retardation, and retinitis pigmentosa [42, 43].

Nephrotic syndrome has been described also in two sisters with CoQ_{10} deficiency and unknown molecular defect(s) [9].

Cerebellar Ataxia

The cerebellar phenotype of CoQ_{10} deficiency is the most common, although frequently secondary, and characterized by cerebellar ataxia and atrophy variably associated with neuropathy, seizures, mental retardation, muscle weakness, hypogonadism, and low levels of CoQ_{10} in fibroblasts [7, 46–52]. Muscle morphology did not show ragged red fibers and lipid storage myopathy in the first reports. Mutations in *COQ8A* (previously named *ADCK3*) cause autosomal recessive cerebellar ataxia 2 (ARCA2), and have been reported in ~40 patients, and therefore represent one of the most common causes of primary CoQ_{10} deficiency, second only after the mutations in *COQ8B* [7, 50–60]. ARCA2 is characterized by a very slowly progressive or apparently stable ataxia associated with other signs of central nervous system involvement, with gait ataxia being the most frequent sign at disease onset. In some patients, hand clumsiness, myoclonus, and choreic movements have also been observed. Individuals rarely present seizures, stroke-like episodes, and developmental delay. In almost half of the patients, involvement of the corticospinal tract is present, but spasticity seldom reaches clinical significance. The majority of ARCA2 patients develop symptoms in childhood or adolescence. Because of the combination of progressive ataxia and acute epileptic encephalopathy with stroke-like episode, together with electrophysiological features of this disorder similar to the polymerase gamma (POLG)-related encephalopathy, it has suggested that *COQ8A* mutations be considered in the differential diagnosis of mitochondrial encephalopathy with POLG-like features [58].

Late onset is quite uncommon. Four patients have been described with an adult-onset form [52, 59, 60]. In two, biochemical analysis disclosed normal CoQ_{10} levels in muscle [52], whereas in the third patient CoQ_{10} level was severely reduced [59], suggesting a lack of correlation between levels of CoQ_{10} in muscle and age of onset and severity of the disease.

Cerebellar ataxia, associated with encephalopathy, generalized tonic-clonic seizures, and cognitive disability was recently described in three siblings carrying mutations in *COQ5* [61].

CoQ_{10} deficiency in cerebellar ataxia is frequently secondary to molecular defects in genes not involved in CoQ_{10} biosynthesis [9]. CoQ_{10} deficiency has been identified in fibroblasts and muscle of patients with ataxia-oculomotor apraxia 1 (AOA1) caused by mutations in the gene encoding aprataxin (APTX) [62–65].

In two patients with adult-onset cerebellar ataxia and CoQ_{10} deficiency in muscle, whole-exome sequencing revealed mutations in *ANO10*, the causative gene for autosomal recessive spinocerebellar ataxia-10 (SCAR10). Both patients presented with slowly progressive ataxia and dysarthria leading to severe disability in the sixth decade. Epilepsy and learning difficulties were also present in one patient, while retinal degeneration and cataract were present in the other [66].

Yubero and colleagues reported a 15-year-old girl with GLUT1 deficiency and reduction of CoQ_{10} levels in muscle, plasma, and skin fibroblasts [67]. However, another study reported normal CoQ_{10} levels in fibroblasts, plasma, and white blood cells of additional patients with GLUT1 deficiency [68].

CoQ_{10} deficiency has been associated also with multiple system atrophy (MSA), a late-onset, sporadic neurodegenerative disorder clinically characterized by autonomic failure, parkinsonism, and cerebellar ataxia [30, 69–71].

The first patients described with CoQ_{10} deficiency and MSA harbored variants in *COQ2* [30], and subsequent studies confirmed that variants in this gene are a genetic risk factor in Japanese patients with MSA with cerebellar ataxia [72]. However, studies in other populations did not confirm this association [73, 74], and others provided evidence of CoQ_{10} deficiency and impaired CoQ biosynthetic pathway in post-mortem cerebellar samples, plasma, and CSF from MSA patients without *COQ2* mutations [69–71].

Isolated Myopathy

Lalani et al. and Horvath et al. described a pure myopathic form of CoQ_{10} deficiency, with lipid storage myopathy and respiratory chain dysfunction [74, 75]. In 2007, Gempel and colleagues found in the patients reported by Horvath and colleagues mutations in the *ETFDH* gene encoding electron-transferring flavoprotein dehydrogenase, which previously had been associated with glutaric aciduria type II (multiple acyl-CoA dehydrogenase deficiency [MADD]) [75, 76]. In that report, all seven patients from five families presented with exercise intolerance, fatigue, proximal myopathy, and elevated serum CK. Muscle histology showed lipid storage and subtle signs of mitochondrial myopathy.

In contrast, other studies reported patients with MADD and *ETFDH* mutations who had normal CoQ_{10} levels in muscle [77, 78].

Diagnostic Tools

Genetic diagnosis of CoQ_{10} deficiency presents some difficulties because of the molecular heterogeneity of this syndrome. A genotype–phenotype correlation is not possible, due to the limited number of patients reported. However, studies in *COQ2* and *COQ8B* mutant human fibroblasts showed that residual CoQ biosynthesis correlates with clinical severity in *COQ2* mutant but not in *COQ8B* mutant cells [79, 80].

In general, patients with infantile presentation of encephalopathy, steroid-resistant nephrotic syndrome, or cerebellar ataxia seem particularly likely to have primary CoQ_{10} deficiency. In the presence of nephrotic syndrome, targeted sequencing of CoQ_{10} biosynthetic genes associated with this syndrome (*PDSS2*, *COQ2*, *COQ6*, *COQ8B*) should be performed, followed by screening of genes encoding proteins known to be involved in CoQ biosynthesis even if they have never been associated with human disease before.

COQ8A should be sequenced in patients with autosomal recessive cerebellar ataxia.

Alternatively or complementarily to exome sequencing, measurement of CoQ_{10} levels in muscle is the gold standard for the diagnosis. Instead, CoQ_{10} can be measured in primary culture skin fibroblasts. Plasma measurement of CoQ_{10} is not accurate for the diagnosis of CoQ_{10} deficiency because it is influenced by the diet. Normally, decreased levels of CoQ_{10} correlate with a decrease in the activities of the CoQ-dependent complexes activities, i.e., complexes I + III (CI + III) and complexes II + III (CII + III) activities, which should be determined in frozen muscle homogenates. However, mild CoQ_{10} deficiency can be associated with normal activities of CI + III, CII + III, or both.

In the presence of low CoQ_{10} levels in cultured skin fibroblasts, defects in CoQ_{10} biosynthetic pathway can be detected by biochemical assays with radiolabelled substrates. Typically, [3H]-mevalonate and [14C]-4HB are used in cell culture, while [3H]-decaprenyl-PP is used in homogenized fibroblast extracts [11, 12, 14]. The combined use of [14C]-4HB and [3H]-decaprenyl-PP may be useful to discriminate defects upstream or downstream of the reaction catalyzed by decaprenyl diphosphate synthase [11, 12]. Unfortunately, multiple steps in the CoQ_{10} biosynthetic pathway cannot be distinguished using the available assays.

Histologically, there are no specific assays for the diagnostic of CoQ deficiency. Nevertheless, ragged red fibers and prominent lipid deposition are present in muscle of patients with myopathic manifestations.

Pathogenesis of the Disease

As mentioned before, CoQ_{10} serves several cellular functions and, consequently, deficiency of CoQ_{10} potentially disrupts multiple vital cellular functions, depending on the severity of the CoQ_{10} deficiency. The residual levels of CoQ_{10} depend on the specific mutation due to the mechanisms of non-sense-mediated mRNA decay, the residual activity of the mutated protein, and/or the consequences in the stability of the CoQ multiprotein complex [79, 81]. Studies of tissues and cells from patients with CoQ_{10} deficiency have revealed multiple pathological consequences. Skeletal muscle biopsies from patients with all clinical forms of CoQ_{10} deficiency have shown variable defects of respiratory chain enzyme activities (complexes I + III and II + III). In addition, muscles from patients with myopathic CoQ_{10} deficiency have revealed signs of apoptosis [5]. Studies of pathogenic mechanisms using cultured fibroblasts from patients have revealed correlations between degree of CoQ_{10} deficiency, oxidative stress, cell growth impairment, and death [82–86]. Evidence of autophagy has been shown in mammalian cells, and in kidney of mice with a homozygous mutation in *Pdss2* ($Pdss2^{kd/kd}$) [87, 88]. Our studies in $Pdss2^{kd/kd}$ mice suggest that autophagy might be triggered by oxidative stress [89], and the roles of oxidative stress and impaired ATP synthesis in the pathogenesis of CoQ deficiency have been confirmed in $Coq9^{R239X}$ mice [90]. On the contrary, several human and murine *in vitro* models of CoQ deficiency suggest that defects in mitochondrial respiration are not detrimental [42, 82–84, 86, 91, 92].

CoQ receives electrons not only from CI and CII but also from different mitochondrial enzymes, and some of these enzymes have been reported to participate in the pathogenesis of CoQ deficiency. Because DHODH participates in the biosynthesis of pyrimidine nucleotides, the increase of growth rate in *COQ2* mutant fibroblasts under supplementation with uridine was attributed to a possible decrease in DHODH activity [93]. Another CoQ-dependent enzyme is SQOR, the first enzyme of sulfide oxidation. Decreased levels and activity of SQOR were demonstrated in human skin fibroblasts carrying different mutations in CoQ biosynthetic genes [94, 95], as well as in two mouse models of CoQ deficiency, $Coq9^{R239X}$ and $Pdss2^{kd/kd}$ mice [94, 95].

Therapeutic Approaches

CoQ_{10} deficiency is one of the few mitochondrial disorders potentially treatable but prompt diagnosis is critical and supplementation with high doses of CoQ_{10} is always recommended, since it is not associated with side effects. However, the response to supplementation depends on the clinical phenotype.

In patients with encephalomyopathy, CoQ_{10} supplementation improved mainly muscle symptoms. In one patient, muscle symptoms and seizures resolved, CK and lactic acid levels normalized, and muscle biopsy showed CoQ_{10} level normalization. In contrast, another patient developed cerebellar ataxia.

Patients with pure myopathy showed dramatic improvements after CoQ_{10} supplementation [76]. Of all the patients reported, six improved with supplementation with CoQ_{10}, while two patients improved with combined treatment of CoQ_{10} and riboflavin.

Nephrotic syndrome is the most responsive to supplementation [17, 27]. However, the mechanisms of action of CoQ_{10} in nephrotic syndrome associated with CoQ deficiency are unclear. Studies in *Pdss2*$^{kd/kd}$ mice, a model of CoQ_{10} deficiency-associated nephrotic syndrome, showed that indeed oral CoQ_{10} supplementation improves survival and kidney disease, but does not increase CoQ_{10} levels in kidney [96].

Response to CoQ_{10} supplementation in patients with cerebellar ataxia is variable. Pineda et al. observed improvement after supplementation in patients with cerebellar ataxia and CoQ_{10} deficiency, independently of the molecular defect [51].

Supplementation with CoQ_{10} was associated with mild, subjective, clinical improvement in patients with cerebellar ataxia associated with mutations in *COQ8A* [7, 50]. Liu reported two affected siblings in their 20s, who presented with cerebellar ataxia, myoclonus, and dysarthria that improved after CoQ_{10} supplementation [57].

Importantly, CoQ_{10} supplementation seems to be beneficial also in cerebellar ataxia associated with secondary CoQ_{10} deficiency. For example, in the three patients with AOA1 described by Musumeci, supplementation with CoQ_{10} was associated with increased strength and energy level, and disappearance of seizures [46]. Dramatic improvement of some neurologic symptoms was described in patients with ANO10 and GLUT 1 deficiency [66, 67].

The multisystemic infantile-onset form of CoQ_{10} deficiency, especially in the presence of encephalopathy, is associated with a worse prognosis than other presentations of CoQ_{10} deficiency, being frequently lethal.

Since the reduced bioavailability of CoQ_{10} and its inability to cross the blood–brain barrier might be accountable for its lack of beneficial effects in patients with encephalopathy, supplementation with the water-soluble short-tail ubiquinone analog idebenone has been attempted but failed [6]. Accordingly, when we compared the effects of CoQ_{10} and idebenone *in vitro* using skin fibroblasts from patients with primary CoQ_{10} deficiency, we observed that idebenone was able to reduce ROS levels and oxidative damage, but it did not increase the ATP levels and ATP/ADP ratio. Mitochondrial bioenergetics was rescued only by CoQ_{10} supplementation, demonstrating the importance of the decaprenyl tail [84].

Based on the variable response to the treatment, some alternative therapies have been tested experimentally with the aim of improving the efficacy of the treatment. A first therapeutic approach was to treat *Coq9*^{R239X} mice, a model of mitochondrial encephalopathy due to CoQ deficiency, with ubiquinol-10 (reduced form of CoQ_{10}) and compare the outcomes with the treatment with ubiquinone-10 (oxidized form of CoQ_{10}), both in water-soluble formulations [97]. While ubiquinol-10 treatment partially increased CoQ-dependent respiratory chain activities in the cerebrum of *Coq9*^{R239X} mice and partially reduced the vacuolization, astrogliosis, and oxidative damage, still 50% of ubiquinol-10-treated *Coq9*^{R239X} mice died at 6 months of age (compared to the 100% of death in the untreated *Coq9*^{R239X} mice) due to the poor absorption and bioavailability of CoQ_{10} together with its low penetration through the blood–brain barrier. The difference in response to the oxidized versus the reduced forms of CoQ_{10} suggests that ubiquinol-10 has better absorption and bioavailability than ubiquinone-10 and, therefore, should be preferentially used for the treatment of CoQ_{10} deficiency. Based on those arguments, ubiquinol-10 was designated by the EMA (EU/3/16/1765) as an orphan drug for the treatment of primary CoQ_{10} deficiency. The results of oral CoQ_{10} supplementation in *Coq9*^{R239X} mice are consistent with studies in humans, where CoQ_{10} deficiency patients with neurological symptoms usually present lower response to CoQ_{10} supplementation.

A novel therapeutic strategy, still in preclinical stage, is the use of analogs of CoQ biosynthetic precursors to bypass defects in CoQ biosynthesis. For example, the hydroxyl group incorporated by COQ7 into the benzoquinone ring is already present in the 2,4-dihydroxybenzoic acid (2,4-diHB) molecule. Therefore, 2,4-diHB is a 4-HB (the natural precursor of CoQ biosynthesis) analog that can be theoretically used in the CoQ biosynthetic pathway in order to bypass a defect of the hydroxylation step catalyzed by COQ7. This strategy was partially successful in *Coq7*-null yeasts [98], as well as in mouse and human fibroblasts with mutations in *COQ7* or *COQ9* [81, 99]. Oral supplementation of 2,4-diHB in *Coq9*^{R239X} mice and *Coq7* conditional KO mice significantly increased the levels of CoQ in kidneys, heart, and muscle [81, 99]. Although in *Coq7* conditional KO mice 2,4-diHB supplementation increased survival [99], the mechanism is not clear, since the cause of death in this model is unknown. Therefore, further studies in *in vivo* models of CoQ deficiency with a well-defined neurological pathology are necessary to understand the mechanism of action of 4-HB analogs.

Other analogs of the precursor 4-HB, such as 3,4-hydroxybenzoic acid or vanillic acid, have been used in *Coq6*-null yeasts expressing human *COQ6* mutations [100, 101], showing an increase in the endogenous CoQ biosynthesis. Thus, 2-methyl-4-hydroxybenzoic acid or 2,3-dimethoxy-4-hydroxybenzoic acid could be theoretically applied in the cases of mutations in *COQ5* or *COQ3*, respectively. Nevertheless, further studies are needed to understand the therapeutic mechanisms of CoQ_{10} and its precursor analogs, to define the most appropriated therapy for each particular biosynthetic step causing CoQ_{10} deficiency and to define the safety use of each particular compound.

References

1. Bentinger M, Tekle M, Dallner G. Coenzyme Q--biosynthesis and functions. Biochem Biophys Res Commun. 2010;396(1):74–9.
2. Ogasahara S, Engel AG, Frens D, Mack D. Muscle coenzyme Q deficiency in familial mitochondrial encephalomyopathy. Proc Natl Acad Sci U S A. 1989;86:2379–82.
3. Sobreira C, Hirano M, Shanske S, Keller RK, Haller RG, Davidson E, et al. Mitochondrial encephalomyopathy with coenzyme Q_{10} deficiency. Neurology. 1997;48:1238–43.
4. Boitier E, Degoul F, Desguerre I, Charpentier C, François D, Ponsot G, et al. A case of mitochondrial encephalomyopathy associated with a muscle coenzyme Q_{10} deficiency. J Neurol Sci. 1998;156:41–6.
5. Di Giovanni S, Mirabella M, Spinazzola A, Crociani P, Silvestri G, Broccolini A, et al. Coenzyme Q_{10} reverses pathological phenotype and reduces apoptosis in familial CoQ_{10} deficiency. Neurology. 2001;57:515–8.
6. Auré K, Benoist JF, Ogier de Baulny H, Romero NB, Rigal O, Lombes A. Progression despite replacement of a myopathic form of coenzyme Q_{10} defect. Neurology. 2004;63:727–9.
7. Mollet J, Delahodde A, Serre V, Chretien D, Schlemmer D, Lombes A, et al. *CABC1* gene mutations cause ubiquinone deficiency with cerebellar ataxia and seizures. Am J Hum Genet. 2008;82:623–30.
8. Salviati L, Trevisson E, Rodriguez Hernandez MA, Casarin A, Pertegato V, Doimo M, et al. Haploinsufficiency of COQ4 causes coenzyme Q_{10} deficiency. J Med Genet. 2012;49:187–91.
9. Emmanuele V, Lopez L, Berardo A, Naini A, Tadesse S, Wen B, et al. Heterogeneity of coenzyme Q_{10} deficiency: patients study and literature review. Arch Neurol. 2012;69:978–83.
10. Hughes BG, Harrison PM, Hekimi S. Estimating the occurrence of primary ubiquinone deficiency by analysis of large-scale sequencing data. Sci Rep. 2017;7(1):17744.
11. López LC, Schuelke M, Quinzii CM, Kanki T, Rodenburg RJ, Naini A, et al. Leigh syndrome with nephropathy and CoQ_{10} deficiency due to decaprenyl diphosphate synthase subunit 2 (PDSS2) mutations. Am J Hum Genet. 2006;79:1125–9.
12. Quinzii C, Naini A, Salviati L, Trevisson E, Navas P, DiMauro S, et al. A mutation in para-

hydroxybenzoate-polyprenyl transferase (COQ2) causes primary coenzyme Q_{10} deficiency. Am J Hum Genet. 2006;78:345–9.
13. Diomedi-Camassei F, Di Giandomenico S, Santorelli FM, Caridi G, Piemonte F, Montini G, et al. COQ2 nephropathy: a newly described inherited mitochondriopathy with primary renal involvement. J Am Soc Nephrol. 2007;18:2773–80.
14. Mollet J, Giurgea I, Schlemmer D, Dallner G, Chretien D, Delahodde A, et al. Prenyldiphosphate synthase, subunit 1 (PDSS1) and OH-benzoate polyprenyltransferase (COQ2) mutations in ubiquinone deficiency and oxidative phosphorylation disorders. J Clin Invest. 2007;117:765–72.
15. Duncan AJ, Bitner-Glindzicz M, Meunier B, Costello H, Hargreaves IP, Lopez LC, et al. A nonsense mutation in COQ9 causes autosomal-recessive neonatal-onset primary coenzyme Q_{10} deficiency: a potentially treatable form of mitochondrial disease. Am J Hum Genet. 2009;84:558–66.
16. Scalais E, Chafai R, Van Coster R, Bindl L, Nuttin C, Panagiotaraki C, et al. Early myoclonic epilepsy, hypertrophic cardiomyopathy and subsequently a nephrotic syndrome in a patient with CoQ10 deficiency caused by mutations in para-hydroxybenzoate-polyprenyl transferase (COQ2). Eur J Paediatr Neurol. 2013;17(6):625–30.
17. Emma F, Salviati L. Mitochondrial cytopathies and the kidney. Nephrol Ther. 2017;13(Suppl 1):S23–8.
18. Brea-Calvo G, Haack TB, Karall D, Ohtake A, Invernizzi F, Carrozzo R, et al. COQ4 mutations cause a broad spectrum of mitochondrial disorders associated with CoQ10 deficiency. Am J Hum Genet. 2015;96(2):309–17.
19. Chung WK, Martin K, Jalas C, Braddock SR, Juusola J, Monaghan KG, et al. Mutations in COQ4, an essential component of coenzyme Q biosynthesis, cause lethal neonatal mitochondrial encephalomyopathy. J Med Genet. 2015;52(9):627–35.
20. Sondheimer N, Hewson S, Cameron JM, Somers GR, Broadbent JD, Ziosi M, et al. Novel recessive mutations in COQ4 cause severe infantile cardiomyopathy and encephalopathy associated with CoQ_{10} deficiency. Mol Genet Metab Rep. 2017;12:23–7.
21. Rahman S, Hargreaves I, Clayton P, Heales S. Neonatal presentation of coenzyme Q_{10} deficiency. J Pediatr. 2001;139:456–8.
22. Heeringa SF, Chernin G, Chaki M, Zhou W, Sloan AJ, Ji Z, et al. COQ6 mutations in human patients produce nephrotic syndrome with sensorineural deafness. J Clin Invest. 2001;121:2013–24.
23. Rötig A, Appelkvist EL, Geromel V, Chretien D, Kadhom N, Edery P, et al. Quinone-responsive multiple respiratory-chain dysfunction due to widespread coenzyme Q_{10} deficiency. Lancet. 2000;356:391–5.
24. Quinzii CM, Loos M. Multisystemic infantile CoQ10 deficiency with renal involvement. In: Mitochondrial case studies: underlying mechanisms and diagnosis. Amsterdam: Elsevier; 2016.
25. Van Maldergem L, Trijbels F, DiMauro S, Sindelar PJ, Musumeci O, Janssen A, et al. Coenzyme Q-responsive Leigh's encephalopathy in two sisters. Ann Neurol. 2002;52:750–4.
26. Salviati L, Sacconi S, Murer L, Zacchello G, Franceschini L, Laverda AM, et al. Infantile encephalomyopathy and nephropathy with CoQ_{10} deficiency: a CoQ_{10}-responsive condition. Neurology. 2005;65:606–8.
27. Montini G, Malaventura C, Salviati L. Early coenzyme Q_{10} supplementation in primary coenzyme Q_{10} deficiency. N Engl J Med. 2008;358:2849–50.
28. Dinwiddie DL, Smith LD, Miller NA, Atherton AM, Farrow EG, Strenk ME, et al. Diagnosis of mitochondrial disorders by concomitant next-generation sequencing of the exome and mitochondrial genome. Genomics. 2013;102(3):148–56.
29. Jakobs BS, van den Heuvel LP, Smeets RJ, de Vries MC, Hien S, Schaible T, et al. A novel mutation in COQ2 leading to fatal infantile multisystem disease. J Neurol Sci. 2013;326(1–2):24–8.
30. Mitsui J, Matsukawa T, Ishiura H, Fukuda Y, Ichikawa Y, Date H, et al. Mutations in COQ2 in familial and sporadic multiple-system atrophy. N Engl J Med. 2013;369(3):233–44.
31. Desbats MA, Lunardi G, Doimo M, Trevisson E, Salviati L. Genetic bases and clinical manifestations of coenzyme Q10 (CoQ 10) deficiency. J Inherit Metab Dis. 2015;38(1):145–56.
32. Cao Q, Li GM, Xu H, Shen Q, Sun L, Fang XY, et al. Coenzyme Q(10) treatment for one child with COQ6 gene mutation induced nephrotic syndrome and literature review. Zhonghua Er Ke Za Zhi. 2017;55(2):135–8.
33. Wang Y, Smith C, Parboosingh JS, Khan A, Innes M, Hekimi S. Pathogenicity of two COQ7 mutations and responses to 2,4-dihydroxybenzoate bypass treatment. J Cell Mol Med. 2017;21(10):2329–43.
34. Freyer C, Stranneheim H, Naess K, Mourier A, Felser A, Maffezzini C, et al. Rescue of primary ubiquinone deficiency due to a novel COQ7 defect using 2,4-dihydroxybensoic acid. J Med Genet. 2015;52(11):779–83.
35. Danhauser K, Herebian D, Haack TB, Rodenburg RJ, Strom TM, Meitinger T, et al. Fatal neonatal encephalopathy and lactic acidosis caused by a homozygous loss-of-function variant in COQ9. Eur J Hum Genet. 2016;24(3):450–4.
36. Aeby A, Sznajer Y, Cavé H, Rebuffat E, Van Coster R, et al. Cardiofaciocutaneous (CFC) syndrome associated with muscular coenzyme Q_{10} deficiency. J Inherit Metab Dis. 2007;30:827.
37. Leshinsky-Silver E, Levine A, Nissenkorn A, Barash V, Perach M, Buzhaker E, et al. Neonatal liver failure and Leigh syndrome possibly due to CoQ-responsive OXPHOS deficiency. Mol Genet Metab. 2003;79:288–93.
38. Machuca E, Benoit G, Nevo F, Tête MJ, Gribouval O, Pawtowski A, et al. Genotype-phenotype

correlations in non-Finnish congenital nephrotic syndrome. J Am Soc Nephrol. 2010;21:1209–17.
39. McCarthy HJ, Bierzynska A, Wherlock M, Ognjanovic M, Kerecuk L, Hegde S, et al. Simultaneous sequencing of 24 genes associated with steroid-resistant nephrotic syndrome. Clin J Am Soc Nephrol. 2013;8(4):637–48.
40. Gigante M, Diella S, Santangelo L, Trevisson E, Acosta MJ, Amatruda M, et al. Further phenotypic heterogeneity of CoQ10 deficiency associated with steroid resistant nephrotic syndrome and novel COQ2 and COQ6 variants. Clin Genet. 2017;92(2):224–6.
41. Park E, Ahn YH, Kang HG, Yoo KH, Won NH, Lee KB, et al. COQ6 mutations in children with steroid-resistant focal segmental glomerulosclerosis and sensorineural hearing loss. Am J Kidney Dis. 2017;70(1):139–44.
42. Ashraf S, Gee HY, Woerner S, Xie LX, Vega-Warner V, Lovric S, et al. ADCK4 mutations promote steroid-resistant nephrotic syndrome through CoQ10 biosynthesis disruption. J Clin Invest. 2013;123(12):5179–89.
43. Korkmaz E, Lipska-Ziętkiewicz BS, Boyer O, Gribouval O, Fourrage C, Tabatabaei M, et al. ADCK4-associated glomerulopathy causes adolescence-onset FSGS. J Am Soc Nephrol. 2016;27(1):63–8.
44. Lolin K, Chiodini BD, Hennaut E, Adams B, Dahan K, Ismaili K. Early-onset of ADCK4 glomerulopathy with renal failure: a case report. BMC Med Genet. 2017;18(1):28.
45. Atmaca M, Gulhan B, Korkmaz E, Inozu M, Soylemezoglu O, Candan C, et al. Follow-up results of patients with ADCK4 mutations and the efficacy of CoQ10 treatment. Pediatr Nephrol. 2017;32(8):1369–75.
46. Musumeci O, Naini A, Slonim AE, Skavin N, Hadjigeorgiou GL, Krawiecki N, et al. Familial cerebellar ataxia with muscle coenzyme Q_{10} deficiency. Neurology. 2001;56:849–55.
47. Lamperti C, Naini A, Hirano M, De Vivo DC, Bertini E, Servidei S, et al. Cerebellar ataxia and coenzyme Q_{10} deficiency. Neurology. 2003;60:1206–8.
48. Gironi M, Lamperti C, Nemni R, Moggio M, Comi G, Guerini FR, et al. Late-onset cerebellar ataxia with hypogonadism and muscle coenzyme Q_{10} deficiency. Neurology. 2004;62:818–20.
49. Artuch R, Brea-Calvo G, Briones P, Aracil A, Galván M, Espinos C, et al. Cerebellar ataxia with coenzyme Q_{10} deficiency: diagnosis and follow-up after coenzyme Q_{10} supplementation. J Neurol Sci. 2006;246:153–8.
50. Lagier-Tourenne C, Tazir M, López LC, Quinzii CM, Assoum M, Drouot N, et al. ADCK3, an ancestral kinase, is mutated in a form of recessive ataxia associated with coenzyme Q_{10} deficiency. Am J Hum Genet. 2008;82:661–72.
51. Pineda M, Montero R, Aracil A, O'Callaghan MM, Mas A, Espinos C, et al. Coenzyme Q(10)-responsive ataxia: 2-year-treatment follow-up. Mov Disord. 2010;25:1262–8.
52. Horvath R, Czermin B, Gulati S, Demuth S, Houge G, Pyle A, et al. Adult-onset cerebellar ataxia due to mutations in CABC1/ADCK3. J Neurol Neurosurg Psychiatry. 2012;83:174–8.
53. Gerards M, van den Bosch B, Calis C, Schoonderwoerd K, van Engelen K, Tijssen M, et al. Nonsense mutations in CABC1/ADCK3 cause progressive cerebellar ataxia and atrophy. Mitochondrion. 2010;10:510–5.
54. Terracciano A, Rnaldo F, Zanni G, D'Amico A, Pastore A, Barresi S, et al. The use of muscle biopsy in the diagnosis of undefined ataxia with cerebellar atrophy in children. Eur J Paediatr Neurol. 2012;16(3):248–56.
55. Mignot C, Apartis E, Durr A, Marques Lourenço C, Charles P, Devos D, et al. Phenotypic variability in ARCA2 and identification of a core ataxic phenotype with slow progression. Orphanet J Rare Dis. 2013;8:173.
56. Blumkin L, Leshinsky-Silver E, Zerem A, Yosovich K, Lerman-Sagie T, Lev D. Heterozygous mutations in the ADCK3 gene in siblings with cerebellar atrophy and extreme phenotypic variability. JIMD Rep. 2014;12:103–7.
57. Liu YT, Hersheson J, Plagnol V, Fawcett K, Duberley KE, Preza E, et al. Autosomal-recessive cerebellar ataxia caused by a novel ADCK3 mutation that elongates the protein: clinical, genetic and biochemical characterisation. Neurol Neurosurg Psychiatry. 2014;85(5):493–8.
58. Hikmat O, Tzoulis C, Knappskog PM, Johansson S, Boman H, Sztromwasser P, et al. ADCK3 mutations with epilepsy, stroke-like episodes and ataxia: a POLG mimic? Eur J Neurol. 2016;23(7):1188–94.
59. Barca E, Musumeci O, Montagnese F, Marino S, Granata F, Nunnari D, et al. Cerebellar ataxia and severe muscle CoQ10 deficiency in a patient with a novel mutation in ADCK3. Clin Genet. 2016;90(2):156–60.
60. Malgireddy K, Thompson R, Torres-Russotto D. A novel CABC1/ADCK3 mutation in adult-onset cerebellar ataxia. Parkinsonism Relat Disord. 2016;33:151–2.
61. Malicdan MCV, Vilboux T, Ben-Zeev B, Guo J, Eliyahu A, Pode-Shakked B, et al. A novel inborn error of the coenzyme Q10 biosynthesis pathway: cerebellar ataxia and static encephalomyopathy due to COQ5 C-methyltransferase deficiency. Hum Mutat. 2018;39(1):69–79.
62. Quinzii CM, Kattah AG, Naini A, Akman HO, Mootha VK, DiMauro S, et al. Coenzyme Q deficiency and cerebellar ataxia associated with an aprataxin mutation. Neurology. 2005;64:539–41.
63. Le Ber I, Dubourg O, Benoist JF, Jardel C, Mochel F, Koenig M, et al. Muscle coenzyme Q_{10} deficiencies in ataxia with oculomotor apraxia 1. Neurology. 2007;68:295–7.

64. Castellotti B, Mariotti C, Rimoldi M, Fancellu R, Plumari M, Caimi S, et al. Ataxia with oculomotor apraxia type1 (AOA1): novel and recurrent aprataxin mutations, coenzyme Q_{10} analyses, and clinical findings in Italian patients. Neurogenetics. 2011;12:193–201.
65. D'Arrigo S, Riva D, Bulgheroni S, Chiapparini L, Castellotti B, Gellera C, et al. Ataxia with oculomotor apraxia type 1 (AOA1): clinical and neuropsychological features in 2 new patients and differential diagnosis. J Child Neurol. 2008;23:895–900.
66. Garcia-Diaz B, Barca E, Balreira A, Lopez LC, Tadesse S, Krishna S, et al. Lack of aprataxin impairs mitochondrial functions via downregulation of the APE1/NRF1/NRF2 pathway. Hum Mol Genet. 2015;24(16):4516–29.
67. Balreira A, Boczonadi V, Barca E, Pyle A, Bansagi B, Appleton M, et al. ANO10 mutations cause ataxia and coenzyme Q_{10} deficiency. J Neurol. 2014;261(11):2192–8.
68. Barca E, Tang M, Kleiner G, Engelstad K, DiMauro S, Quinzii CM, et al. CoQ_{10} deficiency is not a common finding in GLUT1 deficiency syndrome. JIMD Rep. 2016;29:47–52.
69. Barca E, Kleiner G, Tang G, Ziosi M, Tadesse S, Masliah E, et al. Decreased coenzyme Q10 levels in multiple system atrophy cerebellum. J Neuropathol Exp Neurol. 2016;75(7):663–72.
70. Schottlaender LV, Bettencourt C, Kiely AP, Chalasani A, Neergheen V, Holton JL, et al. Coenzyme Q10 levels are decreased in the cerebellum of multiple-system atrophy patients. PLoS One. 2016;11(2):e0149557.
71. Mitsui J, Koguchi K, Momose T, Takahashi M, Matsukawa T, Yasuda T, et al. Three-year follow-up of high-dose ubiquinol supplementation in a case of familial multiple system atrophy with compound heterozygous COQ2 mutations. Cerebellum. 2017;16(3):664–72.
72. Sun Z, Ohta Y, Yamashita T, Sato K, Takemoto M, Hishikawa N, et al. New susceptible variant of COQ2 gene in Japanese patients with sporadic multiple system atrophy. Neurol Genet. 2016;2(2):e54.
73. Sailer A, Scholz SW, Nalls MA, Schulte C, Federoff M, Price TR, et al. A genome-wide association study in multiple system atrophy. Neurology. 2016;87(15):1591–8.
74. Ronchi D, Di Biase E, Franco G, Melzi V, Del Sorbo F, Elia A, et al. Mutational analysis of COQ2 in patients with MSA in Italy. Neurobiol Aging. 2016;45:213.e1–2.
75. Lalani SR, Vladutiu GD, Plunkett K, Lotze TE, Adesina AM, Scaglia F. Isolated mitochondrial myopathy associated with muscle coenzyme Q_{10} deficiency. Arch Neurol. 2005;62:317–20.
76. Horvath R, Schneiderat P, Schoser BG, Gempel K, Neuen-Jacob E, Ploger H, et al. Coenzyme Q_{10} deficiency and isolated myopathy. Neurology. 2006;66:253–5.
77. Gempel K, Topaloglu H, Talim B, Schneiderat P, Schoser BG, Hans VH, et al. The myopathic form of coenzyme Q10 deficiency is caused by mutations in the electron-transferring-flavoprotein dehydrogenase (ETFDH) gene. Brain. 2007;130(Pt 8):2037–44.
78. Liang WC, Ohkuma A, Hayashi YK, López LC, Hirano M, Nonaka I, et al. ETFDH mutations, CoQ_{10} levels, and respiratory chain activities in patients with riboflavin-responsive multiple acyl-CoA dehydrogenase deficiency. Neuromuscul Disord. 2009;19:212–6.
79. Ohkuma A, Noguchi S, Sugie H, Malicdan MC, Fukuda T, Shimazu K, et al. Clinical and genetic analysis of lipid storage myopathies. Muscle Nerve. 2009;39:333–42.
80. Desbats MA, Morbidoni V, Silic-Benussi M, Doimo M, Ciminale V, Cassina M, et al. The COQ2 genotype predicts the severity of coenzyme Q10 deficiency. Hum Mol Genet. 2016;25(19):4256–65.
81. Vazquez Fonseca L, Doimo M, Calderan C, Desbats MA, Acosta MJ, Cerqua C, et al. Mutations in COQ8B (ADCK4) found in patients with steroid-resistant nephrotic syndrome alter COQ8B function. Hum Mutat. 2018;39(3):406–14.
82. Luna-Sánchez M, Díaz-Casado E, Barca E, Tejada MÁ, Montilla-García Á, Cobos EJ, et al. The clinical heterogeneity of coenzyme Q10 deficiency results from genotypic differences in the Coq9 gene. EMBO Mol Med. 2015;7(5):670–87.
83. Quinzii CM, López LC, Von-Moltke J, Naini A, Krishna S, Schuelke M, et al. Respiratory chain dysfunction and oxidative stress correlate with severity of primary CoQ10 deficiency. FASEB J. 2008;22(6):1874–85.
84. Quinzii CM, López LC, Gilkerson RW, Dorado B, Coku J, Naini AB, et al. Reactive oxygen species, oxidative stress, and cell death correlate with level of CoQ10 deficiency. FASEB J. 2010;24(10):3733–43.
85. López LC, Quinzii CM, Area E, Naini A, Rahman S, Schuelke M, et al. Treatment of CoQ(10) deficient fibroblasts with ubiquinone, CoQ analogs, and vitamin C: time- and compound-dependent effects. PLoS One. 2010;5(7):e11897.
86. Quinzii CM, Tadesse S, Naini A, Hirano M. Effects of inhibiting CoQ10 biosynthesis with 4-nitrobenzoate in human fibroblasts. PLoS One. 2012;7(2):e30606.
87. Duberley KE, Heales SJ, Abramov AY, Chalasani A, Land JM, Rahman S, et al. Effect of Coenzyme Q10 supplementation on mitochondrial electron transport chain activity and mitochondrial oxidative stress in Coenzyme Q10 deficient human neuronal cells. Int J Biochem Cell Biol. 2014;50:60–3.
88. Rodríguez-Hernández A, Cordero MD, Salviati L, Artuch R, Pineda M, Briones P, et al. Coenzyme Q deficiency triggers mitochondria degradation by mitophagy. Autophagy. 2009;5(1):19–32.
89. Peng M, Jarett L, Meade R, Madaio MP, Hancock WW, George AL Jr, et al. Mutant prenyltransferase-like mitochondrial protein (PLMP) and

mitochondrial abnormalities in kd/kd mice. Kidney Int. 2004;66(1):20–8.

90. Quinzii CM, Garone C, Emmanuele V, Tadesse S, Krishna S, Dorado B, et al. Tissue-specific oxidative stress and loss of mitochondria in CoQ-deficient Pdss2 mutant mice. FASEB J. 2013;27(2):612–21.
91. García-Corzo L, Luna-Sánchez M, Doerrier C, García JA, Guarás A, Acín-Pérez R, et al. Dysfunctional Coq9 protein causes predominant encephalomyopathy associated with CoQ deficiency. Hum Mol Genet. 2013;22(6):1233–48.
92. Geromel V, Rötig A, Munnich A, Rustin P. Coenzyme Q10 depletion is comparatively less detrimental to human cultured skin fibroblasts than respiratory chain complex deficiencies. Free Radic Res. 2002;36(4):375–9.
93. Wang Y, Hekimi S. Mitochondrial respiration without ubiquinone biosynthesis. Hum Mol Genet. 2013;22(23):4768–83.
94. López-Martín JM, Salviati L, Trevisson E, Montini G, DiMauro S, Quinzii C, et al. Missense mutation of the COQ2 gene causes defects of bioenergetics and de novo pyrimidine synthesis. Hum Mol Genet. 2007;16(9):1091–7.
95. Luna-Sánchez M, Hidalgo-Gutiérrez A, Hildebrandt TM, Chaves-Serrano J, Barriocanal-Casado E, Santos-Fandila Á, et al. CoQ deficiency causes disruption of mitochondrial sulfide oxidation, a new pathomechanism associated with this syndrome. EMBO Mol Med. 2017;9(1):78–95.
96. Ziosi M, Di Meo I, Kleiner G, Gao XH, Barca E, Sanchez-Quintero MJ, et al. Coenzyme Q deficiency causes impairment of the sulfide oxidation pathway. EMBO Mol Med. 2017;9(1):96–111.
97. Saiki R, Lunceford AL, Shi Y, Marbois B, King R, Pachuski J, et al. Coenzyme Q10 supplementation rescues renal disease in Pdss2kd/kd mice with mutations in prenyl diphosphate synthase subunit 2. Am J Physiol Renal Physiol. 2008;295(5):F1535–44.
98. García-Corzo L, Luna-Sánchez M, Doerrier C, Ortiz F, Escames G, Acuña-Castroviejo D, et al. Ubiquinol-10 ameliorates mitochondrial encephalopathy associated with CoQ deficiency. Biochim Biophys Acta. 2014;1842(7):893–901.
99. He CH, Black DS, Allan CM, Meunier B, Rahman S, Clarke CF. Human COQ9 rescues a *coq9* yeast mutant by enhancing coenzyme Q biosynthesis from 4-hydroxybenzoic acid and stabilizing the CoQ-synthome. Front Physiol. 2017;8:463.
100. Wang Y, Oxer D, Hekimi S. Mitochondrial function and lifespan of mice with controlled ubiquinone biosynthesis. Nat Commun. 2015;6:6393.
101. Doimo M, Trevisson E, Airik R, Bergdoll M, Santos-Ocaña C, Hildebrandt F, et al. Effect of vanillic acid on COQ6 mutants identified in patients with coenzyme Q10 deficiency. Biochim Biophys Acta. 2014;1842(1):1–6.

Mitochondrial Depletion Syndromes

Sumit Parikh and Rita Horvath

Introduction

Mitochondrial DNA (mtDNA) depletion syndromes are characterized by a reduced number of mtDNA compared to nuclear DNA in affected tissues [1]. The molecular cause of these clinically very heterogeneous diseases is autosomal recessive mutations in at least 15 nuclear genes involved in nuclear-mitochondrial inter-genomic signaling pathways. The phenotypes for these disorders can be quite varied from isolated ophthalmoplegia to multi-system disease. Almost all of the mtDNA depletion disorders can present with isolated chronic progressive ophthalmoplegia (CPEO). More extensive involvement leads to one of several various phenotypes with a primary myopathic, cardiomyopathic, encephalomyopathic, hepatocerebral, or neurogastrointestinal presentation. These categorizations, while imperfect, provide some structure around which to organize the diverse presentations of mtDNA depletion diseases. Most of these disorders have additional less common presentations, and these phenotypes are discussed within the context of the above categories.

S. Parikh (✉)
Mitochondrial Medicine Center, Neurological Institute, Cleveland Clinic, Cleveland, OH, USA

R. Horvath
Wellcome Trust Centre for Mitochondrial Research, Institute of Genetic Medicine, Newcastle University, Newcastle Upon Tyne, UK

The reason behind the reduced amount of mtDNA in mitochondrial DNA depletion syndromes can be defects in the (1) replication and maintenance of the mtDNA, (2) nucleotide supply and balance, or (3) mitochondrial dynamics and quality control or (4) so far unknown mechanisms [2] (Fig. 1). Although the primary genetic defect is in the nuclear DNA, the clinical presentation is due to the depletion of the mtDNA.

1. The human mitochondrial genome is replicated by polymerase gamma (*POLG*) in concert with other components of the mitochondrial replication machinery (*TWNK, SLC25A4, MGME1, TFAM, DNA2, RNASEH1*). MtDNA depletion in these conditions may be associated with multiple mtDNA deletions and point mutations (*POLG, TWNK, SLC25A4, MGME1, TFAM*). However, some genes affecting mtDNA replication may result only in mtDNA deletions or point mutations in adults (*POLG2, DNA2, RNASEH1*), and the inheritance pattern of these genes may be autosomal dominant or recessive. In this chapter we focus on diseases associated with depletion of mtDNA.
2. Nucleotide balance is critically important for DNA integrity and preventing degeneration. Nucleotide levels are maintained by de novo synthesis or by salvage pathways [3].

M. Mancuso, T. Klopstock (eds.), *Diagnosis and Management of Mitochondrial Disorders*,
https://doi.org/10.1007/978-3-030-05517-2_12

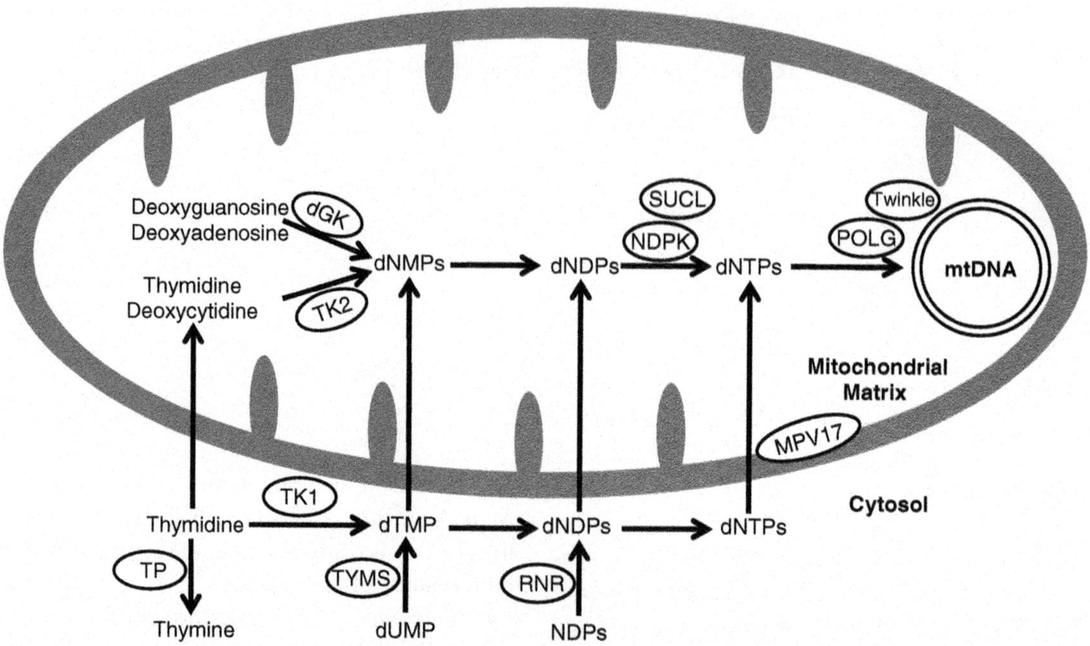

Fig. 1 Adapted with permission from El-Hattab et al. [177]. Schematic presentation of proteins involved in mitochondrial nucleotide pools maintenance and mitochondrial DNA replication. *TK2* mitochondrial thymidine kinase 2 (encoded by *TK2* gene), *dGK* mitochondrial deoxyguanosine kinase (encoded by the *DGUOK* gene), *SUCL* succinyl-CoA ligase (SUCL is composed of an alpha subunit, encoded by *SUCLG1* and a beta subunit, encoded by either *SUCLA2* or *SUCLG2*), *NDPK* nucleoside diphosphate kinase, *POLG* DNA polymerase gamma (POLG is a heterotrimer enzyme composed of one catalytic subunit encoded by *POLG* and two accessory subunits encoded by *POLG2*), *TP* thymidine phosphorylase (encoded by *TYMP* gene), *RNR* ribonucleotide reductase (*RRM2B* encodes the p53-inducible small subunit (p53R2) of the RNR), *dNMP* deoxynucleoside monophosphate, *dNDP* deoxynucleoside diphosphate, *dNTP* deoxynucleoside triphosphate, *NDP* nucleoside diphosphate, *dTMP* deoxythymidine monophosphate, *TK1* cytosolic thymidine kinase 1, *TYMS* thymidylate synthase. The twinkle protein is encoded by *C10orf2* and MPV17 by the *MPV17* gene

Mutations in nuclear genes involved in the maintenance and supply of mitochondrial nucleotide pools have been associated with mtDNA depletion syndromes with different tissue-specific clinical manifestations (*TK2, DGUOK, RRMB2, TYMP, SUCLA2, SUCLG1*).

3. Defects of mtDNA dynamics (*OPA1, MFN2, DRP1*) and quality control (*SPG7, AFG3L2*) can also affect the amount and quality of mtDNA by so far not completely understood pathomechanism [2], and these diseases are more common causes of mtDNA deletions than depletion of mtDNA.
4. Early-onset organ-specific autosomal recessive syndromes due to mutations in genes with miscellaneous pathomechanism (*FBXL4, GFER, ABAT, AGK, SLC25A21*).

The focus of this chapter are diseases with mtDNA depletion.

In this chapter we discuss the clinical presentations and the latest updates in the state-of-the-art diagnosis and treatment of mtDNA maintenance diseases, including the compilation of new genes, new findings on why and how these dysfunctional genes and related proteins lead to the associated severe symptoms, as well as preclinical and clinical evidence on the plausibility of new treatments. The disorders are summarized in Tables 1, 2, and 3.

Table 1 Clinical features of mitochondrial DNA maintenance defects due to abnormalities in mtDNA replication machinery

	Inh.	Onset	MtDNA	Clinical manifestations
Defects in mitochondrial DNA polymerization				
POLG-related Alpers-Huttenlocher syndrome	AR	Early childhood	Depletion	Encephalopathy, neuropathy, and hepatopathy
POLG-related MNGIE	AR	Infancy or childhood	Depletion and multiple deletions	Gastrointestinal dysmotility, myopathy, and neuropathy
POLG-related MEMSA	AR	Young adulthood	Multiple deletions	Epilepsy, myopathy, neuropathy, and ataxia
POLG-related ANS	AR	Young adulthood	Multiple deletions	Ataxia, neuropathy, and encephalopathy
POLG-related ARPEO	AR	Adolescence or young adulthood	Multiple deletions	Ophthalmoplegia
POLG-related ADPEO	AD	Adulthood	Multiple deletions	Ophthalmoplegia and myopathy
POLG2-related myopathic MDMD	AD	Infancy to adulthood	Multiple deletions	Myopathy and ophthalmoplegia
TWNK-related IOSCA	AR	Infancy	Depletion	Ataxia, encephalopathy, and neuropathy
TWNK-related hepatocerebral MDMD	AR	Neonatal period or infancy	Depletion	Encephalopathy and hepatopathy
TWNK-related ADPEO	AD	Early adulthood	Multiple deletions	Ophthalmoplegia and myopathy
TFAM-related hepatocerebral MDMD	AR	Neonatal period	Depletion	Hepatopathy
Defects in mitochondrial nucleases				
RNASEH1-related encephalomyopathic MDMD	AR	Early adulthood	Depletion and multiple deletions	Encephalopathy and myopathy
MGME1-related myopathic MDMD	AR	Childhood or early adulthood	Depletion and multiple deletions	Myopathy
DNA2-related myopathic MDMD	AD	Childhood or early adulthood	Multiple deletions	Myopathy
DNA2-related Seckel syndrome	AR	Birth	NA	Dwarfism

Adapted with permission from El-Hattab et al. [178]

Inh. inheritance, *AR* autosomal recessive, *AD* autosomal dominant, *MDMD* mitochondrial DNA maintenance defects, *MNGIE* mitochondrial neurogastrointestinal encephalopathy, *MEMSA* myoclonic epilepsy myopathy sensory ataxia, *ANS* ataxia-neuropathy spectrum, *ARPEO* autosomal recessive progressive external ophthalmoplegia, *ADPEO* autosomal dominant progressive external ophthalmoplegia, *IOSCA* infantile-onset spinocerebellar ataxia

Myopathic Form (TK2, MGME1)

Both TK2- and MGME1-related mtDNA depletion syndromes present primarily with progressive myopathy as their presenting feature though some patients can develop other neurologic or systemic symptoms.

TK2-Related Disease

Mitochondrial thymidine kinase 2 (TK2) is encoded by the nuclear *TK2* gene and mediates the first step of pyrimidine salvage in the mitochondrial matrix via phosphorylation of nucleosides to nucleotides [4]. Mutations lead to decreased production of pyrimidine nucleotides and secondarily mitochondrial depletion. It is an autosomal recessive (AR) disorder.

TK2-related disorders were first identified in 2001 [5]. The clinical phenotype typically includes a myopathy beginning in infancy though adulthood. The disease often begins in infancy or early childhood after a period of normal development with the onset of fatigue, proximal myopathy, and loss of motor skills. Facial and bulbar weakness develop with altered speech and dysphagia. Cognitive function is

Table 2 Clinical features of mitochondrial DNA maintenance defects due to abnormalities in maintaining a balanced mitochondrial nucleotide pool

MDMD	Inh.	Onset	MtDNA	Clinical manifestations
Defects of mitochondrial nucleotide salvage pathway				
TK2-related myopathic MDMD	AR	Infancy or childhood	Depletion	Myopathy
TK2-related ARPEO	AR	Mid-adulthood	Multiple deletions	Ophthalmoplegia and myopathy
DGUOK-related hepatocerebral MDMD		Neonatal period, infancy, or childhood	Depletion	Hepatopathy and encephalopathy
DGUOK-related myopathic MDMD	AR	Early or mid-adulthood	Multiple deletions	Myopathy
SUCLA2-related encephalomyopathic MDMA	AR	Infancy or early childhood	Depletion	Encephalopathy, myopathy, and elevated MMA
SUCLG1-related encephalomyopathic MDMA	AR	Neonatal period or infancy	Depletion	Encephalopathy, myopathy, and elevated MMA
ABAT-related encephalomyopathic MDMD	AR	Infancy	Depletion	Encephalopathy, myopathy, and elevated GABA
Defects of cytosolic nucleotide metabolism				
TYMP-related MNGIE	AR	Adolescence or early adulthood	Depletion and multiple deletions	Gastrointestinal dysmotility, myopathy, encephalopathy, and neuropathy
RRM2B-related encephalomyopathic MDMD	AR	Neonatal period or infancy	Depletion	Encephalopathy and myopathy
RRM2B-related MNGIE	AR	Early adulthood	Depletion	Gastrointestinal dysmotility, myopathy, encephalopathy, and neuropathy
RRM2B-related ARPEO	AR	Childhood	Multiple deletions	Ophthalmoplegia and myopathy
RRM2B-related ADPEO	AD	Adulthood	Multiple deletions	Ophthalmoplegia and myopathy
Defects of mitochondrial nucleotide import				
SLC25A4-related (*ANT1*) cardiomyopathic MDMD	AR	Early childhood	Multiple deletions	Cardiac and skeletal myopathy
SLC25A4-related (*ANT1*) ADPEO	AD	Adulthood	Multiple deletions	Ophthalmoplegia and myopathy
AGK-related Sengers syndrome	AR	Neonatal period	Depletion	Cardiac and skeletal myopathy and cataract
MPV17-related Navajo neurohepatopathy	AR	Infancy or early childhood	Depletion	Neuropathy and hepatopathy
MPV17-related hepatocerebral MDMD	AR	Neonatal period or infancy	Depletion	Encephalopathy and hepatopathy
MPV17-related neuromyopathic MDMD	AR	Adolescence or young adulthood	Multiple deletions	Neuropathy and myopathy

Adapted with permission from El-Hattab et al. [178]

Inh. inheritance, *AR* autosomal recessive, *AD* autosomal dominant, *MDMD* mitochondrial DNA maintenance defects, *MNGIE* mitochondrial neurogastrointestinal encephalopathy, *ARPEO* autosomal recessive progressive external ophthalmoplegia, *ADPEO* autosomal dominant progressive external ophthalmoplegia, *MMA* methylmalonic acid, *GABA* gamma-aminobutyric acid

generally normal in the classic presentation. Muscle weakness is progressive and rapidly leads to respiratory failure within a few years. Later-onset forms are more insidious in their progression. A mild myopathy that begins in adulthood with a much slower progression has been also described [6].

In contrast, a severe neonatal or early infantile presentation mimicking spinal muscular atrophy can occur with EMG showing findings concerning for motor neuron disease [7, 8]. While not usually associated with an encephalopathy at onset, select young patients have been described with early-onset central nervous system (CNS)

Table 3 Clinical features of mitochondrial DNA maintenance defects due to abnormalities in mitochondria dynamics

MDMD	Inh.	Onset	MtDNA	Clinical manifestations
Defects in mitochondrial dynamics				
OPA1-related ADOA	AD	Childhood or early adulthood	Multiple deletions	Optic atrophy
OPA1-related Behr syndrome	AR	Infancy or early childhood	NA	Optic atrophy, neuropathy, and spinocerebellar degeneration
OPA1-related encephalomyopathic MDMD	AR	Infancy	Depletion	Myopathy, encephalopathy, and optic atrophy
MFN2-related CMT2A	AD	Childhood or early adulthood	NA	Axonal motor neuropathy
MFN2-related ADOA	AD	Early childhood	Multiple deletions	Optic atrophy and neuropathy
FBXL4-related encephalomyopathic MDMD	AR	Neonatal period or infancy	Depletion	Encephalopathy and myopathy

Adapted with permission from El-Hattab et al. [178]
Inh. inheritance, *AR* autosomal recessive, *AD* autosomal dominant, *MDMD* mitochondrial DNA maintenance defects, *ADOA* autosomal dominant optic atrophy, *CMT2A* Charcot-Marie-Tooth neuropathy type 2A

manifestations including seizures and severe cortical atrophy [9, 10]. Hearing loss can occur [11]. A hepato-myopathy presentation has also been seen with elevated transaminases, hepatic enlargement, and mtDNA depletion in the liver [12]. A form leading to isolated CPEO with multiple mtDNA deletions in place of depletion can occur [13].

Creatine kinase (CK) levels are typically elevated at disease onset. Electromyography (EMG) shows myopathy. Muscle histology has shown sarcoplasmic vacuoles, fiber size variation, and increases in connective tissue. There is a mosaic pattern of COX-negative and ragged-red fibers and variable combined mtDNA-dependent respiratory complex deficiency. mtDNA copy number is severely reduced [14].

Care is primarily supportive. Nucleotide bypass therapy originally with deoxycytidine monophosphate and deoxythymidine monophosphate, than with deoxycytidine and deoxythymidine supplementation, is being investigated in patients as a possible treatment for the disease as it has been shown to extend life in TK2-deficient mice [15, 16]. Nucleoside supplementation has been recently tried in some patients in the USA and Spain with success, and a randomized clinical trial will be performed (personal communications with Michio Hirano and Caterina Garone; to be published in ENMC workshop report).

MGME1-Related Disease

The *MGME1* nuclear gene encodes a mitochondrial exonuclease that cleaves single-stranded DNA and DNA or DNA-RNA chimeric oligonucleotides with free nucleic acid ends [17].

Mutations in the gene lead to an autosomal recessive disorder with mtDNA depletion. Only a few patients have been identified thus far with the initial report in 2013 of several members of three families presenting with ptosis, CPEO, progressive myopathy, and muscle atrophy. They developed severe emaciation and respiratory insufficiency. Facial weakness with nasal speech, intellectual disability, microcephaly, ataxia, and intellectual disability were noted in some [17]. A later reported patient also had microcephaly, early-onset progressive ataxia, and cerebellar atrophy potentially making this condition more of an encephalomyopathy [18]. Skeletal muscle shows mtDNA deletion and depletion with variable alterations in mitochondrial respiratory chain enzyme activity and a combination of mtDNA deletions and depletion [17].

Cardiomyopathic Form

Mutations in the *AGK*, *SLC25A4*, and *OPA3* genes can lead to a mtDNA depletion disorder with predominantly a phenotype of myopathy and cardiac involvement. Systemic symptoms can variably occur.

AGK

The nuclear gene *AGK* encodes for a mitochondrially localized protein that phosphorylates acylglycerol to form phosphatidic acid and lysophosphatidic acid [19, 20]. The loss of AGK leads to a decrease in the adenine nucleotide translocator in the inner mitochondrial membrane due to AGK-related impaired phospholipid metabolism in the mitochondria, and potentially the decreased SLC25A4 is responsible for the secondary mtDNA depletion [21]. The clinical presentation of mutations in *AGK* shows similarities with mutations in *SLC25A4*, which can be also due to the mechanistic link between these two genes.

Mutations in the gene lead to autosomal recessive Sengers syndrome. The condition was initially described in 1975 in seven children with congenital cataracts, hypertrophic cardiomyopathy, and muscle biopsy showing mitochondrial ultrastructural abnormalities with bizarre shapes and abnormal cristae along with storage of lipid and glycogen [22]. Additional families were described over the years and linked to *AGK* mutations in 2012 [21, 23].

Patients generally have congenital cataracts and hypertrophic cardiomyopathy, which are the hallmarks of this disease. They may also have delayed motor milestones, hypotonia, and progressive myopathy. Cognition is typically normal though later cognitive decline can occur. Premature ovarian failure has been noted [21, 23].

Lactic acidosis is typically present. Muscle biopsy findings align with the initial reports and show lipid vacuoles, subsarcolemmal accumulation of abnormally shaped mitochondria, and severe mtDNA depletion [23]. Combined mitochondrial complex deficiencies have been noted in the muscle of some but not all patients; normal electron-chain enzymology has also been seen [21, 23].

The clinical course varies with patients passing away in infancy to survival into adulthood. Cardiomyopathy has typically been the cause of death [21, 23]. Cardiac transplantation has been tolerated by a few reported patients [24].

SLC25A4 (ANT1)

The *SLC25A4* gene encodes the mitochondrial adenine nucleotide translocator (ANT1) through which adenosine diphosphate (ADP) is moved into the mitochondrial matrix and adenosine triphosphate (ATP) is moved into the cytoplasm [25]. This isoform of *SLC25A4* is expressed primarily in the heart and skeletal muscle and shows less expression in the kidney and liver [26].

SLC25A4-related disease leads to a broad phenotype ranging from isolated CPEO with or without hypertrophic cardiomyopathy to a severe infant-onset myopathic disease. Mutations in *SLC25A4* were first identified as an autosomal dominant cause of CPEO in adults in 2000 [27]. A more severe infantile-onset phenotype with profound hypotonia, ventilator dependence, occasional cardiomyopathy, and severe-to-profound lactic acidosis with a marked loss of mtDNA copy number in skeletal muscle was later described in patients carrying de novo heterozygous mutations. Epilepsy was sometimes noted. Neuroimaging in these children ranged from normal to showing basal ganglia lesions and/or atrophy [28]. Recessive mutations were shown to lead to multiple mtDNA deletions and adult-onset hypertrophic cardiomyopathy, mild myopathy with exercise intolerance, and lactic acidosis without ophthalmoplegia [29]. Congenital cataracts have been seen [30].

Muscle biopsy in patients shows COX deficiency, lipid accumulation, mitochondrial proliferation, and disorganized cristae [28, 30]. Ragged-red fibers have been noted in patients with autosomal dominant disease [29].

OPA1

The *OPA1* nuclear gene localizes to the inner mitochondrial membrane and encodes for a dynamin-related GTPase that regulates the stability of the mitochondrial network as well as sequestration of proapoptotic cytochrome c oxidase molecules within the mitochondrial cristae spaces [31]. *OPA1* is also needed for mitofusin-mediated mitochondrial fusion [32] and secondarily the exchange of intermitochondrial content with maintenance of a balanced pool of mitochondrial proteins including the enzymes needed for mtDNA synthesis. OPA1-exon4b also supports mtDNA replication by interacting with and regulating the replisome [33]. Disruption leads to impaired fusion, mtDNA depletion, fragmentation of the mitochondrial network, loss of the mitochondrial membrane potential, and disorganization of the cristae followed by cytochrome c release and apoptosis [31, 33].

While mtDNA depletion related disease has only recently been linked to *OPA1* mutations, heterozygous mutations in the gene were linked in 2000 to one of the most common causes of childhood- or adult-onset autosomal dominant optic atrophy with progressive visual loss often leading to legal blindness [34]. The vision loss is typically bilateral, fairly symmetric with temporal pallor of the optic disc due to a loss of central retinal ganglion cells. Typical color vision changes include a loss of blue-yellow or red-green vision.

An optic atrophy "plus" syndrome was later identified in 15–20% of patients with heterozygous missense mutations. Patients had associated bilateral sensorineural deafness beginning in late childhood or early adulthood and a combination of ataxia, myopathy, peripheral neuropathy, and progressive external ophthalmoplegia beginning in their 30s. A single patient with spastic paraparesis and a hereditary spastic paraplegia like presentation was found [35].

Compound heterozygous mutations were shown to lead to Behr syndrome, an autosomal recessive disease with the triad of optic atrophy, spastic paraparesis, and motor neuropathy with onset typically in childhood, often accompanied by some degree of ataxia and ophthalmoparesis [36, 37].

Mitochondrial depletion and a phenotype of a fatal infantile cardioencephalomyopathy were more recently identified in children with homozygous *OPA1* mutations. The siblings initially presented with failure to thrive and generalized neuromuscular weakness and optic atrophy progressing to severe encephalopathy and hypertrophic cardiomyopathy. Mitochondrial respiratory chain complex activity was globally decreased in skeletal muscle [38].

Encephalomyopathies

Mutations in *SUCLG1* and *SUCLA2* were originally reported to cause the encephalomyopathic form of mtDNA depletion; however autosomal recessive mutations in other genes such as *RRM2B*, *TK2*, *OPA1*, and *FBXL4* predominantly cause a disorder with both CNS and muscle involvement, though this is not their common presentation, *TK2* [9, 10] and biallelic *OPA1*-related disease [38].

SUCLG1 and SUCLA2

Mitochondrial succinyl-CoA synthetase (SCS) is located in the mitochondrial matrix and is a heterodimer made up of an α-subunit, SUCLG1, and one of two β-subunit isoforms, SUCLA2 or SUCLG2. SCS catalyzes the reversible conversion of succinyl-CoA and ADP or GDP to succinate and adenosine triphosphate or guanosine triphosphate. The SCS heterodimer also forms a complex with mitochondrial nucleoside diphosphate kinase (NDPK) to allow for conversion of nucleoside diphosphates to nucleoside triphosphates during mitochondrial replication [39, 40].

The *SUCLG1* gene encodes the alpha subunit of SCS [41], while *SUCLA2* encodes one of the two β-subunits.

SUCLG1

Mutations in *SUCLG1* lead to an autosomal recessive mitochondrial depletion syndrome with methylmalonic aciduria [39]. Patients typically present with severe infantile lactic acidosis and encephalomyopathy. Manifestations include severe neonatal hypotonia, failure to thrive, hearing impairment, and profoundly delayed psychomotor development [42]. A relatively milder phenotype has been noted with survival past infancy though the patient described had severe axial hypotonia, no active movements, and atrophic muscles and needed tube feeding and respiratory support via a tracheostomy at age 12 years [43]. Hepatopathy with hepatomegaly and hypertrophic cardiomyopathy can occur. Some may have hypertonia, contractures, rhabdomyolysis, and/or hypoglycemia [44]. A variant phenotype with onset of truncal ataxia at 14 months followed by chorea, hypotonia with weakness, and bilateral and sensorineural hearing loss has been noted. Cognition in this patient appeared to be unaffected at age 11 years [45]. While most patients pass away in early childhood, up to 10% were noted to survive past age 20 years [44].

Elevations in plasma lactate and methylmalonic acid are routinely noted along with mild elevations in urine methylmalonic acid [44]. Methylmalonic elevations are much less than what is seen in primary methylmalonic aciduria. Leigh-like changes have been seen on MRI, predominantly affecting the basal ganglia as well as cortical atrophy and/or a leukoencephalopathy [43, 44]. Muscle studies show moderate to severe mtDNA depletion and variable deficiencies of respiratory chain enzyme activity [42–44].

SUCLA2

Mutations in *SUCLA2* lead to a similar but milder phenotype than *SUCLG1*-related disease. This may be due to *SUCLA2* being predominantly expressed in the brain, heart, and muscle unlike *SUCLG1*, which is ubiquitously expressed [46]. A founder mutation in *SUCLA2* resulted in a frequent occurrence of this disease on the Faroe Islands, enabling a good clinical characterization of the phenotype [44].

Encephalomyopathy with mtDNA depletion and methylmalonic acid excretion and clinical findings similar to patients with *SUCLG1* mutations are typically present [47, 48]. Onset of symptoms is little after the newborn period in *SUCLA2*-related disease with hypotonia with myopathy, dystonia, profound developmental disability, and failure to thrive and deafness. Median survival is much longer at 20 years. Hepatopathy and hypertrophic cardiomyopathy are not typically seen [44].

RRM2B

RRM2B encodes a small subunit of p53-inducible ribonucleotide reductase, responsible for de novo conversion of ribonucleoside diphosphates into the corresponding deoxyribonucleoside diphosphates for DNA synthesis [49]. The enzyme is felt to be unaffected by hypoxic conditions [50].

Mutations lead to an early-onset autosomal recessive disorder with mtDNA depletion or deletion, encephalomyopathy, and at times renal tubulopathy or late-onset autosomal dominant CPEO. The disease typically begins in infancy with hypotonia, muscle weakness, and renal tubulopathy followed by epilepsy. Failure to thrive and respiratory insufficiency can occur. Tubulopathy may be associated with nephrocalcinosis. Death occurs in infancy or early childhood [49, 51–54]. A Kearns-Sayre syndrome phenotype has been noted with onset of disease in later childhood and associated CPEO, myopathy, SNHL, and elevation in CSF protein. Cardiac conduction defects or tubulopathy was not present [55].

A later-onset form of disease with predominantly CPEO has also been described in patients with single heterozygous mutations [53, 56]. These patients may also develop myopathy, bulbar dysfunction, fatigue, SNHL, and GI motility problems though there is minimal to no CNS involvement [57]. A phenotype mimicking mitochondrial neurogastrointestinal encephalopathy (MNGIE) syndrome has also been noted in a patient presenting in adulthood with ophthalmoplegia, ptosis, peripheral neuropathy, and GI dysmotility. Neuroimaging shows white matter and basal ganglia disease [58].

Severe lactic acidosis is often seen in the infant-onset form. Muscle respiratory chain complex activity can be severely decreased. Histology may show subsarcolemmal accumulation of mitochondria and/or cytochrome c oxidase-deficient fibers [49, 52, 53, 57].

FBXL4

FBXL4 encodes an inner mitochondrial membrane protein. While its function is not clearly known, the protein may be integral for the formation of a normal mitochondrial network and maintenance of mtDNA and critical to mitochondrial fusion [59].

FBXL4-related disease is due to biallelic mutations and typically presents in infancy with severe-to-profound global developmental delay and hypotonia with lactic acidosis. Microcephaly, failure to thrive, feeding difficulties, and recurrent intermittent hyperammonemia are often seen. Facial dysmorphism, congenital cataracts, optic atrophy, refractory epilepsy, hypertrophic cardiomyopathy, elevated transaminases, recurrent infections, and renal tubular acidosis can occur [59–62]. Stroke-like episodes have infrequently been described [63].

Lactic acidosis is common in infancy. Neuroimaging may show global cortical atrophy and abnormal supratentorial white matter in most cases and at times a thin corpus callosum and variable involvement of the basal ganglia, thalami, and infratentorial structures [59–62].

Skeletal muscle shows variable defects in mitochondrial respiratory chain enzyme activity and mtDNA depletion [59–62].

Mitochondrial oxodicarboxylate carrier deficiency due to a homozygous mutation in *SLC25A21* led to spinal muscular atrophy-like disease with mitochondrial myopathy and depletion of mtDNA in a child from a consanguineous Pakistani family [64]. The mechanism of mtDNA depletion in this case may be linked to toxic accumulation of oxoadipate and quinolinic acid.

Hepatocerebral Form

mtDNA depletion due to mutations in *DGUOK*, *MPV17*, *POLG*, *C10orf2/TWNK*, and *TFAM* predominantly features with progressive liver and CNS disease. Other less common phenotypes of these disorders are also reviewed. Other mtDNA depletion disorders can also present with hepatopathy and encephalopathy though it is not their most common phenotype. This includes *TK2* [12] and *SUCLG1*-related disease [44].

DGUOK

DGUOK encodes for the mitochondrial deoxyribonucleoside kinase, involved in phosphorylation of purine deoxyribonucleosides and nucleotide salvage [65].

Mutations in DGUOK are linked to an autosomal recessive mtDNA depletion syndrome. The most common phenotype is of early infantile-onset progressive liver failure with hepatomegaly, associated hypoglycemia and jaundice, encephalopathy, hypotonia, myopathy, rotary nystagmus, and lactic acidosis [66, 67].

A phenotype with infant- or childhood-onset milder liver disease, sometimes triggered by viral infections and at times later-onset myopathy and/or CPEO with minimal to no other cortical involvement, has been noted to occur. Later-onset renal involvement with proteinuria and aminoaciduria may occur [68, 69]. A rare patient with reversible liver failure and no neurologic impairment has been described, with 10–15% residual DGUOK enzyme activity noted in tissue analysis [70, 71]. A variant phenotype of isolated noncirrhotic portal hypertension has also been described in individuals with *DGUOK* mutations [72].

Tyrosine or phenylalanine may be elevated on newborn screening samples, without the typical elevation in succinylacetone seen in tyrosinemia type I [73]. Elevated lactate, transaminases, alpha-fetoprotein, and hypoglycemia are commonly seen. Liver and muscle biochemical studies can show variably decreased electron transport chain activity and mtDNA depletion [66, 67]. Liver histology may show cholestasis, microsteatosis, fibrosis, giant cell hepatitis, or cirrhosis. Electron microscopy may show mitochondrial proliferation and abnormal cristae [74].

Liver transplant may be beneficial in selected patients, especially in those with minimal or mild neurologic involvement. Survival after liver transplantation in these patients may be slightly lower or match survival after liver transplantation for other indications [24, 75].

MPV17

The *MPV17* gene produces an inner mitochondrial membrane protein involved in part in the structural preservation of the mitochondrial membrane and maintenance of deoxynucleotide pools, potentially via forming small molecule channels in the inner mitochondrial membrane. The complete function of the protein is not yet fully understood [76–79]. However, recent findings suggest that aberrant ribonucleotide incorporation is a primary abnormality that results in mtDNA depletion and multiple deletions in the liver and brain [80].

Impairment of *MPV17* leads to an autosomal recessive disorder of mtDNA depletion of infantile onset and a condition known as Navajo neurohepatopathy [81, 82]. The common infantile-onset form presents with poor feeding with failure to thrive, hypoglycemia, hypotonia, progressive liver failure, and lactic acidosis [83]. Global developmental disability, hypotonia, and myopathy typically present in infancy though it may begin at a later age. Some develop ataxia, epilepsy, and a mixed sensorimotor polyneuropathy with muscle wasting, decreased reflexes, and loss of sensation in the hands and feet [83–86].

Navajo neurohepatopathy, with a founder effect in the Navajo Native American population, was also found to be due to *MPV17* mutations. The disorder presents with hepatopathy, peripheral neuropathy, painless fractures, acral mutilation, corneal ulceration and scarring, and associated cerebral leukoencephalopathy, failure to thrive, and recurrent metabolic acidosis [82].

As seen in other mtDNA depletion hepatopathies, elevated lactate, transaminases, and alpha-fetoprotein with perturbations in synthetic liver function markers such as glucose, bilirubin, and PT/PTT are seen. CSF lactate levels may also be elevated [83].

Neuroimaging may show a constellation of cortical atrophy, leukoencephalopathy, and infarctions [83]. Isolated signal abnormalities involving the reticular formation of the lower brain stem and within the reticulospinal tracts of the cervicocranial junction have been noted in a single patient [87].

mtDNA depletion of varying degrees of severity is commonly seen – more severely in the liver than muscle. Histopathology may show fatty infiltrates, cirrhosis, fibrosis, loss of hepatocytes and atrophy, cholestasis, and periportal glycogen deposits among other less common findings. Biochemical studies in the liver and muscle may show combined respiratory chain deficiencies [83].

Liver transplant may benefit selected patients though it does not help with the neurological progression. Survival post liver transplant is varied with some patients passing away from multi-organ failure or sepsis and others doing well [24, 88].

POLG

POLG encodes the catalytic subunit of DNA polymerase gamma (POLG), critical for mitochondrial DNA replication and repair [89, 90]. POLG is a heterotrimer, with accessory subunits encoded by *POLG2* [91, 92]. Mutations in *POLG2* have primarily been linked to isolated autosomal dominant CPEO [92].

Mutations in *POLG* lead to mtDNA depletion and deletions and are linked to a variety of partially overlapping phenotypes – most commonly including Alpers-Huttenlocher syndrome (AHS), a myocerebrohepatopathy spectrum (MCHS), autosomal dominant or recessive CPEO, myoclonic epilepsy, myopathy and sensory ataxia (MEMSA), and a disorder leading to an ataxia and neuropathy spectrum (ANS) of disease [93, 94]. Homozygous pathogenic variants located in the linker region of POLG may be with later age of onset and longer survival compared to compound heterozygous mutations [95]. In a large cohort of 68 patients all homozygous for the most common *POLG* variant p.Ala467Thr, a large clinical variability has been shown [96]. The clinical presentation included almost the entire phenotypic spectrum of all known POLG mutations.

A recent paper identified that a complex genomic noncoding locus drives *POLG* expression to its disease-related nervous system regions [97]. The same regulatory locus also expresses two other functional RNAs (*LNC00925* and *MiR9-3*), and *MiR9-3* effects stem cell differentiation and folate metabolism, which defects had been observed in association with *POLG* mutations [97].

AHS was first described in 1931 [98] and linked to *POLG* mutations in 2004 [99]. It is the most severe form of POLG-related disease with an incidence of 1:51000 [100]. The disorder is an autosomal recessive condition leading to an infantile or early childhood onset of developmental disability, intractable epilepsy, and typically progressive liver failure [94, 101]. Children are healthy at birth and show normal development though some may have milder developmental delays prior to an acute worsening. An acute neurological or hepatic decompensation can occur in infancy or childhood, commonly ranging between 1 and 36 months of age. Liver failure can be triggered by exposure to valproic acid [99, 102]. Patients with AHS can less commonly present with new-onset symptoms later in life including in adulthood. The disorder, especially when beginning in infancy, is progressive and typically fatal in childhood though the clinical course may vary. Liver failure can progress rapidly over a few months. Systemic other symptoms also eventually occur including neuropathy, spasticity, ataxia, stroke-like episodes, SNHL, cortical vision loss, and Parkinsonism [94, 101, 103, 104].

Seizures are often the presenting feature of AHS and often focal, progressing to generalized. Epilepsia partialis continua, myoclonic epilepsy, and status epilepticus can be seen, sometimes as the presenting feature [101, 102, 105–108]. Seizures often involve the occipital lobes, and patients may present with headaches and visual complaints including vision loss and auras [109, 110].

Neuroimaging shows variable findings including cortical lesions (often occipital), cortical atrophy, and later involvement of the cerebellum, basal ganglia, thalamus, and brain stem [111]. Lesions in the inferior olivary nuclei may be seen and are associated with palatal myoclonus [107].

Liver histopathology often shows a combination of microvesicular steatosis, hepatocyte dropout, bridging fibrosis or cirrhosis, collapse of liver cell plates, parenchymal lobular architecture, regenerative nodules, oncocytic changes, and bile ductular proliferation [112].

POLG-related MCHS also begins in infancy or early childhood with developmental disability, hypotonia, and failure to thrive. Patients typically have varied additional systemic findings including hepatopathy, neuropathy, epilepsy, renal tubular dysfunction, SNHL, and/or elevations in CSF lactate [103, 113]. Neuroimaging may show cortical atrophy or white matter disease [114, 115].

Patients with MEMSA, due to *biallelic* POLG mutations, develop both central and peripheral (sensory) ataxia in young adulthood, along with sensory neuropathy, distal or proximal myopathy, and myoclonus without ophthalmoplegia. The condition was previously referred to as spinocerebellar ataxia with epilepsy. Epilepsy occurs years later, often focally and then generalizing, and can be refractory to medications [103, 115].

ANS patients also have biallelic *POLG* mutations and typically have central and sensory ataxia with neuropathy and many developing seizures and some ophthalmoplegia. Systemic involvement is seen less often [109, 116, 117]. Symptoms develop in young adulthood. This categorization includes previous categories of mitochondrial recessive ataxia syndrome (MIRAS) and sensory ataxia, neuropathy, dysarthria, and ophthalmoplegia (SANDO). Other findings such as vision impairment, liver dysfunction, migraines, and myoclonus may be present [115, 117–120].

CPEO in patients with *POLG* mutations can occur in isolation due to both heterozygous or biallelic mutations [121]. Patients with biallelic mutations may develop other manifestations of POLG-related disease over time, including myoclonus and neuropathy [119, 122, 123]. The autosomal dominant form of POLG-related CPEO also includes an associated milder myopathy, variable SNHL, neuropathy, ataxia, and cataracts [122, 124].

Less commonly seen phenotypes with *POLG*-related disease include a MNGIE-like presentation, [125], a MELAS-like presentation [126], Parkinsonism [124], a disorder with isolated sensorineural hearing loss, diabetes, cardiomyopathy [101], and isolated premature ovarian failure [127].

Some nonpathogenic variants in *POLG* may predispose patients to reversible valproate-related hepatotoxicity without a risk for developing any other manifestations of *POLG*-related disease [128, 129]. Thus, there may be a role for *POLG* sequencing prior to initiating valproic acid therapy, even in patients without specific POLG-related disease symptoms [108].

There is experimental evidence that VPA triggers increased mitochondrial biogenesis by altering the expression of several mitochondrial genes; however, the capacity of POLG-deficient liver cells to address the increased metabolic rate caused by VPA administration is significantly impaired [130].

Transplantation has been attempted in patients with liver failure due to *POLG*-related disease though patients with AHS may not fare well with an increased morbidity and mortality [24, 107, 115].

C10orf2/TWNK

The *TWNK* gene encodes a mitochondrial protein, Twinkle, which co-localizes with mtDNA in mitochondrial nucleoids [131]. The Twinkle protein is expressed at a high rate in the muscle and pancreas and lower rate in the heart and contains three functional domains including a 3-prime helicase region required for mtDNA replication, a linker region involved in oligomerization into a hexamer required for helicase activity, and a 5-primase domain [131, 132].

Mutations in *TWNK* lead to several phenotypes including hepatocerebral disease, infantile-onset spinocerebellar ataxia (IOCSA), Perrault syndrome, and CPEO [131, 133, 134].

Biallelic mutations lead to severe mtDNA depletion in the brain and liver and infant-onset hypotonia with developmental disability and hepatopathy followed by neurodegeneration, muscle atrophy, and seizures. Failure to thrive can occur [135, 136]. Epilepsy may be refractory and a movement disorder with athetosis may be present [137]. Renal tubulopathy can occur [138]. Nystagmus and ophthalmoplegia can occur. Liver involvement can include cholestasis, coagulopathy, and elevations in transaminases. Neuroimaging may show white matter hyperintensities and cerebellar atrophy. Death typically occurs in early childhood, often by age 3 years [135–137].

IOCSA is an autosomal recessive severe, progressive neurodegenerative disorder predominantly described in Finland. Patients present around a year of age with ataxia, hypotonia, hyporeflexia, and athetosis. This is followed by SNHL and CPEO in school age and optic atrophy, sensory axonal neuropathy, progressive pes cavus, scoliosis, and autonomic dysfunction in the teen years. Affected individuals are no longer independently ambulatory by adolescence. Hypergonadotropic hypogonadism can occur in females. Epilepsy of varying types can develop including status epilepticus and EPC. Migraine-like headaches and severe psychiatric symptom are noted in the adolescent years [139]. Neuroimaging shows progressive atrophy of the cerebellum, brainstem, and spinal cord early on [133, 140]. After the onset of epilepsy, focal stroke-like lesions in a nonvascular distribution have also been described including small cortical to large hemispheric edematous lesions. Cortical atrophy then follows in those with intractable epilepsy [139].

Compound heterozygous mutations in the helicase domain have been linked to Perrault syndrome. Patients present in their adolescent years with primary amenorrhea and SNHL followed by ataxia and a sensory axonal neuropathy [134]. Associated partial atrophy of the vestibulocochlear nerves and decreased gray and increased white matter volumes of the cerebellum have recently been described [141].

Heterozygous mutations with multiple mtDNA deletions have been linked to autosomal dominant PEO [131], and in fact *TWNK* mutations are the most common nuclear genetic causes of pure CPEO. Symptoms may begin in childhood thru the adult years. Fatigue has been reported in half of patients. Less commonly, patients may have additional symptoms including cataracts, diabetes, SNHL, sensory axonal neuropathy, proximal muscle weakness, hypogonadism, and early-onset dementia. Cardiac involvement is less common but can include ventricular hypertrophy and arrhythmias. Late-onset Parkinsonism has been noted in a few patients [132, 142–146]. MRI may show subcortical and periventricular white matter lesions [132].

In patients with mtDNA depletion, *TWNK* mutations lactic acidosis is seen in plasma or CSF. Mitochondrial respiratory chain activity is variably affected. mtDNA content is severely reduced in the muscle and liver. Liver biopsy can show cirrhosis, cholestasis, and steatosis [135, 137, 145].

TFAM

The *TFAM* gene encodes for a mitochondrial transcription factor essential for initiating mtDNA transcription, replication, and nucleoid packaging [147, 148].

Pathogenic mutations in *TFAM* are linked to an autosomal recessive disorder with infantile-onset progressive fatal liver failure. Infants were born with intrauterine growth restriction and developed hepatopathy with elevated transaminases, conjugated hyperbilirubinemia, and hypoglycemia. Liver failure and death occurred in early infancy [148].

mtDNA copy number has been shown to be decreased in patient liver, muscle, and fibroblasts. Liver biopsy shows cirrhosis, micro- and macrovesicular steatosis, and cholestasis. Muscle electron microscopy shows abnormal mitochondrial morphology. Biochemical enzymology in muscle showed increased citrate synthase activity [148].

Neurogastrointestinal Form

Mutations in *TYMP* predominantly lead to an autosomal recessive disorder with MNGIE syndrome and associated mtDNA deletions, depletion, and point mutations [149]. A MNGIE-like phenotype has also been noted in other mtDNA depletion disorders including *RRM2B* [58] and *POLG*-related disease [125, 150] and pseudo-obstruction in select other mitochondrial disorders such as MELAS and MERRF [151–153].

The *TYMP* gene encodes a thymidine phosphorylase (TP) involved in nucleotide salvage by reversibly catalyzing the phosphorylation of thymidine or deoxyuridine to thymine or uracil, respectively [154]. In addition, the protein product inhibits glial cell growth and promotes endothelial cell growth secondarily impacting the development of the central nervous system and blood-brain barrier [155]. The protein is expressed in high levels in the digestive system, brain, spleen, bladder, and lungs [156]. Low TP levels lead to accumulation of thymidine and deoxyuridine and an imbalance of nucleosides with secondary impairment of mtDNA replication.

MNGIE was first described in 1987, [157] though the underlying cause being *TYMP* mutations was identified 10 years later [149]. Patients typically present in their young adult to adult years with slowly progressive GI dysmotility and intestinal pseudo-obstruction [158, 159]. Age of presentation varies between ages 5 months and more than 50 years though the mean reported age is the late teen years [160]. Prior to the onset of GI symptoms, patients are generally healthy though they may have easy fatigue and a thin body habitus. Some symptoms such as CPEO, myopathy, or neuropathy may begin several years prior to the onset of GI disease. Initial worsening may be provoked by an underlying infection. GI symptoms include early satiety, nausea, dysphagia, postprandial emesis, abdominal pain, and recurrent diarrhea [161]. Patients progress to develop cachexia and severe failure to thrive. A mixed sensory and/or axonal polyneuropathy can occur with areflexia, weakness, and painful sensory paresthesias. CPEO and SNHL may be seen. Hypogonadism has been noted in some [162]. A predominantly asymptomatic leukoencephalopathy is seen on neuroimaging that may spare the corpus callosum and is present decades prior to the onset of their GI symptoms [158, 160].

Thymidine phosphorylase activity is reduced in leukocytes and is an accurate diagnostic test along with elevations in plasma thymidine and deoxyuridine [158, 163]. Plasma may show elevated lactate. Spinal fluid analysis may show an increase in protein. Patients may have COX-negative muscle fibers. Single or multiple electron transport chain enzyme activities may be reduced [164]. Muscle and gut biopsies show mtDNA deletions, depletion, or both [158, 159]. Rectal biopsy may show cytoplasmic eosinophilic inclusions in submucosal ganglion cells [165]. Duodenal biopsies may demonstrate focal muscle atrophy, serosal granulomas, and a focal loss of Auerbach's plexus with fibrosis [166].

Therapeutic Implications

There has been a lot of new development in the clinical recognition, diagnosis, and treatment of patients with mtDNA depletion syndromes especially in two diseases: thymidine kinase 2 (TK2) deficiency and mitochondrial neurogastrointestinal encephalomyopathy (MNGIE).

Animal models of the disorders are critical tools for understanding how mutations cause diseases and for testing therapies, some mutant mice (TK2, MNGIE, DGUOK, POLG) and zebrafish (POLG, DGUOK) models available for mtDNA depletion syndromes. Interestingly, several scientific studies of the mouse and cellular models have revealed the importance of balanced pools of the four deoxynucleoside triphosphates needed for mtDNA synthesis: dATP, dGTP, dCTP, and dTTP [167–169]. These four molecules, collectively known as "dNTPs," are the building blocks for the maintenance of mtDNA. Some of these diseases affect genes and proteins involved in dNTP synthesis. For example, TK2 is needed for the synthesis of dTTP and dCTP within mitochondria, and DGUOK is needed for the synthesis of dATP and dGTP in mitochondria. There is accumulated evidence of the potential therapeutic benefits of administration of deoxynucleoside and deoxynucleotides, which are precursors or intermediate molecules needed for dNTP synthesis. The administration of these substances to cells (in vitro) or animal models (in vivo) bypasses the dysfunction of TK2 and dGK and may restore dNTP balance [15, 167–169]. Additional in vitro and in vivo models are required to clarify whether the treatment is also potentially translatable to other mtDNA maintenance diseases.

Based on these laboratory studies, TK2-deficient patients in Europe and North, Central, and South America have been treated with deoxynucleoside and deoxynucleotide therapies under compassionate use protocols with striking and encouraging results (personal communications with Michio Hirano, ENMC workshop paper in preparation). There is a lot to do in this field; first of all full regulatory approvals from the Food and Drug Administration (FDA) and European Medicines Agency (EMA) are required to use deoxynucleosides to treat TK2 deficiency, and a clinical trial must support the efficacy of the product. In contrast to TK2 deficiency, MNGIE has several available therapies; however guidelines were only recently generated.

The deoxynucleoside supplementation therapy for TK2 deficiency is currently being evaluated, and hopefully this will further confirm the benefit of this promising therapy. Regulatory approval will lead to greater availability of the first specific and effective treatment for this disease.

Clearer guidelines will be available (ENMC workshop paper in preparation) to help physicians in choosing the most appropriate option among the innovative therapies for MNGIE. Potential new future clinical trials may test deoxynucleoside therapy for other mtDNA maintenance disorders.

In MNGIE, treatment via dialysis has been attempted in the hopes of clearing excess nucleoside levels; however it did not result in longer-term improvement but improved vomiting and abdominal pain [170, 171]. Transfused platelets, rich in thymidine phosphorylase, may also help to reduce symptoms temporarily [170]. Hematopoietic stem cell transplant (HSCT) has been investigated for MNGIE with some success in partially restoring thymidine phosphorylase activity in the buffy coat and lowering plasma nucleoside levels [172, 173]. However, some patients have not survived the procedure [172, 173]. Post-transplant there is improvement in GI symptoms, fatigue, neuropathy, and muscle strength [174]. However, there is a concern that HSCT does not effectively reduce CSF levels of toxic metabolites and does not reverse the neurologic phenotype or leukoencephalopathy [174, 175]. Liver transplantation seems to be an alternative therapy for MNGIE, which has lower risk and probably similar efficacy as HSCT [176].

TP deficiency represents a particularly favorable situation for a gene therapy approach for several reasons: (1) the correction of a limited number of cells with enough TP activity can be sufficient to clear the systemic overload of nucleosides, as observed in carriers of pathogenic mutations, who are asymptomatic and do not have nucleoside accumulation with levels as low as ≈25% of normal TP activity; (2) the enzyme does not need to be secreted because its substrates are small diffusible water-soluble molecules; and (3) the correction of the molecular defect can be performed in any tissue with sufficient blood flow. AAV vector is currently used in animal models of MNGIE to express human TP in hepatocytes. A single intravenous injection of a liver-targeted AAV2/8 resulted in permanent TP expression in the liver of the mice, normalizing nucleoside metabolism, with no signs of toxicity or hepatocellular damage. These preclinical results suggest that relatively low vector doses could be sufficient for long-term therapeutic nucleoside clearance in MNGIE patients.

Final Remarks

The large variety of clinical syndromes associated with mtDNA depletion makes diagnosis difficult; however we highlighted some clinical hallmarks of these diseases. mtDNA depletion can be only detected in the affected tissues (muscle, liver); therefore even in the era of next-generation sequencing, we may need to perform biopsies in patients when the result of genetic testing is unclear. Diagnosing mtDNA depletion is important because of the possibility of genetic counselling and emerging options for therapy.

References

1. Nogueira C, Almeida LS, Nesti C, Pezzini I, Videira A, Vilarinho L, et al. Syndromes associated with mitochondrial DNA depletion. Ital J Pediatr. 2014;40:34.
2. Viscomi C, Zeviani M. MtDNA-maintenance defects: syndromes and genes. J Inherit Metab Dis. 2017;40(4):587–99.
3. Fasullo M, Endres L. Nucleotide salvage deficiencies, DNA damage and neurodegeneration. Int J Mol Sci. 2015;16(5):9431–49.
4. Johansson M, Karlsson A. Cloning of the cDNA and chromosome localization of the gene for human thymidine kinase 2. J Biol Chem. 1997;272(13):8454–8.
5. Saada A, Shaag A, Mandel H, Nevo Y, Eriksson S, Elpeleg O. Mutant mitochondrial thymidine kinase in mitochondrial DNA depletion myopathy. Nat Genet. 2001;29(3):342–4.
6. Garone C, Taylor RW, Nascimento A, Poulton J, Fratter C, Domínguez-González C, Evans JC, Loos M, Isohanni P, Suomalainen A, Ram D, Hughes MI, McFarland R, Barca E, Lopez Gomez C, Jayawant S, Thomas ND, Manzur AY, Kleinsteuber K, Martin MA, Kerr T, Gorman GS, Sommerville EW, Chinnery PF, Hofer M, Karch C, Ralph J, Cámara Y, Madruga-Garrido M, Domínguez-Carral J, Ortez C, Emperador S, Montoya J, Chakrapani A, Kriger JF, Schoenaker R, Levin B, Thompson JLP, Long Y, Rahman S, Donati MA, DiMauro S, Hirano M. Retrospective natural history of thymidine kinase 2 deficiency. J Med Genet. 2018;55(8):515–21.
7. Pons R, Andreetta F, Wang CH, Vu TH, Bonilla E, DiMauro S, et al. Mitochondrial myopathy simulating spinal muscular atrophy. Pediatr Neurol. 1996;15(2):153–8.
8. Mancuso M, Salviati L, Sacconi S, Otaegui D, Camano P, Marina A, et al. Mitochondrial DNA depletion: mutations in thymidine kinase gene with myopathy and SMA. Neurology. 2002;59(8):1197–202.
9. Lesko N, Naess K, Wibom R, Solaroli N, Nennesmo I, von Dobeln U, et al. Two novel mutations in thymidine kinase-2 cause early onset fatal encephalomyopathy and severe mtDNA depletion. Neuromuscul Disord. 2010;20(3):198–203.
10. Termglinchan T, Hisamatsu S, Ohmori J, Suzumura H, Sumitomo N, Imataka G, et al. Novel TK2 mutations as a cause of delayed muscle maturation in mtDNA depletion syndrome. Neurol Genet. 2016;2(5):e95.
11. Marti R, Nascimento A, Colomer J, Lara MC, Lopez-Gallardo E, Ruiz-Pesini E, et al. Hearing loss in a patient with the myopathic form of mitochondrial DNA depletion syndrome and a novel mutation in the TK2 gene. Pediatr Res. 2010;68(2):151–4.
12. Zhang S, Li FY, Bass HN, Pursley A, Schmitt ES, Brown BL, et al. Application of oligonucleotide array CGH to the simultaneous detection of a deletion in the nuclear TK2 gene and mtDNA depletion. Mol Genet Metab. 2010;99(1):53–7.
13. Paramasivam A, Meena AK, Pedaparthi L, Jyothi V, Uppin MS, Jabeen SA, et al. Novel mutation in C10orf2 associated with multiple mtDNA deletions, chronic progressive external ophthalmoplegia and premature aging. Mitochondrion. 2016;26:81–5.
14. Chanprasert S, Wong LJC, Wang J, Scaglia F. TK2-related mitochondrial DNA depletion syndrome, myopathic form. In: Adam MP, Ardinger HH, Pagon RA, Wallace SE, LJH B, Mefford HC, et al., editors. GeneReviews(R). Seattle, WA: University of Washington, Seattle; 1993. GeneReviews is a registered trademark of the University of Washington, Seattle. All rights reserved.
15. Garone C, Garcia-Diaz B, Emmanuele V, Lopez LC, Tadesse S, Akman HO, et al. Deoxypyrimidine

monophosphate bypass therapy for thymidine kinase 2 deficiency. EMBO Mol Med. 2014;6(8):1016–27.
16. Lopez-Gomez C, Levy RJ, Sanchez-Quintero MJ, Juanola-Falgarona M, Barca E, Garcia-Diaz B, et al. Deoxycytidine and deoxythymidine treatment for thymidine kinase 2 deficiency. Ann Neurol. 2017;81(5):641–52.
17. Kornblum C, Nicholls TJ, Haack TB, Scholer S, Peeva V, Danhauser K, et al. Loss-of-function mutations in MGME1 impair mtDNA replication and cause multisystemic mitochondrial disease. Nat Genet. 2013;45(2):214–9.
18. Hebbar M, Girisha KM, Srivastava A, Bielas S, Shukla A. Homozygous c.359del variant in MGME1 is associated with early onset cerebellar ataxia. Eur J Med Genet. 2017;60(10):533–5.
19. Waggoner DW, Johnson LB, Mann PC, Morris V, Guastella J, Bajjalieh SM. MuLK, a eukaryotic multi-substrate lipid kinase. J Biol Chem. 2004;279(37):38228–35.
20. Bektas M, Payne SG, Liu H, Goparaju S, Milstien S, Spiegel S. A novel acylglycerol kinase that produces lysophosphatidic acid modulates cross talk with EGFR in prostate cancer cells. J Cell Biol. 2005;169(5):801–11.
21. Mayr JA, Haack TB, Graf E, Zimmermann FA, Wieland T, Haberberger B, et al. Lack of the mitochondrial protein acylglycerol kinase causes Sengers syndrome. Am J Hum Genet. 2012;90(2):314–20.
22. Sengers RC, Trijbels JM, Willems JL, Daniels O, Stadhouders AM. Congenital cataract and mitochondrial myopathy of skeletal and heart muscle associated with lactic acidosis after exercise. J Pediatr. 1975;86(6):873–80.
23. Calvo SE, Compton AG, Hershman SG, Lim SC, Lieber DS, Tucker EJ, et al. Molecular diagnosis of infantile mitochondrial disease with targeted next-generation sequencing. Sci Transl Med. 2012;4(118):118ra10.
24. Parikh S, Karaa A, Goldstein A, Ng YS, Gorman G, Feigenbaum A, et al. Solid organ transplantation in primary mitochondrial disease: proceed with caution. Mol Genet Metab. 2016;118(3):178–84.
25. Neckelmann N, Li K, Wade RP, Shuster R, Wallace DC. cDNA sequence of a human skeletal muscle ADP/ATP translocator: lack of a leader peptide, divergence from a fibroblast translocator cDNA, and coevolution with mitochondrial DNA genes. Proc Natl Acad Sci U S A. 1987;84(21):7580–4.
26. Li K, Warner CK, Hodge JA, Minoshima S, Kudoh J, Fukuyama R, et al. A human muscle adenine nucleotide translocator gene has four exons, is located on chromosome 4, and is differentially expressed. J Biol Chem. 1989;264(24):13998–4004.
27. Kaukonen J, Juselius JK, Tiranti V, Kyttala A, Zeviani M, Comi GP, et al. Role of adenine nucleotide translocator 1 in mtDNA maintenance. Science. 2000;289(5480):782–5.
28. Thompson K, Majd H, Dallabona C, Reinson K, King MS, Alston CL, et al. Recurrent de novo dominant mutations in SLC25A4 cause severe early-onset mitochondrial disease and loss of mitochondrial DNA copy number. Am J Hum Genet. 2016;99(4):860–76.
29. Palmieri L, Alberio S, Pisano I, Lodi T, Meznaric-Petrusa M, Zidar J, et al. Complete loss-of-function of the heart/muscle-specific adenine nucleotide translocator is associated with mitochondrial myopathy and cardiomyopathy. Hum Mol Genet. 2005;14(20):3079–88.
30. Echaniz-Laguna A, Chassagne M, Ceresuela J, Rouvet I, Padet S, Acquaviva C, et al. Complete loss of expression of the ANT1 gene causing cardiomyopathy and myopathy. J Med Genet. 2012;49(2):146–50.
31. Olichon A, Baricault L, Gas N, Guillou E, Valette A, Belenguer P, et al. Loss of OPA1 perturbates the mitochondrial inner membrane structure and integrity, leading to cytochrome c release and apoptosis. J Biol Chem. 2003;278(10):7743–6.
32. Cipolat S, Martins de Brito O, Dal Zilio B, Scorrano L. OPA1 requires mitofusin 1 to promote mitochondrial fusion. Proc Natl Acad Sci U S A. 2004;101(45):15927–32.
33. Elachouri G, Vidoni S, Zanna C, Pattyn A, Boukhaddaoui H, Gaget K, et al. OPA1 links human mitochondrial genome maintenance to mtDNA replication and distribution. Genome Res. 2011;21(1):12–20.
34. Delettre C, Lenaers G, Griffoin JM, Gigarel N, Lorenzo C, Belenguer P, et al. Nuclear gene OPA1, encoding a mitochondrial dynamin-related protein, is mutated in dominant optic atrophy. Nat Genet. 2000;26(2):207–10.
35. Yu-Wai-Man P, Griffiths PG, Gorman GS, Lourenco CM, Wright AF, Auer-Grumbach M, et al. Multi-system neurological disease is common in patients with OPA1 mutations. Brain. 2010;133(Pt 3):771–86.
36. Schaaf CP, Blazo M, Lewis RA, Tonini RE, Takei H, Wang J, et al. Early-onset severe neuromuscular phenotype associated with compound heterozygosity for OPA1 mutations. Mol Genet Metab. 2011;103(4):383–7.
37. Pyle A, Ramesh V, Bartsakoulia M, Boczonadi V, Gomez-Duran A, Herczegfalvi A, et al. Behr's syndrome is typically associated with disturbed mitochondrial translation and mutations in the C12orf65 gene. J Neuromuscul Dis. 2014;1(1):55–63.
38. Spiegel R, Saada A, Flannery PJ, Burte F, Soiferman D, Khayat M, et al. Fatal infantile mitochondrial encephalomyopathy, hypertrophic cardiomyopathy and optic atrophy associated with a homozygous OPA1 mutation. J Med Genet. 2016;53(2):127–31.
39. Ostergaard E, Christensen E, Kristensen E, Mogensen B, Duno M, Shoubridge EA, et al. Deficiency of the alpha subunit of succinate-coenzyme A ligase causes fatal infantile lactic acidosis with mitochondrial DNA depletion. Am J Hum Genet. 2007;81(2):383–7.

40. Kowluru A, Tannous M, Chen HQ. Localization and characterization of the mitochondrial isoform of the nucleoside diphosphate kinase in the pancreatic beta cell: evidence for its complexation with mitochondrial succinyl-CoA synthetase. Arch Biochem Biophys. 2002;398(2):160–9.
41. James M, Man NT, Edwards YH, Morris GE. The molecular basis for cross-reaction of an anti-dystrophin antibody with alpha-actinin. Biochim Biophys Acta. 1997;1360(2):169–76.
42. Ostergaard E, Schwartz M, Batbayli M, Christensen E, Hjalmarson O, Kollberg G, et al. A novel missense mutation in SUCLG1 associated with mitochondrial DNA depletion, encephalomyopathic form, with methylmalonic aciduria. Eur J Pediatr. 2010;169(2):201–5.
43. Rouzier C, Le Guedard-Mereuze S, Fragaki K, Serre V, Miro J, Tuffery-Giraud S, et al. The severity of phenotype linked to SUCLG1 mutations could be correlated with residual amount of SUCLG1 protein. J Med Genet. 2010;47(10):670–6.
44. Carrozzo R, Verrigni D, Rasmussen M, de Coo R, Amartino H, Bianchi M, et al. Succinate-CoA ligase deficiency due to mutations in SUCLA2 and SUCLG1: phenotype and genotype correlations in 71 patients. J Inherit Metab Dis. 2016;39(2):243–52.
45. Donti TR, Masand R, Scott DA, Craigen WJ, Graham BH. Expanding the phenotypic spectrum of Succinyl-CoA ligase deficiency through functional validation of a new SUCLG1 variant. Mol Genet Metab. 2016;119(1–2):68–74.
46. Lambeth DO, Tews KN, Adkins S, Frohlich D, Milavetz BI. Expression of two succinyl-CoA synthetases with different nucleotide specificities in mammalian tissues. J Biol Chem. 2004;279(35):36621–4.
47. Ostergaard E, Hansen FJ, Sorensen N, Duno M, Vissing J, Larsen PL, et al. Mitochondrial encephalomyopathy with elevated methylmalonic acid is caused by SUCLA2 mutations. Brain. 2007;130(Pt 3):853–61.
48. Carrozzo R, Dionisi-Vici C, Steuerwald U, Lucioli S, Deodato F, Di Giandomenico S, et al. SUCLA2 mutations are associated with mild methylmalonic aciduria, Leigh-like encephalomyopathy, dystonia and deafness. Brain. 2007;130(Pt 3):862–74.
49. Bourdon A, Minai L, Serre V, Jais JP, Sarzi E, Aubert S, et al. Mutation of RRM2B, encoding p53-controlled ribonucleotide reductase (p53R2), causes severe mitochondrial DNA depletion. Nat Genet. 2007;39(6):776–80.
50. Foskolou IP, Jorgensen C, Leszczynska KB, Olcina MM, Tarhonskaya H, Haisma B, et al. Ribonucleotide reductase requires subunit switching in hypoxia to maintain DNA replication. Mol Cell. 2017;66(2):206–220.e9.
51. Bornstein B, Area E, Flanigan KM, Ganesh J, Jayakar P, Swoboda KJ, et al. Mitochondrial DNA depletion syndrome due to mutations in the RRM2B gene. Neuromuscul Disord. 2008;18(6):453–9.
52. Kollberg G, Darin N, Benan K, Moslemi AR, Lindal S, Tulinius M, et al. A novel homozygous RRM2B missense mutation in association with severe mtDNA depletion. Neuromuscul Disord. 2009;19(2):147–50.
53. Tyynismaa H, Ylikallio E, Patel M, Molnar MJ, Haller RG, Suomalainen A. A heterozygous truncating mutation in RRM2B causes autosomal-dominant progressive external ophthalmoplegia with multiple mtDNA deletions. Am J Hum Genet. 2009;85(2):290–5.
54. Kropach N, Shkalim-Zemer V, Orenstein N, Scheuerman O, Straussberg R. Novel RRM2B mutation and severe mitochondrial DNA depletion: report of 2 cases and review of the literature. Neuropediatrics. 2017;48(6):456–62.
55. Pitceathly RD, Fassone E, Taanman JW, Sadowski M, Fratter C, Mudanohwo EE, et al. Kearns-Sayre syndrome caused by defective R1/p53R2 assembly. J Med Genet. 2011;48(9):610–7.
56. Fratter C, Raman P, Alston CL, Blakely EL, Craig K, Smith C, et al. RRM2B mutations are frequent in familial PEO with multiple mtDNA deletions. Neurology. 2011;76(23):2032–4.
57. Pitceathly RD, Smith C, Fratter C, Alston CL, He L, Craig K, et al. Adults with RRM2B-related mitochondrial disease have distinct clinical and molecular characteristics. Brain. 2012;135(Pt 11):3392–403.
58. Shaibani A, Shchelochkov OA, Zhang S, Katsonis P, Lichtarge O, Wong LJ, et al. Mitochondrial neurogastrointestinal encephalopathy due to mutations in RRM2B. Arch Neurol. 2009;66(8):1028–32.
59. Bonnen PE, Yarham JW, Besse A, Wu P, Faqeih EA, Al-Asmari AM, et al. Mutations in FBXL4 cause mitochondrial encephalopathy and a disorder of mitochondrial DNA maintenance. Am J Hum Genet. 2013;93(3):471–81.
60. Gai X, Ghezzi D, Johnson MA, Biagosch CA, Shamseldin HE, Haack TB, et al. Mutations in FBXL4, encoding a mitochondrial protein, cause early-onset mitochondrial encephalomyopathy. Am J Hum Genet. 2013;93(3):482–95.
61. Huemer M, Karall D, Schossig A, Abdenur JE, Al Jasmi F, Biagosch C, et al. Clinical, morphological, biochemical, imaging and outcome parameters in 21 individuals with mitochondrial maintenance defect related to FBXL4 mutations. J Inherit Metab Dis. 2015;38(5):905–14.
62. El-Hattab AW, Dai H, Almannai M, Wang J, Faqeih EA, Al Asmari A, et al. Molecular and clinical spectra of FBXL4 deficiency. Hum Mutat. 2017;38(12):1649–59.
63. Ebrahimi-Fakhari D, Seitz A, Kolker S, Hoffmann GF. Recurrent stroke-like episodes in FBXL4-associated early-onset mitochondrial encephalomyopathy. Pediatr Neurol. 2015;53(6):549–50.
64. Boczonadi V, King MS, Smith AC, Olahova M, Bansagi B, Roos A, et al. Mitochondrial oxodicarboxylate carrier deficiency is associated with mitochondrial DNA depletion and spinal

muscular atrophy-like disease. Genet Med. 2018;20(10):1224–35.
65. Johansson M, Karlsson A. Cloning and expression of human deoxyguanosine kinase cDNA. Proc Natl Acad Sci U S A. 1996;93(14):7258–62.
66. Mandel H, Szargel R, Labay V, Elpeleg O, Saada A, Shalata A, et al. The deoxyguanosine kinase gene is mutated in individuals with depleted hepatocerebral mitochondrial DNA. Nat Genet. 2001;29(3):337–41.
67. Taanman JW, Kateeb I, Muntau AC, Jaksch M, Cohen N, Mandel H. A novel mutation in the deoxyguanosine kinase gene causing depletion of mitochondrial DNA. Ann Neurol. 2002;52(2):237–9.
68. Dimmock DP, Zhang Q, Dionisi-Vici C, Carrozzo R, Shieh J, Tang LY, et al. Clinical and molecular features of mitochondrial DNA depletion due to mutations in deoxyguanosine kinase. Hum Mutat. 2008;29(2):330–1.
69. Ronchi D, Garone C, Bordoni A, Gutierrez Rios P, Calvo SE, Ripolone M, et al. Next-generation sequencing reveals DGUOK mutations in adult patients with mitochondrial DNA multiple deletions. Brain. 2012;135(Pt 11):3404–15.
70. Ducluzeau PH, Lachaux A, Bouvier R, Duborjal H, Stepien G, Bozon D, et al. Progressive reversion of clinical and molecular phenotype in a child with liver mitochondrial DNA depletion. J Hepatol. 2002;36(5):698–703.
71. Mousson de Camaret B, Taanman JW, Padet S, Chassagne M, Mayencon M, Clerc-Renaud P, et al. Kinetic properties of mutant deoxyguanosine kinase in a case of reversible hepatic mtDNA depletion. Biochem J. 2007;402(2):377–85.
72. Vilarinho S, Sari S, Yilmaz G, Stiegler AL, Boggon TJ, Jain D, et al. Recurrent recessive mutation in deoxyguanosine kinase causes idiopathic noncirrhotic portal hypertension. Hepatology. 2016;63(6):1977–86.
73. Lee NC, Dimmock D, Hwu WL, Tang LY, Huang WC, Chinault AC, et al. Simultaneous detection of mitochondrial DNA depletion and single-exon deletion in the deoxyguanosine gene using array-based comparative genomic hybridisation. Arch Dis Child. 2009;94(1):55–8.
74. Al-Hussaini A, Faqeih E, El-Hattab AW, Alfadhel M, Asery A, Alsaleem B, et al. Clinical and molecular characteristics of mitochondrial DNA depletion syndrome associated with neonatal cholestasis and liver failure. J Pediatr. 2014;164(3):553–9.e1-2.
75. Grabhorn E, Tsiakas K, Herden U, Fischer L, Freisinger P, Marquardt T, et al. Long-term outcomes after liver transplantation for deoxyguanosine kinase deficiency: a single-center experience and a review of the literature. Liver Transpl. 2014;20(4):464–72.
76. Dallabona C, Marsano RM, Arzuffi P, Ghezzi D, Mancini P, Zeviani M, et al. Sym1, the yeast ortholog of the MPV17 human disease protein, is a stress-induced bioenergetic and morphogenetic mitochondrial modulator. Hum Mol Genet. 2010;19(6):1098–107.
77. Lollgen S, Weiher H. The role of the Mpv17 protein mutations of which cause mitochondrial DNA depletion syndrome (MDDS): lessons from homologs in different species. Biol Chem. 2015;396(1):13–25.
78. Antonenkov VD, Isomursu A, Mennerich D, Vapola MH, Weiher H, Kietzmann T, et al. The human mitochondrial DNA depletion syndrome gene MPV17 encodes a non-selective channel that modulates membrane potential. J Biol Chem. 2015;290(22):13840–61.
79. Dalla Rosa I, Camara Y, Durigon R, Moss CF, Vidoni S, Akman G, et al. MPV17 loss causes deoxynucleotide insufficiency and slow DNA replication in mitochondria. PLoS Genet. 2016;12(1):e1005779.
80. Moss CF, Dalla Rosa I, Hunt LE, Yasukawa T, Young R, Jones AWE, et al. Aberrant ribonucleotide incorporation and multiple deletions in mitochondrial DNA of the murine MPV17 disease model. Nucleic Acids Res. 2017;45(22):12808–15.
81. Spinazzola A, Viscomi C, Fernandez-Vizarra E, Carrara F, D'Adamo P, Calvo S, et al. MPV17 encodes an inner mitochondrial membrane protein and is mutated in infantile hepatic mitochondrial DNA depletion. Nat Genet. 2006;38(5):570–5.
82. Karadimas CL, Vu TH, Holve SA, Chronopoulou P, Quinzii C, Johnsen SD, et al. Navajo neurohepatopathy is caused by a mutation in the MPV17 gene. Am J Hum Genet. 2006;79(3):544–8.
83. Uusimaa J, Evans J, Smith C, Butterworth A, Craig K, Ashley N, et al. Clinical, biochemical, cellular and molecular characterization of mitochondrial DNA depletion syndrome due to novel mutations in the MPV17 gene. Eur J Hum Genet. 2014;22(2):184–91.
84. Spinazzola A, Santer R, Akman OH, Tsiakas K, Schaefer H, Ding X, et al. Hepatocerebral form of mitochondrial DNA depletion syndrome: novel MPV17 mutations. Arch Neurol. 2008;65(8):1108–13.
85. Navarro-Sastre A, Martin-Hernandez E, Campos Y, Quintana E, Medina E, de Las Heras RS, et al. Lethal hepatopathy and leukodystrophy caused by a novel mutation in MPV17 gene: description of an alternative MPV17 spliced form. Mol Genet Metab. 2008;94(2):234–9.
86. Kaji S, Murayama K, Nagata I, Nagasaka H, Takayanagi M, Ohtake A, et al. Fluctuating liver functions in siblings with MPV17 mutations and possible improvement associated with dietary and pharmaceutical treatments targeting respiratory chain complex II. Mol Genet Metab. 2009;97(4):292–6.
87. Merkle AN, Nascene DR, McKinney AM. MR imaging findings in the reticular formation in siblings with MPV17-related mitochondrial depletion syndrome. AJNR Am J Neuroradiol. 2012;33(3):E34–5.
88. El-Hattab AW, Li FY, Schmitt E, Zhang S, Craigen WJ, Wong LJ. MPV17-associated hepatocerebral mitochondrial DNA depletion syndrome: new patients and novel mutations. Mol Genet Metab. 2010;99(3):300–8.

89. Bertazzoni U, Scovassi AI, Brun GM. Chick-embryo DNA polymerase gamma. Identity of gamma-polymerases purified from nuclei and mitochondria. Eur J Biochem. 1977;81(2):237–48.
90. Lestienne P. Evidence for a direct role of the DNA polymerase gamma in the replication of the human mitochondrial DNA in vitro. Biochem Biophys Res Commun. 1987;146(3):1146–53.
91. Carrodeguas JA, Theis K, Bogenhagen DF, Kisker C. Crystal structure and deletion analysis show that the accessory subunit of mammalian DNA polymerase gamma, Pol gamma B, functions as a homodimer. Mol Cell. 2001;7(1):43–54.
92. Longley MJ, Clark S, Yu Wai Man C, Hudson G, Durham SE, Taylor RW, et al. Mutant POLG2 disrupts DNA polymerase gamma subunits and causes progressive external ophthalmoplegia. Am J Hum Genet. 2006;78(6):1026–34.
93. Chinnery PF, Zeviani M. 155th ENMC workshop: polymerase gamma and disorders of mitochondrial DNA synthesis, 21-23 September 2007, Naarden, The Netherlands. Neuromuscul Disord. 2008;18(3):259–67.
94. Hikmat O, Tzoulis C, Chong WK, Chentouf L, Klingenberg C, Fratter C, et al. The clinical spectrum and natural history of early-onset diseases due to DNA polymerase gamma mutations. Genet Med. 2017;19(11):1217–25.
95. Anagnostou ME, Ng YS, Taylor RW, McFarland R. Epilepsy due to mutations in the mitochondrial polymerase gamma (POLG) gene: a clinical and molecular genetic review. Epilepsia. 2016;57(10):1531–45.
96. Neeve VC, Samuels DC, Bindoff LA, van den Bosch B, Van Goethem G, Smeets H, et al. What is influencing the phenotype of the common homozygous polymerase-gamma mutation p.Ala467Thr? Brain. 2012;135(Pt 12):3614–26.
97. Nikkanen J, Landoni JC, Balboa D, Haugas M, Partanen J, Paetau A, et al. A complex genomic locus drives mtDNA replicase POLG expression to its disease-related nervous system regions. EMBO Mol Med. 2018;10(1):13–21.
98. Alpers BJ. Diffuse progressive degeneration of the gray matter of the cerebrum. Arch Neurol Psych. 1931;25(3):469–505.
99. Naviaux RK, Nguyen KV. POLG mutations associated with Alpers' syndrome and mitochondrial DNA depletion. Ann Neurol. 2004;55(5):706–12.
100. Darin N, Oldfors A, Moslemi AR, Holme E, Tulinius M. The incidence of mitochondrial encephalomyopathies in childhood: clinical features and morphological, biochemical, and DNA abnormalities. Ann Neurol. 2001;49(3):377–83.
101. Horvath R, Hudson G, Ferrari G, Futterer N, Ahola S, Lamantea E, et al. Phenotypic spectrum associated with mutations of the mitochondrial polymerase gamma gene. Brain. 2006;129(Pt 7):1674–84.
102. Nguyen KV, Ostergaard E, Ravn SH, Balslev T, Danielsen ER, Vardag A, et al. POLG mutations in Alpers syndrome. Neurology. 2005;65(9):1493–5.
103. Cohen BH, Chinnery PF, Copeland WC. POLG-related disorders. In: Pagon RA, Bird TD, Dolan CR, Stephens K, editors. GeneReviews. Seattle, WA: University of Washington, Seattle; 1993.
104. Davidzon G, Greene P, Mancuso M, Klos KJ, Ahlskog JE, Hirano M, et al. Early-onset familial parkinsonism due to POLG mutations. Ann Neurol. 2006;59(5):859–62.
105. Worle H, Kohler B, Schlote W, Winkler P, Bastanier CK. Progressive cerebral degeneration of childhood with liver disease (Alpers Huttenlocher disease) with cytochrome oxidase deficiency presenting with epilepsia partialis continua as the first clinical manifestation. Clin Neuropathol. 1998;17(2):63–8.
106. Naviaux RK, Nyhan WL, Barshop BA, Poulton J, Markusic D, Karpinski NC, et al. Mitochondrial DNA polymerase gamma deficiency and mtDNA depletion in a child with Alpers' syndrome. Ann Neurol. 1999;45(1):54–8.
107. Tzoulis C, Engelsen BA, Telstad W, Aasly J, Zeviani M, Winterthun S, et al. The spectrum of clinical disease caused by the A467T and W748S POLG mutations: a study of 26 cases. Brain. 2006;129(Pt 7):1685–92.
108. Saneto RP, Lee IC, Koenig MK, Bao X, Weng SW, Naviaux RK, et al. POLG DNA testing as an emerging standard of care before instituting valproic acid therapy for pediatric seizure disorders. Seizure. 2010;19(3):140–6.
109. Hakonen AH, Heiskanen S, Juvonen V, Lappalainen I, Luoma PT, Rantamaki M, et al. Mitochondrial DNA polymerase W748S mutation: a common cause of autosomal recessive ataxia with ancient European origin. Am J Hum Genet. 2005;77(3):430–41.
110. Engelsen BA, Tzoulis C, Karlsen B, Lillebo A, Laegreid LM, Aasly J, et al. POLG1 mutations cause a syndromic epilepsy with occipital lobe predilection. Brain. 2008;131(Pt 3):818–28.
111. Smith JK, Mah JK, Castillo M. Brain MR imaging findings in two patients with Alpers' syndrome. Clin Imaging. 1996;20(4):235–7.
112. Nguyen KV, Sharief FS, Chan SS, Copeland WC, Naviaux RK. Molecular diagnosis of Alpers syndrome. J Hepatol. 2006;45(1):108–16.
113. Saneto RP, Cohen BH, Copeland WC, Naviaux RK. Alpers-Huttenlocher syndrome. Pediatr Neurol. 2013;48(3):167–78.
114. Ferrari G, Lamantea E, Donati A, Filosto M, Briem E, Carrara F, et al. Infantile hepatocerebral syndromes associated with mutations in the mitochondrial DNA polymerase-gamma A. Brain. 2005;128(Pt 4):723–31.
115. Wong LJ, Naviaux RK, Brunetti-Pierri N, Zhang Q, Schmitt ES, Truong C, et al. Molecular and clinical genetics of mitochondrial diseases due to POLG mutations. Hum Mutat. 2008;29(9):E150–72.

116. Van Goethem G, Luoma P, Rantamaki M, Al Memar A, Kaakkola S, Hackman P, et al. POLG mutations in neurodegenerative disorders with ataxia but no muscle involvement. Neurology. 2004;63(7):1251–7.
117. Winterthun S, Ferrari G, He L, Taylor RW, Zeviani M, Turnbull DM, et al. Autosomal recessive mitochondrial ataxic syndrome due to mitochondrial polymerase gamma mutations. Neurology. 2005;64(7):1204–8.
118. Fadic R, Russell JA, Vedanarayanan VV, Lehar M, Kuncl RW, Johns DR. Sensory ataxic neuropathy as the presenting feature of a novel mitochondrial disease. Neurology. 1997;49(1):239–45.
119. Van Goethem G, Martin JJ, Dermaut B, Lofgren A, Wibail A, Ververken D, et al. Recessive POLG mutations presenting with sensory and ataxic neuropathy in compound heterozygote patients with progressive external ophthalmoplegia. Neuromuscul Disord. 2003;13(2):133–42.
120. Mancuso M, Filosto M, Bellan M, Liguori R, Montagna P, Baruzzi A, et al. POLG mutations causing ophthalmoplegia, sensorimotor polyneuropathy, ataxia, and deafness. Neurology. 2004;62(2):316–8.
121. Lamantea E, Tiranti V, Bordoni A, Toscano A, Bono F, Servidei S, et al. Mutations of mitochondrial DNA polymerase gamma A are a frequent cause of autosomal dominant or recessive progressive external ophthalmoplegia. Ann Neurol. 2002;52(2):211–9.
122. Van Goethem G, Dermaut B, Lofgren A, Martin JJ, Van Broeckhoven C. Mutation of POLG is associated with progressive external ophthalmoplegia characterized by mtDNA deletions. Nat Genet. 2001;28(3):211–2.
123. Van Goethem G, Mercelis R, Lofgren A, Seneca S, Ceuterick C, Martin JJ, et al. Patient homozygous for a recessive POLG mutation presents with features of MERRF. Neurology. 2003;61(12):1811–3.
124. Luoma P, Melberg A, Rinne JO, Kaukonen JA, Nupponen NN, Chalmers RM, et al. Parkinsonism, premature menopause, and mitochondrial DNA polymerase gamma mutations: clinical and molecular genetic study. Lancet. 2004;364(9437):875–82.
125. Tang S, Dimberg EL, Milone M, Wong LJ. Mitochondrial neurogastrointestinal encephalomyopathy (MNGIE)-like phenotype: an expanded clinical spectrum of POLG1 mutations. J Neurol. 2012;259(5):862–8.
126. Deschauer M, Tennant S, Rokicka A, He L, Kraya T, Turnbull DM, et al. MELAS associated with mutations in the POLG1 gene. Neurology. 2007;68(20):1741–2.
127. Pagnamenta AT, Taanman JW, Wilson CJ, Anderson NE, Marotta R, Duncan AJ, et al. Dominant inheritance of premature ovarian failure associated with mutant mitochondrial DNA polymerase gamma. Hum Reprod. 2006;21(10):2467–73.
128. McFarland R, Hudson G, Taylor RW, Green SH, Hodges S, McKiernan PJ, et al. Reversible valproate hepatotoxicity due to mutations in mitochondrial DNA polymerase gamma (POLG1). Arch Dis Child. 2008;93(2):151–3.
129. Stewart JD, Horvath R, Baruffini E, Ferrero I, Bulst S, Watkins PB, et al. Polymerase gamma gene POLG determines the risk of sodium valproate-induced liver toxicity. Hepatology. 2010;52(5):1791–6.
130. Sitarz KS, Elliott HR, Karaman BS, Relton C, Chinnery PF, Horvath R. Valproic acid triggers increased mitochondrial biogenesis in POLG-deficient fibroblasts. Mol Genet Metab. 2014;112(1):57–63.
131. Spelbrink JN, Li FY, Tiranti V, Nikali K, Yuan QP, Tariq M, et al. Human mitochondrial DNA deletions associated with mutations in the gene encoding Twinkle, a phage T7 gene 4-like protein localized in mitochondria. Nat Genet. 2001;28(3):223–31.
132. Van Hove JL, Cunningham V, Rice C, Ringel SP, Zhang Q, Chou PC, et al. Finding twinkle in the eyes of a 71-year-old lady: a case report and review of the genotypic and phenotypic spectrum of TWINKLE-related dominant disease. Am J Med Genet A. 2009;149A(5):861–7.
133. Nikali K, Suomalainen A, Saharinen J, Kuokkanen M, Spelbrink JN, Lonnqvist T, et al. Infantile onset spinocerebellar ataxia is caused by recessive mutations in mitochondrial proteins Twinkle and Twinky. Hum Mol Genet. 2005;14(20):2981–90.
134. Morino H, Pierce SB, Matsuda Y, Walsh T, Ohsawa R, Newby M, et al. Mutations in Twinkle primase-helicase cause Perrault syndrome with neurologic features. Neurology. 2014;83(22):2054–61.
135. Sarzi E, Goffart S, Serre V, Chretien D, Slama A, Munnich A, et al. Twinkle helicase (PEO1) gene mutation causes mitochondrial DNA depletion. Ann Neurol. 2007;62(6):579–87.
136. Goh V, Helbling D, Biank V, Jarzembowski J, Dimmock D. Next-generation sequencing facilitates the diagnosis in a child with twinkle mutations causing cholestatic liver failure. J Pediatr Gastroenterol Nutr. 2012;54(2):291–4.
137. Hakonen AH, Isohanni P, Paetau A, Herva R, Suomalainen A, Lonnqvist T. Recessive Twinkle mutations in early onset encephalopathy with mtDNA depletion. Brain. 2007;130(Pt 11):3032–40.
138. Prasad C, Melancon SB, Rupar CA, Prasad AN, Nunez LD, Rosenblatt DS, et al. Exome sequencing reveals a homozygous mutation in TWINKLE as the cause of multisystemic failure including renal tubulopathy in three siblings. Mol Genet Metab. 2013;108(3):190–4.
139. Lonnqvist T, Paetau A, Valanne L, Pihko H. Recessive twinkle mutations cause severe epileptic encephalopathy. Brain. 2009;132(Pt 6):1553–62.
140. Hakonen AH, Goffart S, Marjavaara S, Paetau A, Cooper H, Mattila K, et al. Infantile-onset spinocerebellar ataxia and mitochondrial recessive ataxia syndrome are associated with neuronal complex I defect and mtDNA depletion. Hum Mol Genet. 2008;17(23):3822–35.

141. Oldak M, Ozieblo D, Pollak A, Stepniak I, Lazniewski M, Lechowicz U, et al. Novel neuro-audiological findings and further evidence for TWNK involvement in Perrault syndrome. J Transl Med. 2017;15(1):25.
142. Van Goethem G, Lofgren A, Dermaut B, Ceuterick C, Martin JJ, Van Broeckhoven C. Digenic progressive external ophthalmoplegia in a sporadic patient: recessive mutations in POLG and C10orf2/Twinkle. Hum Mutat. 2003;22(2):175–6.
143. Baloh RH, Salavaggione E, Milbrandt J, Pestronk A. Familial parkinsonism and ophthalmoplegia from a mutation in the mitochondrial DNA helicase twinkle. Arch Neurol. 2007;64(7):998–1000.
144. Echaniz-Laguna A, Chanson JB, Wilhelm JM, Sellal F, Mayencon M, Mohr M, et al. A novel variation in the Twinkle linker region causing late-onset dementia. Neurogenetics. 2010;11(1):21–5.
145. Fratter C, Gorman GS, Stewart JD, Buddles M, Smith C, Evans J, et al. The clinical, histochemical, and molecular spectrum of PEO1 (Twinkle)-linked adPEO. Neurology. 2010;74(20):1619–26.
146. Kiferle L, Orsucci D, Mancuso M, Lo Gerfo A, Petrozzi L, Siciliano G, et al. Twinkle mutation in an Italian family with external progressive ophthalmoplegia and parkinsonism: a case report and an update on the state of art. Neurosci Lett. 2013;556:1–4.
147. Parisi MA, Clayton DA. Similarity of human mitochondrial transcription factor 1 to high mobility group proteins. Science. 1991;252(5008):965–9.
148. Stiles AR, Simon MT, Stover A, Eftekharian S, Khanlou N, Wang HL, et al. Mutations in TFAM, encoding mitochondrial transcription factor A, cause neonatal liver failure associated with mtDNA depletion. Mol Genet Metab. 2016;119(1–2):91–9.
149. Nishino I, Spinazzola A, Hirano M. Thymidine phosphorylase gene mutations in MNGIE, a human mitochondrial disorder. Science. 1999;283(5402):689–92.
150. Van Goethem G, Schwartz M, Lofgren A, Dermaut B, Van Broeckhoven C, Vissing J. Novel POLG mutations in progressive external ophthalmoplegia mimicking mitochondrial neurogastrointestinal encephalomyopathy. Eur J Hum Genet. 2003;11(7):547–9.
151. Verny C, Amati-Bonneau P, Letournel F, Person B, Dib N, Malinge MC, et al. Mitochondrial DNA A3243G mutation involved in familial diabetes, chronic intestinal pseudo-obstruction and recurrent pancreatitis. Diabetes Metab. 2008;34(6 Pt 1):620–6.
152. Sekino Y, Inamori M, Yamada E, Ohkubo H, Sakai E, Higurashi T, et al. Characteristics of intestinal pseudo-obstruction in patients with mitochondrial diseases. World J Gastroenterol. 2012;18(33):4557–62.
153. Ng YS, Feeney C, Schaefer AM, Holmes CE, Hynd P, Alston CL, et al. Pseudo-obstruction, stroke, and mitochondrial dysfunction: a lethal combination. Ann Neurol. 2016;80(5):686–92.
154. Usuki K, Saras J, Waltenberger J, Miyazono K, Pierce G, Thomason A, et al. Platelet-derived endothelial cell growth factor has thymidine phosphorylase activity. Biochem Biophys Res Commun. 1992;184(3):1311–6.
155. Asai K, Nakanishi K, Isobe I, Eksioglu YZ, Hirano A, Hama K, et al. Neurotrophic action of gliostatin on cortical neurons. Identity of gliostatin and platelet-derived endothelial cell growth factor. J Biol Chem. 1992;267(28):20311–6.
156. Matsukawa K, Moriyama A, Kawai Y, Asai K, Kato T. Tissue distribution of human gliostatin/platelet-derived endothelial cell growth factor (PD-ECGF) and its drug-induced expression. Biochim Biophys Acta. 1996;1314(1–2):71–82.
157. Bardosi A, Creutzfeldt W, DiMauro S, Felgenhauer K, Friede RL, Goebel HH, et al. Myo-, neuro-, gastrointestinal encephalopathy (MNGIE syndrome) due to partial deficiency of cytochrome-c-oxidase. A new mitochondrial multisystem disorder. Acta Neuropathol. 1987;74(3):248–58.
158. Nishino I, Spinazzola A, Papadimitriou A, Hammans S, Steiner I, Hahn CD, et al. Mitochondrial neurogastrointestinal encephalomyopathy: an autosomal recessive disorder due to thymidine phosphorylase mutations. Ann Neurol. 2000;47(6):792–800.
159. Giordano C, Sebastiani M, De Giorgio R, Travaglini C, Tancredi A, Valentino ML, et al. Gastrointestinal dysmotility in mitochondrial neurogastrointestinal encephalomyopathy is caused by mitochondrial DNA depletion. Am J Pathol. 2008;173(4):1120–8.
160. Hirano M, Nishigaki Y, Marti R. Mitochondrial neurogastrointestinal encephalomyopathy (MNGIE): a disease of two genomes. Neurologist. 2004;10(1):8–17.
161. Garone C, Tadesse S, Hirano M. Clinical and genetic spectrum of mitochondrial neurogastrointestinal encephalomyopathy. Brain. 2011;134(Pt 11):3326–32.
162. Kalkan IH, Tayfur O, Oztas E, Beyazit Y, Yildiz H, Tunc B. A novel finding in MNGIE (mitochondrial neurogastrointestinal encephalomyopathy): hypergonadotropic hypogonadism. Hormones (Athens). 2012;11(3):377–9.
163. Marti R, Spinazzola A, Tadesse S, Nishino I, Nishigaki Y, Hirano M. Definitive diagnosis of mitochondrial neurogastrointestinal encephalomyopathy by biochemical assays. Clin Chem. 2004;50(1):120–4.
164. Vissing J, Ravn K, Danielsen ER, Duno M, Wibrand F, Wevers RA, et al. Multiple mtDNA deletions with features of MNGIE. Neurology. 2002;59(6):926–9.
165. Perez-Atayde AR, Fox V, Teitelbaum JE, Anthony DA, Fadic R, Kalsner L, et al. Mitochondrial neurogastrointestinal encephalomyopathy: diagnosis by rectal biopsy. Am J Surg Pathol. 1998;22(9):1141–7.
166. Teitelbaum JE, Berde CB, Nurko S, Buonomo C, Perez-Atayde AR, Fox VL. Diagnosis and management of MNGIE syndrome in children: case report

and review of the literature. J Pediatr Gastroenterol Nutr. 2002;35(3):377–83.
167. Saada A. Mitochondrial deoxyribonucleotide pools in deoxyguanosine kinase deficiency. Mol Genet Metab. 2008;95(3):169–73.
168. Bulst S, Abicht A, Holinski-Feder E, Muller-Ziermann S, Koehler U, Thirion C, et al. In vitro supplementation with dAMP/dGMP leads to partial restoration of mtDNA levels in mitochondrial depletion syndromes. Hum Mol Genet. 2009;18(9):1590–9.
169. Bulst S, Holinski-Feder E, Payne B, Abicht A, Krause S, Lochmuller H, et al. In vitro supplementation with deoxynucleoside monophosphates rescues mitochondrial DNA depletion. Mol Genet Metab. 2012;107(1–2):95–103.
170. Spinazzola A, Marti R, Nishino I, Andreu AL, Naini A, Tadesse S, et al. Altered thymidine metabolism due to defects of thymidine phosphorylase. J Biol Chem. 2002;277(6):4128–33.
171. Yavuz H, Ozel A, Christensen M, Christensen E, Schwartz M, Elmaci M, et al. Treatment of mitochondrial neurogastrointestinal encephalomyopathy with dialysis. Arch Neurol. 2007;64(3):435–8.
172. Hirano M, Marti R, Casali C, Tadesse S, Uldrick T, Fine B, et al. Allogeneic stem cell transplantation corrects biochemical derangements in MNGIE. Neurology. 2006;67(8):1458–60.
173. Halter J, Schupbach W, Casali C, Elhasid R, Fay K, Hammans S, et al. Allogeneic hematopoietic SCT as treatment option for patients with mitochondrial neurogastrointestinal encephalomyopathy (MNGIE): a consensus conference proposal for a standardized approach. Bone Marrow Transplant. 2011;46(3):330–7.
174. Sicurelli F, Carluccio MA, Toraldo F, Tozzi M, Bucalossi A, Lenoci M, et al. Clinical and biochemical improvement following HSCT in a patient with MNGIE: 1-year follow-up. J Neurol. 2012;259(9):1985–7.
175. Roeben B, Marquetand J, Bender B, Billing H, Haack TB, Sanchez-Albisua I, et al. Hemodialysis in MNGIE transiently reduces serum and urine levels of thymidine and deoxyuridine, but not CSF levels and neurological function. Orphanet J Rare Dis. 2017;12(1):135.
176. Di Giorgio A, Sonzogni A, Picciche A, Alessio G, Bonanomi E, Colledan M, et al. Successful management of acute liver failure in Italian children: a 16-year experience at a referral centre for paediatric liver transplantation. Dig Liver Dis. 2017;49(10):1139–45.
177. El-Hattab AW, Scaglia F. Mitochondrial DNA depletion syndromes: review and updates of genetic basis, manifestations, and therapeutic options. Neurotherapeutics. 2013;10(2):186–98.
178. El-Hattab AW, Craigen WJ, Scaglia F. Mitochondrial DNA maintenance defects. Biochim Biophys Acta. 2017;1863(6):1539–55.

Mitochondrial Neurogastrointestinal Encephalomyopathy Disease (MNGIE)

Shufang Li, Ramon Martí, and Michio Hirano

Introduction

Mitochondrial neurogastrointestinal encephalomyopathy (MNGIE) is a rare autosomal recessive disease caused by primary defects in nuclear gene *TYMP*, which encodes thymidine phosphorylase [1–4]. Deficiency of thymidine phosphorylase causes secondary defects of mitochondrial DNA (mtDNA) [1, 5, 6]. The first patient was described by Okamura and colleagues in 1976 as congenital oculoskeletal myopathy with abnormal muscle and liver mitochondria [7].

MNGIE is a clinically distinct disorder characterized by gastrointestinal (GI) dysmotility, cachexia, extraocular muscle weakness causing ptosis and ophthalmoplegia, predominantly demyelinating peripheral neuropathy, leukoencephalopathy, and mitochondrial abnormalities in skeletal muscle and other affected tissues [8]. The disease is relentlessly progressive, degenerative, and fatal with a poor prognosis [4, 9]. Onset typically ranges from early childhood to early adulthood with the majority (60%) exhibiting manifestations before the age of 20 years [3]. In classical cases, the average age at onset is 17.9 years (range 5 months to 35 years) [3], and the average age at death is 35 years old (range 15–54 years) [3, 4, 9, 10]. There is a small subgroup with late-onset (after age 40 years old) and slower progression [11]. At least 152 patients with MNGIE have been reported [9, 12–51].

Through translational studies of cellular and mouse models as well as analyses of patients, biopsies, and postmortem tissues, the pathomechanism of the disease has been characterized leading to molecularly targeted therapies [4, 52, 53].

Genetic Defects

TYMP Mutations Cause Severe Thymidine Phosphorylase Deficiency

MNGIE is an autosomal recessive inherited disorder which is caused by mutations in the nuclear gene *TYMP* which encodes thymidine phosphorylase (TP) (EC 2.4.2.4.) and is located on chromosome 22q13.33 [54]. TP is a cytoplasmic enzyme and its expression varies in different tissues (Table 1).

S. Li · M. Hirano (✉)
Department of Neurology, H. Houston Merritt Center, Columbia University Medical Center, New York, NY, USA
e-mail: mh29@columbia.edu

R. Martí
Vall d'Hebron Research Institute, Barcelona, Catalonia and CIBERER, Instituto de Salud Carlos III, Madrid, Spain

M. Mancuso, T. Klopstock (eds.), *Diagnosis and Management of Mitochondrial Disorders*, https://doi.org/10.1007/978-3-030-05517-2_13

MNGIE is caused by a variety of pathogenic compound heterozygous or homozygous mutations. While majority of the mutations are loss-of-function *TYMP* point mutations in exons or splice sites [55, 56], single-nucleotide insertions [2], deletions, and duplication mutations [57, 58] have also been observed [59].

Heterozygous mutation carriers of MNGIE are asymptomatic with approximately 35% (222/634) residual TP activity, although the plasma nucleoside levels (Thd and dUrd) are similar to healthy controls (<0.05 μmol/L) (see Tables 2 and 3) [59, 60].

Table 1 TP expression in different tissues

Tissue with high TP expression	Gastrointestinal tract Central and peripheral nervous system Spleen Liver Bladder Leukocytes and in platelets (which accounts for most of the TP activity in human blood and buffy coats) [59, 107, 108]
Tissue with low TP expression	Muscles [8, 109]
Tissue lacking TP expression	Kidney, aorta, and fat tissues [8, 109]

Pathogenesis

TP Deficiency Causes Accumulations of Thd and dUrd in Plasma and Tissues

TP catabolizes pyrimidine nucleosides thymidine (Thd) and deoxyuridine (dUrd) to the bases thymine and uridine [59, 61] plus 2-deoxy 1-phosphate ribose. To assess the effects of TP dysfunction, thymidine and deoxyuridine level in plasma and autopsy tissues have been measured using high-performance liquid chromatography (HPLC) with ultraviolet spectrophotometric or tandem mass spectrometry detection [4, 62]. In contrast to normal controls who have no detectable thymidine or deoxyuridine in plasma (<0.05 μM, n = 20), patients have shown markedly elevated plasma thymidine (Thd) levels (8.6 ± 3.4 μM, mean ± standard deviation), and deoxyuridine (dUrd) (14.2 ± 4.4 μM) [4, 52, 53, 60]. Late-onset MNGIE patients manifest less dramatic elevations of plasma Thd (1.03 ± 0.45) and dUrd (2.9 ± 1.9) and detectable TP activity [11].

Table 2 TP activity in buffy coats in patients and controls [110] and plasma Thd and dUrd in patients and controls [1, 110]

		TP (nmol thymine/h/(mg protein))			Mean (range) (μmol/L)	
Group	*n*	Mean (SD)	Range	*n*	Thd	dUrd
Healthy controls	20	634 (217)	253–1000	20	<0.05	<0.05
TP mutation carriers	14	222 (89)	90–360	14	<0.05	<0.05
MNGIE patients	24	10 (15)	0–46	25	8.6 (3.9–17.7)	14.2 (5.5–24.4)
Late-onset MNGIE	6	103.8 (26.9)	58–132	6	1.4 (0.4–2.1)	1.5 (ND-4.7)

Table 3 Genotype, TP activity, and plasma Thd and dUrd level in six late-onset MNGIE patients

	Genotype		TP (buffy coats) (nmol thymine/h/(mg protein))	Thd (μmol/L)	dUrd (μmol/L)
Patient	Allele 1	Allele 2			
Patient 1 [11]	c.633G>A (p.V208M)	c.931G>C (p.G311R)	105	0.4	1.0
Patient 2 [11]	c.633G>A (p.V208M)	c.605G>C (p.R202T)	89	1.3	ND
Patient 3 [11]	c.457G>A (p.G153S)	c.854T>C (p.L285P)	58	1.4	4.7
Patient 4 [38]	c.1160-1G>A	c.1135G>A (p.E379K)	132	2.1	ND
Patient 5	c.633G>A (p.V208M)	c.607_608insC	116	1.7	1.4
Patient 6	c.633G>A (p.V208M)	c.607_608insC	123	1.7	2.1

Mutations were reported as G2398A (V208M) and G3535C (G311R) in patient 1 and as G2398A (V208M) and G2381C (R202T) in patient 2 [11]

Asymptomatic heterozygous *TYMP* mutation carriers with reduced TP activity (about 35–50% residual activity) have had no detectable thymidine in plasma (n = 14); these findings indicate that 35% residual TP activity is sufficient to eliminate circulating thymidine [4] and deoxyuridine.

In a postmortem study of MNGIE patients (ages at death 29–39 years old; n = 5), tissue levels of Thd and dUrd levels were markedly elevated [8] (Table 4).

Table 4 Increased levels of Thd and dUrd in postmortem tissue of MNGIE patients

	MNGIE patients (ages at death 29–39 years old) (n = 5)	Control tissues
Thd	Range: 1.9–80 pmol/mg-tissue	No detectable nucleosides [8]
dUrd	Range: 3–48 pmol/mg-tissue	No detectable nucleosides [8]
Affected tissues with highest concentrations of Thd and dUrd	Peripheral nerve Small intestine Occipital white matter Liver Kidney Heart	

TP Deficiency Causes Accumulation of Somatic mtDNA Depletion, Multiple Deletions, and Point Mutations in Patients' Tissues and Cells

Multiple deletions, depletion, and site-specific somatic mtDNA point mutations in cultured fibroblasts, blood, and tissues of MNGIE patients [1, 6, 63] are observed. Because mitochondria rely upon the salvage pathway for synthesis of deoxynucleoside triphosphate (dNTP) building blocks for mtDNA replication in postmitotic cells [64–66] and mtDNA lacks an effective mismatch repair system [67, 68], the mitochondrial genome is vulnerable to the toxic effects of excessive Thd [4].

Studies of mouse and cellular models indicate that the elevated levels of Thd and dUrd cause deoxynucleoside triphosphate pool imbalances and mtDNA instability (Fig. 1). In vitro studies also revealed unbalanced mitochondrial dNTP pools and mtDNA depletion or multiple deletions in human fibroblasts and Hela cells exposed to high concentration of Thd in the culture medium (see Table 6) [64, 69–71]. Thymidine phosphorylase/uridine phosphorylase ($Tpp^{-/-}Upp^{-/-}$) double knockout mice show elevated plasma and

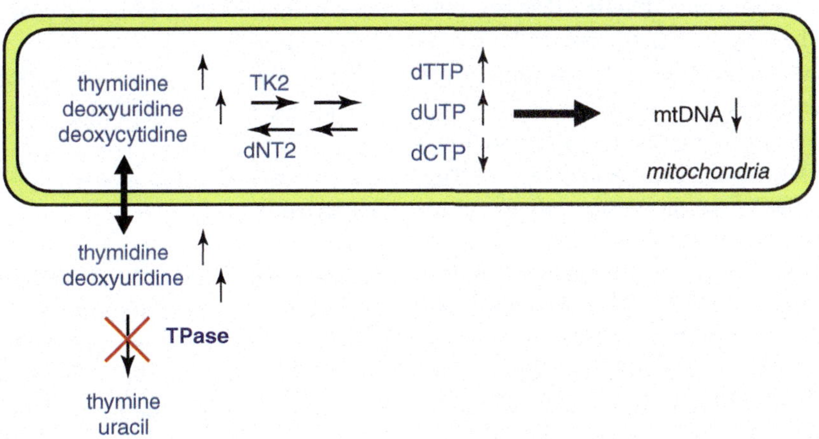

Fig. 1 Molecular pathomechanism of MNGIE. Loss of thymidine phosphorylase (TPase) activity causes toxic accumulations of thymidine and deoxyuridine nucleosides in plasma and tissues and dNTP pool imbalances, which, in turn, impair mtDNA replication [4]

tissue levels of Thd and dUrd, increased deoxythymidine triphosphate (dTTP), and decreased deoxycytidine triphosphate (dCTP) levels in the brain and liver with mild mtDNA depletion and partial deficiency of complex I activity [72]. Further elevations of Thd and dUrd via oral supplementation in $Tpp^{-/-}Upp^{-/-}$ mice produced severe mtDNA depletion, respiratory chain defects, and histopathological defects in the brain and small intestine as well as reduced life span [73]; these findings indicate the pathogenic role of elevated pyrimidine deoxynucleosides in primary TP deficiency.

Clinical Characteristics

Clinical Manifestations

MNGIE is clinically characterized by progressive gastrointestinal dysmotility, cachexia, ptosis, progressive external ophthalmoplegia, leukoencephalopathy, and demyelinating peripheral neuropathy (Table 5). Early development is typically normal. Although the earliest reported age at onset is 5 months, onset is usually between the first and fifth decades. In about 60% of individuals, symptoms begin before the age of 20 years (mean age at onset: 18 years) [3, 9]. The order in which clinical manifestations appear is unpredictable [9]. Prior to the onset of symptoms, many individuals with MNGIE disease may appear to be healthy but usually have a long prodrome of subtle fatigability, mild gastrointestinal symptoms, or thin body habitus.

Due to its variable clinical presentations, MNGIE can be easily overlooked or misdiagnosed with anorexia nervosa, inflammatory bowel disease, or celiac disease [3] due to the prominent gastrointestinal manifestations; myasthenia gravis due to the extraocular and limb muscle weakness [74–76]; or chronic inflammatory demyelinating polyneuropathy (CIPD) or Charcot-Marie-Tooth disease due to the peripheral neuropathy [77, 78]. Family history is consistent with autosomal recessive inheritance with parental consanguinity in many cases.

Clinical Laboratory Findings

Routine clinical blood tests often reveal elevated lactic acid and creatine kinase (CK). Patients may manifest hypertriglyceridemia, particularly on total parenteral nutrition. Serum transaminases may be elevated due to myopathy, hepatopathy, or both.

Brain MRI typically reveals diffuse leukoencephalopathy on T2 and FLAIR image [79]; however, the white matter lesions may be patchy early in the disease course.

Nerve conduction studies and electromyography typically show signs of peripheral neuropathy and myopathy. Although the neuropathy is predominantly demyelinating with slow conduction velocities, axonal involvement is common. Occasionally, the nerve conductions show partial conduction block mimicking CIDP [77].

Muscle biopsies show mitochondrial abnormalities (ragged-red fibers, cytochrome *c* oxidase deficient fibers, or both) in the majority (32/38); however, a few reported patients have lacked these histological hallmarks of mitochondrial myopathy [3, 56] (Table 6). Defects of mitochondrial respiratory chain enzyme activities have been detected in the majority of patients' muscle biopsies including isolated complex IV deficiency and variable combined deficiencies of complexes I and IV or I, III, and IV. Depletion, multiple deletions, and low levels of site-specific point mutations of mtDNA are generally detected in the muscle.

Other frequently observed findings in MNGIE patients are included in Table 7.

Diagnosis

As previously noted, the MNGIE phenotype is defined by the six clinical hallmark manifestations: (1) extraocular muscle weakness, (2) gastrointestinal dysmotility, (3) cachexia, (4) sensorimotor peripheral neuropathy, (5) leukoencephalopathy, and (6) evidence of mitochondrial dysfunction (e.g., lactic acidosis, elevated lactate in the brain, or muscle mitochondrial abnormalities described above). Early in the disease course,

Table 5 Clinical manifestations in MNGIE patients*

Complication/ frequency	Percent as initial manifestation [3]	Manifestations	Pathophysiology	Remarks
Progressive gastrointestinal dysmotility*/(100%) [59, 111–114]	~57%	Gastric and small bowel hypomotility* are invariably present [2, 9, 29] • Poor appetite; early satiety; borborygmi, nausea; dysphagia; gastroesophageal reflux; postprandial emesis; abdominal pain, cramps, and/or distention; chronic diarrhea; constipation; chronic intestinal pseudo-obstruction (CIPO)	• Myogenic (visceral smooth muscle) (enteric myopathy): Mitochondrial DNA depletion, mitochondrial proliferation, and smooth cell atrophy are observed in the external layer of the muscularis propria in the stomach and in the small intestine [9, 111, 115] • Neurogenic (enteric nervous system): Loss of the pacemaker cells that stimulate gut contraction (interstitial cells of Cajal) is also noted in the small bowel [9, 59, 114]. Histologic findings: – Rectal biopsy: eosinophilic cytoplasmic inclusions, representing abnormal mitochondria, in the submucosal ganglion cells [9, 112] – Duodenal pathology: focal muscle atrophy or absence with increased nerve numbers, serosal granulomas, and focal loss of Auerbach's plexus with fibrosis [9, 116]	• Symptoms usually progress slowly over several decades and can affect any part of the GI tract [9] • CIPO in the early disease course is under recognized [9] • A major cause of death and survival is generally related to the severity of these symptoms • Can lead to severe denutrition, anemia, and eventually the necessity for nutritional supportive treatments [111–114] • Despite severe GI dysfunction, serum concentrations of micronutrients, folate, B12, and vitamin E are typically normal [9]
Weight loss, cachexia*				• Weight loss and cachexia coincide with the onset of GI symptoms • The average weight loss is about 15 kg [9, 10] • Affected individuals invariably have a thin body habitus and reduced muscle mass
Ocular* (common) [9, 45, 111, 112]	~19%	• Ptosis*, ophthalmoplegia* or ophthalmoparesis* [9]; • Retinal pigmentary changes, glaucoma, optic nerve atrophy [9, 45, 111, 112]		• The abnormalities are usually first noted by a health-care provider since the individuals with MNGIE disease are often unaware of the eye movement defect because of the absence of symptoms like diplopia [9] • CPEO phenotype is often present [59]

(continued)

Table 5 (continued)

Complication/ frequency	Percent as initial manifestation [3]	Manifestations	Pathophysiology	Remarks
PNS*/(100%) [9, 77, 113–115]	~14%	• Paresthesias – Stocking-glove distribution – Described as tingling, numbness, or even pain • Weakness – Symmetric and distal – Lower extremities are more prominently – Foot drop, as well as clawed hands may occur – Unilateral or bilateral	• Sensorimotor peripheral neuropathy*: The neuropathy is demyelinating in all cases and about half also have axonal neuropathy – The segmental demyelination is hypothesized to be caused by the uneven distribution of mtDNA abnormalities (*depletion, single-nucleotide variants,* deletions, duplications) along the nerve. Areas with the highest concentration of these pathogenic variants may be predisposed to demyelination [9]. Reduced sensory motor conduction, loss of myelin sheaths in lumbar and brachial plexus [9, 59, 77, 113–115] – Since Schwann cell provide nutrients and structural support for peripheral neurons, with the progression of the demyelination, the axonal neuropathy is also observed in the clinic	• All individuals with MNGIE disease have peripheral neuropathy • Some MNGIE cases are misdiagnosed with chronic inflammatory demyelinating polyneuropathy [9] • The severity of the neuropathic symptoms often fluctuates during the early stages of the disease • Electrodiagnostic features – Decreased motor and sensory nerve conduction velocities – Prolonged F-wave latency – Partial conduction block – Myopathic changes are common [9, 59]
CNS [42, 51, 79, 116–120]		• Leukoencephalopathy*(usually asymptomatic) • Spasticity is not present • Intellectual disability is rare • Dementia can be a rare late feature of the disease [9, 42]	• Asymptomatic leukoencephalopathy* – Diffusely abnormal brain white matter (increased FLAIR or T2-weighted signal) on brain MRI – Relative sparing of the corpus callosum is reported in some individuals [9, 121] – Although magnetic resonance spectroscopy (MRS) can show increases in lactate within the white matter, it is not a sensitive diagnostic test [9] • Pattern on brain MRI indicative of vasogenic cerebral edema and glial cell dysfunction	• In the absence of leukoencephalopathy, MNGIE disease is very unlikely [9] • The correlation is debatable between: – The extent of these brain MRI signal alterations – Age, clinical severity, CNS involvement, or the biochemical and genetic profiles of MNGIE patients

Skeletal muscle [5, 9, 36, 56, 90]	~5%	Proximal myopathy	• mtDNA molecular alterations and abnormal respiratory chain enzymes in skeletal muscles	• Two cases with classical clinical presentation of MNGIE were reported without skeletal muscle involvement. Both cases showed identical homozygous splice-acceptor site mutation in TYMP gene (c.215-1G>C), which may suggest a genotype-phenotype correlation
Auditory (61%) [9, 59, 122, 123]		Hearing loss*	• Dysfunction of cranial nerve and auditory cortex atrophy of the stria vascularis in the cochlea Early-onset sensorineural hearing loss involving either the cochlea or eighth cranial nerve	• Hearing loss is common among patients (in 61% of patients) • Satisfactory results were obtained soon following cochlear implantation in MNGIE patients [59]
Others [9, 18, 124]		• Endocarditis • Cardiomyopathy • Psoriasis • Anemia • Endocrine – Short status – Diabetes mellitus – Hypergonadotropic Hypogonadism [27] – Hypogonadotropic Hypogonadism [9, 42] – Hypothyroidism • Hepatic manifestation – Active hepatic cirrhosis with increased liver enzymes and macrovesicular steatosis • Spontaneous abdominal esophageal perforation • Diverticula, – May become infected (diverticulitis) or perforate, causing peritonitis, which may be fatal		Rare complications • Short stature as seen in many mitochondrial diseases and partly as a complication of failure to thrive [59]

CIPO chronic intestinal obstruction, *CPEO* chronic progressive external ophthalmoplegia, *CNS* central nervous system, *PNPs* polyneuropathies, *: major clinical feature of the disease.

Table 6 Clinical laboratory findings in MNGIE patients from the literature

Blood		Normochromic normocytic anemia [41]; chronic iron deficiency anemia [94] and hypocholesterolemia were detected [42, 44]; inflammatory anemia [39], elevated blood leukocyte level
	Electrolyte	Hypokalemia, hypocalcemia, hypomagnesemia, hypoalbuminemia [44, 46]
	Nutrition	Reduction of vitamin B6 and vitamin E [44], copper [44], zinc [44, 51]
	Metabolism	Elevated lactate/pyruvate ratio [30, 36], elevated pyruvic acid [34, 36, 44], mild hyperlactaciduria accompanied by increased urinary excretion of the Krebs cycle intermediates, like fumarate, aconitate, and 3-methylglutaconic aciduria [46] Mild generalized hyperaminoaciduria; the excretion of ethylmalonic acid (EMA) and creatine was slightly elevated [37] Elevated LDH [44, 49], hypertriglyceridemia [34], elevated GGT [34]
	Positive serology [13]	Anti-tissue transglutaminase and anti-endomysial antibodies and compatible histology [13] (Marsh 3)
GI	Abdominal ultrasound	Last ileal loop wall thickness [14], hepatomegaly and hepatosteatosis [34], steatosis hepatis [51]
	Abdominal X-ray	Dilated stomach, small bowel loops [30], and a hypotonic bowel with reduced motility up until the last ileal loop [14] and jejunal diverticulosis [46]
	Barium study	Dilated stomach and duodenum and diffuse thickening of the small intestinal wall [30]. Dilatation of the duodenal cap and segment up to the level of papilla [21, 50]. Excess of gastric fluid and gastroptosis [43]
	CT scan	Mild thickening of the terminal ileum [44]; stomach and small bowel dilation and thickening [39], along with few mildly enlarged iliac and mesenteric lymph nodes [30]; gross hepatosplenomegaly with marked hepatic steatosis and nodularity [41]
	The upper endoscopy	Features of reflux esophagitis [44] and pangastritis [18]. Fluid residue in the stomach, enlarged duodenal bulb, grossly dilated and tortuous second segment of the duodenum with effaced folds and residue [21]. Diffuse thickening of the small intestinal wall following diluted barium ingestion. The mucosal folds could not be observed clearly [33]
	Esophagogastroduodenoscopy and histology	Duodenal lymphocytic infiltrate and "focal" villous atrophy [13, 49]
	Esophageal manometry	Decreased lower esophageal sphincter pressure, low amplitude esophageal contractions [21]
	The gastric emptying scintigraphy	Gastroduodenal transit was severely reduced [14, 31]
	The colonoscopy	Narrowed ileocaecal valve [44]
	Biopsy	Showed non-specific chronic inflammation in the small intestine and a positive *Helicobacter pylori* chronic gastritis [42]
	Histology	Foamy cells in the intestinal wall [51]
Brain	EEG	Bilateral intermittent delta activity; isolated spikes and/or sharp waves localized in right temporal region and less evident in left temporal region [38]
	CT scan	Diffuse white matter hypodensity [39] involving frontal, parietal, and occipital cortex without any focal lesion [30]
	Spectroscopic study	Modest reduction in peak of N-acetylaspartate [14]
Vision	Visual evoked potential studies	Prolonged P100 latency [38]
	Neuro-ophthalmologic	Revealed retinitis pigmentosa [39], mild chorioretinal atrophy [34]
Heart	Echocardiogram	Mitral valve prolapse [21, 51] and in some cases indicated left ventricular noncompaction, left ventricular false tendons [31], sinus rhythm, and incomplete right bundle branch block [51]

Table 6 (continued)

Hearing	Audio	Unilateral or bilateral sensorineural hearing impairment was evident on pure tone audiometry [49]. Audiometry showed bilateral neurosensory deafness [36]; subclinical, bilateral, sensorineural hearing loss [38]
Endocrine	Hypogonadism	Increased FSH level and decreased total testosterone [18] have been observed. Hypogonadotropic hypogonadism: elevated follicle stimulation hormone and elevated luteinizing hormone elevated, while testosterone serum concentrations were decreased [42]. A spermogram showed oligospermia [42]
Other	Electron microscopy	Enlarged mitochondria with vacuolation and blurring of cristae [30]. Observation confirmed lipid storage, a mild increase in glycogen-like granules and unremarkable mitochondria [36]
	Biopsy	Enzyme histochemistry glycogen accumulation [42]
	Autopsy	Megamitochondria were observed by light microscopy in submucosal and myenteric ganglion cells and in smooth muscle cells of muscularis mucosae and muscularis propria, along the entire gastrointestinal tract from the esophagus to the rectum [25]

Table 7 Specialized laboratory findings in MNGIE patients

Urinary Thd and dUrd accumulation [80, 125, 126]	These compounds are not detectable in controls or in individuals who are heterozygous for a TYMP pathogenic variant [6, 110, 125, 126]	
Lactic acidemia and hyperalaninemia	Common	
Lactic acidosis	Unusual but is more likely to occur in the presence of renal or hepatic impairment	
Elevated protein levels in CSF	Typically 60–100 mg/dL (normal range 15–45 mg/dL) [77]	
Deficiency of mitochondrial respiratory chain enzymes	Mainly complex I and IV [9, 127]	
mtDNA analysis	May reveal acquired deletions, depletions, or point mutations [6, 75]	
Mitochondrial dysfunction	Histologic abnormalities of a mitochondrial myopathy	Ragged-red fibers (Gomori trichrome)
		Defects in single or multiple OXPHOS enzyme complexes The most common is in cytochrome c oxidase (complex IV)
		Note: Normal muscle histopathology can be observed [56]
	Acquired mitochondrial DNA (mtDNA) deletions/duplications detected in any tissue	By Southern blot analysis and long-range PCR
	Mitochondrial DNA depletion	Detected by quantitation of mtDNA relative to nuclear DNA
	Site-specific mtDNA single-nucleotide variants	Detected in the blood and tissues [8]

Lactic acidemia: increased serum concentration of lactate without a change in the pH [9]
Lactic acidosis: increased serum lactate concentration associated with a decrease in blood pH [9]

some of the clinical features may be absent rendering the diagnosis challenging.

The gold standard for diagnosis is the identification of biallelic pathogenic *TYMP* variants, which are often detected in *TYMP* gene sequencing, mitochondrial disease gene panels or whole exome sequencing. More than 60 *TYMP* mutations have been identified, and occasional new variants of uncertain significance (VUS) have been detected. To assess potential pathogenicity of such *TYMP* VUSs, functional testing of TP activity in buffy coat or measurement of serum or plasma levels of Thd and dUrd can be very useful. In classical MNGIE patients, TP activity in buffy coat of is less than 8% of the control mean (634 nmol thymine formed/h/mg protein) with marked elevation of plasma levels of Thd (>3 μM, normal <0.05) and dUrd (>5 μM, normal <0.05) [59]. In late-onset MNGIE, buffy coat TP activity is less severely diminished (<18% of the control mean) and increased of plasma levels of Thd and dUrd compared to the typical patients [2, 60].

The unambiguous severe reduction of TP activity and consequent blood accumulation of Thd and dUrd in all MNGIE patients provides a very robust method for the biochemical screening for patients with clinical features suggestive of MNGIE. Analyzing TP activity in buffy coat and plasma Thd and dUrd concentrations is the easiest way to confirm the diagnosis. The screening of urine to detect Thd and dUrd may be also useful, but precautions should be taken to prevent bacterial growth in the sample; otherwise, in vitro catabolism of Thd and dUrd via bacterial TP can lead to underestimation of urinary excretion. For both plasma and urine samples, Thd and dUrd concentrations can be easily assessed by HPLC-UV, or HPLC-MS/MS. There is complete concordance between nucleoside accumulation and reduced TP activity in buffy coat. Only in cases where TP dysfunction is first observed and confirms the diagnosis of MNGIE, *TYMP* may to be sequenced to identify the pathogenic mutations [60].

Genotype-Phenotype Correlations

While numerous *TYMP* mutations have been linked to the typical MNGIE phenotype, the c.622G>A (p.Val208Met) variant has been identified in two of four published late-onset cases with milder TP deficiency described above [11, 38]. We have identified this variant in two additional unpublished late-onset MNGIE patients (Hirano, personal communication).

Treatment

Current Treatments for MNGIE

Dialysis to Eliminate Deoxynucleosides

Our preliminary MNGIE study indicated that therapies like dialysis to eliminate the toxic nucleosides thymidine and deoxyuridine from the blood of patients could be effective treatments for the disease [52, 53, 80]. Unfortunately, hemodialysis was ineffective as a long-term treatment in one patient [80]. Peritoneal dialysis has been used in two patients; one showed improvement in gastrointestinal symptoms (vomiting, anorexia, abdominal pain, and diarrhea) with weight gain [43], and the other reported decreased hand numbness [22]. However, the first patient did not show neurological improvements despite continuing peritoneal dialysis for 3 years [43], and the second patient had recurrence of elevated nucleoside levels after 15 months of continuous ambulatory peritoneal dialysis [22].

AHSCT for MNGIE

AHSCT has been successfully applied to other rare metabolic diseases caused by enzyme deficiencies [81, 82]. AHSCT appears to be effective in purine nucleoside phosphorylase (PNP) deficiency which biochemically parallels MNGIE caused by loss-of-function mutations in the *PNP* gene and lead to purine nucleoside accumulations [4]. The disease presents with immunological and neurological dysfunction, and AHSCT can restore the immune system and may stabilize neurological functions [77, 83] and also have positive result in patients with Hurler syndrome and lysosomal storage diseases.

Prior to performing AHSCT in MNGIE patients, we administered platelets (which contain abundant TP) to two patients [84]. In both individuals, plasma thymidine levels were reduced for 24–48 h. The transient effects of platelet infusions suggest that permanent TP replacement therapy through AHSCT could be an effective treatment for MNGIE.

Of the first 24 patients who underwent AHSCT, nine were alive (median 3.9 years) after successful transplants [85]. All show normalization of blood TPase activity and reductions of plasma thymidine and deoxyuridine to barely detectable levels; clinical improvements observed in all seven patients who were alive more than 2 years posttransplant. However, the severely compromised medical condition of MNGIE patients led to an unacceptably high mortality;

nine died of transplant-related complications (including two after a second transplant due to graft failure) and six died of disease progression. Survival was associated with two defined pre-transplant characteristics: human leukocyte antigen (HLA) match (10/10 versus <10/10) and disease characteristics (liver disease, history of gastrointestinal pseudo-obstruction, or both). Thus, AHSCT should only be considered for MNGIE patients at an early disease stage (e.g., before hepatopathy and intestinal pseudo-obstruction) and only if an HLA 10/10 (preferably related) donor is available. A standardize AHSCT protocol has been recommended [85, 86].

Orthotopic Liver Transplantation

Liver transplantation has been proposed as an alternative therapeutic strategy for treatment of MNGIE patients [87]. Because orthotopic liver transplantation (OLT) does not require a pre-transplant conditioning regimen, it may be less risky and better tolerated by MNGIE patients than AHSCT. Recently, OLT was successfully applied in a severely affected, 25-year-old MNGIE patient [16]. Marked reductions of plasma deoxynucleosides, slightly increased mtDNA level in muscle, reduced brain lactate, and slight improvements in leg strength and quality of life were observed for 13 months post-OLT. However, this approach requires matched organ donors, which are limited, and imposes significant risks of transplantation-related complications and long-term immunosuppression. Further data are needed regarding risks and long-term outcomes of OLT in MNGIE before this therapy can be recommended.

Enzyme Replacement Therapy

Enzyme replacement therapy (ERT) is a reliable, well-tolerated approach to replace the deficient enzyme in a variety of lysosomal storage disorders including Gaucher, Pompe, Fabry, and Sly diseases [88]. For MNGIE, approaches were developed to encapsulate TP in order to prolong the half-life of circulatory TP enzyme and reduce immunogenic reactions. These include polymeric nanoparticles [89] and erythrocytes as nucleoside permeable vehicles to deliver TP, which can reduce Thd and dUrd [41, 90]. The therapeutic value of erythrocyte-encapsulated TP (EE-TP) has been documented in one patient who showed partial (~60%) reductions of circulating Thd and dUrd and clinical improvements in ability to walk and climb, recovery of sensation, and mitigation of numbness in the hands and feet after 23 months of multiple cycles of approximately monthly EE-TP infusions [90]. This therapeutic approach is limited as it requires frequent EE-TP infusions that must be administered a specialized center and may not sufficiently reduce deoxynucleoside levels. Although not a permanent therapy for MNGIE, EE-TP may be a bridge to more effective and lasting treatments.

Preclinical Experimental Approaches Toward Therapy

Inhibition of Renal Nucleoside Reabsorption

After *TYMP* mutations were identified as the cause of MNGIE [2], the first biochemical studies on TP deficiency in MNGIE patients showed that plasma Thd is freely ultrafiltratable, but its renal clearance is low compared with the clearance of creatinine, indicating that most of the filtered nucleoside is reabsorbed [53]. This provides a potential pharmacological strategy to reduce nucleoside accumulation by blocking renal dThd and dUrd reabsorption, thereby increasing their urinary elimination. The kinetics and pharmacological properties of nucleoside transporters have been studied, and several drugs can inhibit the function of these carriers [91, 92]. The main challenge for this approach is to find drugs that selectively inhibit deoxypyrimidine reabsorption, without disturbing the renal transport of other compounds. Animal models would be a useful tool to study this approach with different candidate drugs.

Increase of Deoxycytidine Availability

Evidence that dCTP depletion is responsible for Thd-induced mtDNA depletion in MNGIE has been observed in cellular and animal models [72, 93]. Therefore, increasing dCTP availability is expected to prevent mtDNA depletion, as suggested by the fact that deoxycytidine supplementation prevents mtDNA depletion induced by Thd in cultured fibroblasts [93]. Depletion of mtDNA is probably the main factor contributing to mitochondrial dysfunction and the clinical phenotype in MNGIE. We proposed that administration of deoxycytidine and/or an inhibitor of its catabolism could be a potential pharmacological treatment for MNGIE. However, the metabolic interconnections between cytosolic and mitochondrial pathways involved in nucleotide metabolism need to be carefully considered when choosing the best way to provide this precursor. Deoxycytidine supply alone would have a rather undesired biochemical effect, i.e., the additional increase of dUrd, its first catabolic product via cytidine deaminase [94]. Thus, the combination with cytidine deaminase inhibitors would be advisable, but care must be taken to ensure that such inhibitors do not have additional undesired effects, as they would interfere with normal physiological cytidine and deoxycytidine deamination. In any case, deoxycytidine supply and/or inhibition of its catabolism would only prevent dCTP depletion, but would not reduce Thd and dUrd overload. Therefore, this strategy has been proposed as a maintenance treatment before a more enduring alternative can be applied to patients.

TP Polymeric Nanoreactors

An alternate strategy to provide enzyme replacement was based on the use of polymeric nanoreactors. This strategy has only been tested in preclinical settings and is based on the infusion of TP-loaded nanoparticles incorporating a nucleoside transporter which allows the transport of the substrates Thd and dUrd and products of the reaction to be exchanged across the capsule wall. In vitro experiments demonstrated that the nanoreactors were enzymatically active and stable in blood serum at 37 °C, and did not produce cytotoxicity when incubated with hepatocytes nor induce an inflammatory response when tested ex vivo or after intraperitoneal administration in mice [89, 95]. Further investigations are needed to confirm the feasibility of this approach, which would work by means of periodic infusions of the nanoreactor preparations, according to the half-life in patient's blood.

Gene Therapy

The use of gene therapy for MNGIE was proposed and investigated some years ago because this disease a particularly good candidate for this advanced therapy. MNGIE is a monogenic disorder, and there is no need for a specific target organ because TP deficiency can be corrected in any tissue as long as the treatment provides sufficient TP activity to effectively clear the nucleosides and to prevent their systemic accumulation. These are small water-soluble molecules that readily diffuse across plasma membranes through dedicated transporters; therefore the enzyme does not need to be secreted. Based on this, and considering that currently available treatments present significant risks to the patients, gene therapy may be a good alternative to them.

Two different preclinical gene therapy approaches for MNGIE have been investigated. The first, a lentiviral vector (LV) targeted to hematopoietic progenitors, aims at restoring TP activity in blood cells. The second, an adeno-associated vector (AAV) transcriptionally targeted to the liver. Both strategies have been investigated in preclinical settings using both cultured cells from MNGIE patients and the murine model of the disease, the *Tymp*/*Upp1* double knockout (dKO) mouse, which recapitulates the biochemical imbalances of the disease [96].

LV-Mediated Hematopoietic Stem Cell Gene Therapy (HSCGT)

The proof of concept that gene therapy is able to correct the biochemical imbalances of MNGIE was obtained using a LV targeted to hematopoietic stem cells. This approach was used in cultured TP-deficient B-lymphoblastoid cells obtained from MNGIE patients and in sublethally myeloablated mice and demonstrated that the transduction of the human *TYMP* gene can restore TP function and dThd and dUrd homeostasis both in vitro and in vivo [97]. The follow-up study of the treated mice has confirmed that the effects of the treatment are maintained in the long-term [98]. The use of LV-carrying *TYMP* under different promoters has been further studied [99], and the results confirm and expand the first results, supporting the notion that gene therapy is a feasible strategy for MNGIE.

Although LV-mediated HSCGT could overcome some of the limitations and risks associated with AHSCT or liver transplantation, it generates new potential risks that cannot be ignored. This strategy requires reinfusion of autologous hematopoietic progenitors after ex vivo transduction with the LV, which requires myelosuppression, which would pose some risks for patients. In fact, this procedure is associated with some reductions in survival curves of treated mice, which have been observed in both studies [98, 99], especially when mice were followed for more than 18 months after treatment [98].

AAV-Mediated Liver-Directed Gene Therapy

The use of AAV may reduce the risks associated with the ex vivo-based LV-mediated HSCGT. AAV vectors predominantly remain as episomes in the host cells; a very small percentage can integrate into the host genome, but there is no evidence that AAV vectors can be oncogenic in humans, at least under the conditions normally used in gene therapy clinical trials [100, 101]. AAV-mediated liver-directed gene therapy vectors have demonstrated efficacy for patients with factor IX deficiency hemophilia [102, 103]. In these studies the serotype 8 (AAV8), which has a high tropism for the liver, was used. The preclinical testing of this strategy in the murine model of MNGIE, using AAV8 in combination with the liver-specific thyroxine-binding globulin protein (TBG) promoter, improved the previous results obtained in the hematopoietic approach. The rationale of the AAV-mediated liver-directed gene therapy was to provide to the liver enough TP activity to act as effective clearing organ for Thd and dUrd nucleosides. A single intravenous injection of the vector resulted in permanent therapeutic TP expression in the liver of the KO mice and normalized nucleoside and mitochondrial nucleotide homeostasis in this animal model. Doses between 10^{12} and 10^{13} vector genomes/kg resulted in reductions to normal or slightly below normal nucleoside levels in virtually all mice treated [104]. Despite the non-integrative nature of AAV, the effect was sustained (with a negligible decrease in TP activity) and fully effective on nucleoside homeostasis for at least 21 months at a dose of 2×10^{12} vg/kg [105]. These results further support the feasibility of gene therapy for MNGIE and open the possibility to initiate formal clinical studies to demonstrate the efficacy of this strategy in a clinical setting.

AAV-Mediated GT or HSCGT

Both LV-mediated HSCGT and AAV-mediated liver-directed gene therapy have demonstrated to be similarly effective in preclinical settings. The non-integrative nature of AAV vectors makes them safer than LV but limits their use to nondividing tissues. In dividing cells, the copy number of the transgene present in non-integrated episomes is gradually diluted, and the therapeutic effect would be reduced in non-quiescent tissues over time. By contrast, LV replicates as the cells divide because they are integrated in the genome, but episomal AAVs do not replicate; the copy number dilutes as cells divide. However, as indicated above, risks derived from partial myelosuppression and ex vivo transduction are significant, and this procedure has been associated with a reduction in the animals' life span in preclinical studies [98, 99]. On the other hand, although AAV8 therapy is in principle a safer approach, it should be noted that a significant percentage of patients would not be eligible because of the presence of neutralizing anti-capsid antibodies in their sera due to a previous contact with the virus; for anti-AAV8 antibodies, the prevalence is 38% [106]. In addition, liver dysfunction is another exclusion criterion for this strategy. The above-mentioned potential dilution of the effect over the life of the patients could be also an AAV-related issue.

It could be therefore proposed that the first and safer gene therapy option would be a liver-directed therapy using AAV, but efforts should be made to increase the safety of LV-HSCT in order to provide an alternative for patients who are not eligible for the liver-directed AAV.

References

1. Hirano M, et al. Mitochondrial neurogastrointestinal encephalomyopathy (MNGIE): clinical, biochemical, and genetic features of an autosomal recessive mitochondrial disorder. Neurology. 1994;44:721–7.
2. Nishino I, Spinazzola A, Hirano M. Thymidine phosphorylase gene mutations in MNGIE, a human mitochondrial disorder. Science. 1999;283:689–92. https://doi.org/10.1126/science.283.5402.689.
3. Garone C, Tadesse S, Hirano M. Clinical and genetic spectrum of mitochondrial neurogastrointestinal encephalomyopathy. Brain. 2011;134:3326–32. https://doi.org/10.1093/brain/awr245.
4. Hirano M, Garone C, Quinzii CM. CoQ10 deficiencies and MNGIE: two treatable mitochondrial disorders. Biochim Biophys Acta Gen Subj. 2012;1820:625–31. https://doi.org/10.1016/j.bbagen.2012.01.006.
5. Papadimitriou A, et al. Partial depletion and multiple deletions of muscle mtDNA in familial MNGIE syndrome. Neurology. 1998;51:1086–92.
6. Nishigaki Y, MartÌ R, Copeland WC, Hirano M. Site-specific somatic mitochondrial DNA point mutations in patients with thymidine phosphorylase deficiency. J Clin Invest. 2003;111:1913–21. https://doi.org/10.1172/JCI17828.
7. Okamura K, Santa T, Nagae K, Omae T. Congenital oculoskeletal myopathy with abnormal muscle and liver mitochondria. J Neurol Sci. 1976;27:79–91. https://doi.org/10.1016/0022-510X(76)90236-7.
8. Valentino ML, et al. Thymidine and deoxyuridine accumulate in tissues of patients with mitochondrial neurogastrointestinal encephalomyopathy (MNGIE). FEBS Lett. 2007;581:3410–4. https://doi.org/10.1016/j.febslet.2007.06.042.
9. Hirano M. In: Adam MP, et al., editors. GeneReviewsÆ. Seattle, WA: University of Washington, Seattle; 1993.
10. Nishino I, et al. Mitochondrial neurogastrointestinal encephalomyopathy: an autosomal recessive disorder due to thymidine phosphorylase mutations. Ann Neurol. 2000;47:792–800.
11. MartÌ R, et al. Late-onset MNGIE due to partial loss of thymidine phosphorylase activity. Ann Neurol. 2005;58:649–52. https://doi.org/10.1002/ana.20615.
12. Röeben B, et al. Hemodialysis in MNGIE transiently reduces serum and urine levels of thymidine and deoxyuridine, but not CSF levels and neurological function. Orphanet J Rare Dis. 2017;12:135. https://doi.org/10.1186/s13023-017-0687-0.
13. Imperatore N, Tortora R, Gerbino N, Caporaso N, Rispo A. Mitochondrial neurogastrointestinal encephalomyopathy (MNGIE) mimicking refractory celiac disease. Dig Liver Dis. 2017;49:1061–2. https://doi.org/10.1016/j.dld.2017.04.017.
14. Demaria F, et al. Mitochondrial neurogastrointestinal encephalomyopathy presenting as anorexia nervosa. J Adolesc Health. 2016;59:729–31. https://doi.org/10.1016/j.jadohealth.2016.08.012.
15. Wang H-F, et al. A novel thymidine phosphorylase mutation in a Chinese MNGIE patient. Acta Neurol Belg. 2017;117:259–67. https://doi.org/10.1007/s13760-016-0701-7.
16. De Giorgio R, et al. Liver transplantation for mitochondrial neurogastrointestinal encephalomyopathy. Ann Neurol. 2016;80:448–55. https://doi.org/10.1002/ana.24724.
17. Casarez VQ, Zavala AM, Owusu-Agyemang P, Hagan K. Anesthetic management of a child with mitochondrial neurogastrointestinal encephalopathy. Case Rep Anesthesiol. 2015;2015:453714. https://doi.org/10.1155/2015/453714.
18. Kalkan IH, et al. Spontaneous abdominal esophageal perforation in a patient with mitochondrial neurogastrointestinal encephalomyopathy. Acta Clin Belg. 2015;70:44–5. https://doi.org/10.1179/2295333714Y.0000000053.
19. Grechanina IB. [Mitochondrial neurogastrointestinal encephalopathy syndrome]. Likars'ka Sprava. 2014;11:146–8.
20. Benureau A, et al. LíencÈphalomyopathie neurogastro-intestinale mitochondriale†: un tableau díanorexie mentale atypique. Arch PÈdiatr. 2014;21:1370–4. https://doi.org/10.1016/j.arcped.2014.08.006.
21. Dreznik Y, Gutman M, Weiss B, Nevler A. Mitochondrial neuro-gastrointestinal encephalomyopathy presenting with recurrent bowel perforations and intra-abdominal abscesses. J Gastrointest Surg. 2014;18:2054–6. https://doi.org/10.1007/s11605-014-2589-y.
22. Ariaudo C, et al. Mitochondrial neurogastrointestinal encephalomyopathy treated with peritoneal dialysis and bone marrow transplantation. J Nephrol. 2015;28:125–7. https://doi.org/10.1007/s40620-014-0069-9.
23. Suh BC, et al. Compound heterozygous mutations of TYMP as underlying causes of mitochondrial neurogastrointestinal encephalomyopathy (MNGIE). Mol Med Rep. 2013;8:17–22. https://doi.org/10.3892/mmr.2013.1479.
24. Mihaylova V, et al. Possible toxicity of tuberculostatic agents in a patient with a novel TYMP mutation leading to mitochondrial neurogastrointestinal encephalomyopathy. J Neurogenet. 2013;27:19–22. https://doi.org/10.3109/01677063.2013.778256.
25. Perez-Atayde AR. Diagnosis of mitochondrial neurogastrointestinal encephalopathy disease in gastrointestinal biopsies. Hum Pathol. 2013;44:1440–6. https://doi.org/10.1016/j.humpath.2012.12.005.
26. Hussein E. Non-myeloablative bone marrow transplant and platelet infusion can transiently improve the clinical outcome of mitochondrial neurogastrointestinal encephalopathy: a case report. Transfus Apher Sci. 2013;49:208–11. https://doi.org/10.1016/j.transci.2013.01.014.
27. Kalkan IH, et al. A novel finding in MNGIE (mitochondrial neurogastrointestinal encephalomyopathy): hypergonadotropic hypogonadism. Hormones (Athens, Greece). 2012;11:377–9.

28. Cardaioli E, et al. A new thymidine phosphorylase mutation causing elongation of the protein underlies mitochondrial neurogastrointestinal encephalomyopathy. J Neurol. 2012;259:172–4. https://doi.org/10.1007/s00415-011-6113-y.
29. Ibáñez C, Fernández-González I. Anestesia de urgencia en paciente adulto con sÌndrome de MNGIE. Rev Esp Anestesiol Reanim. 2011;58:585–7. https://doi.org/10.1016/S0034-9356(11)70144-X.
30. Patel J, et al. An interesting case of intestinal pseudo-obstruction: MNGIE. Trop Gastroenterol. 2011;32:138–41.
31. Li J-N, et al. Successful cochlear implantation in a patient with MNGIE syndrome. Acta Otolaryngol. 2011;131:1012–6. https://doi.org/10.3109/00016489.2011.579623.
32. Torres-Torronteras J, et al. A novel nonstop mutation in TYMP does not induce nonstop mRNA decay in a MNGIE patient with severe neuropathy. Hum Mutat. 2011;32:E2061–8. https://doi.org/10.1002/humu.21447.
33. Oztas E, et al. Chronic intestinal pseudo-obstruction and neurological manifestations in early adulthood: considering MNGIE syndrome in differential diagnosis. J Gastrointestin Liver Dis. 2010;19:195–7.
34. Bariş Z, Eminoğlu T, Dalgiç B, Tümer L, Hasanoğlu A. Mitochondrial neurogastrointestinal encephalomyopathy (MNGIE): case report with a new mutation. Eur J Pediatr. 2010;169:1375–8. https://doi.org/10.1007/s00431-010-1237-0.
35. Petcharunpaisan S, Castillo M. Multiple cranial nerve enhancement in mitochondrial neurogastrointestinal encephalomyopathy. J Comput Assist Tomogr. 2010;34:247–8. https://doi.org/10.1097/RCT.0b013e3181c71d48.
36. Cardaioli E, et al. A second MNGIE patient without typical mitochondrial skeletal muscle involvement. Neurol Sci. 2010;31:491–4. https://doi.org/10.1007/s10072-010-0225-5.
37. Bakker JA, Schlesser P, Smeets HJM, Francois B, Bierau J. Biochemical abnormalities in a patient with thymidine phosphorylase deficiency with fatal outcome. J Inherit Metab Dis. 2010;33:139–43. https://doi.org/10.1007/s10545-010-9049-y.
38. Massa R, et al. Late-onset MNGIE without peripheral neuropathy due to incomplete loss of thymidine phosphorylase activity. Neuromuscul Disord. 2009;19:837–40. https://doi.org/10.1016/j.nmd.2009.08.013.
39. Laforce R, et al. A novel TYMP mutation in a French Canadian patient with mitochondrial neurogastrointestinal encephalomyopathy. Clin Neurol Neurosurg. 2009;111:691–4. https://doi.org/10.1016/j.clineuro.2009.05.005.
40. Taanman J-W, et al. Characterization of a novel TYMP splice site mutation associated with mitochondrial neurogastrointestinal encephalomyopathy (MNGIE). Neuromuscul Disord. 2009;19:151–4. https://doi.org/10.1016/j.nmd.2008.11.002.
41. Moran NF, Bain MD, Muqit MMK, Bax BE. Carrier erythrocyte entrapped thymidine phosphorylase therapy for MNGIE. Neurology. 2008;71:686–8. https://doi.org/10.1212/01.wnl.0000324602.97205.ab.
42. Carod-Artal FJ, et al. Cognitive dysfunction and hypogonadotropic hypogonadism in a Brazilian patient with mitochondrial neurogastrointestinal encephalomyopathy and a novel ECGF1 mutation. Eur J Neurol. 2007;14:581–5. https://doi.org/10.1111/j.1468-1331.2007.01720.x.
43. Yavuz H, et al. Treatment of mitochondrial neurogastrointestinal encephalomyopathy with dialysis. Arch Neurol. 2007;64:435–8. https://doi.org/10.1001/archneur.64.3.435.
44. Peedikayil MC, Kagevi EI, Abufarhaneh E, Alsayed MD, Alzahrani HA. Mitochondrial neurogastrointestinal encephalomyopathy treated with stem cell transplantation: a case report and review of literature. Hematol Oncol Stem Cell Ther. 2015;8:85–90. https://doi.org/10.1016/j.hemonc.2014.12.001.
45. Vinciguerra C, et al. Eye movement changes in mitochondrial neurogastrointestinal encephalomyopathy (MNGIE). J Neurol Sci. 2015;350:107–9. https://doi.org/10.1016/j.jns.2015.01.031.
46. Vondráčková A, et al. Large copy number variations in combination with point mutations in the TYMP and SCO2 genes found in two patients with mitochondrial disorders. Eur J Hum Genet. 2014;22:431–4. https://doi.org/10.1038/ejhg.2013.148.
47. Libernini L, et al. Mitochondrial neurogastrointestinal encephalomyopathy: novel pathogenic mutations in thymidine phosphorylase gene in two Italian brothers. Neuropediatrics. 2012;43:201–8. https://doi.org/10.1055/s-0032-1315431.
48. Filosto M, et al. Pitfalls in diagnosing mitochondrial neurogastrointestinal encephalomyopathy. J Inherit Metab Dis. 2011;34:1199–203. https://doi.org/10.1007/s10545-011-9332-6.
49. Çoban G, et al. Mitochondrial neurogastrointestinal encephalomyopathy: imaging and clinical findings in three patients. Diagn Interv Radiol (Ankara, Turkey). 2013;19:191–4. https://doi.org/10.5152/dir.2013.008.
50. Nalini A, Gayathri N. Mitochondrial neurogastrointestinal encephalopathy in an Indian family with possible manifesting carriers of heterozygous TYMP mutation. J Neurol Sci. 2011;309:131–5. https://doi.org/10.1016/j.jns.2011.06.052.
51. Schüpbach WM, et al. Mitochondrial neurogastrointestinal encephalomyopathy in three siblings. J Neurol. 2007;254:146–53. https://doi.org/10.1007/s00415-006-0255-3.
52. Mart R, Nishigaki Y, Hirano M. Elevated plasma deoxyuridine in patients with thymidine phosphorylase deficiency. Biochem Biophys Res Commun. 2003;303:14–8. https://doi.org/10.1016/S0006-291X(03)00294-8.
53. Spinazzola A, et al. Altered thymidine metabolism due to defects of thymidine phosphorylase. J Biol

Chem. 2002;277:4128–33. https://doi.org/10.1074/jbc.M111028200.
54. Stenman G, et al. Regional localization of the human platelet-derived endothelial cell growth factor (ECGF1) gene to chromosome 22q13. Cytogenet Cell Genet. 1992;59:22–3. https://doi.org/10.1159/000133191.
55. Stenson PD, et al. The human gene mutation database: building a comprehensive mutation repository for clinical and molecular genetics, diagnostic testing and personalized genomic medicine. Hum Genet. 2014;133:1–9. https://doi.org/10.1007/s00439-013-1358-4.
56. Szigeti K, et al. MNGIE with lack of skeletal muscle involvement and a novel TP splice site mutation. J Med Genet. 2004;41:125–9. https://doi.org/10.1136/jmg.2003.013789.
57. Blazquez A, et al. Increased muscle nucleoside levels associated with a novel frameshift mutation in the thymidine phosphorylase gene in a Spanish patient with MNGIE. Neuromuscul Disord. 2005;15:775–8. https://doi.org/10.1016/j.nmd.2005.07.008.
58. Gamez J, et al. A novel thymidine phosphorylase mutation in a Spanish MNGIE patient. J Neurol Sci. 2005;228:35–9. https://doi.org/10.1016/j.jns.2004.09.034.
59. Yadak R, et al. Mitochondrial neurogastrointestinal encephalomyopathy caused by thymidine phosphorylase enzyme deficiency: from pathogenesis to emerging therapeutic options. Front Cell Neurosci. 2017;11:31. https://doi.org/10.3389/fncel.2017.00031.
60. MartÌ R, et al. Definitive diagnosis of mitochondrial neurogastrointestinal encephalomyopathy by biochemical assays. Clin Chem. 2004;50:120–4. https://doi.org/10.1373/clinchem.2003.026179.
61. Friedkin M, Roberts D. The enzymatic synthesis of nucleosides. II. Thymidine and related pyrimidine nucleosides. J Biol Chem. 1954;207:257–66.
62. Sun Q. Urine pyrimidine metabolite determination by HPLC tandem mass spectrometry. Methods Mol Biol (Clifton, N.J.). 2016;1378:237–42. https://doi.org/10.1007/978-1-4939-3182-8_25.
63. Nishigaki Y, MartÌ R, Hirano M. ND5 is a hot-spot for multiple atypical mitochondrial DNA deletions in mitochondrial neurogastrointestinal encephalomyopathy. Hum Mol Genet. 2004;13:91–101. https://doi.org/10.1093/hmg/ddh010.
64. Ferraro P, et al. mitochondrial deoxynucleotide pools in quiescent fibroblasts a possible model for mitochondrial neurogastrointestinal encephalomyopathy (MNGIE). J Biol Chem. 2005;280:24472–80. https://doi.org/10.1074/jbc.M502869200.
65. Bestwick RK, Mathews CK. Unusual compartmentation of precursors for nuclear and mitochondrial DNA in mouse L cells. J Biol Chem. 1982;257:9305–8.
66. Bogenhagen D, Clayton D. A. Thymidylate nucleotide supply for mitochondrial DNA synthesis in mouse L cells. Effect of 5 fluorodeoxyuridine and methotrexate in thymidine kinase plus and thymidine kinase minus cells. J Biol Chem. 1976;251:2938–44.
67. Croteau DL, Stierum RH, Bohr VA. Mitochondrial DNA repair pathways. Mutat Res DNA Repair. 1999;434:137–48. https://doi.org/10.1016/S0921-8777(99)00025-7.
68. Hirano M, MartÌ R, Vilà MR, Nishigaki Y. Mitochondrial function and biogenesis topics in current genetics. Berlin: Springer; 2004. p. 177–200.
69. Song S, Wheeler LJ, Mathews CK. Deoxyribonucleotide pool imbalance stimulates deletions in HeLa cell mitochondrial DNA. J Biol Chem. 2003;278:43893–6. https://doi.org/10.1074/jbc.C300401200.
70. Pontarin G, et al. Mitochondrial DNA depletion and thymidine phosphate pool dynamics in a cellular model of mitochondrial neurogastrointestinal encephalomyopathy. J Biol Chem. 2006;281:22720–8. https://doi.org/10.1074/jbc.M604498200.
71. Cámara Y, et al. Administration of deoxyribonucleosides or inhibition of their catabolism as a pharmacological approach for mitochondrial DNA depletion syndrome. Hum Mol Genet. 2014;23:2459–67. https://doi.org/10.1093/hmg/ddt641.
72. LÛpez LC, et al. Unbalanced deoxynucleotide pools cause mitochondrial DNA instability in thymidine phosphorylase-deficient mice. Hum Mol Genet. 2009;18:714–22. https://doi.org/10.1093/hmg/ddn401.
73. Garcia-Diaz B, et al. Deoxynucleoside stress exacerbates the phenotype of a mouse model of mitochondrial neurogastrointestinal encephalopathy. Brain J Neurol. 2014;137:1337–49. https://doi.org/10.1093/brain/awu068.
74. Rickards H, Prendergast M, Booth IW. Psychiatric presentation of Crohn's disease: diagnostic delay and increased morbidity. Br J Psychiatry. 1994;164:256–61. https://doi.org/10.1192/bjp.164.2.256.
75. Teitelbaum JE, et al. Diagnosis and management of MNGIE syndrome in children: case report and review of the literature. J Pediatr Gastroenterol Nutr. 2002;35:377–83.
76. MartÌn MA, et al. Lack of gastrointestinal symptoms in a 60-year-old patient with MNGIE. Neurology. 2004;63:1536–7.
77. Bedlack RS, et al. MNGIE neuropathy: five cases mimicking chronic inflammatory demyelinating polyneuropathy. Muscle Nerve. 2004;29:364–8. https://doi.org/10.1002/mus.10546.
78. Said G, Lacroix C. Primary and secondary vasculitic neuropathy. J Neurol. 2005;252:633–41. https://doi.org/10.1007/s00415-005-0833-9.
79. Millar WS, Lignelli A, Hirano M. MRI of five patients with mitochondrial neurogastrointestinal encephalomyopathy. AJR Am J Roentgenol. 2004;182:1537–41. https://doi.org/10.2214/ajr.182.6.1821537.
80. la Marca G, et al. Pre- and post-dialysis quantitative dosage of thymidine in urine and plasma of a MNGIE patient by using HPLC-ESI-MS/MS. J Mass

Spectrom. 2006;41:586–92. https://doi.org/10.1002/jms.1013.
81. Boelens JJ, Prasad VK, Tolar J, Wynn RF, Peters C. Current international perspectives on hematopoietic stem cell transplantation for inherited metabolic disorders. Pediatr Clin N Am. 2010;57:123–45. https://doi.org/10.1016/j.pcl.2009.11.004.
82. Lachmann R. Treatments for lysosomal storage disorders. Biochem Soc Trans. 2010;38:1465–8. https://doi.org/10.1042/BST0381465.
83. Delicou S, et al. Successful HLA-identical hematopoietic stem cell transplantation in a patient with purine nucleoside phosphorylase deficiency. Pediatr Transplant. 2007;11:799–803. https://doi.org/10.1111/j.1399-3046.2007.00772.x.
84. Lara MC, et al. Infusion of platelets transiently reduces nucleoside overload in MNGIE. Neurology. 2006;67:1461–3. https://doi.org/10.1212/01.wnl.0000239824.95411.52.
85. Halter JP, et al. Allogeneic haematopoietic stem cell transplantation for mitochondrial neurogastrointestinal encephalomyopathy. Brain J Neurol. 2015;138:2847–58. https://doi.org/10.1093/brain/awv226.
86. Halter J, et al. Allogeneic hematopoietic SCT as treatment option for patients with mitochondrial neurogastrointestinal encephalomyopathy (MNGIE): a consensus conference proposal for a standardized approach. Bone Marrow Transplant. 2011;46:330–7. https://doi.org/10.1038/bmt.2010.100.
87. Boschetti E, et al. Liver as a source for thymidine phosphorylase replacement in mitochondrial neurogastrointestinal encephalomyopathy. PLoS One. 2014;9:e96692. https://doi.org/10.1371/journal.pone.0096692.
88. Wilcox AJ, Choy J, Bustamante C, Matouschek A. Effect of protein structure on mitochondrial import. Proc Natl Acad Sci. 2005;102:15435–40. https://doi.org/10.1073/pnas.0507324102.
89. De Vocht C, et al. Assessment of stability, toxicity and immunogenicity of new polymeric nanoreactors for use in enzyme replacement therapy of MNGIE. J Control Release. 2009;137:246–54. https://doi.org/10.1016/j.jconrel.2009.03.020.
90. Bax BE, et al. Clinical and biochemical improvements in a patient with MNGIE following enzyme replacement. Neurology. 2013;81:1269–71. https://doi.org/10.1212/WNL.0b013e3182a6cb4b.
91. Cass CE, et al. Nucleoside transporters of mammalian cells. Pharm Biotechnol. 1999;12:313–52.
92. Van Aubel RA, Masereeuw R, Russel FG. Molecular pharmacology of renal organic anion transporters. Am J Physiol Renal Physiol. 2000;279:F216–32. https://doi.org/10.1152/ajprenal.2000.279.2.F216.
93. Gonzalez-Vioque E, Torres-Torronteras J, Andreu AL, Marti R. Limited dCTP availability accounts for mitochondrial DNA depletion in mitochondrial neurogastrointestinal encephalomyopathy (MNGIE). PLoS Genet. 2011;7:e1002035. https://doi.org/10.1371/journal.pgen.1002035.
94. Ebrahem Q, Mahfouz RZ, Ng KP, Saunthararajah Y. High cytidine deaminase expression in the liver provides sanctuary for cancer cells from decitabine treatment effects. Oncotarget. 2012;3:1137–45. https://doi.org/10.18632/oncotarget.597.
95. De Vocht C, et al. Polymeric nanoreactors for enzyme replacement therapy of MNGIE. J Control Release. 2010;148:e19–20. https://doi.org/10.1016/j.jconrel.2010.07.011.
96. Lopez LC, et al. Unbalanced deoxynucleotide pools cause mitochondrial DNA instability in thymidine phosphorylase-deficient mice. Hum Mol Genet. 2009;18:714–22. https://doi.org/10.1093/hmg/ddn401.
97. Torres-Torronteras J, et al. Hematopoietic gene therapy restores thymidine phosphorylase activity in a cell culture and a murine model of MNGIE. Gene Ther. 2011;18:795–806. https://doi.org/10.1038/gt.2011.24.
98. Torres-Torronteras J, et al. Long-Term restoration of thymidine phosphorylase function and nucleoside homeostasis using hematopoietic gene therapy in a murine model of mitochondrial neurogastrointestinal encephalomyopathy. Hum Gene Ther. 2016;27:656–67. https://doi.org/10.1089/hum.2015.160.
99. Yadak R, et al. Preclinical Efficacy and safety evaluation of hematopoietic stem cell gene therapy in a mouse Model of MNGIE. Mol Ther Methods Clin Dev. 2018;8:152–65. https://doi.org/10.1016/j.omtm.2018.01.001.
100. Donsante A, et al. Observed incidence of tumorigenesis in long-term rodent studies of rAAV vectors. Gene Ther. 2001;8:1343–6. https://doi.org/10.1038/sj.gt.3301541.
101. Gauttier V, et al. No tumour-initiating risk associated with scAAV transduction in newborn rat liver. Gene Ther. 2013;20:779–84. https://doi.org/10.1038/gt.2013.7.
102. Nathwani AC, et al. Long-term safety and efficacy of factor IX gene therapy in hemophilia B. N Engl J Med. 2014;371:1994–2004. https://doi.org/10.1056/NEJMoa1407309.
103. Nienhuis AW, Nathwani AC, Davidoff AM. Gene therapy for hemophilia. Hum Gene Ther. 2016;27:305–8. https://doi.org/10.1089/hum.2016.018.
104. Torres-Torronteras J, et al. Gene therapy using a liver-targeted AAV vector restores nucleoside and nucleotide homeostasis in a murine model of MNGIE. Mol Ther. 2014;22:901–7. https://doi.org/10.1038/mt.2014.6.
105. Torres-Torronteras J, et al. Long-term sustained effect of liver-targeted adeno-associated virus gene therapy for mitochondrial neurogastrointestinal encephalomyopathy. Hum Gene Ther. 2018;29:708–18. https://doi.org/10.1089/hum.2017.133.
106. Boutin S, et al. Prevalence of serum IgG and neutralizing factors against adeno-associated virus (AAV) types 1, 2, 5, 6, 8, and 9 in the healthy population: implications for gene therapy using AAV vec-

tors. Hum Gene Ther. 2010;21:704–12. https://doi.org/10.1089/hum.2009.182.
107. Fukami MH, Salganicoff L. Isolation and properties of human platelet mitochondria. Blood. 1973;42:913–8.
108. Shaw T, Smillie RH, Miller AE, MacPhee DG. The role of blood platelets in nucleoside metabolism: regulation of platelet thymidine phosphorylase. Mutat Res. 1988;200:117–31.
109. Fox SB, et al. Platelet-derived endothelial cell growth factor/thymidine phosphorylase expression in normal tissues: an immunohistochemical study. J Pathol. 1995;176:183–90. https://doi.org/10.1002/path.1711760212.
110. Marti R, et al. Definitive diagnosis of mitochondrial neurogastrointestinal encephalomyopathy by biochemical assays. Clin Chem. 2004;50:120–4. https://doi.org/10.1373/clinchem.2003.026179.
111. Threlkeld AB, et al. Ophthalmic involvement in myo-neuro-gastrointestinal encephalopathy syndrome. Am J Ophthalmol. 1992;114:322–8. https://doi.org/10.1016/S0002-9394(14)71799-4.
112. Barboni P, et al. Ocular findings in mitochondrial neurogastrointestinal encephalomyopathy: a case report. Graefes Arch Clin Exp Ophthalmol. 2004;242:878–80. https://doi.org/10.1007/s00417-004-0914-y.
113. Simon DK, O'Leary DD. Relationship of retinotopic ordering of axons in the optic pathway to the formation of visual maps in central targets. J Comp Neurol. 1991;307:393–404. https://doi.org/10.1002/cne.903070305.
114. Menezes MP, Ouvrier RA. Peripheral neuropathy associated with mitochondrial disease in children. Dev Med Child Neurol. 2012;54:407–14. https://doi.org/10.1111/j.1469-8749.2012.04271.x.
115. Finkenstedt A, et al. MNGIE syndrome: liver cirrhosis should be ruled out prior to bone marrow transplantation. JIMD Rep. 2013;10:41–4. https://doi.org/10.1007/8904_2012_199.
116. Barragán-Campos HM, et al. Brain magnetic resonance imaging findings in patients with mitochondrial cytopathies. Arch Neurol. 2005;62:737–42. https://doi.org/10.1001/archneur.62.5.737.
117. Scaglia F, Wong L-JC, Vladutiu GD, Hunter JV. Predominant cerebellar volume loss as a neuroradiologic feature of pediatric respiratory chain defects. AJNR Am J Neuroradiol. 2005;26:1675–80.
118. Schiffmann R, van der Knaap MS. Invited article: an MRI-based approach to the diagnosis of white matter disorders. Neurology. 2009;72:750–9. https://doi.org/10.1212/01.wnl.0000343049.00540.c8.
119. Salsano E, et al. Adult-onset leukodystrophies from respiratory chain disorders: do they exist? J Neurol. 2013;260:1617–23. https://doi.org/10.1007/s00415-013-6844-z.
120. Scarpelli M, et al. The role of brain MRI in mitochondrial neurogastrointestinal encephalomyopathy. Neuroradiol J. 2013;26:520–30. https://doi.org/10.1177/197140091302600505.
121. Vissing J, et al. Multiple mtDNA deletions with features of MNGIE. Neurology. 2002;59:926–9.
122. Yasumura S, Aso S, Fujisaka M, Watanabe Y. Cochlear implantation in a patient with mitochondrial encephalopathy, lactic acidosis and stroke-like episodes syndrome. Acta Otolaryngol. 2003;123:55–8.
123. Craven L, et al. Mitochondrial DNA disease: new options for prevention. Hum Mol Genet. 2011;20:R168–74. https://doi.org/10.1093/hmg/ddr373.
124. Yolcu M, Yolcu C, Kaya Z, Cakmak EO, Sezen Y. Endocarditis in mitochondrial neurogastrointestinal encephalomyopathy (MNGIE) syndrome: the first in the literature. J Clin Diagn Res. 2014;8:SD01–2. https://doi.org/10.7860/JCDR/2014/9528.5016.
125. Fairbanks LD, Marinaki AM, Carrey EA, Hammans SR, Duley JA. Deoxyuridine accumulation in urine in thymidine phosphorylase deficiency (MNGIE). J Inherit Metab Dis. 2002;25:603–4.
126. Marti R, et al. Mitochondrial neurogastrointestinal encephalomyopathy and thymidine metabolism: results and hypotheses. Mitochondrion. 2002;2:143–7.
127. Debouverie M, et al. MNGIE syndrome in 2 siblings. Rev Neurol. 1997;153:547–53.

Mitochondrial Neurodegenerative Disorders I: Parkinsonism and Cognitive Deficits

Yi Shiau Ng, Nichola Z. Lax, Laurence A. Bindoff, and Doug M. Turnbull

Introduction

Idiopathic Parkinson's disease (IPD) is the most common movement disorder in the adult population, with the estimated prevalence of over 2% in the age group of over 65 years old [1]. Patients with IPD present with a unilateral/asymmetrical onset of symptoms characterised by resting tremor, bradykinesia and rigidity together with postural instability. In addition, IPD shows a persistent response to dopamine treatment even though increased dosage is often required as the disease advances.

The pathological hallmarks of IPD are the presence of alpha-synuclein containing Lewy bodies (LBs) and loss of dopaminergic neurons in the substantia nigra of the midbrain. While age is recognised as the major risk factor for IPD, environmental and genetic factors are implicated in the pathogenesis of IPD and intensely researched over the last few decades. The role of mitochondrial dysfunction has attracted a lot of interest in the research field following the initial observation of 1-methyl-4-phenyl-1,2,3,6-tetrahydropyridine (MPTP) toxicity leading to the development of Parkinsonism and complex I deficiency in the 1980s [2], and the experiment of chronic exposure of rotenone (known complex I inhibitor) producing Parkinsonian features in rats [3] further supported the link of complex I deficiency and dopaminergic neuronal loss. The advent of genetic sequencing technology facilitated the discovery of higher level of qualitative defect of mitochondrial DNA, multiple deletions, in the substantia nigra neurons of IPD patients, compared to the age-matched controls [4]. In 2004, the Finnish research group published a seminal paper directly linking Parkinsonism to multiple mtDNA deletions secondary to the deficiency of mitochondrial polymerase gamma (POLG) [5], the essential enzyme responsible for the replication and maintenance of mitochondrial DNA in mammals. The association of Parkinsonism and *POLG* mutations has subsequently been observed and hence validated in multiple pedigrees independently [6–8]. More recently, nuclear genes involved in mitochondrial dynamics and mitochondrial quality control have been implicated in the neurodegeneration of familial Parkinsonism [9].

In this chapter, we begin with an overview of the oxidative phosphorylation system and features of mitochondrial DNA, followed by the

Y. S. Ng (✉) · N. Z. Lax · D. M. Turnbull (✉)
Wellcome Centre for Mitochondrial Research, Institute of Neuroscience, Newcastle University, Newcastle Upon Tyne, UK
e-mail: Yi.Ng@newcastle.ac.uk; doug.turnbull@newcastle.ac.uk

L. A. Bindoff
Department of Clinical Medicine (K1), University of Bergen, Bergen, Norway

Department of Neurology, Haukeland University Hospital, Bergen, Norway

M. Mancuso, T. Klopstock (eds.), *Diagnosis and Management of Mitochondrial Disorders*,
https://doi.org/10.1007/978-3-030-05517-2_14

description of salient clinical features, molecular genetics and neuropathological findings of primary mitochondrial disorders that have a known association of Parkinsonism. The roles of mitochondrial dynamics and mitophagy will also be discussed.

Oxidative Phosphorylation, Mitochondrial DNA and Primary Mitochondrial Disorders

The oxidative phosphorylation system (OXPHOS) consists of five enzymatic complexes located in the mitochondrial inner membrane (MIM). The mitochondrial respiratory chain is constituted of first four complexes (complex I, II, III and IV), while the fifth complex (complex V), also known as ATP synthase, drives the synthesis of ATP from ADP. Electron movement along the respiratory chain is coupled with the transfer of protons across the MIM to create an electrochemical gradient (the proton motive force); this provides energy that is harnessed by the ATPase to synthesise ATP [10]. Organs with high-energy demand such as the brain, heart and skeletal muscle are particularly susceptible to the perturbation of OXPHOS and are frequently affected in mitochondrial disorders [11].

Mitochondria are the only cellular organelles that contain an extranuclear genome (mitochondrial DNA, mtDNA); mtDNA is present in multiple copies (hundreds to thousands) per cell and inherited only from the mother. Each mitochondrial genome comprises 37 genes: 13 genes that encode the subunits of OXPHOS, 22 transfer RNAs and two ribosomal RNAs. The rest of the OXPHOS components, all the assembly factors and ancillary proteins, the proteins involved in replication and maintenance of mtDNA and all other functions are under the control of nuclear genome [12].

Mitochondrial disease is an umbrella term for diseases that arise due to defects in either mtDNA or nuclear genes. These diseases comprise a diverse range of clinical phenotypes in which central nervous system involvement such as developmental delay, seizures, ataxia, early-onset dementia and extrapyramidal movement disorders is often evident both alone and among patients manifesting with severe multisystem disease [13].

One of the conventional classifications divides mitochondrial diseases based on the molecular defects between primary and secondary mtDNA disorders. Primary mtDNA defects encompass pathogenic mtDNA point mutations, such as m.3243A>G (*MT-TL1*), m.8334A>G (*MT-TK*) and single, large-scale deletions in mtDNAs. The majority of the pathogenic mtDNA point mutations and single, large-scale mtDNA deletions are present in a heteroplasmic state in which mutated and wild-type mtDNA exist in the same cell. Some mutations are more often homoplasmic, i.e. all mtDNAs are mutated, such as the m.11778G>A in *MT-ND4* that causes Leber hereditary optic neuropathy (LHON). Almost all single, large-scale mtDNA deletions arise sporadically (<5% are transmitted from mother) [14], while many common pathogenic mtDNA mutations are maternally inherited. Interestingly, a recent study suggested that around a quarter of rare pathogenic mtDNA variants were de novo mutations with a low risk of transmission [15].

Secondary mtDNA abnormalities can be subdivided into qualitative defects (multiple mtDNA deletions) and quantitative defect (reduction in the copy number of mtDNA/mtDNA depletion). These secondary mtDNA abnormalities are caused by defects in nuclear genes involved in maintenance of mitochondria or mtDNA integrity and follow the Mendelian pattern of inheritance.

Association of Pathogenic mtDNA Mutations and Parkinsonism

The prevalence of primary mtDNA mutations is approximately 1 in 5000 in the adult population [16]. While over 300 pathogenic mtDNA variants have been identified, several such as m.3243A>G, the three common LHON point mutations (m.3460G>A, m.11778G>A and m.14487T>C), and single, large-scale mtDNA deletions account for the majority of mtDNA disease [16]. These mutations can cause isolated complex I deficiency or multiple respiratory chain deficiency (affecting complexes I, III, IV) and result in a wide spectrum of clinical phenotypes that includes well-known variants such as mitochondrial encephalomyopathy, lactic acidosis and stroke-like episodes (MELAS), myoclonic epilepsy and ragged-red fibres (MERRF), Kearns-Sayre syndrome and Leigh syndrome as well as non-syndromic multisystem involvement.

Since the first discovery of primary mtDNA mutations in 1988 [17, 18], only a few case reports have associated mtDNA mutations with Parkinsonism. These include m.11778G>A in *MT-ND6* [19, 20], a heteroplasmic 4 bp deletion in *MT-CYB* [21] and m.8344A>G in *MT-TK* [22]. Furthermore, Parkinsonism has not been observed in several national cohort studies of common mtDNA mutations [23–25], suggesting the association with primary mtDNA mutations is more likely to be serendipitous [9]. An Italian study also failed to demonstrate the connection of m.8344A>G mutation in 159 patients with IPD [26]. In addition, neuropathological studies have not identified an increase in mtDNA mutations in substantia nigra of patients with IPD compared to controls [27]. Based on these findings, it would suggest that primary mtDNA point mutations do not play a role in the pathogenesis of IPD.

MtDNA Maintenance Nuclear Genes, Multiple Deletions and Parkinsonism

The enzyme polymerase gamma (POLG) is the DNA polymerase responsible for the synthesis and repair of mtDNA. It consists of a catalytic subunit (encoded by *POLG*) and two accessory subunits (encoded by *POLG2*). Genetic defects in *POLG* can result in both mtDNA depletion and multiple deletions [28]. In 2004, a Finnish research group reported compelling evidence showing the co-segregation of Parkinsonism, chronic progressive external ophthalmoplegia (CPEO), multiple deletions in mtDNA and heterozygous *POLG* mutations [5]. The onset of unilateral Parkinsonism ranged from 36 to 75 years and was preceded by CPEO, premature ovarian failure in females and peripheral neuropathy. Two patients underwent PET scanning that showed a reduction of [^{18}F]beta-CFT uptake in striatum. Neuropathological studies also revealed a severe loss of pigmented neurons in the substantia nigra, but Lewy bodies and alpha-synuclein inclusions were absent. Good response to levodopa was documented in these patients. All families had a heterozygous *POLG* mutation, and the authors speculated that Parkinsonism might be a unique feature of mutations in the polymerase domain. Subsequently, compound heterozygous *POLG* mutations (variants located in the polymerase and linker domains) were also identified in two sisters manifesting in their early 20s with Parkinsonism and neuropathy but without CPEO [6].

In a large, national cohort UK study, Parkinsonism accounted for 43% of all extrapyramidal movement disorders in patients with mitochondrial disease, making it the most common extrapyramidal movement disorders identified in this population. The most common genetic defect associated with Parkinsonism is *POLG* mutations (four out of five patients harboured recessive mutations) [29].

The link between POLG deficiency and substantia nigra neuronal loss is not, however, straightforward. In a study of both post-mortem samples and living patients with *POLG* mutations [30], massive loss of neurons in the SN was found, even in a child below the age of 12 months. Moreover, single neuron analysis showed depletion of mtDNA with a threshold of ca. 40%. DAT scan studies of living patients with *POLG* mutations also showed abnormal tracer uptake starting between 20 and 30 years of age, and the older the patient, the more severe the DAT scan abnormality became [30]. Despite the loss of neurons and DAT scan abnormality being much more severe than seen in idiopathic PD, none of the patients in this study had clinical features of Parkinsonism. Further, studies to ascertain if this was a general phenomenon in mitochondrial defects showed that patients with primary mtDNA mutations (single deletions, m.3243A>G) did not show this, while patients with mutations in Twinkle did. This suggested that the disturbance was due to a defect in mtDNA homoeostasis and subsequent studies confirmed that patients with idiopathic PD did indeed lack the normal compensatory increase in mtDNA copy number (that potentially helps restrict the effects of increasing mtDNA damage) seen in non-affected individuals (see later) [27].

Other nuclear defects causing multiple mtDNA deletions have also been associated with CPEO and Parkinsonism (Table 1), but only mutations in *TWNK* and *OPA1* have been reported in more than two families. *TWNK* (previously also known as *PEO1/c10orf2*) encodes the twinkle helicase, and the heterozygous *TWNK* mutations usually cause a mild form of mitochondrial disorder characterised by CPEO and multiple DNA deletions [31, 32]. Parkinsonism reported in pedigrees with heterozygous *TWNK* mutations has an onset between 40 and 80 years and typically developed at least 10 years after the manifestation of CPEO [33]. Asymmetrical reduction of the dopamine uptake in striatum on DAT scan has recently been reported in Parkinsonism associated with *TWNK* mutations [30]. The severity of Parkinsonism appeared to be mild, and levodopa treatment was not required in several cases [34, 35]. According to a neuropathological study of six patients (*POLG*-related Parkinsonism and CPEO ($n = 2$), *POLG*-related MIRAS ($n = 2$), *TWNK*-related adPEO ($n = 1$) and *TWNK*-related IOSCA ($n = 1$)), severe, widespread complex I deficiency was present in the substantia nigra (SN) of all patients [36]. Moreover, severe atrophy of mesencephalon and severe loss of SN pigment neurons were identified in two patients with *POLG*-related Parkinsonism compared to the others without Parkinsonism [36, 37]. The authors concluded that complex I deficiency in SN was simply the consequence of mtDNA deletions and/or depletion and challenged the mechanistic link of complex I deficiency and pathogenesis of Parkinsonism.

Mitochondrial Dynamics, Mitophagy and Mitochondrial Quality Control

Mitochondria are dynamic organelles that can fuse and divide according to the metabolic demands and physiological states of the cell. A number of highly conserved guanosine triphosphatase (GTPase) proteins regulate fusion and fission in mitochondria. Mitofusin 1 and 2 (Mfn1 and Mfn2) mediate fusion in the outer membrane and optic atrophy 1 (Opa1) in the inner membrane. The main result of fusion is the formation of an interconnected network which helps to maintain a healthy mitochondrial population [38]. Mitochondrial fission, in contrast, creates smaller mitochondria which in turn facilitate mitochondrial transport, accelerating cell proliferation, or the degradation of damaged mitochondria, a process known as mitophagy [39]. The key mediators for promoting mitochondrial fission are dynamin-related protein 1 (DRP1), FIS1, OPA3 and GDAP1 [40]. The fission events generate two subsets of daughter mitochondria with either increased or decreased membrane potential. The daughter mitochondria with higher membrane potential would fuse back into the mitochondrial network, whereas the depolarised daughter mitochondria are unable to proceed to the fusion process and are removed by mitophagy [41].

Mutations in *OPA1* are one of the most common genetic defects of dominant optic atrophy (>50%) [42]. In contrast to the subacute onset, rapid visual loss in LHON due to mtDNA point mutations, individuals who harbour a heterozygous OPA1 mutation typically present with a childhood-onset, progressive visual failure that is often accompanied by other neurological features including ataxia, neuropathy, myopathy, deafness, CPEO and CNS demyelination mimicking multiple sclerosis [43–46]. COX-deficient muscle fibres and multiple mtDNA deletions are common findings in the muscle biopsies of patients with OPA1 mutations [47], demonstrating the importance of OPA1 in mtDNA maintenance although its precise role is not clear [43, 45]. Carelli and colleagues reported the first

Table 1 The association of Parkinsonism and genetic defects causing mitochondrial disorders

Gene	Protein	Inheritance	Clinical features	Age of Parkinsonism	DAT scan findings	Response to levodopa	References
POLG	Catalytic subunit of polymerase gamma (replication and maintenance of mtDNA)	AD AR	CPEO, neuropathy, ataxia, epilepsy, premature ovarian failure	40–65	Both symmetrical and asymmetrical reductions of striatal uptake were reported	Yes	[5–7, 29, 35, 100–104]
TWNK	Twinkle helicase	AD	CPEO	40–70	Bilateral reduced uptake in putamen	Variable	[30, 33–35, 105]
OPA1	Mitochondrial dynamin-like GTPase	AD	Dominant optic atrophy, CPEO, neuropathy	40–70	Both symmetrical and asymmetrical reductions of striatal uptake were reported	Variable	[48–50]
POLG2	Accessory subunits of polymerase gamma	AD	Ataxia, neuropathy, dementia, seizures, CPEO	50–70	Not known	Variable	[106]
DGUOK	Deoxyguanosine kinase	AR	Ptosis, hyperCKaemia, and a wide range of unusual symptoms	67	Asymmetrical reduction of uptake in putamen	No	[107]
MPV17	MPV17 (function not well characterised)	AR	CPEO, neuropathy, myopathy, diabetes, deafness, gut dysmotility	65	Not known	Not known	[108]
AFG3L2	AFG3-like matrix AAA peptidase subunit 2	AR	SCA28, CPEO	Not known	Not known	Not known	[109]
SPG7	Paraplegin	AR	HSP, CPEO	55	Reduced uptake on putamen	Not known	[57]
RRM2B	p53-R2	AD	CPEO, myopathy, neuropathy, SNHL	50	Normal	Not known	[29]
SDHA	Succinate dehydrogenase complex flavoprotein subunit A	AD	Ataxia, bilateral optic atrophy, restless leg syndrome	50s	Reduced striatal uptake in one out of two patients	Poor	[29, 110]

All genes listed above have been associated with multiple mtDNA deletions in the muscle biopsies except *SDHA*. Parkinsonism has been reported in three or more family pedigrees with *POLG*, *TWNK* and *OPA1* mutations. *AD* autosomal dominant, *AR* autosomal recessive, *CPEO* chronic progressive external ophthalmoplegia, *HSP* hereditary spastic paraplegia, *SCA* spinocerebellar ataxia, *SNHL* sensorineural hearing loss association of heterozygous *OPA1* mutations and CPEO, Parkinsonism and dementia in two large Italian families in 2015 [48]. Intriguingly, optic neuropathy and visual failure were not the prominent features in their patients. Six individuals presented with CPEO, myopathy, neuropathy and ataxia in the 30–40s and developed asymmetrical Parkinsonism and dementia later in life. Abnormal DAT scan with asymmetrical dopamine uptake was observed. The response to levodopa was variable. Multiple DNA deletions were identified in the muscle biopsies, and heterozygous mutations c.1462G>A and c.1484C>T in *OPA1* were identified in these two families, respectively. Fibroblast study revealed impaired ATP synthesis, fragmented mitochondria, increased autophagy and mitophagy. Two other case reports of heterozygous *OPA1* mutations associated with Parkinsonism [49, 50] provided further evidence of the putative link of mitochondrial fusion, mtDNA stability and the pathogenesis of Parkinsonism.

The mitochondrial protease AFG3L2 plays a crucial role in the intra-mitochondrial quality control system. AFG3L2 forms homo-oligomeric complexes or hetero-oligomeric hexamers with the homologous subunit paraplegin (encoded by *SPG7*) to constitute the *m*-AAA (matrix-ATPase associated with various cellular activities) protease in the inner mitochondrial membrane [51, 52]. This ATP-dependent proteolytic complex degrades misfolded proteins such as structural subunits of mitochondrial respiratory chain and controls ribosome assembly [52]. Mutations in *AFG3L2* cause autosomal dominant cerebellar ataxia (SCA28), and a recent case series described the spectrum of clinical features associated with SCA28 to include cerebellar ataxia, ophthalmoplegia, ptosis, nystagmus and dysarthria, and interestingly, three patients exhibited Parkinsonism (12%). Furthermore, multiple mtDNA deletions have been detected in the muscle biopsy of two patients who harboured a heterozygous mutation in *AFG3L2* [53]. Mutations in *SPG7* are one of the most common causes of recessive cerebellar ataxia [54, 55], and both complex I deficiency [51] and multiple mtDNA deletions [56] have been detected in patients with *SPG7* mutations. Pedroso and coworkers reported a 55-year-old female who developed progressive gait disorder, CPEO, symmetrical Parkinsonism and abnormal DAT scan [57]. Whole-exome sequencing identified compound heterozygous mutations in *SPG7* in this patient [57]. While the mechanistic link of mitochondrial housekeeping functions of AFG3L2 and paraplegin and the pathogenesis of Parkinsonism are possible, further longitudinal, clinical studies are required to confirm the phenotypic association of Parkinsonism with these genetic defects.

Mitochondrial Dysfunction in Other Familial Parkinsonism

Approximately 5% of Parkinson's disease has a monogenic aetiology. Increasing evidence shows that genetic defects linked to familial Parkinsonism, especially *PARK2*, *PINK1*, *DJ-1* and *HTRA2*, are also associated with mitochondrial impairment [58]. The kinase PTEN-induced putative kinase protein 1 (PINK1) accumulates in the damaged or depolarised mitochondria, leading to the recruitment E3 ubiquitin ligase parkin (encoded by *PARK2*) from the cytosol, ubiquitination of mitochondrial proteins and eventually the degradation of mitochondria by lysosomes [59]. Mutations in *PARK2* have emerged as the most common cause of early-onset (<40 years old), autosomal recessive Parkinson's disease which has a slowly progressive course, excellent levodopa responsiveness, selective dopaminergic neuronal loss in the substantia nigra and no formation of Lewy body in the brain [60]. The clinical features of *PINK1-associated parkinsonism* may be indistinguishable from IPD, with the onset age typically less than 45 years old, good response to levodopa and slow disease progression [61, 62]. Mechanistic studies in *Drosophila* mutants clearly demonstrated that PINK1 and parkin are crucial for maintaining mtDNA integrity and that parkin functions downstream of PINK1 [63, 64]. Mutations in both PINK1 and parkin cause similar phenotypes in *Drosophila*, including dopaminergic neurodegeneration, altered mitochondrial morphology in muscle and brain and reductions in mtDNA levels and mtDNA-encoded structural subunits. Complex I deficiency has also been reported in both parkin-mutant and PINK1-mutant fibroblasts of humans [65, 66].

Relationship Between Mitochondrial Dysfunction and Idiopathic Parkinson's Disease: Insights into Potential Mechanisms from Neuropathological Studies

IPD is characterised by selective and progressive degeneration of dopaminergic neurons from the substantia nigra pars compacta (SNpc). Approximately 31% of SNpc neurons are lost prior to the onset of motor symptoms in patients with IPD [67, 68]. The neuropathological hallmark of IPD is characterised by accumulation of proteinaceous deposits within the neuronal soma and their processes, termed Lewy bodies (LBs) and Lewy neurites, respectively. These bodies are composed mainly of alpha-synuclein, ubiquitin, neurofilaments and molecular chaperones.

Mitochondrial Respiratory Chain Impairments

Mitochondrial dysfunction was implicated in the pathogenesis of IPD by the discovery that a synthetic opiate, MPTP, can penetrate the blood-brain barrier (BBB) and be converted to the toxin MPP^+. MPP^+ is actively taken up by the Dopa uptake system and selectively accumulates in dopaminergic neurons where it further accumulates in mitochondria and inhibits mitochondrial complex I (NADPH ubiquinone oxidoreductase) causing severe SNpc neuron loss and Parkinsonism [2, 69]. The first human neuropathological studies positing a link between mitochondrial dysfunction and IPD were performed in the late 1980s where post-mortem samples from individuals with IPD revealed downregulation of specific complex I subunits within the SNpc [70, 71]. Further histochemical evidence of cytochrome *c* oxidase (COX; complex IV) activity relative to succinate dehydrogenase (SDH; complex II) activity within frozen midbrain sections revealed 3% of SNpc neurons are COX-deficient relative to 1% of age-matched control neurons [72].

To determine whether complex I deficiencies are specific only to the SN, a recent study has evaluated complex I subunit NDUFB8 expression in prefrontal cortex, hippocampus, putamen, cerebellum and pons and using a semi-quantitative analysis revealed higher levels of complex I deficient neurons throughout the CNS [73]. This suggests that respiratory chain deficiency is not restricted to the SNpc neurons in IPD.

Accumulation of Mitochondrial DNA Deletions

The discovery that high levels of mtDNA deletions are present in various brain regions in patients with IPD provided further evidence of the central role that mitochondrial dysfunction plays in the pathogenesis [4, 74]. Typically high levels of mtDNA deletion exist in areas of the brain, such as the caudate, putamen and substantia nigra, where dopamine metabolism is most active [75]. Laser capture microdissection of single SNpc neurons revealed a mixture of multiple mtDNA deletions accumulating with normal ageing but were also abundant in IPD and clonally expanded in surviving COX-deficient dopaminergic neurons [72, 76]. Recent ultra-deep mapping of neuronal mtDNA deletions has revealed approximately 38 distinct mtDNA deletions coexisting within each SNpc neurons from IPD, ranging in size from 113 to 8048 bp. Generally 1–4 deleted mtDNA species will present at high enough levels detectable by PCR; the remainder is present only at low frequencies which are in agreement with the ongoing formation of de novo mtDNA deletions [77]. These studies were fundamental in proving a direct link between mtDNA damage and a functional deficit in mitochondria.

Mapping of mtDNA deletions reveals that the majority of deletions can be localised to major arc, the region between the origins of replication of heavy and light strands [78, 79]. The mechanisms underpinning their formation are not clear; however, mtDNA deletions are thought to arise spontaneously at microhomologous sites of short base repeats due either to errors in replication and/or repair [80, 81]. Once formed, a proportion of mtDNA deletions can undergo clonal expansion, but again the mechanisms promoting expansion are not known [79].

MtDNA Point Mutations

Molecular analysis of laser microcapture dissected neurons from individuals with IPD confirms that mtDNA point mutations occur only at very low levels and therefore are unlikely to play a role in the pathogenesis [82]. Development of ultra-deep sequencing of SNpc neurons from IPD and age-matched controls did not reveal any significant differences in single-nucleotide variants (SNVs) distribution and the ratio of mtDNA transitions to transversions [27].

Altered mtDNA Content

Combined multiple-label immunofluorescence and single-cell laser capture microdissection of individual SNpc neurons revealed downregulated expression of mitochondrial respiratory chain subunits of complexes I and II in ~50% of neurons (Fig. 1a). Complex I deficient neurons also exhibit decreased mitochondrial transcription factor A (TFAM) and TFB2M expression levels and fewer mtDNA copies. Occasional complex IV deficiencies were detected but only in those neurons that harboured decreased complex I expression [83]. MtDNA copy number appears to increase with age in control SNpc neurons, and this correlates with the level of mtDNA deletion in each neuron. In IPD, mtDNA deletions accumulate to higher levels (IPD mean = 40.2 ± 20.0%, controls mean = 31.5 ± 19.5%), and while mtDNA content in neurons appeared comparable to controls, the rate of age-related copy number increase with age was much lower. Given the levels of mtDNA deletions that accumulate in SN neurones, this results in a relative depletion of the wild-type mtDNA pool. Mitochondrial biogenesis was assessed in this study. Using immunohistochemical labelling of peroxisome proliferator-activated receptor gamma co-activator (PGC-1alpha) revealed no detectable differences in expression between control and IPD; however, this analysis did not take into consideration post-translational modifications [27]. The authors suggested that it is likely that changes in mtDNA homeostatic control might play an important role in the pathogenesis of IPD.

Alpha-synuclein Pathology and Mitochondrial Dysfunction

Since aggregation of alpha-synuclein inclusions is the pathological hallmark of IPD, there have been a number of studies investigating how this protein aggregates and, once aggregated, how this impacts on the survival of neurons with or without mitochondrial impairments. Numerous cell culture studies suggest that mitochondria and alpha-synuclein interact directly with one another. One such study interrogated the toxic effects of alpha-synuclein on mitochondria by coculturing alpha-synuclein monomers and oligomers with neuronal cell lines that harboured a mutation affecting either complex I or IV of the mitochondrial respiratory chain versus a wild-type control. Results suggested that in wild-type neurons, the aggregation of alpha-synuclein exerted toxic effects by inhibiting complex I leading to cell death. Intriguingly however in complex I deficient neurons, the aggregation of alpha-synuclein did not worsen the phenotype, and neurons did not undergo an increased rate of cell death [84]. Human neuropathological studies reveal that Lewy pathology is significantly less prevalent in complex I deficient in SNpc neurons [73], and in fact alpha-synuclein inclusions in neurons are present in neurons demonstrating high expression levels of mitochondrial respiratory chain proteins [85].

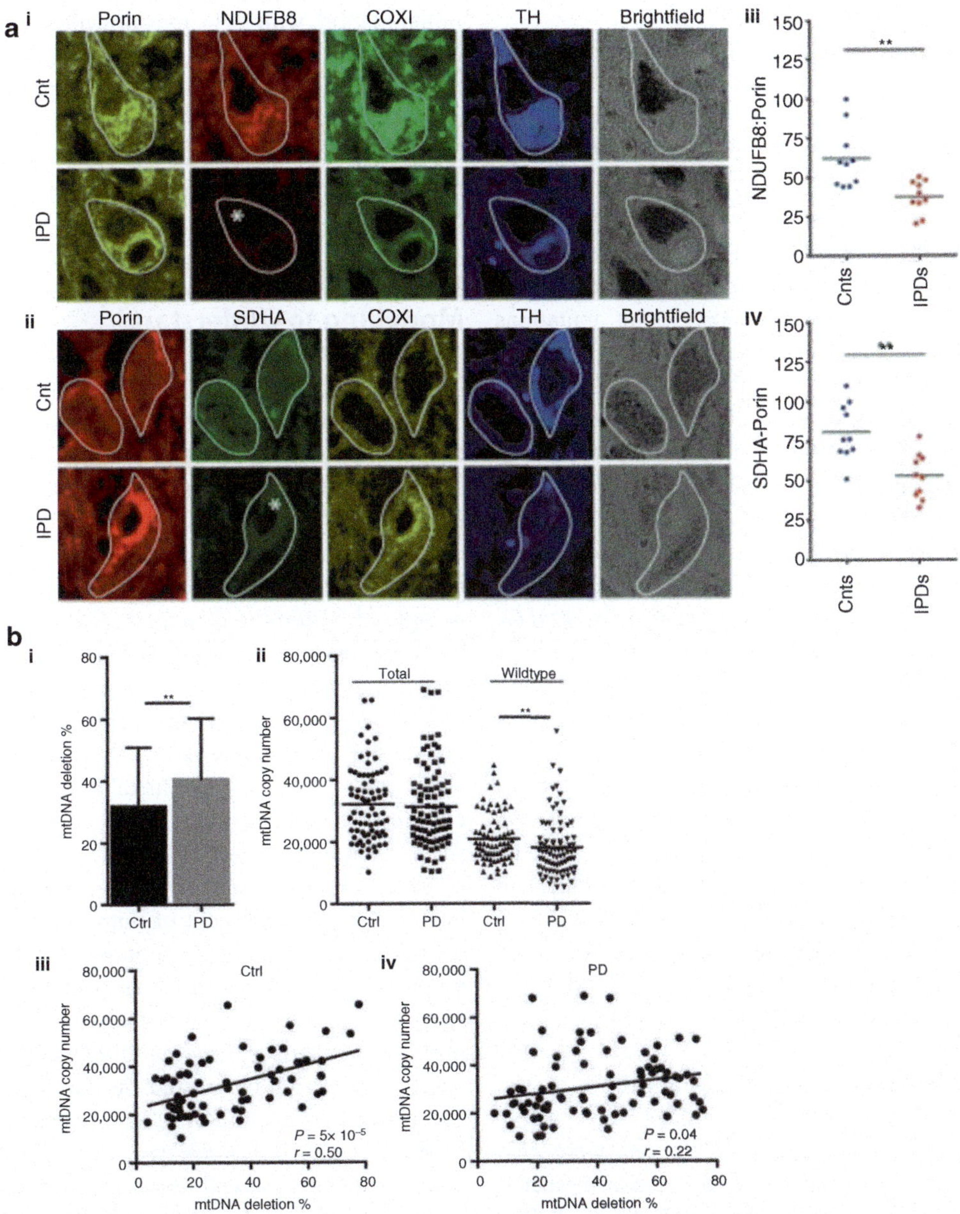

Fig. 1 Mitochondrial respiratory chain defects and impaired mtDNA maintenance in dopaminergic SNpc neurons in IPD. The abundances of subunits of respiratory chain complexes I and II are downregulated despite maintenance of mitochondrial mass in dopaminergic SNpc neurons from IPD patients relative to controls (Cnt) (**a**). Epifluorescence microscopy following quadruple-label immunofluorescence indicated reduced levels of complex I subunit NDUFB8 (i) and complex II subunit SDHA (ii) in IPD neurons and which densitometric analysis confirmed a significant decrease in NDUFB8:porin (iii, $P < 0.01$) and SDHA:porin (iv, $P < 0.01$) ratios in IPD neurons (Adapted from Grunewald et al., Ann Neurol., 2016). Molecular analyses of single dopaminergic SNpc neurons from individuals with IPD ($n = 84$ neurons from 10 individuals) and age-matched controls ($n = 74$ neurons from 10 individuals) reveal changes in mtDNA quality and quantity (**b**). The levels of mtDNA deletion are significantly higher in IPD compared with controls (i, $P = 0.004$; Mann–Whitney *U* test). Error bars show s.d. Total mtDNA copy number is similar in IPD and controls, but the levels of wild-type mtDNA are significantly decreased in IPD (ii, $P = 0.006$; Mann–Whitney *U* test). Bars show mean. Linear regression analysis of neuronal mtDNA copy number plotted against deletion levels reveals that the correlation between mtDNA copy number and deletion is poor in IPD (iv, $P = 0.04$, $r = 0.22$) compared with controls (iii, $P = 5 \times 10^{-5}$, $r = 0.50$; Pearson correlation) (Adapted from Dolle et al., Nature Comm, 2018)

Parkinsonism-Related Neuropathology in Mitochondrial Disease

Primary Mitochondrial Disorders

A neuropathological investigation of the SNpc was performed in six adult patients with primary mtDNA disease (two patients with each of the m.3243A>G and m.8344A>G point mutations and two patients with single, large-scale mtDNA deletions) and five patients with biallelic *POLG* mutations. All those with mtDNA mutations showed no features of Parkinsonism, while one with *POLG* mutations did show Parkinsonism. No alpha-synuclein pathology was seen in the SNpc in patients harbouring primary mtDNA mutations, but LBs, neurites and cytoplasmic granular staining were detected in 2/5 patients with *POLG*-related disease. High levels of neuronal complex I deficiencies were detected in patients harbouring a single large-scale mtDNA deletion and in patients harbouring *POLG* mutations and m.8344A>G mutation, while those patients with the common m.3243A>G mutation had complex I deficiencies comparable to control neurons. The level of complex I deficiency did not correlate with either SNpc cell loss or accumulation of alpha-synuclein pathology which was similar to that observed in IPD SNpc neurons [73, 86].

POLG-Related Encephalopathies

In a recent study, mtDNA deletions were also found in single-laser capture microdissected SNpc neurons from patients harbouring *POLG* mutations that were very similar to those seen in IPD implying a shared mechanism for the formation of mtDNA deletions [85]. Neuropathological assessment of patients harbouring *POLG* and *TWNK* (*C10orf2*) mutations revealed extensive neuronal loss without alpha-synuclein or LBs within SNpc neurons, while surviving neurons demonstrated a preferential complex I deficiency [36]. Another study of patients with *POLG* mutations demonstrated severe nigrostriatal degeneration accompanied by astrogliosis and inflammation with selective downregulation of complex I subunits and decreased mtDNA in remaining neurons [87]. In both studies, the degree of nigrostriatal degeneration did not correlate with clinical signs of Parkinsonism suggesting that other pathological mechanisms contribute to the development of symptoms.

Modelling to Understand Mechanisms

The idea that complex I deficiency within the SNpc might play a central role in the pathogenesis of IPD spurred the generation of a mouse model which featured selective knock out of complex I subunit NDUFS4 in dopaminergic neurons. In this mouse model, the inactivation of complex I within the dopaminergic neurons was not sufficient to cause a Parkinsonism phenotype or degeneration of the SNpc neurons. However this mouse did reveal changes in dopamine metabolism, with impaired dopamine release and high levels of dopamine metabolites. Primary cultures of neurons taken from this mouse showed a sensitivity to MPTP [88].

The MitoPark mouse is a dopaminergic neuron-specific knock out of mitochondrial transcription factor A (TFAM), a protein essential for mtDNA expression and maintenance, which provides genetic evidence that primary mitochondrial respiratory chain defects within dopaminergic neurons result in Parkinsonism-like phenotype. The mice have an adult-onset neurodegeneration, progressive clinical course, earlier onset and more severe and extensive cell death in the SNpc, with responsiveness to L-DOPA [89, 90]. There was no recruitment of parkin to mtDNA-depleted mitochondria in dopaminergic neurons [91].

Finally, the PD-mito-pst1 mouse model shows similar behavioural and biochemical phenotype to the MitoPark mouse. This mouse model is generated by the expression of a mitochondrial-targeted endonuclease, known as mito-pst1 which induced double-strand breaks in dopaminergic neurons. The formation of rearranged and depleted mtDNA causes respiratory chain deficiencies and perturbed mitochondrial membrane potential with dopaminergic neurons. The mice show a slower progression than that of the MitoPark mice; approximately 60% of SNpc neurons are lost by 9 months of age; and the onset of motor symptoms precedes degeneration of the SNpc neurons suggesting dopaminergic axonal loss and dopamine depletion in the striatum [92].

Neurodegenerative Changes Associated with Cognitive Impairment

Although cognitive decline is a recognised symptom in patients with mitochondrial disease, there is a paucity of clinical studies systematically reviewing cognitive impairments in these patients. This may be because cognitive decline and dementia often occur together with multiple neurological deficits, including stroke-like episodes (Fig. 2a), epilepsy and cerebellar ataxia, reflecting the multifaceted aetiology of mitochondrial disease, and the emergence of certain symptoms, such as seizures, may worsen cognition. Cognitive impairment is a feature of *POLG*-related disease and progressively worsens as the atrophy and necrotic lesions accumulate. In a study of patients with *POLG* mutations before they had developed the aggressive form of the disease, cognitive testing using intelligence test (WAIS), memory tests and a comprehensive neuropsychological test battery showed significant cognitive dysfunction [93]. Their mean verbal IQ (84.3) was significantly better than performance IQ (71.8) ($t = 5.23$, $P = 0.001$).

One of the major distinctions between mitochondrial disease and other neurodegenerative disorders associated with dementia has been the absence of protein inclusions or aggregates. These are often considered the neuropathological hallmarks of neurodegenerative disease. The accumulation of amyloid has, however, been found in an experimental model of a rare mitochondrial disease caused by mutations in the pitrilysin metallopeptidase 1 (PITRM1). This protease is thought to degrade the signal peptides of proteins imported into mitochondria, and mutation in the gene was associated with an early-onset disorder with cognitive problems, ataxia and psychiatric features [94]. Mice with a knockout of this gene on one allele showed the accumulation of amyloid beta gradually in the

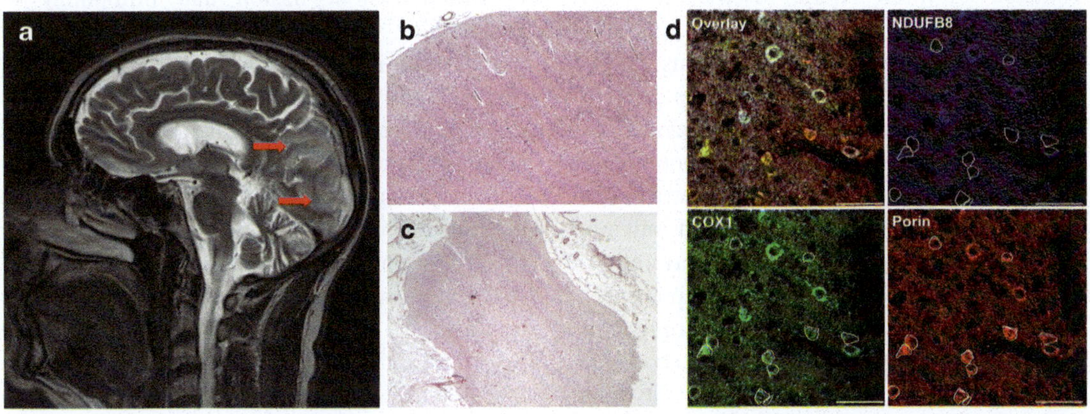

Fig. 2 Neurodegeneration in primary mitochondrial disorders are characterised by neuronal respiratory chain impairments, neuronal cell loss and formation of necrotic lesions throughout the CNS. T2 sagittal MRI head shows stroke-like lesions involving occipital and parietal lobes, generalised cerebral and cerebellar atrophy in a patient who harbours the m.3243A>G mutation (**a**). Neuronal cell loss ranging from diffuse neuronal dropout from cortical layers (**b**, ×4 magnification) to extensive neuronal cell loss within focal necrotic lesions affecting the cortical ribbon (**c**, ×2 magnification) in patients harbouring the m.3243A>G mutation. A mosaic pattern of mitochondrial respiratory chain complex I subunit NDUFB8 expression is observed in neurons in occipital cortex in patients harbouring the m.3243A>G mutation (**d**). Outlined neurons show downregulated NDUFB8 expression with varying levels of complex IV subunit COX1 expression and preserved mitochondrial mass (porin). Scale bar = 100 μm

brain. Whether this is also true of the human disease, and what Aβ is doing inside mitochondria, has yet to be established, but this at least points to a potential link between abnormal protein accumulation and mitochondrial dysfunction.

The most common neuropathological findings in patients with mitochondrial disease are brain atrophy, neuronal cell loss, focal necrosis affecting the neocortex and cerebellar cortex, presence of mitochondrial respiratory chain deficiencies in surviving neurons and astrogliosis. There are two processes that contribute to these neuropathological features in mitochondrial disease: (1) chronic neurodegenerative processes with the gradual attrition of neurons and atrophy of the cerebrum and cerebellum (Fig. 2b) and (2) acute neurodegenerative processes with the development of necrotic foci within the cortex throughout the brain (Fig. 2c) which are often identified as T2-weighted hyperintensities on MRI (Fig. 2a). It is likely that deterioration in cognition may be attributed to both pathways which impinge on neural network activity and connectivity throughout the brain.

The appearance of multiple, large foci of neuronal necrosis affecting the neocortex and cerebellum is a common neuropathological finding in patients with mitochondrial disease, particularly in those harbouring the m.3243A>G mutation in *MT-TL* and biallelic *POLG* mutations [95–97]. These areas of chronic degeneration are ischaemic-like in appearance with evidence of almost complete neuronal cell dropout, microvacuolation of the neuropil and subcortical white matter and increased astrogliosis and inflammation. It is certainly feasible that deterioration in cognition might be attributed to the presence of necrotic foci which encroach on multiple neuronal circuits involved in cognitive processing. Adjacent normal-appearing cortex typically shows a mosaic pattern of mitochondrial respiratory chain subunit expression, and predominantly neurons show downregulation of subunits of complex I (Fig. 2d).

Recent neuropathological studies have shown changes in neuronal populations in patients affected by either mtDNA or nDNA mutations which could contribute to cognitive dysfunction in mitochondrial disease. A loss of calbindin-positive neurons from the hippocampal without neuronal loss has been described and also loss of cortical inhibitory interneurons and complex I and IV deficiencies in surviving interneurons which could certainly contribute to impaired network activity in the brain [98, 99].

Conclusions

Parkinsonism typically develops after the manifestation of CPEO or other complex neurological phenotypes in mitochondrial disorders due to nuclear defects of mtDNA maintenance. Multiple mtDNA deletions and mitochondrial complex I deficiency are present in both groups of idiopathic Parkinson's disease and mitochondrial genetic disorders manifesting with Parkinsonism, suggesting mitochondrial dysfunction is a shared common pathway of dopaminergic neuronal death. Furthermore, the discovery of causal genetic defects in familial Parkinsonism and other inherited neurodegenerative disorders, such as Charcot-Marie-Tooth neuropathy and dominant optic atrophy, have demonstrated the importance of balanced mitochondrial fusion, fission and mitophagy in maintaining neuronal functions. Cognitive impairment is multifactorial in mitochondrial diseases and is challenging to study clinically due to the presence of other neurological deficits such as stroke-like episodes, epilepsy and cerebellar dysfunction, which all can contribute to neurodegeneration. Better elucidation of mtDNA homoeostasis and mitochondrial quality control will be crucial in developing new treatment strategies for primary mitochondrial disorders and a wide array of neurodegenerative diseases in future.

References

1. de Lau LM, Breteler MM. Epidemiology of Parkinson's disease. Lancet Neurol. 2006;5(6):525–35.
2. Langston JW, Ballard P, Tetrud JW, Irwin I. Chronic parkinsonism in humans due to a product of meperidine-analog synthesis. Science. 1983;219(4587):979–80.

3. Betarbet R, Sherer TB, MacKenzie G, Garcia-Osuna M, Panov AV, Greenamyre JT. Chronic systemic pesticide exposure reproduces features of Parkinson's disease. Nat Neurosci. 2000;3(12):1301–6.
4. Ikebe S, Tanaka M, Ohno K, Sato W, Hattori K, Kondo T, Mizuno Y, Ozawa T. Increase of deleted mitochondrial DNA in the striatum in Parkinson's disease and senescence. Biochem Biophys Res Commun. 1990;170(3):1044–8.
5. Luoma P, Melberg A, Rinne JO, Kaukonen JA, Nupponen NN, Chalmers RM, Oldfors A, Rautakorpi I, Peltonen L, Majamaa K, Somer H, Suomalainen A. Parkinsonism, premature menopause, and mitochondrial DNA polymerase gamma mutations: clinical and molecular genetic study. Lancet. 2004;364(9437):875–82.
6. Davidzon G, Greene P, Mancuso M, Klos KJ, Ahlskog JE, Hirano M, DiMauro S. Early-onset familial parkinsonism due to pol γ mutations. Ann Neurol. 2006;59(5):859–62.
7. Mancuso M, Filosto M, Oh SJ, DiMauro S. A novel polymerase gamma mutation in a family with ophthalmoplegia, neuropathy, and Parkinsonism. Arch Neurol. 2004;61(11):1777–9.
8. Remes AM, Hinttala R, Kärppä M, Soini H, Takalo R, Uusimaa J, Majamaa K. Parkinsonism associated with the homozygous W748S mutation in the pol γ1 gene. Parkinsonism Relat Disord. 2008;14(8):652–4.
9. Giannoccaro MP, La Morgia C, Rizzo G, Carelli V. Mitochondrial DNA and primary mitochondrial dysfunction in Parkinson's disease. Mov Disord. 2017;32(3):346–63.
10. Alston CL, Rocha MC, Lax NZ, Turnbull DM, Taylor RW. The genetics and pathology of mitochondrial disease. J Pathol. 2017;241(2):236–50.
11. Gorman GS, Chinnery PF, DiMauro S, Hirano M, Koga Y, McFarland R, Suomalainen A, Thorburn DR, Zeviani M, Turnbull DM. Mitochondrial diseases. Nat Rev Dis Primers. 2016;2:16080.
12. Lightowlers RN, Taylor RW, Turnbull DM. Mutations causing mitochondrial disease: what is new and what challenges remain? Science. 2015;349(6255):1494–9.
13. McFarland R, Taylor RW, Turnbull DM. A neurological perspective on mitochondrial disease. Lancet Neurol. 2010;9(8):829–40.
14. Chinnery PF, DiMauro S, Shanske S, Schon EA, Zeviani M, Mariotti C, Carrara F, Lombes A, Laforet P, Ogier H, Jaksch M, Lochmüller H, Horvath R, Deschauer M, Thorburn DR, Bindoff LA, Poulton J, Taylor RW, Matthews JNS, Turnbull DM. Risk of developing a mitochondrial DNA deletion disorder. Lancet. 2004;364(9434):592–6.
15. Sallevelt SC, de Die-Smulders CE, Hendrickx AT, Hellebrekers DM, de Coo IF, Alston CL, Knowles C, Taylor RW, McFarland R, Smeets HJ. De novo mtDNA point mutations are common and have a low recurrence risk. J Med Genet. 2017;54(2):73–83.
16. Gorman GS, Schaefer AM, Ng Y, Gomez N, Blakely EL, Alston CL, Feeney C, Horvath R, Yu-Wai-Man P, Chinnery PF, Taylor RW, Turnbull DM, McFarland R. Prevalence of nuclear and mitochondrial DNA mutations related to adult mitochondrial disease. Ann Neurol. 2015;77(5):753–9.
17. Wallace DC, Singh G, Lott MT, Hodge JA, Schurr TG, Lezza AM, Elsas LJ 2nd, Nikoskelainen EK, Mitochondrial DNA. Mutation associated with Leber's hereditary optic neuropathy. Science. 1988;242(4884):1427–30.
18. Holt IJ, Harding AE, Morgan-Hughes JA. Deletions of muscle mitochondrial DNA in patients with mitochondrial myopathies. Nature. 1988;331(6158):717–9.
19. Simon DK, Pulst SM, Sutton JP, Browne SE, Beal MF, Johns DR. Familial multisystem degeneration with parkinsonism associated with the 11778 mitochondrial DNA mutation. Neurology. 1999;53(8):1787–93.
20. Nikoskelainen EK, Marttila RJ, Huoponen K, Juvonen V, Lamminen T, Sonninen P, Savontaus ML. Leber's "plus": neurological abnormalities in patients with Leber's hereditary optic neuropathy. J Neurol Neurosurg Psychiatry. 1995;59(2):160–4.
21. De Coo IF, Renier WO, Ruitenbeek W, Ter Laak HJ, Bakker M, Schagger H, Van Oost BA, Smeets HJ. A 4-base pair deletion in the mitochondrial cytochrome b gene associated with parkinsonism/MELAS overlap syndrome. Ann Neurol. 1999;45(1):130–3.
22. Horvath R, Kley RA, Lochmuller H, Vorgerd M. Parkinson syndrome, neuropathy, and myopathy caused by the mutation A8344G (MERRF) in tRNALys. Neurology. 2007;68(1):56–8.
23. Nesbitt V, Pitceathly RDS, Turnbull DM, Taylor RW, Sweeney MG, Mudanohwo EE, Rahman S, Hanna MG, McFarland R. The UK MRC Mitochondrial disease patient cohort study: clinical phenotypes associated with the m.3243A>G mutation—implications for diagnosis and management. J Neurol Neurosurg Psychiatry. 2013;84(8):936–8.
24. Mancuso M, Orsucci D, Angelini C, Bertini E, Carelli V, Comi GP, Donati A, Minetti C, Moggio M, Mongini T, Servidei S, Tonin P, Toscano A, Uziel G, Bruno C, Ienco EC, Filosto M, Lamperti C, Catteruccia M, Moroni I, Musumeci O, Pegoraro E, Ronchi D, Santorelli FM, Sauchelli D, Scarpelli M, Sciacco M, Valentino ML, Vercelli L, Zeviani M, Siciliano G. The m.3243A>G mitochondrial DNA mutation and related phenotypes. A matter of gender? J Neurol. 2014;261:504–10.
25. Mancuso M, Orsucci D, Angelini C, Bertini E, Carelli V, Comi GP, Minetti C, Moggio M, Mongini T, Servidei S, Tonin P, Toscano A, Uziel G, Bruno C, Caldarazzo Ienco E, Filosto M, Lamperti C, Martinelli D, Moroni I, Musumeci O, Pegoraro E, Ronchi D, Santorelli FM, Sauchelli D, Scarpelli M, Sciacco M, Spinazzi M, Valentino ML, Vercelli L, Zeviani M, Siciliano G. Phenotypic heterogeneity of the 8344A>G mtDNA "MERRF" mutation. Neurology. 2013;80(22):2049–54.
26. Mancuso M, Nesti C, Petrozzi L, Orsucci D, Frosini D, Kiferle L, Bonuccelli U, Ceravolo R, Murri L, Siciliano G. The mtDNA A8344G "MERRF" mutation is not a common cause of sporadic Parkinson

disease in Italian population. Parkinsonism Relat Disord. 2008;14(4):381–2.
27. Dolle C, Flones I, Nido GS, Miletic H, Osuagwu N, Kristoffersen S, Lilleng PK, Larsen JP, Tysnes OB, Haugarvoll K, Bindoff LA, Tzoulis C. Defective mitochondrial DNA homeostasis in the substantia nigra in Parkinson disease. Nat Commun. 2016;7:13548.
28. Cohen BH, Chinnery PF, Copeland WC. pol γ-related disorders. 2010 Mar 16 [Updated 2014 Dec 18]. In: Pagon RA, Adam MP, Ardinger HH, et al., editors. GeneReviews® [Internet]. Seattle, WA: University of Washington, Seattle; 1993–2016. Available from: http://www.ncbi.nlm.nih.gov/books/NBK26471/.
29. Martikainen MH, Ng YS, Gorman GS, Alston CL, Blakely EL, Schaefer AM, Chinnery PF, Burn DJ, Taylor RW, McFarland R, Turnbull DM. Clinical, genetic, and radiological features of extrapyramidal movement disorders in mitochondrial disease. JAMA Neurol. 2016;73(6):668–74.
30. Tzoulis C, Schwarzlmuller T, Biermann M, Haugarvoll K, Bindoff LA. Mitochondrial DNA homeostasis is essential for nigrostriatal integrity. Mitochondrion. 2016;28:33–7.
31. Spelbrink JN, Li FY, Tiranti V, Nikali K, Yuan QP, Tariq M, Wanrooij S, Garrido N, Comi G, Morandi L, Santoro L, Toscano A, Fabrizi GM, Somer H, Croxen R, Beeson D, Poulton J, Suomalainen A, Jacobs HT, Zeviani M, Larsson C. Human mitochondrial DNA deletions associated with mutations in the gene encoding twinkle, a phage T7 gene 4-like protein localized in mitochondria. Nat Genet. 2001;28(3):223–31.
32. Fratter C, Gorman GS, Stewart JD, Buddles M, Smith C, Evans J, Seller A, Poulton J, Roberts M, Hanna MG, Rahman S, Omer SE, Klopstock T, Schoser B, Kornblum C, Czermin B, Lecky B, Blakely EL, Craig K, Chinnery PF, Turnbull DM, Horvath R, Taylor RW. The clinical, histochemical, and molecular spectrum of PEO1 (Twinkle)-linked adPEO. Neurology. 2010;74(20):1619–26.
33. Baloh RH, Salavaggione E, Milbrandt J, Pestronk A. Familial parkinsonism and ophthalmoplegia from a mutation in the mitochondrial DNA helicase twinkle. Arch Neurol. 2007;64(7):998–1000.
34. Kiferle L, Orsucci D, Mancuso M, Lo Gerfo A, Petrozzi L, Siciliano G, Ceravolo R, Bonuccelli U. Twinkle mutation in an Italian family with external progressive ophthalmoplegia and parkinsonism: a case report and an update on the state of art. Neurosci Lett. 2013;556:1–4.
35. Brandon BR, Diederich NJ, Soni M, Witte K, Weinhold M, Krause M, Jackson S. Autosomal dominant mutations in pol γ and C10orf2: association with late onset chronic progressive external ophthalmoplegia and Parkinsonism in two patients. J Neurol. 2013;260(7):1931–3.
36. Palin EJ, Paetau A, Suomalainen A. Mesencephalic complex I deficiency does not correlate with parkinsonism in mitochondrial DNA maintenance disorders. Brain. 2013;136(Pt 8):2379–92.
37. Palin EJH, Hakonen AH, Korpela M, Paetau A, Suomalainen A. Mitochondrial recessive ataxia syndrome mimicking dominant spinocerebellar ataxia. J Neurol Sci. 2012;315(1–2):160–3.
38. Detmer SA, Chan DC. Functions and dysfunctions of mitochondrial dynamics. Nat Rev Mol Cell Biol. 2007;8(11):870–9.
39. Archer SL. Mitochondrial dynamics—Mitochondrial fission and fusion in human diseases. N Engl J Med. 2013;369(23):2236–51.
40. Burte F, Carelli V, Chinnery PF, Yu-Wai-Man P. Disturbed mitochondrial dynamics and neurodegenerative disorders. Nat Rev Neurol. 2015;11(1):11–24.
41. Twig G, Elorza A, Molina AJ, Mohamed H, Wikstrom JD, Walzer G, Stiles L, Haigh SE, Katz S, Las G, Alroy J, Wu M, Py BF, Yuan J, Deeney JT, Corkey BE, Shirihai OS. Fission and selective fusion govern mitochondrial segregation and elimination by autophagy. EMBO J. 2008;27(2):433–46.
42. Yu-Wai-Man P, Votruba M, Moore AT, Chinnery PF. Treatment strategies for inherited optic neuropathies: past, present and future. Eye (Lond). 2014;28(5):521–37.
43. Amati-Bonneau P, Valentino ML, Reynier P, Gallardo ME, Bornstein B, Boissiere A, Campos Y, Rivera H, de la Aleja JG, Carroccia R, Iommarini L, Labauge P, Figarella-Branger D, Marcorelles P, Furby A, Beauvais K, Letournel F, Liguori R, La Morgia C, Montagna P, Liguori M, Zanna C, Rugolo M, Cossarizza A, Wissinger B, Verny C, Schwarzenbacher R, Martin MA, Arenas J, Ayuso C, Garesse R, Lenaers G, Bonneau D, Carelli V. OPA1 mutations induce mitochondrial DNA instability and optic atrophy 'plus' phenotypes. Brain. 2008;131(Pt 2):338–51.
44. Yu-Wai-Man P, Griffiths PG, Gorman GS, Lourenco CM, Wright AF, Auer-Grumbach M, Toscano A, Musumeci O, Valentino ML, Caporali L, Lamperti C, Tallaksen CM, Duffey P, Miller J, Whittaker RG, Baker MR, Jackson MJ, Clarke MP, Dhillon B, Czermin B, Stewart JD, Hudson G, Reynier P, Bonneau D, Marques W, Lenaers G, McFarland R, Taylor RW, Turnbull DM, Votruba M, Zeviani M, Carelli V, Bindoff LA, Horvath R, Amati-Bonneau P, Chinnery PF. Multi-system neurological disease is common in patients with OPA1 mutations. Brain. 2010;133(3):771–86.
45. Hudson G, Amati-Bonneau P, Blakely EL, Stewart JD, He L, Schaefer AM, Griffiths PG, Ahlqvist K, Suomalainen A, Reynier P, McFarland R, Turnbull DM, Chinnery PF, Taylor RW. Mutation of OPA1 causes dominant optic atrophy with external ophthalmoplegia, ataxia, deafness and multiple mitochondrial DNA deletions: a novel disorder of mtDNA maintenance. Brain. 2008;131(Pt 2):329–37.
46. Yu-Wai-Man P, Spyropoulos A, Duncan HJ, Guadagno JV, Chinnery PF. A multiple sclerosis-like disorder in patients with OPA1 mutations. Ann Clin Transl Neurol. 2016;3(9):723–9.
47. Yu-Wai-Man P, Sitarz KS, Samuels DC, Griffiths PG, Reeve AK, Bindoff LA, Horvath R, Chinnery

PF. OPA1 mutations cause cytochrome c oxidase deficiency due to loss of wild-type mtDNA molecules. Hum Mol Genet. 2010;19(15):3043–52.
48. Carelli V, Musumeci O, Caporali L, Zanna C, La Morgia C, Del Dotto V, Porcelli AM, Rugolo M, Valentino ML, Iommarini L, Maresca A, Barboni P, Carbonelli M, Trombetta C, Valente EM, Patergnani S, Giorgi C, Pinton P, Rizzo G, Tonon C, Lodi R, Avoni P, Liguori R, Baruzzi A, Toscano A, Zeviani M. Syndromic parkinsonism and dementia associated with OPA1 missense mutations. Ann Neurol. 2015;78(1):21–38.
49. Lynch DS, Loh SHY, Harley J, Noyce AJ, Martins LM, Wood NW, Houlden H, Plun-Favreau H. Nonsyndromic Parkinson disease in a family with autosomal dominant optic atrophy due to OPA1 mutations. Neurol Genet. 2017;3(5):e188.
50. Jonikas M, Madill M, Mathy A, Zekoll T, Zois CE, Wigfield S, Kurzawa-Akanbi M, Browne C, Sims D, Chinnery PF, Cowley SA, Tofaris GK. Stem cell modeling of mitochondrial Parkinsonism reveals key functions of OPA1. Ann Neurol. 2018;83(5):915–25.
51. Atorino L, Silvestri L, Koppen M, Cassina L, Ballabio A, Marconi R, Langer T, Casari G. Loss of m-AAA protease in mitochondria causes complex I deficiency and increased sensitivity to oxidative stress in hereditary spastic paraplegia. J Cell Biol. 2003;163(4):777–87.
52. Koppen M, Metodiev MD, Casari G, Rugarli EI, Langer T. Variable and tissue-specific subunit composition of mitochondrial m-AAA protease complexes linked to hereditary spastic paraplegia. Mol Cell Biol. 2007;27(2):758–67.
53. Gorman GS, Pfeffer G, Griffin H, Blakely EL, Kurzawa-Akanbi M, Gabriel J, Sitarz K, Roberts M, Schoser B, Pyle A, Schaefer AM, McFarland R, Turnbull DM, Horvath R, Chinnery PF, Taylor RW. Clonal expansion of secondary mitochondrial DNA deletions associated with spinocerebellar ataxia type 28. JAMA Neurol. 2015;72(1):106–11.
54. Pfeffer G, Pyle A, Griffin H, Miller J, Wilson V, Turnbull L, Fawcett K, Sims D, Eglon G, Hadjivassiliou M, Horvath R, Nemeth A, Chinnery PF. SPG7 mutations are a common cause of undiagnosed ataxia. Neurology. 2015;84(11):1174–6.
55. Choquet K, Tetreault M, Yang S, La Piana R, Dicaire MJ, Vanstone MR, Mathieu J, Bouchard JP, Rioux MF, Rouleau GA, Boycott KM, Majewski J, Brais B. SPG7 mutations explain a significant proportion of French Canadian spastic ataxia cases. Eur J Hum Genet. 2016;24(7):1016–21.
56. Wedding IM, Koht J, Tran GT, Misceo D, Selmer KK, Holmgren A, Frengen E, Bindoff L, Tallaksen CM, Tzoulis C. Spastic paraplegia type 7 is associated with multiple mitochondrial DNA deletions. PLoS One. 2014;9(1):e86340.
57. Pedroso JL, Vale TC, Bueno FL, Marussi VHR, Amaral L, Franca MC Jr, Barsottini OG. SPG7 with parkinsonism responsive to levodopa and dopaminergic deficit. Parkinsonism Relat Disord. 2018;47:88–90.
58. Larsen SB, Hanss Z, Kruger R. The genetic architecture of mitochondrial dysfunction in Parkinson's disease. Cell Tissue Res. 2018;373(1):21–37.
59. Youle RJ, Narendra DP. Mechanisms of mitophagy. Nat Rev Mol Cell Biol. 2011;12(1):9–14.
60. Matsumine H, Saito M, Shimoda-Matsubayashi S, Tanaka H, Ishikawa A, Nakagawa-Hattori Y, Yokochi M, Kobayashi T, Igarashi S, Takano H, Sanpei K, Koike R, Mori H, Kondo T, Mizutani Y, Schaffer AA, Yamamura Y, Nakamura S, Kuzuhara S, Tsuji S, Mizuno Y. Localization of a gene for an autosomal recessive form of juvenile Parkinsonism to chromosome 6q25.2-27. Am J Hum Genet. 1997;60(3):588–96.
61. Valente EM, Bentivoglio AR, Dixon PH, Ferraris A, Ialongo T, Frontali M, Albanese A, Wood NW. Localization of a novel locus for autosomal recessive early-onset parkinsonism, PARK6, on human chromosome 1p35-p36. Am J Hum Genet. 2001;68(4):895–900.
62. Valente EM, Abou-Sleiman PM, Caputo V, Muqit MM, Harvey K, Gispert S, Ali Z, Del Turco D, Bentivoglio AR, Healy DG, Albanese A, Nussbaum R, Gonzalez-Maldonado R, Deller T, Salvi S, Cortelli P, Gilks WP, Latchman DS, Harvey RJ, Dallapiccola B, Auburger G, Wood NW. Hereditary early-onset Parkinson's disease caused by mutations in PINK1. Science. 2004;304(5674):1158–60.
63. Park J, Lee SB, Lee S, Kim Y, Song S, Kim S, Bae E, Kim J, Shong M, Kim JM, Chung J. Mitochondrial dysfunction in Drosophila PINK1 mutants is complemented by parkin. Nature. 2006;441(7097):1157–61.
64. Clark IE, Dodson MW, Jiang C, Cao JH, Huh JR, Seol JH, Yoo SJ, Hay BA, Guo M. Drosophila pink1 is required for mitochondrial function and interacts genetically with parkin. Nature. 2006;441(7097):1162–6.
65. Mortiboys H, Thomas KJ, Koopman WJ, Klaffke S, Abou-Sleiman P, Olpin S, Wood NW, Willems PH, Smeitink JA, Cookson MR, Bandmann O. Mitochondrial function and morphology are impaired in parkin-mutant fibroblasts. Ann Neurol. 2008;64(5):555–65.
66. Rakovic A, Grunewald A, Seibler P, Ramirez A, Kock N, Orolicki S, Lohmann K, Klein C. Effect of endogenous mutant and wild-type PINK1 on Parkin in fibroblasts from Parkinson disease patients. Hum Mol Genet. 2010;19(16):3124–37.
67. Fearnley JM, Lees AJ. Ageing and Parkinson's disease: substantia nigra regional selectivity. Brain. 1991;114(Pt 5):2283–301.
68. Ma SY, Roytta M, Rinne JO, Collan Y, Rinne UK. Correlation between neuromorphometry in the substantia nigra and clinical features in Parkinson's disease using disector counts. J Neurol Sci. 1997;151(1):83–7.
69. Langston JW, Ballard PA Jr. Parkinson's disease in a chemist working with 1-methyl-4-phenyl-1,2,5,6-tetrahydropyridine. N Engl J Med. 1983;309(5):310.

70. Mizuno Y, Ohta S, Tanaka M, Takamiya S, Suzuki K, Sato T, Oya H, Ozawa T, Kagawa Y. Deficiencies in complex I subunits of the respiratory chain in Parkinson's disease. Biochem Biophys Res Commun. 1989;163(3):1450–5.
71. Hattori N, Tanaka M, Ozawa T, Mizuno Y. Immunohistochemical studies on complexes I, II, III, and IV of mitochondria in Parkinson's disease. Ann Neurol. 1991;30(4):563–71.
72. Bender A, Krishnan KJ, Morris CM, Taylor GA, Reeve AK, Perry RH, Jaros E, Hersheson JS, Betts J, Klopstock T, Taylor RW, Turnbull DM. High levels of mitochondrial DNA deletions in substantia nigra neurons in aging and Parkinson disease. Nat Genet. 2006;38(5):515–7.
73. Flones IH, Fernandez-Vizarra E, Lykouri M, Brakedal B, Skeie GO, Miletic H, Lilleng PK, Alves G, Tysnes OB, Haugarvoll K, Dolle C, Zeviani M, Tzoulis C. Neuronal complex I deficiency occurs throughout the Parkinson's disease brain, but is not associated with neurodegeneration or mitochondrial DNA damage. Acta Neuropathol. 2018;135(3):409–25.
74. Ozawa T, Tanaka M, Ikebe S, Ohno K, Kondo T, Mizuno Y. Quantitative determination of deleted mitochondrial DNA relative to normal DNA in parkinsonian striatum by a kinetic PCR analysis. Biochem Biophys Res Commun. 1990;172(2):483–9.
75. Soong NW, Hinton DR, Cortopassi G, Arnheim N. Mosaicism for a specific somatic mitochondrial DNA mutation in adult human brain. Nat Genet. 1992;2(4):318–23.
76. Kraytsberg Y, Kudryavtseva E, McKee AC, Geula C, Kowall NW, Khrapko K. Mitochondrial DNA deletions are abundant and cause functional impairment in aged human substantia nigra neurons. Nat Genet. 2006;38(5):518–20.
77. Nido GS, Dolle C, Flones I, Tuppen HA, Alves G, Tysnes OB, Haugarvoll K, Tzoulis C. Ultradeep mapping of neuronal mitochondrial deletions in Parkinson's disease. Neurobiol Aging. 2018;63:120–7.
78. Bender A, Schwarzkopf RM, McMillan A, Krishnan KJ, Rieder G, Neumann M, Elstner M, Turnbull DM, Klopstock T. Dopaminergic midbrain neurons are the prime target for mitochondrial DNA deletions. J Neurol. 2008;255(8):1231–5.
79. Reeve AK, Krishnan KJ, Elson JL, Morris CM, Bender A, Lightowlers RN, Turnbull DM. Nature of mitochondrial DNA deletions in substantia nigra neurons. Am J Hum Genet. 2008;82(1):228–35.
80. Krishnan KJ, Reeve AK, Samuels DC, Chinnery PF, Blackwood JK, Taylor RW, Wanrooij S, Spelbrink JN, Lightowlers RN, Turnbull DM. What causes mitochondrial DNA deletions in human cells? Nat Genet. 2008;40(3):275–9.
81. Shoffner JM, Lott MT, Voljavec AS, Soueidan SA, Costigan DA, Wallace DC. Spontaneous Kearns-Sayre/chronic external ophthalmoplegia plus syndrome associated with a mitochondrial DNA deletion: a slip-replication model and metabolic therapy. Proc Natl Acad Sci U S A. 1989;86(20):7952–6.
82. Reeve AK, Krishnan KJ, Taylor G, Elson JL, Bender A, Taylor RW, Morris CM, Turnbull DM. The low abundance of clonally expanded mitochondrial DNA point mutations in aged substantia nigra neurons. Aging Cell. 2009;8(4):496–8.
83. Grunewald A, Rygiel KA, Hepplewhite PD, Morris CM, Picard M, Turnbull DM. Mitochondrial DNA depletion in respiratory chain-deficient Parkinson disease neurons. Ann Neurol. 2016;79(3):366–78.
84. Reeve AK, Ludtmann MH, Angelova PR, Simcox EM, Horrocks MH, Klenerman D, Gandhi S, Turnbull DM, Abramov AY. Aggregated alpha-synuclein and complex I deficiency: exploration of their relationship in differentiated neurons. Cell Death Dis. 2015;6:e1820.
85. Reeve AK, Park TK, Jaros E, Campbell GR, Lax NZ, Hepplewhite PD, Krishnan KJ, Elson JL, Morris CM, McKeith IG, Turnbull DM. Relationship between mitochondria and alpha-synuclein: a study of single substantia nigra neurons. Arch Neurol. 2012;69(3):385–93.
86. Reeve A, Meagher M, Lax N, Simcox E, Hepplewhite P, Jaros E, Turnbull D. The impact of pathogenic mitochondrial DNA mutations on substantia nigra neurons. J Neurosci. 2013;33(26):10790–801.
87. Tzoulis C, Tran GT, Schwarzlmuller T, Specht K, Haugarvoll K, Balafkan N, Lilleng PK, Miletic H, Biermann M, Bindoff LA. Severe nigrostriatal degeneration without clinical parkinsonism in patients with polymerase gamma mutations. Brain. 2013;136(Pt 8):2393–404.
88. Sterky FH, Hoffman AF, Milenkovic D, Bao B, Paganelli A, Edgar D, Wibom R, Lupica CR, Olson L, Larsson NG. Altered dopamine metabolism and increased vulnerability to MPTP in mice with partial deficiency of mitochondrial complex I in dopamine neurons. Hum Mol Genet. 2012;21(5):1078–89.
89. Ekstrand MI, Galter D. The MitoPark mouse - an animal model of Parkinson's disease with impaired respiratory chain function in dopamine neurons. Parkinsonism Relat Disord. 2009;15(Suppl 3):S185–8.
90. Ekstrand MI, Terzioglu M, Galter D, Zhu S, Hofstetter C, Lindqvist E, Thams S, Bergstrand A, Hansson FS, Trifunovic A, Hoffer B, Cullheim S, Mohammed AH, Olson L, Larsson NG. Progressive parkinsonism in mice with respiratory-chain-deficient dopamine neurons. Proc Natl Acad Sci U S A. 2007;104(4):1325–30.
91. Sterky FH, Lee S, Wibom R, Olson L, Larsson NG. Impaired mitochondrial transport and Parkin-independent degeneration of respiratory chain-deficient dopamine neurons in vivo. Proc Natl Acad Sci U S A. 2011;108(31):12937–42.
92. Pickrell AM, Pinto M, Hida A, Moraes CT. Striatal dysfunctions associated with mitochondrial DNA damage in dopaminergic neurons in a mouse model of Parkinson's disease. J Neurosci. 2011;31(48):17649–58.

93. Gramstad A, Bindoff LA, Lillebo A, Tzoulis C, Engelsen BA. Neuropsychological performance in patients with pol γ1 mutations and the syndrome of mitochondrial spinocerebellar ataxia and epilepsy. Epilepsy Behav. 2009;16(1):172–4.
94. Brunetti D, Torsvik J, Dallabona C, Teixeira P, Sztromwasser P, Fernandez-Vizarra E, Cerutti R, Reyes A, Preziuso C, D'Amati G, Baruffini E, Goffrini P, Viscomi C, Ferrero I, Boman H, Telstad W, Johansson S, Glaser E, Knappskog PM, Zeviani M, Bindoff LA. Defective PITRM1 mitochondrial peptidase is associated with Abeta amyloidotic neurodegeneration. EMBO Mol Med. 2016;8(3):176–90.
95. Betts J, Jaros E, Perry RH, Schaefer AM, Taylor RW, Abdel-All Z, Lightowlers RN, Turnbull DM. Molecular neuropathology of MELAS: level of heteroplasmy in individual neurones and evidence of extensive vascular involvement. Neuropathol Appl Neurobiol. 2006;32(4):359–73.
96. Lax NZ, Pienaar IS, Reeve AK, Hepplewhite PD, Jaros E, Taylor RW, Kalaria RN, Turnbull DM. Microangiopathy in the cerebellum of patients with mitochondrial DNA disease. Brain. 2012;135(Pt 6):1736–50.
97. Tzoulis C, Tran GT, Coxhead J, Bertelsen B, Lilleng PK, Balafkan N, Payne B, Miletic H, Chinnery PF, Bindoff LA. Molecular pathogenesis of polymerase gamma-related neurodegeneration. Ann Neurol. 2014;76(1):66–81.
98. Emmanuele V, Garcia-Cazorla A, Huang HB, Coku J, Dorado B, Cortes EP, Engelstad K, De Vivo DC, Dimauro S, Bonilla E, Tanji K. Decreased hippocampal expression of calbindin D28K and cognitive impairment in MELAS. J Neurol Sci. 2012;317(1–2):29–34.
99. Lax NZ, Grady J, Laude A, Chan F, Hepplewhite PD, Gorman G, Whittaker RG, Ng Y, Cunningham MO, Turnbull DM. Extensive respiratory chain defects in inhibitory interneurones in patients with mitochondrial disease. Neuropathol Appl Neurobiol. 2016;42(2):180–93.
100. Hudson G, Schaefer AM, Taylor RW, Tiangyou W, Gibson A, Venables G, Griffiths P, Burn DJ, Turnbull DM, Chinnery PF. Mutation of the linker region of the polymerase γ-1 (pol γ1) gene associated with progressive external ophthalmoplegia and parkinsonism. Arch Neurol. 2007;64(4):553–7.
101. Delgado-Alvarado M, de la Riva P, Jimenez-Urbieta H, Gago B, Gabilondo A, Bornstein B, Rodriguez-Oroz MC. Parkinsonism, cognitive deficit and behavioural disturbance caused by a novel mutation in the polymerase gamma gene. J Neurol Sci. 2015;350(1–2):93–7.
102. Invernizzi F, Varanese S, Thomas A, Carrara F, Onofrj M, Zeviani M. Two novel pol γ1 mutations in a patient with progressive external ophthalmoplegia, levodopa-responsive pseudo-orthostatic tremor and parkinsonism. Neuromuscul Disord. 2008;18(6):460–4.
103. Remes AM, Hinttala R, Karppa M, Soini H, Takalo R, Uusimaa J, Majamaa K. Parkinsonism associated with the homozygous W748S mutation in the pol γ1 gene. Parkinsonism Relat Disord. 2008;14(8): 652–4.
104. Mukai M, Sugaya K, Matsubara S, Cai H, Yabe I, Sasaki H, Nakano I. Familial progressive external ophthalmoplegia, parkinsonism and polyneuropathy associated with pol γ1 mutation. Clin Neurol. 2014;54(5):417–22.
105. Martin-Negrier ML, Sole G, Jardel C, Vital C, Ferrer X, Vital A. TWINKLE gene mutation: report of a French family with an autosomal dominant progressive external ophthalmoplegia and literature review. Eur J Neurol. 2011;18(3):436–41.
106. Van Maldergem L, Besse A, De Paepe B, Blakely EL, Appadurai V, Humble MM, Piard J, Craig K, He L, Hella P, Debray FG, Martin JJ, Gaussen M, Laloux P, Stevanin G, Van Coster R, Taylor RW, Copeland WC, Mormont E, Bonnen PE. pol γ2 deficiency causes adult-onset syndromic sensory neuropathy, ataxia and parkinsonism. Ann Clin Transl Neurol. 2017;4(1):4–14.
107. Caporali L, Bello L, Tagliavini F, La Morgia C, Maresca A, Di Vito L, Liguori R, Valentino ML, Cecchin D, Pegoraro E, Carelli V. DGUOK recessive mutations in patients with CPEO, mitochondrial myopathy, parkinsonism and mtDNA deletions. Brain. 2018;141(1):e3.
108. Garone C, Rubio JC, Calvo SE, Naini A, Tanji K, Dimauro S, Mootha VK, Hirano M. MPV17 mutations causing adult-onset multisystemic disorder with multiple Mitochondrial DNA deletions. Arch Neurol. 2012;69(12):1648–51.
109. Cagnoli C, Stevanin G, Brussino A, Barberis M, Mancini C, Margolis RL, Holmes SE, Nobili M, Forlani S, Padovan S, Pappi P, Zaros C, Leber I, Ribai P, Pugliese L, Assalto C, Brice A, Migone N, Durr A, Brusco A. Missense mutations in the AFG3L2 proteolytic domain account for approximately 1.5% of European autosomal dominant cerebellar ataxias. Hum Mutat. 2010;31(10): 1117–24.
110. Birch-Machin MA, Taylor RW, Cochran B, Ackrell BA, Turnbull DM. Late-onset optic atrophy, ataxia, and myopathy associated with a mutation of a complex II gene. Ann Neurol. 2000;48(3):330–5.

Mitochondrial Neurodegenerative Disorders II: Ataxia, Dystonia and Leukodystrophies

Enrico Bertini and Shamima Rahman

Mitochondrial Ataxias

Ataxia is one of the most frequent symptoms of mitochondrial disease across all age groups and may be cerebellar in origin, or sensory, or a combination of the two (spinocerebellar). Clinical features of cerebellar ataxia may include nystagmus, dysarthria, intention tremor with past-pointing, dysdiadochokinesia, head titubation and truncal and gait ataxia. Sensory ataxia is characterised by unsteadiness exacerbated by a loss of visual cues, i.e. a positive Romberg's sign. In one study, 9% of patients with ataxia caused by mitochondrial disease were reported to present with isolated ataxia [1], but more often ataxia is part of a complex neurological or multisystem disorder.

The mitochondrial ataxias may be considered in three groups: mitochondrial DNA (mtDNA)-encoded mitochondrial ataxia syndromes, nuclear-encoded mitochondrial ataxia syndromes and multisystem disorders in which ataxia is part of a more complex phenotype. It is often only when non-neurological symptoms and signs are present in combination with neurological manifestations including ataxia, dystonia and leukodystrophies that the possibility of a mitochondrial disorder is suspected.

E. Bertini (✉)
Unit of Neuromuscular and Neurodegenerative Disorders, Department of Neurosciences, Bambino Gesu' Children's Research Hospital IRCCS, Rome, Italy
e-mail: enricosilvio.bertini@opbg.net

S. Rahman
Mitochondrial Research Group, UCL Great Ormond Street Institute of Child Health, London, UK

Metabolic Unit, Great Ormond Street Hospital NHS Foundation Trust, London, UK

mtDNA-Encoded Ataxia Syndromes

Single mtDNA deletion disorders are associated with a clinical continuum ranging from infantile-onset Pearson syndrome (sideroblastic anaemia with/without pancreatic exocrine insufficiency) to late-onset progressive external ophthalmoplegia (PEO), with an intermediary phenotype of the Kearns-Sayre syndrome (KSS) [2]. KSS is traditionally defined as a triad of onset before age 20 years with PEO and retinitis pigmentosa, together with at least one of the following additional features: cardiac conduction block, elevated cerebrospinal fluid (CSF) protein or cerebellar ataxia. Typical associated findings include sensorineural hearing loss (SNHL), seizures and pyramidal signs. Ataxia is frequently a presenting feature in KSS and PEO-plus, occurring in approaching 50% of patients in one large French series [3]. Ragged-red fibres are found in muscle biopsy, together with variable deficiencies of oxidative phosphorylation (OXPHOS) enzymes.

M. Mancuso, T. Klopstock (eds.), *Diagnosis and Management of Mitochondrial Disorders*,
https://doi.org/10.1007/978-3-030-05517-2_15

A mitochondrial phenotype that strongly resembles a spinocerebellar ataxia is the syndrome of neurogenic muscle weakness, ataxia and retinitis pigmentosa (NARP) caused by mutations (m.8993T>C or T>G and m.9176T>C or T>G) in the mitochondrial *MT-ATP6* gene encoding a subunit of complex V, the ATP synthase [4]. These mutations are associated with NARP when present at moderately high loads but cause maternally inherited Leigh syndrome (subacute necrotizing encephalomyelopathy) when present at loads of >90% [4].

Although ataxia is not present in the acronym of MERRF (myoclonic epilepsy ragged-red fibres), ataxia is one of the most frequent complaints of affected patients. Ataxia affects 35–45% of patients with MERRF and correlates more closely with myoclonus than epilepsy, leading to the suggestion that MERRF should be redefined as a myoclonic ataxia rather than a myoclonic epilepsy [5]. The MERFF phenotype is most commonly associated with the m.8344A>G mutation in the *MTTK* gene but has also been linked to a number of other mtDNA mutations, including mutations in the following genes: *MTTL1*, *MTTH*, *MTTS1*, *MTTS2*, *MTTF and MTTP* (www.mitomap.org). Ataxia may also be seen in patients with mitochondrial encephalomyopathy with lactic acidosis and stroke-like episodes (MELAS) syndrome caused by the m.3243A>G mutation in *MTTL1* [6].

Nuclear-Encoded Ataxia Syndromes

Several mitochondrial phenotypes can strongly resemble cerebellar or a spinocerebellar ataxia.

POLG-Related Disorders

Mutations of *POLG*, encoding the catalytic subunit of DNA polymerase gamma responsible for replicating mtDNA, represent the most frequent nuclear gene cause of mitochondrial disease and are a frequent cause of ataxia, accounting for 11% of unexplained ataxia in one sizeable cohort. *POLG*-related disorders comprise a continuum of overlapping phenotypes and should be suspected in individuals with combinations of the following clinical features (depending on the age of onset): hypotonia, developmental delay, seizures, movement disorders, myopathy, ataxia, hepatopathy, peripheral neuropathy, episodic psychomotor regression, psychiatric illness and endocrinopathy (diabetes mellitus, premature ovarian failure) [7]. Syndromic presentations of ataxia related to autosomal recessive (AR) *POLG* mutations include myoclonic epilepsy myopathy sensory ataxia, commonly abbreviated to MEMSA. The signs and symptoms of MEMSA typically appear during young adulthood, and this condition was previously defined as spinocerebellar ataxia with epilepsy (SCAE) [8]. Another *POLG*-related syndrome with prominent ataxia is the ataxia neuropathy spectrum (ANS) which includes entities previously known as mitochondrial recessive ataxia syndrome (MIRAS) and sensory ataxia neuropathy dysarthria and ophthalmoplegia (SANDO) [8].

IOSCA

Infantile-onset spinocerebellar ataxia (IOSCA) is a Finnish heritage disorder caused by biallelic mutations in *TWNK* encoding a helicase required for mtDNA replication. *TWNK* encodes a mitochondrial protein structurally similar to hexameric ring helicases that co-localises with mtDNA in mitochondrial nucleoids [9]. Affected individuals typically present after a normal first year with ataxia, hypotonia and sensory neuropathy leading to hyporeflexia [10]. Other clinical features include athetosis, SNHL, ophthalmoplegia, intractable epilepsy and liver dysfunction. AR mutations in *TWNK* also occur in non-Finnish populations, causing mitochondrial DNA depletion syndrome 7 (MTDPS7) characterised by a severe hepatocerebral phenotype, with neonatal lactic acidosis (increased serum and CSF lactate) and truncal hypotonia with peripheral hypertonia, mild liver insufficiency, psychomotor retardation, seizures and peripheral neuropathy, leading to death in early childhood [11].

ARCA2

Early-onset ataxias (EOAs) are a highly heterogeneous group of degenerative and metabolic diseases, manifesting in childhood after a *disease-free interval*, and are predominantly caused by recessive mutations in genes with pleiotropic, multisystemic manifestations frequently accompanied by global atrophy of the cerebellum [12]. A typical EOA is caused by a defect in *COQ8A (ADCK3)* that leads to impaired biogenesis of coenzyme Q_{10} (CoQ_{10}), a mobile electron carrier and fundamental component of the mitochondrial OXPHOS machinery [13, 14]. Studies in mice and yeast models revealed that COQ8 possesses evolutionarily conserved ATPase activity, interacts with lipid CoQ intermediates and is activated by binding to membranes containing cardiolipin and by phenolic compounds that resemble CoQ pathway intermediates [15, 16]. Secondary CoQ_{10} deficiency has also been reported in oculomotor ataxia type I caused by aprataxin mutations [17].

Friedreich Ataxia

Friedreich ataxia (FRDA) is the most frequent autosomal recessive ataxia. Onset is usually before age 25 years with a mean age of around 10 years [18]. Symptoms of gait ataxia related to a combination of spinocerebellar degeneration and peripheral neuropathy leading to loss of proprioception are characteristically associated with dysarthria, muscle weakness, lower limb spasticity, scoliosis, bladder dysfunction, absent lower limb reflexes and loss of position and vibration sense with a positive Romberg sign. About 30% of individuals with FRDA have hypertrophic cardiomyopathy, and overall around 60% have heart disorders. Moreover, 10–30% have diabetes mellitus, and about a quarter of patients have an 'atypical' presentation with later onset or retained tendon reflexes or with cardiomyopathy preceding the ataxia. The genetic cause of FRDA is an unstable GAA trinucleotide repeat expansion in intron 1 of the *FXN* gene encoding the protein frataxin. In about 95% of affected individuals, the GAA expansion is homozygous, while the remaining patients carry a GAA expansion on one allele and an inactivating mutation in the coding region of the other allele. Lower levels of the corresponding mRNA transcript and protein correlate with the longer the GAA expansion. Frataxin has a role in the synthesis of iron-sulphur clusters, and the decrease of frataxin is responsible for impaired biogenesis of mitochondrial OXPHOS enzyme complexes I, II, III and the Krebs cycle enzyme aconitase, as well as increased mitochondrial and cytosolic iron accumulation, leading to susceptibility to oxidative damage [19].

ARSACS

Autosomal recessive spastic ataxia of Charlevoix-Saguenay (ARSACS) is caused by mutations of *SACS* encoding sacsin, a protein that has been implicated in the ubiquitin-proteasome system, in Hsp70 chaperone machinery and in mitochondrial network organisation [20–22]. Investigation of sacsin deficiency in a knockout mouse model demonstrated abnormalities of the neurofilament cytoskeleton and mitochondrial dynamics as the underlying pathophysiological basis of ARSACS [23]. Clinical manifestations generally start between the first and third decade, with gait disturbance and walking difficulties, while early signs of cerebellar ataxia include dysarthria and nystagmus. The spasticity is progressive and eventually dominates the clinical picture, and onset of the peripheral neuropathy generally occurs later with distal amyotrophy and deep sensory disturbances (impaired vibration sense); nerve conduction velocity is reduced, and retinal hypermyelination (without vision loss) is a frequent feature in ARSACS patients and may be detected with optical coherence tomography (OCT). Although this condition was originally identified as a founder disorder in Quebec, it has since been reported in several other countries, particularly in the Mediterranean area and in Japan [24].

ARSAL

Autosomal recessive spastic ataxia with leukoencephalopathy (ARSAL) or SPAX3 is a condition reported so far in French Canadian families and is related to biallelic mutations in *MARS2* encoding the mitochondrial methionyl-tRNA synthetase [25]. Age at onset is reportedly variable, ranging from 2 to 59 years, and all patients have an ataxic gait and spasticity with no evidence of a peripheral neuropathy. Other variable but frequent manifestations included dysarthria (74%), dystonic positioning (57%), mild horizontal nystagmus (44%), scoliosis (35%) and mild hearing impairment (13%). The disease is slowly progressive. Neuroimaging showed cerebellar atrophy and some signs of cerebral atrophy, and about half had nonspecific focal white matter changes in periventricular and deep white matter regions [25].

Other Mitochondrial Ataxias

Ataxia has been reported in association with dozens of mitochondrial gene defects, including disorders of OXPHOS subunits and their assembly, and defects of mtNA maintenance, mitochondrial translation, mitochondrial membrane lipids, homeostasis and dynamics (Table 1). Cerebellar ataxia is a frequent feature of Leigh syndrome, particularly with *SURF1* mutations, and affected 50% of cases in one large cohort [26]. Pyruvate dehydrogenase (PDH) deficiency caused by X-linked *PDHA1* mutations usually presents as congenital lactic acidosis or Leigh syndrome in infancy, but milder mutations may cause an episodic ataxia syndrome triggered by carbohydrate ingestion [27]. Mitochondrial spinocerebellar ataxias include mutations of *AFG3L2* (SCA28) and *SPG7,* which encode components of the mitochondrial AAA protease complex involved in protein homeostasis [28]. Most recently mutations in the complex IV assembly factor COA7 have been reported to cause spinocerebellar ataxia with peripheral neuropathy [29].

Table 1 Genetic causes of mitochondrial ataxia

Disease mechanism	Biochemical defect	Examples of gene defects
OXPHOS subunits and assembly factors	Complex I	*MT-ND1,3,5,6* [mat], *NDUFA1,13, NDUFS1,2,7,8, NDUFV1, NDUFAF2,5,6, ACAD9, NUBPL* [AR]
	Complex II	*SDHA* [AR]
	Complex III	*MT-CYB* [mat], *UQCRQ, TTC19, LYRM7* [AR]
	Complex IV	*MT-CO1* [mat], *COX6B1, NDUFA4, SURF1, COA7, COX10, COX15, COX20, CEP89* [AR]
	Complex V	*MT-ATP6,8* [mat], *TMEM70* [AR]
mtDNA maintenance	Multiple (complexes I, III, IV and V)	*POLG, TWNK, RRM2B, MGME1, FBXL4* [AR]
Mitochondrial translation	Multiple (variably affect complexes I, III, IV and V)	*MTO1, AARS2, MARS2, RARS2, LRPPRC,* [AR]
Cofactor biosynthesis	Multiple (variable)	*COQ8A, COQ6* [AR]
Mitochondrial import	Multiple (variably affect complexes I, III, IV and V)	*TIMM8A* [X-linked]
Mitochondrial membrane lipids, homeostasis and dynamics	Multiple (variable)	*SERAC1, CLPB, OPA1* [AR]
Pyruvate metabolism	Pyruvate dehydrogenase	*PDHA1* [X-linked], *PDHB, PDHX, DLAT, DLD* [AR]
Miscellaneous	Variable	*SLC19A3* [AR]

Pontocerebellar Hypoplasia

RARS2 Mutations

Pontocerebellar hypoplasia (PCH) syndromes are a group of disorders that can be defined by the neuroimaging appearance of marked hypoplasia of the pons and cerebellum. PCH type 6 (PCH6) is known to be related to biallelic mutations in *RARS2*, encoding the mitochondrial arginyl–transfer RNA (tRNA) synthetase [30]. PCH6 usually presents shortly after birth with intractable seizures and lactic acidosis with variable OXPHOS deficiencies [31, 32]. Most affected children have severe developmental delay and do not achieve ambulation, but the first author has managed a milder case who at 5 years walks with an ataxic gait and has mild microcephaly and moderate intellectual disability (EB, unpublished observation).

Mitochondrial Dystonias

Dystonia is a frequent symptom in mitochondrial disease and may be isolated or part of a more complex neurological syndrome. Dystonia is a genetically heterogeneous movement disorder characterised by abnormal twisting postures and movements that may be induced by specific, sometimes complex, tasks. Although isolated dystonia has been reported in mitochondrial disease, more commonly it is associated with other features suggestive of an underlying mitochondrial disorder.

Leigh Syndrome Spectrum

By far the most frequent cause of mitochondrial dystonia is Leigh syndrome or subacute necrotising encephalomyelopathy. Dystonia was reported in almost 50% of a multinational cohort of 130 children with Leigh syndrome [33]. Affected children typically present in the first year of life, after a period of normal development, with developmental regression variably associated with symptoms and signs of basal ganglia and brainstem dysfunction, including dystonia, feeding and swallowing difficulties, vomiting, nystagmus, ophthalmoplegia, optic atrophy and breathing abnormalities. The disease is characterised by progressive neurodegeneration, with stepwise episodes of neurological deterioration interspersed by unpredictable periods of stability. The median age of death was 2.4 years in one large cohort but varies between different gene defects [26, 33]. Some patients may survive into the third or even the fourth decade, and adult-onset disease is also recognised. The syndrome is biochemically and genetically heterogeneous and has been linked to approaching 90 different gene defects, including defects of OXPHOS complexes and assembly factors, mtDNA maintenance, mitochondrial transport, cofactor biosynthesis and pyruvate dehydrogenase complex deficiency [34, 35].

Leber Hereditary Optic Neuropathy

Leber hereditary optic neuropathy (LHON) is usually caused by one of three common homoplasmic mtDNA mutations (m.3460G>A, m.11778G>A and m.14484T>C) affecting subunits of complex I and is typically an isolated optic neuropathy disorder with a male predominance. However, some less frequently reported LHON mutations are commonly associated with dystonia, particularly the heteroplasmic m.14459G>A mutation. Individuals with high mutation loads of m.14459G>A typically have a Leigh-like disorder with dystonia starting in early childhood and only later develop visual disturbance.

Neurodegeneration with Brain Iron Accumulation

Neurodegeneration with brain iron accumulation (NBIA) is a genetically heterogeneous disorder, and some of the gene defects affect mitochondrially localised proteins, specifically *PANK2*, encoding pantothenate kinase which is involved in mitochondrial coenzyme-A biosynthesis, and *C19Orf12*, encoding a protein of currently unknown function [36]. PKAN (pantothenate kinase-associated neurodegeneration) is the most common NBIA, and affected patients with *PANK2* mutations typically present with early-onset dystonia. Atypical PKAN cases may present later, in the second or third decade, with speech and psychiatric difficulties, and later develop dystonia and spasticity. MPAN (caused by *C19Orf12* mutations) is rare (birth prevalence <1 in 1 million) and presents with gait disturbance related to spasticity and dystonia, with onset ranging from childhood to early adulthood, with typically slow progression and survival into adult life. NBIA disorders are characterised by T2-weighted hypodensities of the basal ganglia on brain MRI, because of iron accumulation, and in the case of PKAN, there may be associated T2-hyperintensities within the globus pallidus

Table 2 Genetic causes of mitochondrial dystonia

Disease mechanism	Biochemical defect	Examples of gene defects
OXPHOS subunits and assembly factors	Complex I	*MT-ND1,3,4,6* [mat], *NDUFA1,9,10,12, NDUFS1,2,3,4,7,8, NDUFV1, NDUFAF2,4,5, ACAD9, FOXRED1* [AR]
	Complex II	*SDHA* [AR]
	Complex III	*UQCRQ, BCS1L, TTC19* [AR]
	Complex IV	*MT-CO3* [mat], *NDUFA4, SURF1, SCO2, COX15, COX20, FASTKD2, PET100* [AR]
	Complex V	*MT-ATP6* [mat], *ATP5A1* [AR]
mtDNA maintenance	Multiple (complexes I, III, IV and V)	*POLG, SUCLA2, SUCLG1, MPV17, FBXL4, ABAT, SAMHD1* [AR]
Mitochondrial translation	Multiple (variably affect complexes I, III, IV and V)	*MTO1, GTPBP3, GFM1, TFSM, AARS2, CARS2, EARS2, MARS2, NARS2, PARS2, RARS2, LRPPRC, TACO1, TRIT1, GUF1* [AR]
Cofactor biosynthesis	Multiple (variable)	*PDSS2, COQ2, COQ8A, COQ9, NFU1, LIPT1, MECR* [AR]
Mitochondrial import	Multiple (variably affect complexes I, III, IV and V)	*TIMM8A* [X-linked], *GFER* [AR]
Mitochondrial membrane lipids, homeostasis and dynamics	Multiple (variable)	*SERAC1, CLPB, OPA1* [AR]
Pyruvate metabolism	Pyruvate dehydrogenase	*PDHA1* [X-linked], *PDHB* [AR]
Miscellaneous	Variable	*HIBCH, ECHS1, PNPT1* [AR]

leading to a characteristic 'eye of the tiger' appearance.

Other Mitochondrial Dystonias

Deafness-dystonia-optic neuronopathy (Mohr-Tranebjaerg) syndrome is an X-linked disorder of mitochondrial protein import caused by *TIMM8A* mutations. The syndrome is characterised by early-onset hearing loss in affected males, usually progressing to profound deafness by the end of the first decade, associated with teenage-onset slowly progressive dystonia or ataxia, and visual impairment related to optic atrophy in the third decade [37]. Variable behavioural and psychiatric manifestations have been reported in childhood, as well as dementia starting in the fifth decade. Occasionally females may be affected, with mild hearing loss and focal dystonia.

Dystonia may also be a feature of KSS, MERRF, *POLG* disease and disorders of CoQ_{10} biosynthesis such as *COQ8A* mutations. There is a growing list of causes of mitochondrial dystonias, with underlying disease mechanisms including disordered OXPHOS enzyme complex assembly, and impaired mtDNA maintenance, mitochondrial translation, cofactor biosynthesis and mitochondrial import, pyruvate dehydrogenase deficiency and toxic damage to the OXPHOS system in two disorders of valine degradation, HIBCH and ECHS1 deficiencies (Table 2).

Mitochondrial Leukodystrophies

Leukodystrophies are a genetically heterogeneous and growing list of disorders, with mitochondrial leukodystrophies becoming an increasingly significant subgroup of these conditions [38]. Moreover, certain mitochondrial leukodystrophies may be defined and recognised by suggestive neuroimaging patterns linked to specific gene defects, which may expedite diagnosis. In other mitochondrial encephalomyopathies, a prominent white matter abnormality can also be associated with the involvement of other subsystems of the brain, most frequently the basal ganglia such as in KSS [39]. Here we will specifically address the primary mitochondrial diseases that clinically and on neuroimaging manifest with a leukoencephalopathy, underscoring the importance of MRI pattern recognition for preliminary assessment.

It is well established that neuroimaging is of pivotal importance for a preliminary differential diagnosis in the increasingly heterogeneous group of leukodystrophies and that a subset of these conditions are characterised by cystic changes and vacuolization of the white matter on MRI [40]. Mitochondrial leukodystrophies are typically recognisable on MRI because they are frequently cavitating disorders of the white matter. The best known form of cavitating leukodystrophy that has similarities with the mitochondrial leukoencephalopathies is vanishing white matter (VWM) disease, an autosomal recessive leukodystrophy caused by mutations in any of five genes encoding subunits of the translation initiation factor EIF-2B [40]. The MRI pattern in both conditions is consistent with vacuolization changes, but in VWM leukodystrophy, the white matter abnormal signal involves the subcortical U-fibres as well, while subcortical U-fibres are generally spared in mitochondrial leukodystrophies, which also frequently have a hyperintense outer rim in FLAIR-weighted images (Fig. 1).

mtDNA-Encoded Mitochondrial Leukodystrophies

Several syndromic disorders related to defects of mtDNA-encoded genes, namely, maternally inherited Leigh syndrome, KSS and MELAS syndrome, are known to occasionally have prominent cerebral white matter involvement, but in these cases, associated abnormalities of the basal ganglia and brainstem are an almost constant finding. MRI features of KSS frequently show a characteristic pattern, involving hyperintensity of the basal ganglia, thalamus, subcortical cerebral white matter (affecting U-fibres and internal capsule) and corpus callosum as well as the cerebellar white matter and brainstem, particularly in T2 and FLAIR images [39]. Cerebral folate deficiency has been reported in KSS, and it has been suggested that the severity of the white matter abnormalities correlates with CSF 5-methyltetrahydrofolate levels [39]. White matter lesions have occasionally been described in LHON [41], and there is a single report of a severe cavitating leukoencephalopathy in a child with the m.8344A>G mutation usually associated with MERRF [42].

Nuclear-Encoded Mitochondrial Leukodystrophies

Disorders of OXPHOS Complexes and Their Assembly

Mitochondrial leukoencephalopathies may present with characteristic recognisable neuroimaging patterns associated with specific genetic defects but may also be defined by biochemical

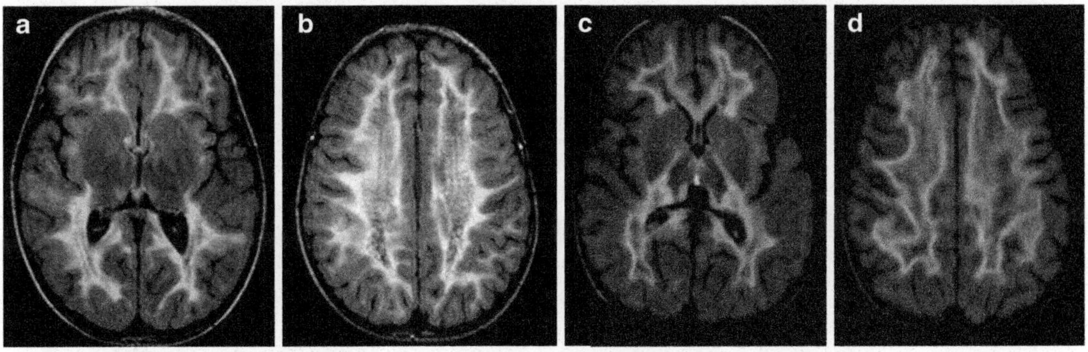

Fig. 1 Axial FLAIR-weighted brain MR images comparing features of two vacuolating leukodystrophies: a patient with vanishing white matter leukodystrophy (VWM) (**a**, **b**) with a patient affected by a mitochondrial leukodystrophy with complex II deficiency and biallelic mutations in *SDHAF1* (**c**, **d**). In VWM there is characteristically no sparing of the subcortical U-fibres (**a**, **b**), while they are mostly spared in most vacuolating mitochondrial leukodystrophies such as *SDHAF1*-related leukodystrophy. Moreover the hyperintense outer rim is particularly well marked in the FLAIR-weighted images of this *SDHAF1*-related leukodystrophy and in most vacuolating mitochondrial leukodystrophies

defects of the OXPHOS enzyme complexes. Mutations of OXPHOS subunits and assembly factors are a frequent cause of mitochondrial leukodystrophy, particularly associated with isolated deficiencies of complexes I, II and IV. Isolated complex I deficiency is the most frequently encountered defect of mitochondrial energy metabolism and may be caused by mutations of mtDNA- or nuclear-encoded subunits or of assembly factors (the latter are all nuclear encoded) [43]. Clinical presentations are heterogeneous and include fatal infantile lactic acidosis, progressive encephalocardiomyopathy, Leigh syndrome and leukodystrophy [43]. Leukoencephalopathy appears to be especially frequent in patients harbouring mutations in *NDUFS1* or *NDUFV1* and is frequently a progressive cavitating leukoencephalopathy which may be mistaken for VWM leukoencephalopathy (Fig. 2) [43]. Recently a cavitating leukodystro-

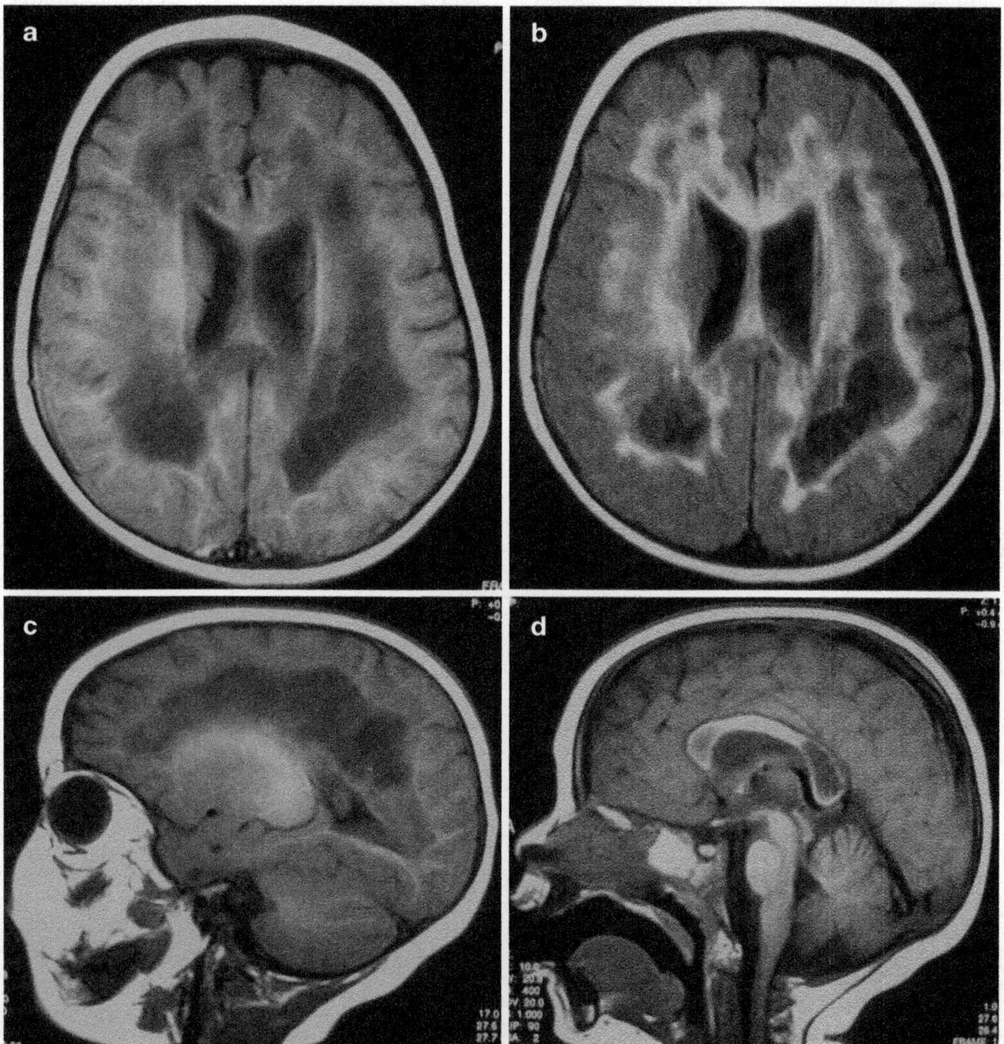

Fig. 2 Set of neuroimages of a 2-year-old girl harbouring homozygous mutations in *NDUFS1* with a biochemical defect of complex I in muscle. **a** is a T1-weighted axial image; **b** is a corresponding FLAIR-weighted axial image to show T1 hypointensity and hyperintense rim in the FLAIR-weighted images; and **c** and **d** are, respectively, T1 parasagittal and T1 sagittal images to show hypointensity of the white matter corresponding to vacuolization (**c**) and cavitations of the corpus callosum (**d**)

phy has also been described in a patient with a defect of the complex I assembly factor NDUFAF3 [44]. The cavitating leukoencephalopathy in this patient showed in addition bilaterally symmetrical hyperintensity in the substantia nigra, medial thalamic nuclei and basal nuclei. Mutations of *NUBPL*, encoding an iron-sulphur cluster assembly factor for complex I, are associated with a complex I deficient encephalopathy with a characteristic MRI pattern involving abnormalities of the cerebellar cortex, deep cerebral white matter and corpus callosum [45].

Mutations in two of the four complex II subunits, SDHA and SDHB, have been reported to cause childhood onset leukoencephalopathy and isolated complex II deficiency [46], but the most frequent leukodystrophy with complex II deficiency is related to mutations in *SDHAF1* [47], one of four known assembly factors of complex II. The leukodystrophy with *SDHAF1* mutations leads to progressive cavitation of the white matter that is characteristic of several mitochondrial leukodystrophies (Fig. 1) and also abnormal T2 hyperintensity in the middle cerebellar peduncles [48, 49]. MRS may be used to demonstrate succinate accumulation in the brains of patients with *SDHA*, *SDHB* and *SDHAF1* mutations [49]. Recently SDHAF1 was demonstrated to have a role in transferring Fe-S clusters to the SDHB subunit [50].

A single leukodystrophy with complex III deficiency has been reported to date, related to mutations in *LYRM7*, encoding mitochondrial LYR motif-containing protein 7, an assembly factor for complex III [51]. Distinctive magnetic resonance imaging features, including progressive signal abnormalities with multifocal small cavitations in the periventricular and deep cerebral white matter, were reported in four patients from three unrelated families [51].

Severe cystic leukoencephalopathy was linked to recessive mutations in a complex IV (cytochrome *c* oxidase, COX) subunit COX6B1 in two brothers with bilateral, symmetrical MRI signal abnormalities involving the frontal, parietal and occipital white matter, as well as the corpus callosum [52]. Severe deficits of COX as a result of recessive mutations in the assembly factor SURF1 usually cause classical Leigh syndrome, but in a minority of cases were associated with leukodystrophy (Fig. 3) [26, 53]. Severe leukodystrophy has also been linked to recessive mutations in another COX assembly factor, COA7, associated with a slowly progressive neurodegenerative disorder with onset of psychomotor delay at around 1 year of age, leukoencephalopathy on brain imaging and a mixed axonal demyelinating sensorimotor neuropathy [54]. A cavitating leukodystrophy with COX deficiency and a recognisable phenotype has also been described with AR mutations in *APOPT1* encoding apoptogenic protein 1 (Fig. 4) [55].

Disorders of Iron-Sulphur Cluster Biosynthesis

Leukodystrophies caused by defects of Fe-S cluster assembly factors constitute a new class of AR mitochondrial disease frequently presenting with white matter abnormalities and multiple respiratory chain deficiencies. These have been classified as Mitochondrial Multiple Dysfunction Syndromes (MMDS) particularly impairing activities of complex I, complex II and complex III. So far, five classes of MMDS have been defined, according to the gene involved in the disease: MMDS1 (*NFU1*), MMDS2 (*BOLA3*), MMDS3 (*IBA57*), MMDS4 (*ISCA2*) and MMDS5 (*ISCA1*) [56]. A common feature of all these MMDS is the frequent presence of hyperglycinaemia (because the gene products are needed for synthesis of the mitochondrial glycine cleavage system) and leukodystrophy as a predominant feature, especially for the *NFU1*, *IBA57*, *ISCA2* and *ISCA1* gene defects [56–59]. Recently AR *BOLA3* mutations were reported to cause a severe leukoencephalopathy followed by good clinical recovery associated with partial resolution of MRI changes [60]. So far there does not appear to be a clearly recognisable MRI phenotype, although *NFU1* and *IBA57* mutations represent further causes of cavitating leukoencephalopathies [61, 62].

Disorders of mtDNA Maintenance

Defects of mtDNA maintenance may be classified broadly in two groups: defects of the

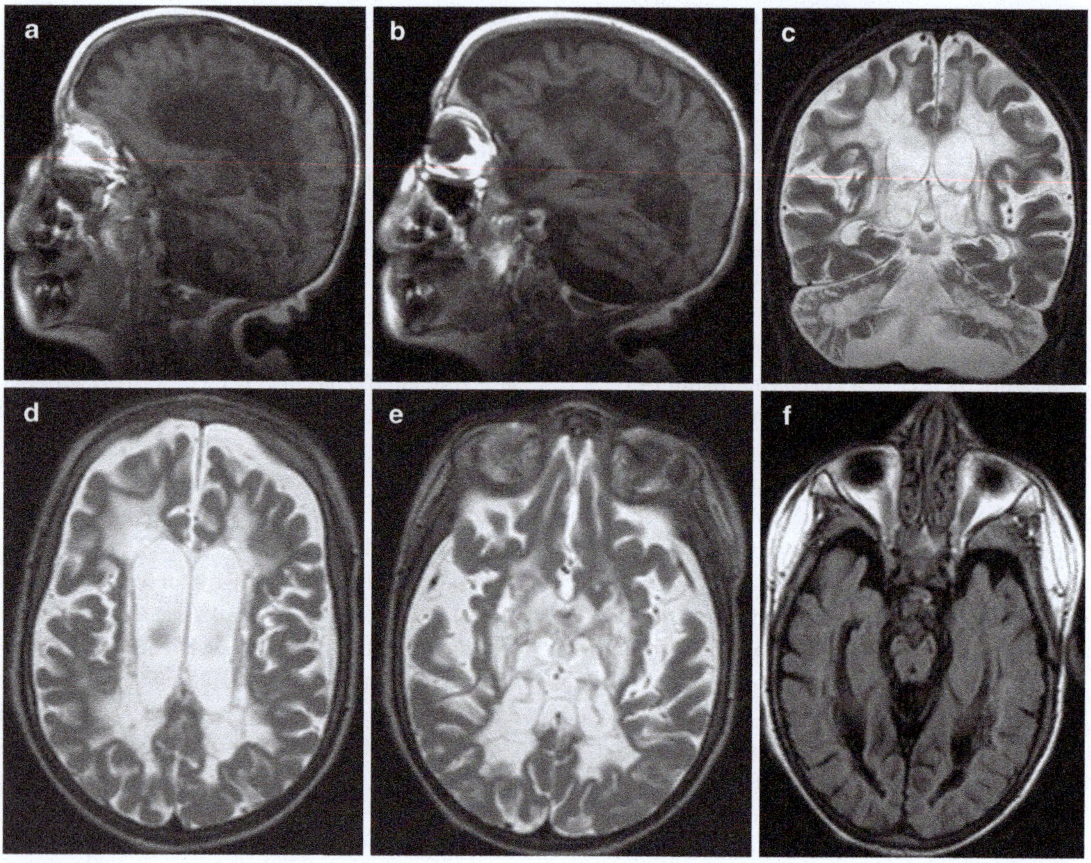

Fig. 3 Neuroimaging of a 10-year-old boy with homozygous biallelic mutations in *SURF1*. **a** and **b** are T1 sagittal images; **c** is a coronal T2-weighted image; **d** and **e** are axial T2-weighted images; and **f** is a T1-weighted axial image. Although the white matter in this patient is particularly and diffusely involved, there is in addition a clear and severe involvement of the cortical grey matter, as well as symmetrical basal ganglia involvement typical of Leigh syndrome

mitochondrial replication fork (e.g. *POLG*, *TWNK* mutations) and disorders of nucleoside metabolism [63]. These disorders are characterised at a molecular level by progressive depletion of the mtDNA and/or accumulation of multiple mtDNA deletions. Mitochondrial neurogastrointestinal encephalomyopathy (MNGIE) caused by mutations in the *TYMP* gene encoding thymidine phosphorylase is characteristically associated with a leukoencephalopathy resulting from CNS demyelination. The leukoencephalopathy is typically relatively asymptomatic, and the predominant clinical features are peripheral neuropathy and severe gastrointestinal disturbance leading to episodes of pseudo-obstruction and extreme cachexia, ptosis and distal muscle weakness, especially in the lower limbs [64]. Navajo neurohepatopathy is caused by a homozygous founder mutation in the *MPV17* gene [65]. Clinical features include liver disease, peripheral neuropathy, corneal anaesthesia and scarring, acral mutilation and leukoencephalopathy. Patients with infantile-onset hepatocerebral mtDNA depletion syndrome caused by *MPV17* mutations may die of liver failure before developing MRI changes, but leukodystrophy has been reported in some infants with hepatocerebral mtDNA depletion associated with MPV17 deficiency [66]. Mutations of *FBXL4* are associated with a multisystem mtDNA depletion disorder

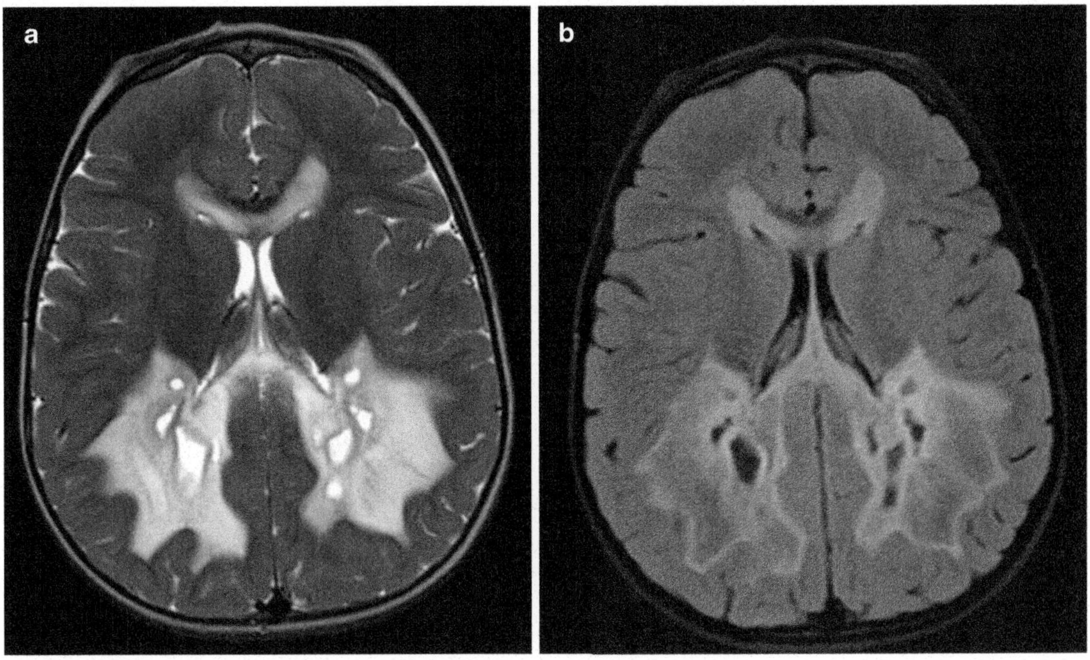

Fig. 4 Axial T2 (**a**)- and FLAIR (**b**)-weighted images of a 3-year-old patient harbouring biallelic mutations in *APOPT1* and biochemical defect of complex IV in muscle. The cavitating lesions are typically located in the posterior areas symmetrically, with a hyperintense rim that is clearly evident in the FLAIR-weighted image

including growth failure, microcephaly, hyperammonaemia, seizures and characteristic facial features, and there may be white matter abnormalities and cerebral atrophy on MRI brain [67]. Other mtDNA depletion syndromes associated with leukodystrophy are mutations in *SUCLA2* and *SUCLG1* [68, 69], encoding succinyl-CoA ligase, a Krebs cycle enzyme that is thought to contribute to mitochondrial nucleoside salvage by stabilising the nucleoside diphosphate kinase [70]. AR mutations in *POLG* typically affect the grey matter, causing Alpers disease in late infancy/early childhood, but leukodystrophy has occasionally been reported in childhood onset *POLG* disease [71, 72].

Defects of Mitochondrial Aminoacyl-tRNA Synthetases

A growing group of mitochondrial leukodystrophies with highly characteristic neuroimaging features are disorders of the mitochondrial aminoacyl-tRNA synthetases, ancient proteins that play essential roles in mitochondrial translation. Defects of some of these genes show MRI recognisable forms of site-specific leukodystrophies such as leukoencephalopathy with brainstem and spinal cord involvement and lactate elevation (LBSL) and leukoencephalopathy with thalamus and brainstem involvement and high lactate (LTBL). LBSL is caused by mutations of *DARS2* encoding the mitochondrial aspartyl-tRNA synthetase and is characterised by slowly progressive cerebellar ataxia, spasticity owing to pyramidal involvement and sensory abnormalities related to neurodegeneration of the corticospinal tracts and dorsal columns. The main MRI features are abnormalities in the cerebral white matter (sparing U-fibres), dorsal columns, corticospinal tracts, pyramids, cerebellar peduncles, intraparenchymal tract of the V cranial nerve, posterior arm of the internal capsule and splenium of the corpus callosum [73]. LTBL is caused by mutations in *EARS2* encoding the mitochondrial glutamyl-tRNA synthetase [74]. This disease is characterised by an early-onset leukoencephalopathy with a biphasic clinical course; the disorder may be fatal in infancy [75], but in other cases, there is progressive improvement during childhood [74]. EARS2 deficiency is hallmarked by unique MRI features involving the deep cerebral white matter (but consistently sparing the periventricular rim), corpus callosum, thalamus, basal ganglia, midbrain, pons, medulla oblongata and cerebellar white matter [74]. Mutations in *AARS2* encoding the mitochondrial alanyl-tRNA synthetase were initially reported to cause a fatal infantile cardiomyopathy [76] but subsequently have also been associated with an adult-onset disorder with a highly specific leukoencephalopathy with striking involvement of left-right connections, descending tracts and cerebellar atrophy, associated with psychiatric manifestations and ovarian failure in all female patients, but with notable absence of cardiomyopathy [77]. Mutations of *MARS2* encoding the methionyl-tRNA synthetase cause the syndrome of ARSAL, as discussed above, in which there is frequent white matter involvement [25], while mutations of *WARS2* encoding the mitochondrial tryptophanyl-tRNA synthetase have recently been reported to present with a severe infantile-onset leukoencephalopathy [78].

Other Disorders of Mitochondrial Translation

There are two reports describing four individuals with a severe infantile encephalopathy with a very similar MRI pattern of macrocystic leukodystrophy and micropolygyria, with a combined defect of complexes I and IV in muscle biopsy, caused by biallelic mutations in *TUFM*, encoding the mitochondrial elongation factor Tu [79, 80]. The most recent leukodystrophy related to a defect of a protein involved in mitochondrial translation, RMND1, has been described in more than ten individuals who had a characteristic MRI including temporal lobe swelling, with cystic evolution, and multifocal confluent subcortical white matter changes [81]. All had SNHL and hypotonia, while renal impairment, lactic acidosis and seizures were also frequent findings.

Table 3 Genetic causes of mitochondrial leukodystrophies

Disease mechanism	Biochemical defect	Examples of gene defects
OXPHOS subunits and assembly factors	Complex I	*NDUFS1, NDUFV1, NDUFA2, NDUFAF3, NUBPL* [AR]
	Complex II	*SDHA, SDHB, SDHAF1* [AR]
	Complex III	*LYRM7* [AR]
	Complex IV	*COX6B1, SURF1 COA7, APOPT1* [AR]
mtDNA maintenance	Multiple (complexes I, III, IV and V)	*TYMP, MPV17, FBXL4, SUCLA2, SUCLG1, POLG, TWNK* [AR]
Mitochondrial translation	Multiple (variably affect complexes I, III, IV and V)	*DARS2, EARS2, AARS2, MARS2, WARS2, TUFM, RMND1* [AR]
Disorders of iron-sulphur cluster biosynthesis	Multiple (complexes I, II and III)	*NFU1, ISCA1, ISCA2, IBA57, BOLA3* [AR]
Miscellaneous	Variable	*MICU2, ECHS1, DARS* [AR]

Other Mitochondrial Leukodystrophies

Other rare causes of mitochondrial leukoencephalopathy are highlighted in Table 3 and include mutations of *MICU2*, encoding part of the mitochondrial calcium uniporter complex [82], and ECHS1 deficiency, a disorder of valine degradation leading to toxic damage to OXPHOS enzymes, which may present as a vacuolating leukoencephalopathy [83]. Defects of some of the cytosolic aminoacyl-tRNA synthetases may also mimic mitochondrial leukoencephalopathies, for example, mutations in *DARS* and *RARS*, encoding the cytosolic aspartyl and arginyl-tRNA synthetases, respectively, cause a hypomyelinating leukodystrophy [84, 85].

Conclusions

We have described three topics related to neurodegeneration, namely, ataxia, dystonia and leukodystrophy, in the broadening area of mitochondrial medicine [86]. Each of these topics needs experience and expertise in integrating different disciplines to achieve a definitive molecular genetic diagnosis. Interpretation of clinical and neuroimaging data is very important in the preliminary assessment, but these results must be combined with information from clinical chemistry and (when needed) histopathology and biochemistry of muscle and fibroblasts derived from the affected patient. Rapid advances in molecular genetics have accelerated genetic diagnosis, but next-generation sequencing methods yield a multitude of genetic variants that need to be validated by clinical, biochemical and neuroimaging biomarkers before assigning a final diagnosis.

Acknowledgments This work was supported by a Great Ormond Street Hospital Children's Charity Research Leadership Award (V1260) to SR and by the NIHR Great Ormond Street Hospital Biomedical Research Centre. We also acknowledge research grant funding from the Italian Ministry of Health Ricerca Corrente to EB and from the Lily Foundation to SR. We thank Joyeeta Rahman for her assistance with literature searches.

References

1. Bargiela D, Shanmugarajah P, Lo C, Blakely EL, Taylor RW, Horvath R, et al. Mitochondrial pathology in progressive cerebellar ataxia. Cerebellum Ataxias. 2015;2:16.
2. Pitceathly RD, Rahman S, Hanna MG. Single deletions in mitochondrial DNA – molecular mechanisms and disease phenotypes in clinical practice. Neuromuscul Disord. 2012;22(7):577–86.
3. Aure K, Ogier de Baulny H, Laforet P, Jardel C, Eymard B, Lombes A. Chronic progressive ophthalmoplegia with large-scale mtDNA rearrangement: can we predict progression? Brain. 2007;130(Pt 6):1516–24.
4. Thorburn DR, Rahman J, Rahman S. Mitochondrial DNA-associated leigh syndrome and NARP. In: Adam MP, Ardinger HH, Pagon RA, Wallace SE, LJH B, Stephens K, et al., editors. GeneReviews((R)). Seattle, WA: University of Washington, Seattle; 1993. University of Washington, Seattle. GeneReviews is a registered trademark of the University of Washington, Seattle. All rights reserved.
5. Mancuso M, Orsucci D, Angelini C, Bertini E, Carelli V, Comi GP, et al. Phenotypic heterogeneity of the 8344A>G mtDNA "MERRF" mutation. Neurology. 2013;80(22):2049–54.
6. Petruzzella V, Zoccolella S, Amati A, Torraco A, Lamberti P, Carnicella F, et al. Cerebellar ataxia as atypical manifestation of the 3243A>G MELAS mutation. Clin Genet. 2004;65(1):64–5.
7. Rahman S, Copeland WC POLG-related disorders and neurological manifestations. Nat Rev Neurol. 2018. https://doi.org/10.1038/s41582-018-0101-0.
8. Cohen BH, Chinnery PF, Copeland WC. POLG-related disorders. 2010 Mar 16 [updated 2018 Mar 1]. In: Adam MP, Ardinger HH, Pagon RA, Wallace SE, Bean LJH, Stephens K, Amemiya A, editors. GeneReviews® [Internet]. Seattle: University of Washington, Seattle; 1993–2019. http://www.ncbi.nlm.nih.gov/books/NBK26471/
9. Spelbrink JN, Li FY, Tiranti V, Nikali K, Yuan QP, Tariq M, et al. Human mitochondrial DNA deletions associated with mutations in the gene encoding Twinkle, a phage T7 gene 4-like protein localized in mitochondria. Nat Genet. 2001;28(3):223–31.
10. Nikali K, Suomalainen A, Saharinen J, Kuokkanen M, Spelbrink JN, Lonnqvist T, et al. Infantile onset spinocerebellar ataxia is caused by recessive mutations in mitochondrial proteins Twinkle and Twinky. Hum Mol Genet. 2005;14(20):2981–90.
11. Sarzi E, Goffart S, Serre V, Chretien D, Slama A, Munnich A, et al. Twinkle helicase (PEO1) gene mutation causes mitochondrial DNA depletion. Ann Neurol. 2007;62(6):579–87.
12. Wolf NI, Koenig M. Progressive cerebellar atrophy: hereditary ataxias and disorders with spinocerebellar degeneration. Handb Clin Neurol. 2013;113: 1869–78.
13. Lagier-Tourenne C, Tazir M, Lopez LC, Quinzii CM, Assoum M, Drouot N, et al. ADCK3, an ancestral kinase, is mutated in a form of recessive ataxia associated with coenzyme Q10 deficiency. Am J Hum Genet. 2008;82(3):661–72.
14. Mollet J, Delahodde A, Serre V, Chretien D, Schlemmer D, Lombes A, et al. CABC1 gene mutations cause ubiquinone deficiency with cerebellar ataxia and seizures. Am J Hum Genet. 2008;82(3):623–30.
15. Stefely JA, Licitra F, Laredj L, Reidenbach AG, Kemmerer ZA, Grangeray A, et al. Cerebellar ataxia and coenzyme Q deficiency through loss of unorthodox kinase activity. Mol Cell. 2016;63(4):608–20.
16. Reidenbach AG, Kemmerer ZA, Aydin D, Jochem A, McDevitt MT, Hutchins PD, et al. Conserved lipid and small-molecule modulation of COQ8 reveals regulation of the ancient kinase-like UbiB family. Cell Chem Biol. 2018;25(2):154–65.e11.
17. Quinzii CM, Kattah AG, Naini A, Akman HO, Mootha VK, Dimauro S, et al. Coenzyme Q deficiency and cerebellar ataxia associated with an aprataxin mutation. Neurology. 2005;64(3):539–41.
18. Bidichandani SI, Delatycki MB. Friedreich ataxia. In: Adam MP, Ardinger HH, Pagon RA, Wallace SE, LJH B, Stephens K, et al., editors. GeneReviews((R)). Seattle, WA: University of Washington, Seattle; 1993. University of Washington, Seattle. GeneReviews is a

registered trademark of the University of Washington, Seattle. All rights reserved.
19. Rotig A, de Lonlay P, Chretien D, Foury F, Koenig M, Sidi D, et al. Aconitase and mitochondrial iron-sulphur protein deficiency in Friedreich ataxia. Nat Genet. 1997;17(2):215–7.
20. Engert JC, Berube P, Mercier J, Dore C, Lepage P, Ge B, et al. ARSACS, a spastic ataxia common in northeastern Quebec, is caused by mutations in a new gene encoding an 11.5-kb ORF. Nat Genet. 2000;24(2):120–5.
21. Parfitt DA, Michael GJ, Vermeulen EG, Prodromou NV, Webb TR, Gallo JM, et al. The ataxia protein sacsin is a functional co-chaperone that protects against polyglutamine-expanded ataxin-1. Hum Mol Genet. 2009;18(9):1556–65.
22. Bradshaw TY, Romano LE, Duncan EJ, Nethisinghe S, Abeti R, Michael GJ, et al. A reduction in Drp1-mediated fission compromises mitochondrial health in autosomal recessive spastic ataxia of Charlevoix Saguenay. Hum Mol Genet. 2016;25(15): 3232–44.
23. Lariviere R, Gaudet R, Gentil BJ, Girard M, Conte TC, Minotti S, et al. Sacs knockout mice present pathophysiological defects underlying autosomal recessive spastic ataxia of Charlevoix-Saguenay. Hum Mol Genet. 2015;24(3):727–39.
24. Takiyama Y. Sacsinopathies: sacsin-related ataxia. Cerebellum (London, England). 2007;6(4):353–9.
25. Bayat V, Thiffault I, Jaiswal M, Tetreault M, Donti T, Sasarman F, et al. Mutations in the mitochondrial methionyl-tRNA synthetase cause a neurodegenerative phenotype in flies and a recessive ataxia (ARSAL) in humans. PLoS Biol. 2012;10(3):e1001288.
26. Wedatilake Y, Brown RM, McFarland R, Yaplito-Lee J, Morris AA, Champion M, et al. SURF1 deficiency: a multi-centre natural history study. Orphanet J Rare Dis. 2013;8:96.
27. Debray FG, Lambert M, Gagne R, Maranda B, Laframboise R, MacKay N, et al. Pyruvate dehydrogenase deficiency presenting as intermittent isolated acute ataxia. Neuropediatrics. 2008;39(1):20–3.
28. Patron M, Sprenger HG, Langer T. m-AAA proteases, mitochondrial calcium homeostasis and neurodegeneration. Cell Res. 2018;28(3):296–306.
29. Higuchi Y, Okunushi R, Hara T, Hashiguchi A, Yuan J, Yoshimura A, et al. Mutations in COA7 cause spinocerebellar ataxia with axonal neuropathy. Brain. 2018;141(6):1622–36.
30. Edvardson S, Shaag A, Kolesnikova O, Gomori JM, Tarassov I, Einbinder T, et al. Deleterious mutation in the mitochondrial arginyl-transfer RNA synthetase gene is associated with pontocerebellar hypoplasia. Am J Hum Genet. 2007;81(4):857–62.
31. Glamuzina E, Brown R, Hogarth K, Saunders D, Russell-Eggitt I, Pitt M, et al. Further delineation of pontocerebellar hypoplasia type 6 due to mutations in the gene encoding mitochondrial arginyl-tRNA synthetase, RARS2. J Inherit Metab Dis. 2012;35(3):459–67.
32. Cassandrini D, Cilio MR, Bianchi M, Doimo M, Balestri M, Tessa A, et al. Pontocerebellar hypoplasia type 6 caused by mutations in RARS2: definition of the clinical spectrum and molecular findings in five patients. J Inherit Metab Dis. 2013;36(1):43–53.
33. Sofou K, De Coo IF, Isohanni P, Ostergaard E, Naess K, De Meirleir L, et al. A multicenter study on Leigh syndrome: disease course and predictors of survival. Orphanet J Rare Dis. 2014;9:52.
34. Lake NJ, Compton AG, Rahman S, Thorburn DR. Leigh syndrome: one disorder, more than 75 monogenic causes. Ann Neurol. 2016;79(2):190–203.
35. Rahman J, Noronha A, Thiele I, Rahman S. Leigh map: a novel computational diagnostic resource for mitochondrial disease. Ann Neurol. 2017;81(1):9–16.
36. Di Meo I, Tiranti V. Classification and molecular pathogenesis of NBIA syndromes. Eur J Paediatr Neurol. 2018;22(2):272–84.
37. Tranebjaerg L. Deafness-dystonia-optic neuronopathy syndrome. In: Adam MP, Ardinger HH, Pagon RA, Wallace SE, LJH B, Stephens K, et al., editors. GeneReviews((R)). Seattle, WA: University of Washington, Seattle; 1993. University of Washington, Seattle. GeneReviews is a registered trademark of the University of Washington, Seattle. All rights reserved.
38. Morato L, Bertini E, Verrigni D, Ardissone A, Ruiz M, Ferrer I, et al. Mitochondrial dysfunction in central nervous system white matter disorders. Glia. 2014;62(11):1878–94.
39. Serrano M, Garcia-Silva MT, Martin-Hernandez E, O'Callaghan MM, Quijada P, Martinez-Aragon A, et al. Kearns-Sayre syndrome: cerebral folate deficiency, MRI findings and new cerebrospinal fluid biochemical features. Mitochondrion. 2010;10(5):429–32.
40. van der Knaap MS, Pronk JC, Scheper GC. Vanishing white matter disease. Lancet Neurol. 2006;5(5):413–23.
41. Wong LJ. Mitochondrial syndromes with leukoencephalopathies. Semin Neurol. 2012;32(1):55–61.
42. Biancheri R, Rossi D, Cassandrini D, Rossi A, Bruno C, Santorelli FM. Cavitating leukoencephalopathy in a child carrying the mitochondrial A8344G mutation. AJNR Am J Neuroradiol. 2010;31(9):E78–9.
43. Fassone E, Rahman S. Complex I deficiency: clinical features, biochemistry and molecular genetics. J Med Genet. 2012;49(9):578–90.
44. Ishiyama A, Muramatsu K, Uchino S, Sakai C, Matsushima Y, Makioka N, et al. NDUFAF3 variants that disrupt mitochondrial complex I assembly may associate with cavitating leukoencephalopathy. Clin Genet. 2018;93(5):1103–6.
45. Kevelam SH, Rodenburg RJ, Wolf NI, Ferreira P, Lunsing RJ, Nijtmans LG, et al. NUBPL mutations in patients with complex I deficiency and a distinct MRI pattern. Neurology. 2013;80(17):1577–83.
46. Alston CL, Davison JE, Meloni F, van der Westhuizen FH, He L, Hornig-Do HT, et al. Recessive germline SDHA and SDHB mutations causing leukodystrophy

electrical abnormalities (arrhythmias and conduction system disease) and vary in severity from asymptomatic to severe forms, complicated by HF and/or sudden cardiac death (SCD) [14]. Additionally, diseases of the vasculature and autonomic system dysfunction are also possible as cardiovascular manifestations of MID.

Mitochondrial cardiomyopathy usually occurs as part of the multi-organ involvement of MID—fitting or not into an established clinical syndrome (syndromic or non-syndromic MID); yet notably, it may be encountered in the absence of known MID, of which it may be the first or sole clinical manifestation [16–20].

Table 1 summarizes syndromic and non-syndromic MID in which cardiac involvement is described. Among these, syndromic MID manifesting with cardiomyopathy include (among others) the following: chronic progressive external ophthalmoplegia (***CPEO***), Kearns–Sayre syndrome (***KSS***), mitochondrial encephalomyopathy with lactic acidosis and stroke-like

Table 1 Cardiac manifestations in primary mitochondrial disorders

Mitochondrial disease	Gene (s)	Cardiac manifestations
Syndromic MID		
Kearns–Sayre syndrome	*mtDNA single deletion*	AV block, bundle branch block, intraventricular conduction defects DCM SCD
CPEO	Multiple genes involved	AV block Concentric remodeling, myocardial fibrosis
MELAS	*MTTL1 (m.3242A>G in 80% cases), MIDND1*	**HCM**, DCM, LVNC Sinus node dysfunction, AV block, intraventricular conduction defects, WPW SCD
MERRF	*MTTK (m.8344A>G in 80% cases), MTTF, MTTL1, MTTI, MTTP*	HCM, DCM, histiocytoid cardiomyopathy WPW SCD
NARP	*MTATP6*	HCM Conduction defects
Leigh syndrome	*MTATP6, MTTL1, MTTK, MTTW, MTTV, MTND1, MTND2, MTND3, MTND4, MTND5, MTND6, TCO3*	**HCM**, DCM
MNGIE	*TYMP*	HCM (mild), bundle branch block
Respiratory chain complex deficiencies		
Complex I	*Subunit mtDNA genes: MTND1, MTND2, MTND4, MTND5, TND6* *Subunit nDNA genes: NDUFV1, NDUFV2, NDUFS1, NDUFS2, NDUFS3, NDUFS4, NDUFS6, NDUFS7, NDUFS8, NDUFA2, NDUFA11, NDUFAF3, NDUFA10, NDUFB3, NDUFB9, and NDUFA1* *Assembly genes: NDUFAF2, NDUFAF4, NDUFAF5, NUBPL, NDUFAF1, FOXRED1, ACAD9*	**HCM**, DCM, LVNC, WPW
Complex II	*Subunit genes: SDHA, SDHD*	HCM, DCM, LVNC
Complex III	*MTCYB*	HCM, DCM, histiocytoid cardiomyopathy

(continued)

Table 1 (continued)

Mitochondrial disease	Gene (s)	Cardiac manifestations
Complex IV	*Subunit mtDNA genes:* *MTCO1, MTCO2, MTCO3* *Subunit nDNA genes:* *COX6B1* *Assembly factors: COX10, COX14, COX15, COX20, SCO1, SCO2, COA3, COA5*	HCM, DCM, histiocytoid cardiomyopathy
Complex V	*TMEM70* *Subunit mtDNA genes: MT-ATP5E, MT-ATP8*	HCM, LVNC
CoQ10 deficiency		
Coenzyme Q10 deficiency	*COQ2, COQ4, COQ6, COQ7, COQ9, ADCK3, PDSS1, PDSS2*	HCM
Disorders characterized by 3-methylglutaconic aciduria (3-MGA)		
Barth syndrome	*TAZ*	HCM, DCM, LVNC, endocardial fibroelastosis Ventricular arrhythmias SCD
DCM and ataxia syndrome	*DNAJC19*	DCM, LVNC Long QT interval
TMEM70 associated 3-MGA	*TMEM70*	HCM
Sengers syndrome	*AGK*	HCM
Disorders of mitochondrial iron metabolism		
Friedreich ataxia	*FXN*	HCM
Disorders of β-oxidation and carnitine metabolism		
Primary carnitine deficiency	*SLC22A5*	DCM, HCM, arrhythmias, conduction defects
CPTII deficiency	*CPT2*	DCM, HCM, arrhythmias, conduction defects, SCD
CACT deficiency	*SLC25A20*	DCM, HCM, arrhythmias, conduction defects, SCD
VLCADD	*ACADVL*	HCM, DCM, arrhythmias, conduction defects
LCHAD/MTP deficiency	*HADHA*	HCM, DCM, arrhythmias, conduction defects
MADD	*ETFDH, ETFA, ETFB*	HCM, DCM, arrhythmias, conduction defects, SCD

Modified according to [14, 16]; additional references [99, 100]
CPEO chronic progressive external ophthalmoplegia, *MELAS* mitochondrial encephalomyopathy, lactic acidosis, and stroke-like episodes, *MERRF* myoclonic epilepsy with ragged red fibers, *NARP* neurogenic muscle weakness with sensory neuropathy, ataxia, and pigmentary retinopathy, *MNGIE* mitochondrial neurogastrointestinal encephalopathy, *CPTII* carnitine palmitoyl-transferase II, *CACT* carnitine-acylcarnitine translocase, *VLCADD* very long chain acyl-coenzyme Q dehydrogenase deficiency, *LCHAD*/MTP longchain 3-hydroxyacyl-coenzyme A dehydrogenase/mitochondrial trifunctional protein, *MADD* multiple acyl-coenzyme Q dehydrogenase deficiency (glutaric aciduria type II), *AV* atrioventricular, *HCM* hypertrophic cardiomyopathy, *DCM* dilated cardiomyopathy, *LVNC* left ventricular noncompaction cardiomyopathy, *WPW* Wolf–Parkinson–White syndrome, *SCD* sudden cardiac death

episodes (***MELAS***), myoclonic epilepsy with ragged red fibers (***MERRF***), neurogenic weakness with ataxia and retinitis pigmentosa (***NARP***), mitochondrial neurogastrointestinal encephalopathy (***MNGIE***), and ***Barth*** and ***Leigh syndromes*** [1, 14, 16]. Nevertheless, even within the same syndrome, symptom severity and the number of organs affected can vary greatly between individuals as well as in time for the same individual [16, 21]. For example, in a report including patients with the mutation *m.8344A>G* (associated with MERRF syndrome), "myocardiomyopathy" was the most frequent clinical feature, whereas half of them did not show signs of central nervous system involvement even in late stages of the disease [16, 21].

Cardiomyopathy Phenotypes/ Myocardial Abnormalities

The most common manifestation of myocardial involvement in MID is represented by a hypertrophic cardiomyopathy phenotype (HCM) [1, 14]. Additionally, dilated (DCM), restrictive, left ventricular non-compaction (LVNC) and histiocytoid cardiomyopathy phenotypes were described in these patients [1, 14]. The rare finding of ***histiocytoid cardiomyopathy*** or ***Purkinje fiber dysplasia*** seems to be encountered only in MID and is histologically characterized by morphological and functional abnormalities of cardiomyocytes and Purkinje cells with a cytoplasm like in histiocyte foam cells, which contain a huge amount of glycogen and lipids [22–24].

Among different MID, ***MELAS*** syndrome with the most common underlying mutation—*m.3243A>G*—is most strongly associated with cardiomyopathy [25]. Several studies using transthoracic echocardiography report LV hypertrophy in 23% of children and in up to 56% of adults with MELAS syndrome [5, 26, 27]. In a smaller MID series using cardiovascular magnetic resonance (CMR), 9 out of 11 ***MELAS/ MELAS-like*** patients included presented LV hypertrophy with or without LV systolic dysfunction, 67% of them showing a concentric pattern (Fig. 2) [7]. Moreover, the concentric remodeling encountered in *m.3243A>G* carriers correlated with the presence of LV longitudinal systolic dysfunction in CMR and with a higher mutation load [28]. Additionally, by means of late gadolinium enhancement (LGE) CMR, myocardial fibrosis with a unique, focally accentuated, and diffusely distributed pattern can be depicted in these patients [7, 8, 13]. Notably, LV hypertrophy was the only parameter independently associated with occurrence of HF and cardiac death in patients carrying the *m.3243A>G* mutation [4]. DCM, as primary manifestation or secondary to HCM, is also reported in ***MELAS*** but less commonly as HCM [5, 11, 29].

A tendency toward concentric LV remodeling or overt LVH was described also in ***CPEO*** [7, 8, 30]. In ***KSS*** patients, on the other hand, progressive conduction disturbances are usually present (see further), and only a few cases of cardiomyopathy—either left ventricular dysfunction or DCM—have been reported in literature [31–33]. In a recent CMR study, LGE with a predominantly nonischemic intramural pattern involving the inferolateral wall was encountered in 30% of adults with ***CPEO/KSS*** (Fig. 3) [7]. Interestingly, despite high prevalence of patients with cardiac symptoms (50%), the detection of fibrosis on CMR did not correlate with ECG or cardiac biomarker abnormalities and was the only pathologic finding in half of the patients [7, 8].

In a small study which included patients carrying the common ***MERRF*** syndrome mutation *m.8344A>G*, myocardial abnormalities on echocardiography comprising LV dilatation or hypertrophy with or without systolic dysfunction were found altogether in 44% of patients. Moreover, cardiomyopathy was associated with an increased risk of cardiac death due to HF [34]. In another study with similar echocardiographic findings, LGE with a nonischemic, subepicardial, and intramural distribution in the basal inferolateral LV wall was found as an early sign of cardiac involvement, also in ***MERRF*** [21]. Histiocytoid cardiomyopathy was reported in an infant carrying the common ***MERRF*** mutation *m.8344A>G* [35].

Cardiomyopathy, mostly hypertrophic as well as dilated, is described in 10% of the patients with ***Leigh syndrome***, the most common infantile MID [9, 36–38]. About 50% of affected individuals die by age 3, most often as a result of cardiorespiratory failure [39]. Interestingly, cardiac disease was twice as prevalent in patients with mtDNA mutations compared with nuclear DNA mutations [38]. HCM was described also in ***NARP***, another syndromic MID with symptom onset in early childhood [40]. HCM, even requiring heart transplantation, is described also in children with ***Sengers syndrome*** [3].

Cardiomyopathy, manifesting as LV hypertrophy and/or ventricular dilation with or without endocardial fibroelastosis, is the most common feature of the X-linked ***Barth syndrome***, with onset within the first year of life in >70% of cases [41]. Moreover, approximately 50% of patients present prominent LV trabeculations, suggesting LVNC [42, 43]. Data from the Pediatric Cardiomyopathy Registry of the USA suggest that 3–5% of young boys with cardiomyopathy turn out to have ***Barth syndrome*** [42]. In ***Barth syndrome***, cardiomyopathy follows a typical undulating course, with improvement during childhood and subsequent progressive late dilation in a subset of the population [9, 42, 44]. Thus, 14% of the 151 patients worldwide

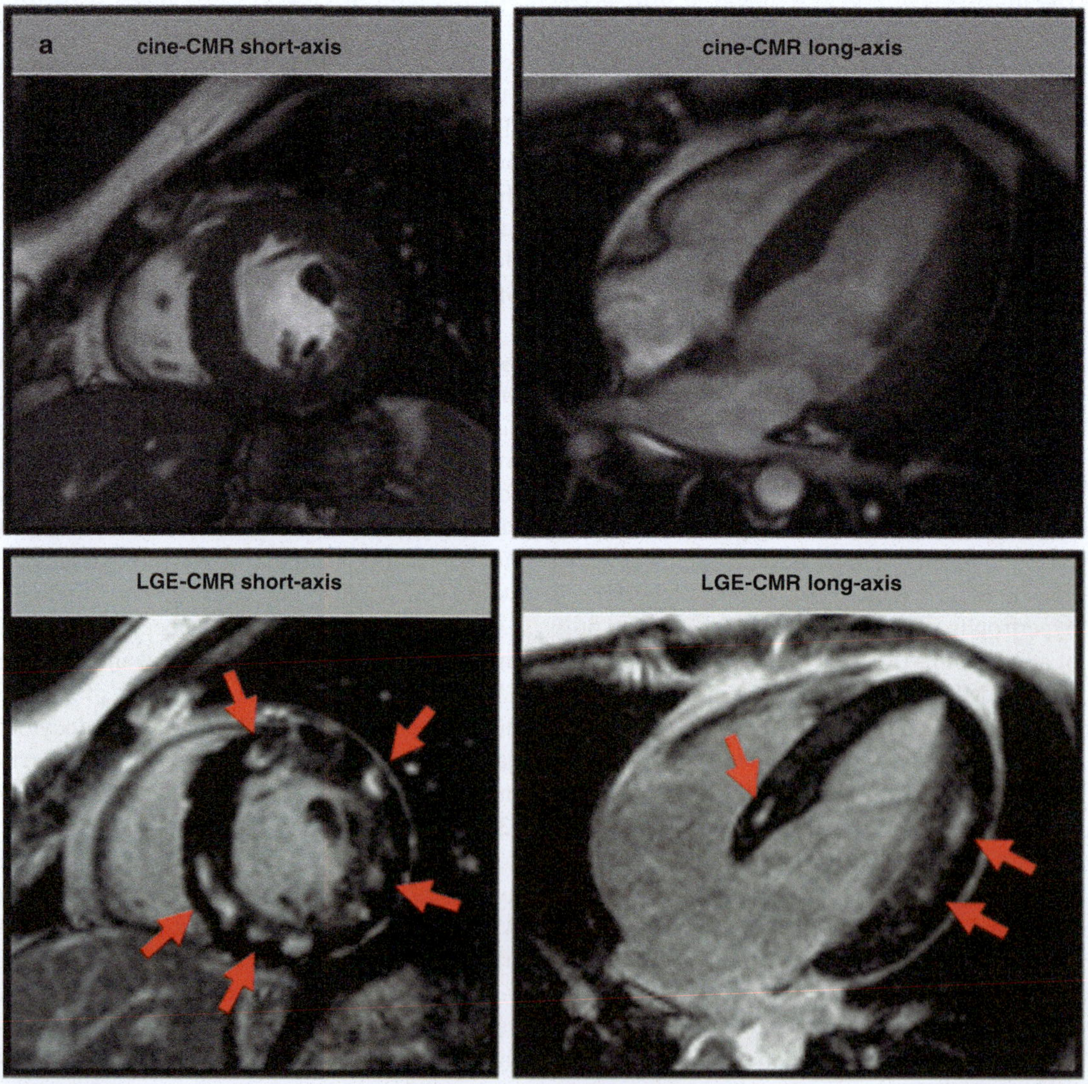

Fig. 2 (**a**) Short- and long-axis CMR images in female patient with a MELAS-like mitochondrial disorder. Red arrows indicate the areas of myocardial fibrosis detected in late gadolinium enhancement (LGE) images. (**b**) Short- and long-axis CMR images in the younger brother of the female patient also suffering from the same MELAS-like mitochondrial disorder

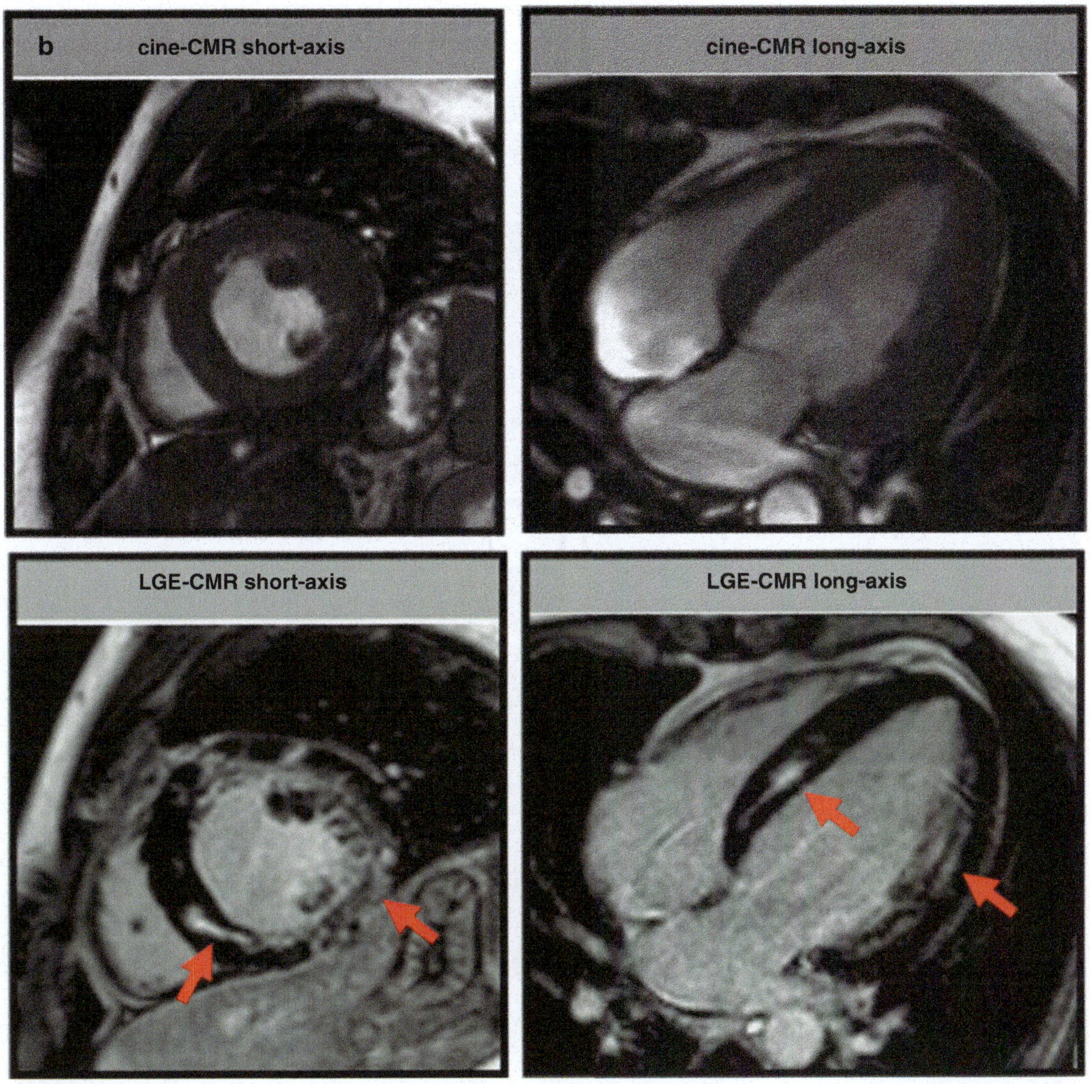

Fig. 2 (continued)

included in the Barth Foundation Registry ended up requiring cardiac transplantation [42]. In another more recent study from the UK, 26% of the 27 patients included underwent cardiac transplantation before the age of 5. The same study suggests a good long-term prognosis after the first 5 years of life [45].

Cardiac manifestations are also described in ***MNGIE*** syndrome and include mild ventricular hypertrophy and bundle branch block [14]. HCM has been described in case reports also in ***COQ2-, COQ4-, and COQ9-related CoQ10 deficiencies***, usually associating encephalopathy, myopathy, and other severe system manifestations and having pre- or neonatal onset of disease [46].

Moreover, ***Friedreich ataxia*** represents another genetic disorder that is characterized by intramitochondrial iron accumulation. Based on a CMR study, patients with FA were found to have a reduced myocardial perfusion reserve and the presence of myocardial fibrosis without (or prior to) a significant LV hypertrophy and prior to clinical heart failure symptoms [47].

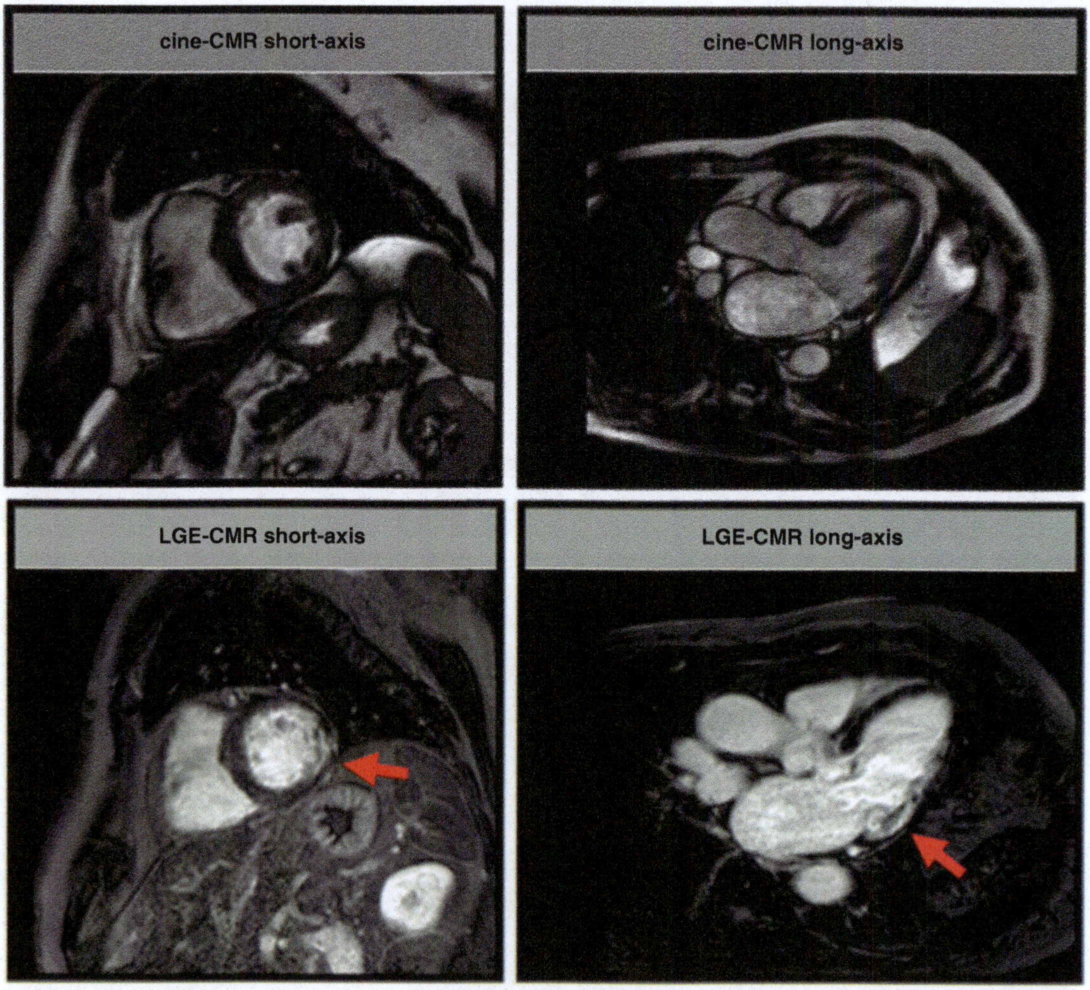

Fig. 3 Short- and long-axis CMR images in a male patient with CPEO. Red arrows indicate the areas of myocardial fibrosis detected in late gadolinium enhancement (LGE) images

Rhythm and Conduction System Abnormalities

Table 1 includes rhythm and conduction system abnormalities described in syndromic and non-syndromic MID. Syndromic MID in which arrhythmias are particularly encountered comprise ***KSS***, ***MELAS***, and ***Leigh*** syndromes [48]. However, depending on the stage of disease, arrhythmias may occur in most patients with MID suffering from cardiomyopathy (Fig. 4) [1]. In a study including adult MID patients, arrhythmias were found in 22% of cases, while another study reported rhythm or conduction abnormalities in 8% of children with MID and cardiac symptoms [1, 49, 50].

Conduction defects with progressive, often unpredictable course, including intraventricular conduction abnormalities, bundle branch block, and varying degrees of AV block, represent a hallmark of ***KSS syndrome*** [1, 31, 51]. Electrophysiological studies (EP) in KSS patients show normal sinus node recovery and atrial to His times but prolonged His to ventricle conduction intervals. However, the incremental value of a routine EP study in KSS patients remains unclear [52, 53]. In a study following 67 KSS patients over 10 years, 32% developed conduc-

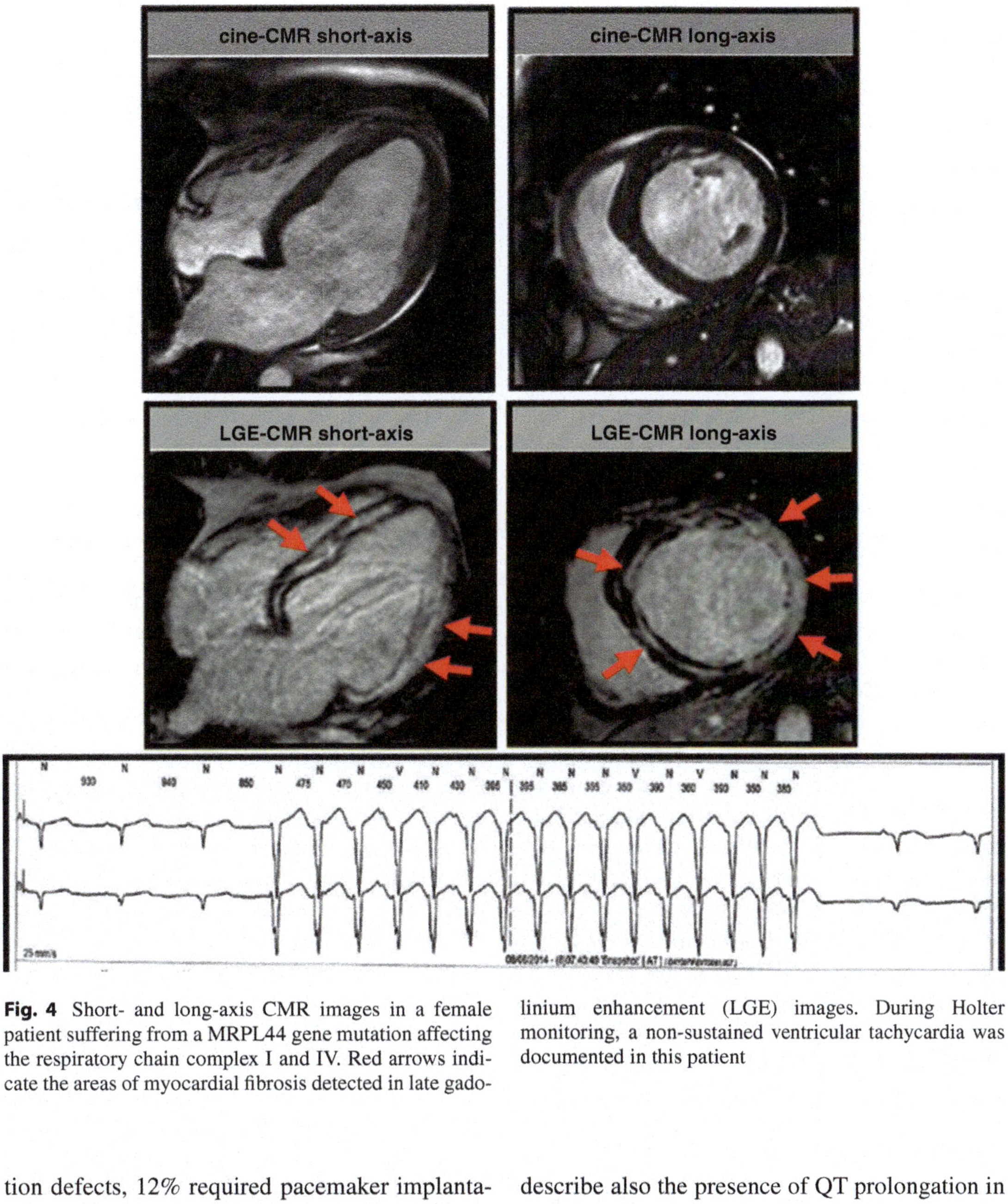

Fig. 4 Short- and long-axis CMR images in a female patient suffering from a MRPL44 gene mutation affecting the respiratory chain complex I and IV. Red arrows indicate the areas of myocardial fibrosis detected in late gadolinium enhancement (LGE) images. During Holter monitoring, a non-sustained ventricular tachycardia was documented in this patient

tion defects, 12% required pacemaker implantation, and 5% suffered SCD [31]. In another series following 35 KSS patients for an average time of 10 years, 31% developed AV blocks, and in 31% a pacemaker was implanted, while 6 patients experienced syncope, 5 had a resuscitated cardiac arrest, and 4 died of SCD [54]. Ventricular arrhythmias represented by bradycardia-related polymorphic ventricular tachycardia are reported in a few ***KSS*** patients [1, 52]. Several case reports describe also the presence of QT prolongation in ***KSS syndrome*** [55, 56].

Conduction system abnormalities, such as sinus node dysfunction, AV, or intraventricular conduction defects, were reported also in several ***MELAS*** cases [1, 4, 26, 57]. Interestingly, one study found preexcitation (Wolff–Parkinson–White syndrome) in 18% of patients carrying the ***MELAS***-associated mutation, *m.3243A>G* [4]. Tachyarrhythmia represented by atrial fibrillation and non-sustained ventricular tachycardia are also reported in a few MELAS patients, usually in association with LV hypertrophy [26]. Sudden death may occur in the presence of *m.3243A>G*, and it was described in 26% of mutation carriers as well as in patients with ***MELAS*** [4, 5, 58]. The large Medical Research Council Center Mitochondrial Disease Patient Cohort, based on data from *n* = 209 *m.3243A>G* carriers followed up for 6 years, estimated an incidence rate of sudden death of 2.4 per 1000 person-years, suggesting that this could be an underestimated cause of death in young, asymptomatic adults [59]. Wolff–Parkinson–White syndrome was also described in 17% of a study group of 18 patients carrying the ***MERRF***-associated mutation (*m.8344A>G*) and in 22% of an earlier published, larger ***MERRF*** cohort [34, 60].

Regarding MID in the pediatric population, clinical manifestations of ***NARP*** syndrome include also cardiac conduction abnormalities [39]. In patients with ***Barth syndrome***, ventricular arrhythmias are reported [44, 61]. Spencer et al. documented ventricular arrhythmias in 7 out of the 34 Barth syndrome patients examined [43, 61]. In a later publication with a larger study group, 13% of 70 patients underwent ICD implantation [44]. There are data suggesting that ventricular arrhythmias seem to occur predominantly in older rather than in small children and are not necessarily related to the presence or severity of cardiomyopathy [61]. SCD occurring within families is also described in ***Barth syndrome*** [61, 62].

Mitochondrial Vasculopathy

A primary ***mitochondrial vasculopathy*** due to direct involvement of blood vessels, mainly arteries, by the MID is also described and comprises clinical or subclinical ***micro- and macroangiopathy***. Clinical manifestations of ***microangiopathy*** involve the nervous system and include leucoencephalopathy, migraine-like headache, stroke-like episodes, and peripheral retinopathy [63].

Macroangiopathy is a rare manifestation of MID and seems to involve the aorta and cerebral arteries [63]. A single study by Brunetti–Pierri et al. reports ***aortic root dilation*** in ten patients with non-syndromic MID [64]. It is unknown whether this is associated with an increased risk of aortic dissection [63]. ***Dilation of the cerebral arteries*** is even rarer with only two cases reported: one case illustrates an ectatic basilary artery with suspected MID and the other a pseudoaneurysm of the internal carotid artery in association with MELAS [65, 66]. ***Spontaneous dissection of the carotid artery*** was described in a few patients so far, all carriers of the *m.3243A>G* mutation [67]. Additionally, there is one report of a ***spontaneous thoracic aorta rupture*** in a girl with MELAS syndrome and histological signs of severe mitochondrial aortopathy together with a high mutation load in the aorta [68]. Though not systematically investigated, there are indications that ***premature atherosclerosis*** might occur more frequently in patients with MID, particularly in the absence of classical risk factors [1, 63, 69, 70]. In addition, vasculopathy may be a secondary manifestation of MID due to organ involvement causing diabetes, hyperlipidemia, and arterial hypertension [63].

Pulmonary arterial hypertension (PAH) is cited, though only based on a limited number of cases, as a very rare manifestation of both syndromic and non-syndromic MID. The mechanism of this association remains unclear [1]. Three patients—two children and one adult, associating PAH with the MELAS mutation m.A3243A>G—have been described [1, 71]. PAH is also part of the extremely rare ***HUPRA syndrome*** (hyperuricemia, pulmonary hypertension, renal failure in infancy and alkalosis), caused by a mutation in the SARS2 gene, which encodes the mitochondrial seryl-tRNA synthetase. There are only three cases of HUPRA syndrome cited so far (all infants) [72]. Severe persistent PAH in the newborn in association with neonatal hypotonia, HCM, facial dysmorphism, severe lactic acidosis, hyperammonemia, and 3-methylglutaconic aciduria is reported as a frequent manifestation of ***complex V deficiency*** caused by a defect in the nuclear gene ***TMEM70***

[73]. Further, PAH has been described in association with poor growth, microcephaly, and multiple linear skin defects in a child with ***complex IV deficiency*** due to a mutation in the COX7B gene [74]. Lastly, PAH can also be encountered in some syndromic or non-syndromic MID secondary to organ involvement with consecutive severe dysfunction, such as severe liver disease or ventilatory impairment [71].

Autonomic Dysfunction

Primary mitochondrial neuropathy involving the autonomic nervous system may be present in patients with MID [1]. Particularly carriers of the mutation *m.3243A>G* have a high prevalence of autonomic dysfunction symptoms, including ***orthostatic intolerance*** in up to 28% of cases [75]. In a series of 22 MID patients in whom the cardiovascular parasympathetic and sympathetic function as well as heart rate variability were extensively investigated, 46% showed definite and 36% moderate autonomic involvement, while only 18% presented symptoms of autonomic dysfunction [76]. In another study that examined 28 patients with the mutation *m.3243A>G*, heart rate variability abnormalities were noted independently to other manifestations of disease, suggesting a primary mitochondrial autonomic system dysfunction [77]. Moreover, there is evidence that in MID, skeletal myopathy is characterized by an enhanced ergoreflex sensitivity, and this is associated with a higher incidence of cardiac involvement, exercise intolerance, and sympathetic activation [78].The ergoreflex is a neuromuscular reflex regulating ventilatory and autonomic responses to exercise. In chronic HF, for example, increased ergoreflex sensitivity was associated with a worse clinical status and abnormal cardiorespiratory reflex control, independently of clinical severity [79]. Currently, it is yet unclear whether MID patients without symptoms suggesting an autonomic involvement should be routinely screened for subclinical cardiovascular autonomic dysfunction [76].

Secondary Mitochondrial Dysfunction in Cardiovascular Disease

Besides primary genetic MID, which are rare diseases, there is strong evidence that perturbations of mitochondrial morphology and function are involved in the pathogenesis of more common, acquired cardiovascular diseases such as hypertension, atherosclerosis, ischemic heart disease, or heart failure [80]. Moreover, there is increasing evidence that "natural" nonpathogenic mtDNA polymorphisms could be associated with changes in mitochondrial function and may influence individual susceptibility to cardiovascular disease [25]. This rather complex topic is beyond the purpose of the current chapter, yet as future direction, a better understanding of mitochondrial genetics and function is expected to open avenues toward novel therapeutic strategies in the abovementioned cardiovascular diseases [80].

Diagnostic Approach and Management of Mitochondrial Heart Involvement

Since possible cardiac manifestations of mitochondrial disease comprise (1) heart failure symptoms due to systolic and/or diastolic functional impairment, (2) conduction abnormalities as well as ventricular arrhythmias such as higher-degree AV blocks and ventricular tachycardia, and (3) sudden cardiac death, diagnostic and therapeutic approaches have to consider not only functional and structural abnormalities but also electric disturbances.

The clinical course and disease severity differ between young patients and adults with MID: severe disease manifestations with profound metabolic abnormalities mostly occur in infants and young children and demonstrate a quickly progressive disease course, whereas adult patients with a late onset of mild-to-moderate symptoms show a more benign and slowly progressive disease manifestation. Certain triggers and/or constellations such as severe infections, malnutrition, surgery, or even pregnancy may cause a rapid deterioration of both the general condition and the cardiac performance [30].

Obviously, a close collaboration between experienced neurologists, cardiologists, and geneticists (and other specialists, e.g., ophthalmologist) is required in order to adequately address different organ involvements in such complex multi-organ disorders. Noteworthy, the following recommendation was mentioned in a recently published scientific statement from the American Heart Association (AHA) regarding the management of cardiac involvement associated with neuromuscular diseases [81]:

- *All neurologists diagnosing and managing NMDs should work to identify either a cardiologist with expertise in these conditions or at minimum a collaborative electrophysiologist or heart failure specialist, depending on the condition being evaluated (Class I; Level of Evidence B).*

However, since cardiac disease and subsequent cardiac symptoms may represent the first clinical manifestation of several MID, an experienced cardiologist with awareness of multisystem disorders and of red flags that are characteristic for some mitochondriopathies may already diagnose the underlying mitochondrial disease and spare the patient going through or continue an unnecessary odyssey [82]. For example, patients with KSS are characterized by ophthalmoplegia (particularly ptosis) and retinopathy from a neurological point of view. On the other hand, KSS patients are predisposed to suffer from atrioventricular conduction defects that can be quickly progressive in individual cases, potentially resulting in higher-degree AV blocks and clinical signs of bradycardia such as dizziness, syncope, and even sudden cardiac death. Therefore, a cardiologist has to consider KSS in a young patient presenting with the combination of an eye disorder and cardiac conduction abnormalities. In contrast, MELAS patients are characterized by hardness of hearing, stroke-like episodes in their history, and elevated blood lactate levels. Such patients typically demonstrate hypertrophied left ventricles and are prone to rapid cardiac decompensations and/or ventricular arrhythmias. Hence, MELAS and MELAS-like syndromes need to be considered by cardiologists in patients with hearing loss, seizures, and signs of hypertrophic cardiomyopathy.

General Recommendations Regarding the Diagnosis of Cardiac Disease

After taking a thorough patient history with a major focus on (1) neuromuscular symptoms, (2) heart failure symptoms, (3) potential arrhythmic events, and (4) the family history, a physical examination with a careful assessment of signs of heart failure (ankle edema, lung crackles, swollen jugular veins, and/or auscultation of S3 and S4 gallop) should be performed. Baseline laboratory work-up should include a complete blood count, electrolyte levels, creatine kinase (CK and CK-MB), troponin T or I, renal/liver/thyroid parameters, blood glucose and hemoglobin A1c, as well as lactate and pyruvate (a lactate-to-pyruvate ratio >20 is considered abnormal). Considering the observation that troponin T concentrations are regularly elevated in most patients with skeletal myopathies due to a suggested cross-reaction of the troponin T immunoassay with skeletal muscle troponin isoforms, the measurement of troponin I—that is more heart muscle specific—should be preferred in patients with MID [27]. Thereafter, a resting ECG and a thorough thoracic echocardiography study are mandatory. A conventional echocardiography should be performed as the first-line imaging tool in order to quickly assess anatomic and functional parameters such as ventricle diameter or systolic/diastolic LV function.

The diagnostic armamentarium for the work-up of cardiomyopathies has increased greatly over the past years. Today, noninvasive imaging modalities such as CMR allow a detailed and comprehensive work-up of cardiomyopathies and enable the noninvasive and safe diagnosis of the underlying origin in various cardiovascular diseases [83, 84]. Noteworthy, in a recent CMR study comprising patients with different forms of

MID, CMR was superior to ECG as well as to the measurement of cardiac biomarkers regarding the detection of cardiomyopathy for both the whole study group and individual subgroups [7]. Obviously, ECG abnormalities are quite common and are sometimes seen early in the disease course, but they are mostly unspecific [85]. Moreover, ECG abnormalities did not relate to the functional and/or structural CMR findings in CPEO/KSS, and there was only a weak relationship in MELAS/MELAS-like patients [7]. Nevertheless, in a recent large-scale study by Wahbi et al. that comprised 260 patients with genetically proven MID, MACE were independently predicted (among others) by an intraventricular conduction block documented in the resting ECG [5].

Considering available data and the unique diagnostic capabilities of CMR [8, 83], we suggest that a CMR study should be part of the diagnostic approach of cardiomyopathy in patients with mitochondrial disease. In this context, the recently published ESC guidelines for the management of hypertrophic cardiomyopathy also address mitochondrial diseases such as MELAS and suggest to perform a CMR study at initial presentation—if local expertise in this technique is available [86]. Therefore, CMR should be considered in all patients with MID (in particular in those with LV hypertrophy) at their baseline assessment—if local expertise and individual patient characteristics permit it. Moreover, CMR follow-up studies in patients with MID and the presence of pathological CMR results (particularly with presence of LGE and/or impaired systolic function) and potentially progressive disease (particularly those with MELAS and MELAS-like disease) should be considered every 6–12 months, while a follow-up study every 4–5 years will be sufficient in (adult) patients without involvement of the heart muscle. Nevertheless, regular Holter monitoring (at least once a year and even more frequently in the case of abnormal ECG findings) is required also in those patients with normal CMR results, since electric disturbances may be present without detectable functional and/or structural abnormalities (Fig. 5).

In addition to the aforementioned issues, invasive endomyocardial biopsy (EMB) techniques have been optimized and allow a safe and targeted sampling of biopsy specimens from both the LV and RV myocardia with sophisticated postprocedural techniques, allowing a comprehensive histopathological work-up of such specimens with subsequent exact diagnosis [87, 88]. However, such a sophisticated but also expensive array of techniques forces the clinician to use these tools carefully and rationally. In order to achieve a straightforward diagnosis in a patient with suspected cardiomyopathy, a holistic and systematic approach with a stepwise targeted selection of appropriate diagnostic techniques is required [84].

In spite of the availability of novel and promising noninvasive diagnostic approaches (such as CMR), "invasive" endomyocardial biopsy still constitutes the gold standard for the definitive diagnosis of a specific cardiomyopathy. Keeping major limitations of the EMB procedure in mind (such as the "sampling error," the invasiveness of the procedure with a non-neglectable risk of complication and the respective guideline restrictions with respect to performing one or serial biopsies in patients with preserved LV systolic function), a CMR-targeted sampling of myocardial samples with a subsequent work-up of the obtained specimens by an experienced pathologist may help in individual cases to obtain the underlying diagnosis and/or to rule out other (e.g., inflammatory) cardiac diseases [88]. Work-up of EMB samples in the case of suspected mitochondrial disease should not only include light microscopy for the assessment of structural changes but also histochemistry as well as electron microscopy in order to accurately assess specific findings such as "cytochrome oxidase-negative fibers" (due to disturbances in the respiratory chain that can be detected by histochemistry), "ragged red fibers" (subsarcolemmal accumulation of mitochondria that may be detected using a modified Gomori trichrome staining), or the presence of swollen mitochondria with irregular cristae (nonfunctional, however, enlarged mitochondria that can be depicted by electron microscopy) (Fig. 6).

Fig. 5 Suggested algorithm for the cardiac management of patients with mitochondrial disorders

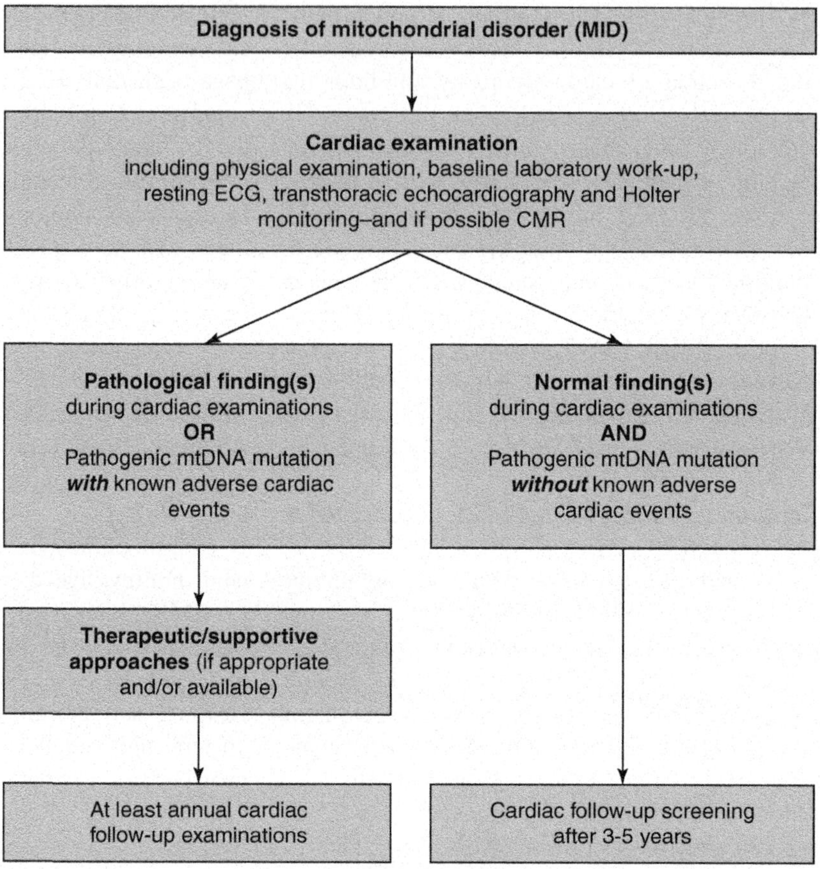

Moreover, spectrophotometric assays that are routinely performed in the case of skeletal muscle biopsies in order to assess disturbances in the respiratory chain function as well as mitochondrial genome screening (e.g., for mtDNA deletions) can also be applied to fresh-frozen EMB samples [89]; however, respective data regarding cardiac samples are quite limited, and specific cardiac criteria have therefore not been defined [87].

General Recommendations Regarding the Management of Cardiac Disease

Evidence-based data regarding therapeutic implementations for the treatment of cardiac disease in patients with MID are quite limited. Therefore, current treatment strategies focus on relieving symptoms and avoiding mitochondrial stress factors. However, different promising therapeutic approaches were successfully tested in preclinical animal models of MID and small-sized human studies, but the respective evidence is not sufficient to draw any valid conclusions for a broad clinical application [80].

Patients with MID have different nutritional requirements and therefore should receive an age-appropriate diet and energy intake [90]. However, the cardiac benefit of such an approach (e.g., evaluation of the nutritional state by interpretation of the skeletal muscle biochemistry in patients with a suspected oxidative phosphorylation defect) is not well-known, and respective data regarding the effect on cardiac disease are missing.

Regular exercise training is reasonable not only in patients with mitochondrial disorders but actually in almost all patients with cardiovascular diseases. In a small-sized study, the authors assessed the effects of exercise training and

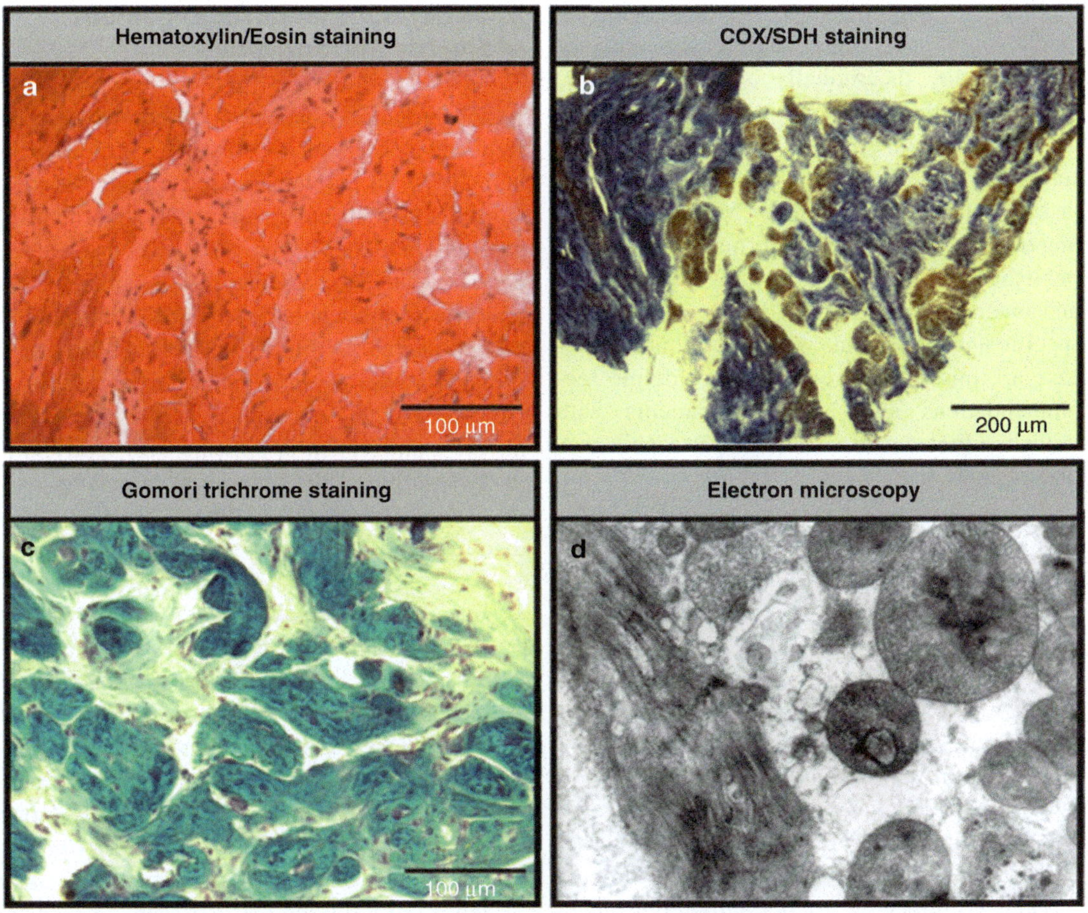

Fig. 6 Endomyocardial biopsy (EMB) images of a patient with a MELAS-like mitochondrial disorder: (**a**) Hematoxylin/eosin staining illustrating hypertrophic cardiomyocytes with disproportional cell sizes and intercellular areas of fibrosis. (**b**) Combined cytochrome c oxidase (COX) and succinate dehydrogenase (SDH) staining indicating COX deficiency in some cardiomyocytes. (**c**) Modified Gomori trichrome staining demonstrating irregular-shaped cardiomyocytes and increased areas of intercellular fibrosis. (**d**) Electron microscopy image showing an excessive number of swollen mitochondria with variability in size and shape and abnormal morphology

detraining in eight patients with single, large-scale mtDNA deletions [91]. They could show that only 14 weeks of exercise training significantly improved tolerance of submaximal exercise and peak capacity for work, oxygen utilization, and skeletal muscle oxygen extraction with no change in the level of deleted mtDNA. This improvement prevailed when exercise training was continued for an additional 14 weeks. Moreover, stopping of training (detraining) resulted in loss of physiological adaptation to baseline capacity with no overall change in mutation load. Hence, one may expect beneficial effects of training on physiological outcome and quality of life that (unfortunately) quickly disappear after stopping exercise training.

Specific Issues in the Management of Functional and/or Structural Cardiac Abnormalities

In patients with mitochondrial disease and a rather hypertrophic pattern of cardiomyopathy (e.g., MELAS or MELAS-like patients), ß-blockers, angiotensin-converting enzyme (ACE) inhibitors, and angiotensin receptor blockers may theoretically help to (at least) slow down the progression of cardiomyopathy—as was shown in etiologically different forms of HCM [86]. Noteworthy, mitochondrial diseases such as MELAS and MELAS-like are mentioned as specific HCM forms in the recently published "2014 ESC guidelines on diagnosis and management of HCM." Hence, as long as specific data on patients with mitochondrial disease are missing, current HCM guideline recommendations also apply to patients with mitochondrial disease and a hypertrophic cardiac phenotype.

Although specific data on heart failure medications such as ACE inhibitors, ß-blockers, and diuretics in patients with mitochondrial disease are lacking, the following AHA recommendations should be considered [81]:

- *The use of an ACE inhibitor or ARB in the setting of a reduced EF is recommended for all NMDs (Class I; Level of Evidence B).*
- *Given the balance of human data regarding the use of β-adrenergic blockade in DMD/BMD and, to a lesser extent, other neuromuscular disorders, the use of β-adrenergic blockade in the setting of any NMD with a reduced EF is recommended (Class I; Level of Evidence B).*
- *Without other indication (e.g., arrhythmia), the use of β-adrenergic blockade in the absence of reduced EF as therapy to delay or prevent onset of dilated cardiomyopathy is currently not recommended (Class III; Level of Evidence C).*
- *Patients with NMD and fluid retention associated with ventricular dysfunction should be treated with diuretic agents to achieve a euvolemic state (Class I; Level of Evidence C).*
- *Aspirin or low-dose anticoagulation therapy may be considered for patients with BTHS and non-compaction phenotype (Class IIb; Level of Evidence C).*

Specific Issues in the Management of Electric Abnormalities

Atrioventricular conduction abnormalities are frequently observed in some MID such as KSS and CPEO. In individual cases, a rapid progression of atrioventricular conduction abnormalities resulting in higher-degree AV blocks and sudden cardiac death was described [92]—although the majority of mitochondrial patients with first- or second-degree AV blocks do not show any progression over years and even decades. Nevertheless, the current *2015 ESC Guidelines for the management of patients with ventricular arrhythmias and the prevention of sudden cardiac death* specifically address neuromuscular disorders and state that:

- *Permanent pacemaker implantation is recommended in patients with neuromuscular diseases and third-degree or advanced second-degree AV block at any anatomical level (Class I, Level of Evidence B).*
- *Permanent pacemaker implantation may be considered in patients with Kearns–Sayre syndrome with any degree of AV block (including first-degree) in consideration of the risk of rapid progression (Class IIb, Level of Evidence B).*
- *Patients with neuromuscular disorders who have ventricular arrhythmias are treated in the same way as patients without neuromuscular disorders (Class I, Level of Evidence C).*

Similar to other genetic cardiomyopathies, e.g., HCM, the presence and CMR-based detection of nonischemic myocardial scars may play an additional prognostic role in the risk stratification of patients with MID (particularly in MELAS and MELAS-like patients) [86, 93]. Available data suggest that MELAS patients have a high incidence of cardiac death as well as ventricular arrhythmia and heart failure events that are primarily related to LV hypertrophy [3]. Preliminary CMR data in MELAS/MELAS-like patients point to a rather disproportionately extensive pattern of myocardial fibrosis compared to the degree of LV hypertrophy [7, 13]. Therefore, it may be expected that CMR-based detection of myocardial fibrosis in these patients could have a superior prognostic value than in other non-mitochondrial diseases that are also associated with LV hypertrophy. However, according prognostic data in patients with mitochondrial disease are so far missing.

Although EP studies in KSS patients showed prolonged His to ventricle conduction intervals in some patients, the diagnostic value of a routine EP study remains unclear not only in KSS patients but also other forms of MID [52, 53]. Hence, the indication and potential benefit in performing an EP study has to be evaluated after careful consideration of the individual findings.

In spite of lacking data regarding the use of oral anticoagulation in patients with mitochondrial disease, the following AHA recommendation should be considered [81]:

- *Thrombosis prophylaxis in children with NMDs, normal systolic ventricular function, and AF/atrial flutter may be considered, with type of therapy determined based on the individual patient's thrombosis risk (Class IIb; Level of Evidence C).*

Moreover, it should be kept in mind that class I, II, or IV anti-arrhythmic medications can further increase peripheral muscular weakness in patients with mitochondrial diseases [94]. Hence, the decision to use such agents should be carefully evaluated considering individual patient characteristics and needs.

Supportive Therapy of Mitochondrial Disorders with Heart Involvement (Data About Effects of Diet, CoQ10, Exercise, etc. on Cardiac Involvement)

Supportive therapeutic strategies in patients with mitochondrial disorders comprise the use of (mostly dietary) supplements such as coenzyme Q10, L-carnitine, riboflavin, creatine, folate, and vitamin C and E. Unfortunately, evidence-based data supporting the use of the aforementioned supplements are either scarce or completely missing. In a very comprehensive systematic review by Chinnery et al. that was already performed in 2006, the authors reviewed 678 abstracts, and only 6 of them fulfilled their predefined entry criteria (defined as randomized controlled trials and quasi-randomized trials comparing pharmacological treatments) [95]. Two of those trials studied the effects of coenzyme Q10: Whereas one study reported a "subjective" improvement and a significant increase in a global scale of muscle strength, the other trial did not show any benefit. Two other trials used creatine: one trial reported improved measures of muscle strength and post-exercise lactate, but the other trial reported no benefit. Finally, one trial of dichloroacetate showed an improvement in secondary outcome measures of mitochondrial metabolism, and one trial using dimethylglycine showed no significant effect. Hence, the authors correctly argued that there was no clear evidence supporting the broad use of any intervention in mitochondrial disorders.

Recently (in 2013), the same authors repeated their systematic approach and identified 1039 publications on treatments for mitochondrial diseases [96]. However, only 35 of those publications included observations on more than five patients. Moreover, the authors observed that those reports suggesting a positive outcome on the basis of a biomarker of unproven clinical significance were more common in non-randomized and non-blinded studies, suggesting a publication bias toward positive but poorly executed studies.

A temporary enthusiasm spread out in the neuromuscular community some years ago, when idebenone (a synthetic variant of coenzyme Q10) was used in patients with Friedreich's ataxia and showed a significant reduction in LV hypertrophy in addition to an improvement in cardiac function—in spite of having no effect on the progression of ataxia [97]. Unfortunately, in a subsequent clinical trial including 70 pediatric patients with

Friedreich's ataxia, idebenone did not decrease LV hypertrophy or improve cardiac function after a 6-month treatment period [98]. Hence, a general recommendation of an idebenone-based therapy is neither possible for patients with Friedreich's ataxia nor for other forms of mitochondrial disease.

Taken together, the evidence for using supportive therapeutic strategies in patients with mitochondrial disorders such as coenzyme Q10, L-carnitine, riboflavin, creatine, and others is quite limited and mostly based on individual case studies. Obviously, this does not preclude a clinical benefit in an individual patient, and individual approaches need to be pursued due to the lack of evidence-based therapeutic strategies. However, an evidence-based recommendation for the broad use of dietary supplements is not possible.

Importantly, the use of certain drugs and medications may impair mitochondrial function and therefore result in adverse and/or deteriorating effects. Therefore, the following drugs should not be used in patients with mitochondrial disease: metformin, statins, propofol, valproic acid, erythromycin, azithromycin, streptomycin, tetracycline, chloramphenicol, and aminoglycosides.

Special Considerations: Surgery (Metabolic Stress), Heart Transplantation

Special care is needed in the case of general anesthesia required for specific interventions or surgeries, since some agents may lead to a prolonged and/or intensified effect in patients with mitochondrial diseases and are therefore contraindicated in these patients (e.g., propofol).

The following recommendations were mentioned in a recently published scientific statement from the American Heart Association (AHA) regarding the management of cardiac involvement associated with neuromuscular diseases [81]:

- *Cardiac evaluation should be performed before anesthesia or sedation in any patient with NMD at risk for cardiac involvement. For those with a history or symptoms suggestive of cardiac involvement, cardiac evaluation should be in close proximity (3–6 months) to the anesthesia/sedation event (Class I; Level of Evidence C).*
- *For NMD patients believed to be at increased cardiac risk during surgery, cardiac monitoring by an anesthesiologist experienced in the care of patients with NMDs should occur during major surgery, and the procedure should take place in a center with appropriate intensive care facilities (Class I; Level of Evidence C).*

Furthermore, heart transplantation is a touchy and controversial issue in patients with mitochondrial disease and advanced cardiomyopathy. In principle, heart transplantation is not recommended in patients with (advanced) multi-system diseases—although some case reports suggest successful heart transplantation. Hence, the great majority of patients with mitochondrial disease will not be suitable for heart transplantation. Only those patients presenting with an isolated cardiomyopathy but without other severe organ manifestations may be considered even for heart transplantation.

Conclusions and Outlook

Frequent clinical signs in mitochondrial disorders are (among others) ptosis, proximal myopathy, fatigue, exercise intolerance, encephalopathy, and ataxia—but also cardiac disease. Previous studies mainly based on ECG recordings, echocardiography, and/or CMR have revealed different forms of cardiomyopathy such as HCM, DCM, or LVNC (manifesting at variable age) and suggested varying incidences based on the respective subform of MID. Importantly, a significantly higher mortality was documented in those patients with MID and proof of cardiomyopathy compared to those without signs of cardiac involvement. Moreover, cardiac death was identified as the main cause of mortality in several MID studies. Hence, early identification of those patients with mitochondrial disease who are either prone to cardiac involvement or already suffering from cardiac disease is of clinical importance.

Fortunately, noninvasive imaging modalities such as CMR allow a detailed and comprehensive work-up of cardiomyopathies and enable a non-invasive and safe diagnosis of the underlying origin also in MID patients today. Unfortunately, causal therapeutic strategies are still lacking for patients with MID and cardiac involvement. Nevertheless, e.g., device therapies can be particularly helpful (and prolong life) in MID patients with arrhythmias—in case of early and timely diagnosis of the underlying cardiac disease. Novel therapeutic approaches for the successful prevention and/or treatment of cardiac disease are highly desired for those MID patients with a severe and rapidly progressive cardiac involvement.

References

1. Finsterer J, Kothari S. Cardiac manifestations of primary mitochondrial disorders. Int J Cardiol. 2014;177(3):754–63.
2. Barends M, Verschuren L, Morava E, Nesbitt V, Turnbull D, McFarland R. Causes of death in adults with mitochondrial disease. JIMD Rep. 2016;26:103–13.
3. Holmgren D, Wahlander H, Eriksson BO, Oldfors A, Holme E, Tulinius M. Cardiomyopathy in children with mitochondrial disease; clinical course and cardiological findings. Eur Heart J. 2003;24(3):280–8.
4. Malfatti E, Laforet P, Jardel C, Stojkovic T, Behin A, Eymard B, Lombes A, Benmalek A, Becane HM, Berber N, Meune C, Duboc D, Wahbi K. High risk of severe cardiac adverse events in patients with mitochondrial m.3243A>G mutation. Neurology. 2013;80(1):100–5.
5. Wahbi K, Bougouin W, Behin A, Stojkovic T, Becane HM, Jardel C, Berber N, Mochel F, Lombes A, Eymard B, Duboc D, Laforet P. Long-term cardiac prognosis and risk stratification in 260 adults presenting with mitochondrial diseases. Eur Heart J. 2015;36(42):2886–93.
6. Bates MG, Bourke JP, Giordano C, d'Amati G, Turnbull DM, Taylor RW. Cardiac involvement in mitochondrial DNA disease: clinical spectrum, diagnosis, and management. Eur Heart J. 2012;33(24):3023–33.
7. Florian A, Ludwig A, Stubbe-Drager B, Boentert M, Young P, Waltenberger J, Rosch S, Sechtem U, Yilmaz A. Characteristic cardiac phenotypes are detected by cardiovascular magnetic resonance in patients with different clinical phenotypes and genotypes of mitochondrial myopathy. J Cardiovasc Magn Reson. 2015;17:40.
8. Yilmaz A, Gdynia HJ, Ponfick M, Rosch S, Lindner A, Ludolph AC, Sechtem U. Cardiovascular magnetic resonance imaging (CMR) reveals characteristic pattern of myocardial damage in patients with mitochondrial myopathy. Clin Res Cardiol. 2012;101(4):255–61.
9. Towbin JA, Jefferies JL. Cardiomyopathies due to left ventricular noncompaction, mitochondrial and storage diseases, and inborn errors of metabolism. Circ Res. 2017;121(7):838–54.
10. Lopaschuk GD, Ussher JR, Folmes CD, Jaswal JS, Stanley WC. Myocardial fatty acid metabolism in health and disease. Physiol Rev. 2010;90(1):207–58.
11. Hsu YH, Yogasundaram H, Parajuli N, Valtuille L, Sergi C, Oudit GY. MELAS syndrome and cardiomyopathy: linking mitochondrial function to heart failure pathogenesis. Heart Fail Rev. 2016;21(1):103–16.
12. Gurrieri C, Kivela JE, Bojanic K, Gavrilova RH, Flick RP, Sprung J, Weingarten TN. Anesthetic considerations in mitochondrial encephalomyopathy, lactic acidosis, and stroke-like episodes syndrome: a case series. Can J Anaesth. 2011;58(8):751–63.
13. Jose T, Gdynia HJ, Mahrholdt H, Vohringer M, Klingel K, Kandolf R, Bornemann A, Yilmaz A. CMR gives clue to "ragged red fibers" in the heart in a patient with mitochondrial myopathy. Int J Cardiol. 2011;149(1):e24–7.
14. El-Hattab AW, Scaglia F. Mitochondrial cardiomyopathies. Front Cardiovasc Med. 2016;3:25.
15. El-Hattab AW, Scaglia F. Mitochondrial cytopathies. Cell Calcium. 2016;60(3):199–206.
16. Brunel-Guitton C, Levtova A, Sasarman F. Mitochondrial diseases and cardiomyopathies. Can J Cardiol. 2015;31(11):1360–76.
17. Marin-Garcia J, Goldenthal MJ, Ananthakrishnan R, Pierpont ME. The complete sequence of mtDNA genes in idiopathic dilated cardiomyopathy shows novel missense and tRNA mutations. J Card Fail. 2000;6(4):321–9.
18. Merante F, Tein I, Benson L, Robinson BH. Maternally inherited hypertrophic cardiomyopathy due to a novel T-to-C transition at nucleotide 9997 in the mitochondrial tRNA(glycine) gene. Am J Hum Genet. 1994;55(3):437–46.
19. Santorelli FM, Tanji K, Manta P, Casali C, Krishna S, Hays AP, Mancini DM, DiMauro S, Hirano M. Maternally inherited cardiomyopathy: an atypical presentation of the mtDNA 12S rRNA gene A1555G mutation. Am J Hum Genet. 1999;64(1):295–300.
20. Shin WS, Tanaka M, Suzuki J, Hemmi C, Toyooka T. A novel homoplasmic mutation in mtDNA with a single evolutionary origin as a risk factor for cardiomyopathy. Am J Hum Genet. 2000;67(6):1617–20.

21. Catteruccia M, Sauchelli D, Della MG, Primiano G, Cuccagna C, Bernardo D, Leo M, Camporeale A, Sanna T, Cianfoni A, Servidei S. "Myo-cardiomyopathy" is commonly associated with the A8344G "MERRF" mutation. J Neurol. 2015;262(3):701–10.
22. Bregel' LV, Belozerov I, Ogloblina ML, Golubev SS, Zemchenko OA, Pavlenok KN, Antoshkina EP, Bochkareva AK, Popod'ko TN. [Histiocytoid cardiomyopathy in an infant]. Kardiologiia. 2012;52(7):93–6.
23. Finsterer J. Histiocytoid cardiomyopathy: a mitochondrial disorder. Clin Cardiol. 2008;31(5):225–7.
24. Finsterer J, Stollberger C. Is mitochondrial disease the common cause of histiocytoid cardiomyopathy and non-compaction? Int J Legal Med. 2009;123(6):507–8.
25. Bray AW, Ballinger SW. Mitochondrial DNA mutations and cardiovascular disease. Curr Opin Cardiol. 2017. https://doi.org/10.1097/HCO.0000000000000383.
26. Majamaa-Voltti K, Peuhkurinen K, Kortelainen ML, Hassinen IE, Majamaa K. Cardiac abnormalities in patients with mitochondrial DNA mutation 3243A>G. BMC Cardiovasc Disord. 2002;2:12.
27. Scaglia F, Towbin JA, Craigen WJ, Belmont JW, Smith EO, Neish SR, Ware SM, Hunter JV, Fernbach SD, Vladutiu GD, Wong LJ, Vogel H. Clinical spectrum, morbidity, and mortality in 113 pediatric patients with mitochondrial disease. Pediatrics. 2004;114(4):925–31.
28. Bates MG, Hollingsworth KG, Newman JH, Jakovljevic DG, Blamire AM, MacGowan GA, Keavney BD, Chinnery PF, Turnbull DM, Taylor RW, Trenell MI, Gorman GS. Concentric hypertrophic remodelling and subendocardial dysfunction in mitochondrial DNA point mutation carriers. Eur Heart J Cardiovasc Imaging. 2013;14(7):650–8.
29. Fayssoil A. Heart diseases in mitochondrial encephalomyopathy, lactic acidosis, and stroke syndrome. Congest Heart Fail. 2009;15(6):284–7.
30. Limongelli G, Tome-Esteban M, Dejthevaporn C, Rahman S, Hanna MG, Elliott PM. Prevalence and natural history of heart disease in adults with primary mitochondrial respiratory chain disease. Eur J Heart Fail. 2010;12(2):114–21.
31. Sehgal S, Choudhry S, Debelenko L, L'Ecuyer T. Dilated cardiomyopathy with cardiogenic shock in a child with Kearns-Sayre syndrome. BMJ Case Rep. 2016;16:2016.
32. Tranchant C, Mousson B, Mohr M, Dumoulin R, Welsch M, Weess C, Stepien G, Warter JM. Cardiac transplantation in an incomplete Kearns-Sayre syndrome with mitochondrial DNA deletion. Neuromuscul Disord. 1993;3(5–6):561–6.
33. Channer KS, Channer JL, Campbell MJ, Rees JR. Cardiomyopathy in the Kearns-Sayre syndrome. Br Heart J. 1988;59(4):486–90.
34. Wahbi K, Larue S, Jardel C, Meune C, Stojkovic T, Ziegler F, Lombes A, Eymard B, Duboc D, Laforet P. Cardiac involvement is frequent in patients with the m.8344A>G mutation of mitochondrial DNA. Neurology. 2010;74(8):674–7.
35. Vallance HD, Jeven G, Wallace DC, Brown MD. A case of sporadic infantile histiocytoid cardiomyopathy caused by the A8344G (MERRF) mitochondrial DNA mutation. Pediatr Cardiol. 2004;25(5):538–40.
36. Brecht M, Richardson M, Taranath A, Grist S, Thorburn D, Bratkovic D. Leigh syndrome caused by the MT-ND5 m.13513G>A mutation: a case presenting with WPW-like conduction defect, cardiomyopathy, hypertension and Hyponatraemia. JIMD Rep. 2015;19:95–100.
37. Hadzsiev K, Maasz A, Kisfali P, Kalman E, Gomori E, Pal E, Berenyi E, Komlosi K, Melegh B. Mitochondrial DNA 11777C>A mutation associated Leigh syndrome: case report with a review of the previously described pedigrees. NeuroMolecular Med. 2010;12(3):277–84.
38. Sofou K, de Coo IFM, Ostergaard E, Isohanni P, Naess K, De ML, Tzoulis C, Uusimaa J, Lonnqvist T, Bindoff LA, Tulinius M, Darin N. Phenotype-genotype correlations in Leigh syndrome: new insights from a multicentre study of 96 patients. J Med Genet. 2018;55(1):21–7.
39. Thorburn DR, Rahman J, Rahman S. Mitochondrial DNA-associated Leigh syndrome and NARP. In: Adam MP, Ardinger HH, Pagon RA, Wallace SE, Bean LJH, Stephens K, Amemiya A, editors. GeneReviews® [Internet]. Seattle: University of Washington, 1993–2019. 2003 Oct 30.
40. Tesarova M, Hansikova H, Hlavata A, Klement P, Houst'kova H, Houstek J, Zeman J. [Variation in manifestations of heteroplasmic mtDNA mutation 8993 T>G in two families]. Cas Lek Cesk. 2002;141(17):551–4.
41. Ferreira C, Thompson R, Vernon H. Barth syndrome. In: Adam MP, Ardinger HH, Pagon RA, Wallace SE, Bean LJH, Stephens K, Amemiya A, editors. GeneReviews® [Internet]. Seattle: University of Washington, 1993–2019. 2014 Oct 9.
42. Clarke SL, Bowron A, Gonzalez IL, Groves SJ, Newbury-Ecob R, Clayton N, Martin RP, Tsai-Goodman B, Garratt V, Ashworth M, Bowen VM, McCurdy KR, Damin MK, Spencer CT, Toth MJ, Kelley RI, Steward CG. Barth syndrome. Orphanet J Rare Dis. 2013;8:23.
43. Spencer CT, Bryant RM, Day J, Gonzalez IL, Colan SD, Thompson WR, Berthy J, Redfearn SP, Byrne BJ. Cardiac and clinical phenotype in Barth syndrome. Pediatrics. 2006;118(2):e337–46.
44. Roberts AE, Nixon C, Steward CG, Gauvreau K, Maisenbacher M, Fletcher M, Geva J, Byrne BJ, Spencer CT. The Barth syndrome registry: distinguishing disease characteristics and growth data from a longitudinal study. Am J Med Genet A. 2012;158A(11):2726–32.
45. Kang SL, Forsey J, Dudley D, Steward CG, Tsai-Goodman B. Clinical characteristics and outcomes of cardiomyopathy in Barth syndrome: the UK experience. Pediatr Cardiol. 2016;37(1):167–76.

46. Salviati L, Trevisson E, Doimo M, Navas P. Primary coenzyme Q10 deficiency; 1993.
47. Raman SV, Phatak K, Hoyle JC, Pennell ML, McCarthy B, Tran T, Prior TW, Olesik JW, Lutton A, Rankin C, Kissel JT, Al-Dahhak R. Impaired myocardial perfusion reserve and fibrosis in Friedreich ataxia: a mitochondrial cardiomyopathy with metabolic syndrome. Eur Heart J. 2011;32(5):561–7.
48. Finsterer J, Stollberger C, Keller H. Arrhythmia-related workup in hereditary myopathies. J Electrocardiol. 2012;45(4):376–84.
49. Yaplito-Lee J, Weintraub R, Jamsen K, Chow CW, Thorburn DR, Boneh A. Cardiac manifestations in oxidative phosphorylation disorders of childhood. J Pediatr. 2007;150(4):407–11.
50. Zhang LH, Fang LG, Cheng ZW, Fang Q. [Cardiac manifestations of patients with mitochondrial disease]. Zhonghua Xin Xue Guan Bing Za Zhi. 2009;37(10):892–5.
51. Charles R, Holt S, Kay JM, Epstein EJ, Rees JR. Myocardial ultrastructure and the development of atrioventricular block in Kearns-Sayre syndrome. Circulation. 1981;63(1):214–9.
52. Kabunga P, Lau AK, Phan K, Puranik R, Liang C, Davis RL, Sue CM, Sy RW. Systematic review of cardiac electrical disease in Kearns-Sayre syndrome and mitochondrial cytopathy. Int J Cardiol. 2015;181:303–10.
53. Polak PE, Zijlstra F, Roelandt JR. Indications for pacemaker implantation in the Kearns-Sayre syndrome. Eur Heart J. 1989;10(3):281–2.
54. Khambatta S, Nguyen DL, Beckman TJ, Wittich CM. Kearns-Sayre syndrome: a case series of 35 adults and children. Int J Gen Med. 2014;7:325–32.
55. Karanikis P, Korantzopoulos P, Kountouris E, Dimitroula V, Patsouras D, Pappa E, Siogas K. Kearns-Sayre syndrome associated with trifascicular block and QT prolongation. Int J Cardiol. 2005;101(1):147–50.
56. Rashid A, Kim MH. Kearns-Sayre syndrome: association with long QT syndrome? J Cardiovasc Electrophysiol. 2002;13(2):184–5.
57. Reato S, Sparta S, D'Este D. Intraventricular conduction disturbances and paroxysmal atrioventricular block in a young patient with MELAS. J Cardiovasc Med (Hagerstown). 2015;16(Suppl 2):S100–3.
58. Majamaa-Voltti K, Turkka J, Kortelainen ML, Huikuri H, Majamaa K. Causes of death in pedigrees with the 3243A>G mutation in mitochondrial DNA. J Neurol Neurosurg Psychiatry. 2008;79(2):209–11.
59. Ng YS, Grady JP, Lax NZ, Bourke JP, Alston CL, Hardy SA, Falkous G, Schaefer AG, Radunovic A, Mohiddin SA, Ralph M, Alhakim A, Taylor RW, McFarland R, Turnbull DM, Gorman GS. Sudden adult death syndrome in m.3243A>G-related mitochondrial disease: an unrecognized clinical entity in young, asymptomatic adults. Eur Heart J. 2016;37(32):2552–9.
60. DiMauro S, Hirano M, Kaufmann P, Tanji K, Sano M, Shungu DC, Bonilla E, DeVivo DC. Clinical features and genetics of myoclonic epilepsy with ragged red fibers. Adv Neurol. 2002;89:217–29.
61. Spencer CT, Byrne BJ, Gewitz MH, Wechsler SB, Kao AC, Gerstenfeld EP, Merliss AD, Carboni MP, Bryant RM. Ventricular arrhythmia in the X-linked cardiomyopathy Barth syndrome. Pediatr Cardiol. 2005;26(5):632–7.
62. Mazurova S, Tesarova M, Magner M, Houstkova H, Hansikova H, Augustinova J, Tomek V, Vondrackova A, Zeman J, Honzik T. Novel mutations in the TAZ gene in patients with Barth syndrome. Prague Med Rep. 2013;114(3):139–53.
63. Finsterer J, Zarrouk-Mahjoub S. Mitochondrial vasculopathy. World J Cardiol. 2016;8(5):333–9.
64. Brunetti-Pierri N, Pignatelli R, Fouladi N, Towbin JA, Belmont JW, Craigen WJ, Wong LJ, Jefferies JL, Scaglia F. Dilation of the aortic root in mitochondrial disease patients. Mol Genet Metab. 2011;103(2):167–70.
65. Finsterer J, Bastovansky A. Dilative Arteriopathy and Leucencephalopathy as manifestations of a neurometabolic disease. Open Neurol J. 2015;9:28–31.
66. Ryther RC, Cho-Park YA, Lee JW. Carotid dissection in mitochondrial encephalomyopathy with lactic acidosis and stroke-like episodes. J Neurol. 2011;258(5):912–4.
67. Mancuso M, Montano V, Orsucci D, Peverelli L, Caputi L, Gambaro P, Siciliano G, Lamperti C. Mitochondrial m.3243A>G mutation and carotid artery dissection. Mol Genet Metab Rep. 2016;9:12–4.
68. Tay SH, Nordli DR Jr, Bonilla E, Null E, Monaco S, Hirano M, DiMauro S. Aortic rupture in mitochondrial encephalopathy, lactic acidosis, and stroke-like episodes. Arch Neurol. 2006;63(2):281–3.
69. Finsterer J, Mahjoub SZ. Primary mitochondrial arteriopathy. Nutr Metab Cardiovasc Dis. 2012;22(5):393–9.
70. Iizuka T, Goto Y, Miyakawa S, Sato M, Wang Z, Suzuki K, Hamada J, Kurata A, Sakai F. Progressive carotid artery stenosis with a novel tRNA phenylalanine mitochondrial DNA mutation. J Neurol Sci. 2009;278(1–2):35–40.
71. Barclay AR, Sholler G, Christodolou J, Shun A, Arbuckle S, Dorney S, Stormon MO. Pulmonary hypertension – a new manifestation of mitochondrial disease. J Inherit Metab Dis. 2005;28(6):1081–9.
72. Belostotsky R, Ben-Shalom E, Rinat C, Becker-Cohen R, Feinstein S, Zeligson S, Segel R, Elpeleg O, Nassar S, Frishberg Y. Mutations in the mitochondrial seryl-tRNA synthetase cause hyperuricemia, pulmonary hypertension, renal failure in infancy and alkalosis, HUPRA syndrome. Am J Hum Genet. 2011;88(2):193–200.
73. Catteruccia M, Verrigni D, Martinelli D, Torraco A, Agovino T, Bonafe L, D'Amico A, Donati MA, Adorisio R, Santorelli FM, Carrozzo R, Bertini E, Dionisi-Vici C. Persistent pulmonary arterial hypertension in the newborn (PPHN): a frequent

manifestation of TMEM70 defective patients. Mol Genet Metab. 2014;111(3):353–9.
74. Indrieri A, van Rahden VA, Tiranti V, Morleo M, Iaconis D, Tammaro R, D'Amato I, Conte I, Maystadt I, Demuth S, Zvulunov A, Kutsche K, Zeviani M, Franco B. Mutations in COX7B cause microphthalmia with linear skin lesions, an unconventional mitochondrial disease. Am J Hum Genet. 2012;91(5):942–9.
75. Parsons T, Weimer L, Engelstad K, Linker A, Battista V, Wei Y, Hirano M, DiMauro S, De Vivo DC, Kaufmann P. Autonomic symptoms in carriers of the m.3243A>G mitochondrial DNA mutation. Arch Neurol. 2010;67(8):976–9.
76. Di LR, Musumeci O, de GC, Recupero A, Grimaldi P, Messina C, Coglitore S, Vita G, Toscano A. Evidence of cardiovascular autonomic impairment in mitochondrial disorders. J Neurol. 2007;254(11):1498–503.
77. Majamaa-Voltti K, Majamaa K, Peuhkurinen K, Makikallio TH, Huikuri HV. Cardiovascular autonomic regulation in patients with 3243A>G mitochondrial DNA mutation. Ann Med. 2004;36(3):225–31.
78. Giannoni A, Aimo A, Mancuso M, Piepoli MF, Orsucci D, Aquaro GD, Barison A, De MD, Taddei C, Cameli M, Raglianti V, Siciliano G, Passino C, Emdin M. Autonomic, functional, skeletal muscle, and cardiac abnormalities are associated with increased ergoreflex sensitivity in mitochondrial disease. Eur J Heart Fail. 2017;19(12):1701–9.
79. Ponikowski PP, Chua TP, Francis DP, Capucci A, Coats AJ, Piepoli MF. Muscle ergoreceptor overactivity reflects deterioration in clinical status and cardiorespiratory reflex control in chronic heart failure. Circulation. 2001;104(19):2324–30.
80. Dominic EA, Ramezani A, Anker SD, Verma M, Mehta N, Rao M. Mitochondrial cytopathies and cardiovascular disease. Heart. 2014;100(8):611–8.
81. Feingold B, Mahle WT, Auerbach S, Clemens P, Domenighetti AA, Jefferies JL, Judge DP, Lal AK, Markham LW, Parks WJ, Tsuda T, Wang PJ, Yoo SJ. Management of cardiac involvement associated with neuromuscular diseases: a scientific statement from the American Heart Association. Circulation. 2017;136(13):e200–31.
82. Rapezzi C, Arbustini E, Caforio AL, Charron P, Gimeno-Blanes J, Helio T, Linhart A, Mogensen J, Pinto Y, Ristic A, Seggewiss H, Sinagra G, Tavazzi L, Elliott PM. Diagnostic work-up in cardiomyopathies: bridging the gap between clinical phenotypes and final diagnosis. A position statement from the ESC working group on myocardial and pericardial diseases. Eur Heart J. 2013;34(19):1448–58.
83. Messroghli DR, Moon JC, Ferreira VM, Grosse-Wortmann L, He T, Kellman P, Mascherbauer J, Nezafat R, Salerno M, Schelbert EB, Taylor AJ, Thompson R, Ugander M, van Heeswijk RB, Friedrich MG. Clinical recommendations for cardiovascular magnetic resonance mapping of T1, T2, T2* and extracellular volume: a consensus statement by the Society for Cardiovascular Magnetic Resonance (SCMR) endorsed by the European Association for Cardiovascular Imaging (EACVI). J Cardiovasc Magn Reson. 2017;19(1):75.
84. Yilmaz A, Sechtem U. Diagnostic approach and differential diagnosis in patients with hypertrophied left ventricles. Heart. 2014;100(8):662–71.
85. Baik R, Chae JH, Lee YM, Kang HC, Lee JS, Kim HD. Electrocardiography as an early cardiac screening test in children with mitochondrial disease. Korean J Pediatr. 2010;53(5):644–7.
86. Elliott PM, Anastasakis A, Borger MA, Borggrefe M, Cecchi F, Charron P, Hagege AA, Lafont A, Limongelli G, Mahrholdt H, McKenna WJ, Mogensen J, Nihoyannopoulos P, Nistri S, Pieper PG, Pieske B, Rapezzi C, Rutten FH, Tillmanns C, Watkins H. 2014 ESC guidelines on diagnosis and management of hypertrophic cardiomyopathy: the Task Force for the Diagnosis and Management of Hypertrophic Cardiomyopathy of the European Society of Cardiology (ESC). Eur Heart J. 2014;35(39):2733–79.
87. Bernier FP, Boneh A, Dennett X, Chow CW, Cleary MA, Thorburn DR. Diagnostic criteria for respiratory chain disorders in adults and children. Neurology. 2002;59(9):1406–11.
88. Yilmaz A, Kindermann I, Kindermann M, Mahfoud F, Ukena C, Athanasiadis A, Hill S, Mahrholdt H, Voehringer M, Schieber M, Klingel K, Kandolf R, Bohm M, Sechtem U. Comparative evaluation of left and right ventricular endomyocardial biopsy: differences in complication rate and diagnostic performance. Circulation. 2010;122(9):900–9.
89. Rustin P, Chretien D, Bourgeron T, Wucher A, Saudubray JM, Rotig A, Munnich A. Assessment of the mitochondrial respiratory chain. Lancet. 1991;338(8758):60.
90. Morava E, Rodenburg R, van Essen HZ, De VM, Smeitink J. Dietary intervention and oxidative phosphorylation capacity. J Inherit Metab Dis. 2006;29(4):589.
91. Taivassalo T, Gardner JL, Taylor RW, Schaefer AM, Newman J, Barron MJ, Haller RG, Turnbull DM. Endurance training and detraining in mitochondrial myopathies due to single large-scale mtDNA deletions. Brain. 2006;129(Pt 12):3391–401.
92. Tveskov C, Angelo-Nielsen K. Kearns-Sayre syndrome and dilated cardiomyopathy. Neurology. 1990;40(3 Pt 1):553–4.
93. Ismail TF, Jabbour A, Gulati A, Mallorie A, Raza S, Cowling TE, Das B, Khwaja J, Alpendurada FD, Wage R, Roughton M, McKenna WJ, Moon JC, Varnava A, Shakespeare C, Cowie MR, Cook SA, Elliott P, O'Hanlon R, Pennell DJ, Prasad SK. Role of late gadolinium enhancement cardiovascular magnetic resonance in the risk stratification of hypertrophic cardiomyopathy. Heart. 2014;100(23):1851–8.

94. Merino JL, Peinado R. Arrhythmias associated with neuromuscular disorders. Card Electrophysiol Rev. 2002;6(1–2):132–5.
95. Chinnery P, Majamaa K, Turnbull D, Thorburn D. Treatment for mitochondrial disorders. Cochrane Database Syst Rev. 2006;1:CD004426.
96. Pfeffer G, Horvath R, Klopstock T, Mootha VK, Suomalainen A, Koene S, Hirano M, Zeviani M, Bindoff LA, Yu-Wai-Man P, Hanna M, Carelli V, McFarland R, Majamaa K, Turnbull DM, Smeitink J, Chinnery PF. New treatments for mitochondrial disease-no time to drop our standards. Nat Rev Neurol. 2013;9(8):474–81.
97. Buyse G, Mertens L, Di SG, Matthijs I, Weidemann F, Eyskens B, Goossens W, Goemans N, Sutherland GR, Van Hove JL. Idebenone treatment in Friedreich's ataxia: neurological, cardiac, and biochemical monitoring. Neurology. 2003;60(10):1679–81.
98. Lagedrost SJ, Sutton MS, Cohen MS, Satou GM, Kaufman BD, Perlman SL, Rummey C, Meier T, Lynch DR. Idebenone in Friedreich ataxia cardiomyopathy-results from a 6-month phase III study (IONIA). Am Heart J. 2011;161(3):639–45.
99. Bonnet D, Martin D, Pascale DL, Villain E, Jouvet P, Rabier D, Brivet M, Saudubray JM. Arrhythmias and conduction defects as presenting symptoms of fatty acid oxidation disorders in children. Circulation. 1999;100(22):2248–53.
100. Finsterer J, Stollberger C, Maeztu C. Sudden cardiac death in neuromuscular disorders. Int J Cardiol. 2016;203:508–15.

Diagnostic Approach to Mitochondrial Diseases

Rita Horvath and Patrick F. Chinnery

The first genetically defined mitochondrial disorders were identified in the late 1980s and early 1990s. Mitochondrial DNA deletions and point mutations were identified in patients with a wide range of phenotypes, in large part because the 16.5 kb size of the mtDNA was experimentally tractable. Progress in discovering nuclear gene defects in mitochondrial diseases was slow initially, and limited by available technology, which required multiple affected individuals from the same family [1, 2]. While mutations in the same mitochondrial disease gene (mtDNA or nuclear) can give rise to different clinical phenotypes, the same clinical picture can be caused by a large number of genes affecting mitochondrial function, involved in different pathways [3]. In some patients, there is a clinically recognizable phenotype, which is easily available for direct testing of frequent causes of mitochondrial disease (m.3243A>G and mutations causing Leber hereditary optic neuropathy); however, in the majority of patients, the clinical phenotype is less characteristic or suggests a wide range of possible candidate genes (e.g. Leigh syndrome). In this context, screening all of the implicated genes was technically demanding in the routine diagnostic laboratory before the availability of next-generation sequencing (Fig. 1) [4]. The detection of larger number of patients with the more common gene defects enabled genotype/phenotype correlations in some forms of mitochondrial disease (*POLG*, *RRM2B*, *PEO1*, *SURF1*, *RRM2B*, etc.) [5–8]. Some additional non-invasive clinical investigations such as serum biomarkers (lactate, FGF21, GDF15) [9] or imaging studies (MRI, MRS) [10] have been developed to help confirm the diagnosis of a mitochondrial disease, but they rarely point to a definite molecular diagnosis. However, the role of these biomarkers in measuring disease progression is less clear, and much could be gained through well-designed longitudinal studies of genotyped cohorts using these modalities [9].

Histochemical and biochemical respiratory chain (RC) complex defects in skeletal muscle are hallmarks of mitochondrial disease, and a muscle biopsy has been used to underpin the diagnosis for over 20 years, particularly in adults. Muscle involvement can arise from mutations in nuclear or mtDNA genes, and the association with distinctive histopathological hallmarks makes the muscle an excellent postmitotic surrogate for the study of many multisystem mitochondrial disorders [11]. The histological and histochemical examination of serially sectioned

R. Horvath (✉)
John Van Geest Centre for Brain Repair and MRC Mitochondrial Biology Unit, Department of Clinical Neurosciences, University of Cambridge, Cambridge Biomedical Campus, Cambridge, UK
e-mail: rh732@medschl.cam.ac.uk

P. F. Chinnery
MRC Mitochondrial Biology Unit, Department of Clinical Neurosciences, University of Cambridge, Cambridge Biomedical Campus, Cambridge, UK

M. Mancuso, T. Klopstock (eds.), *Diagnosis and Management of Mitochondrial Disorders*,
https://doi.org/10.1007/978-3-030-05517-2_17

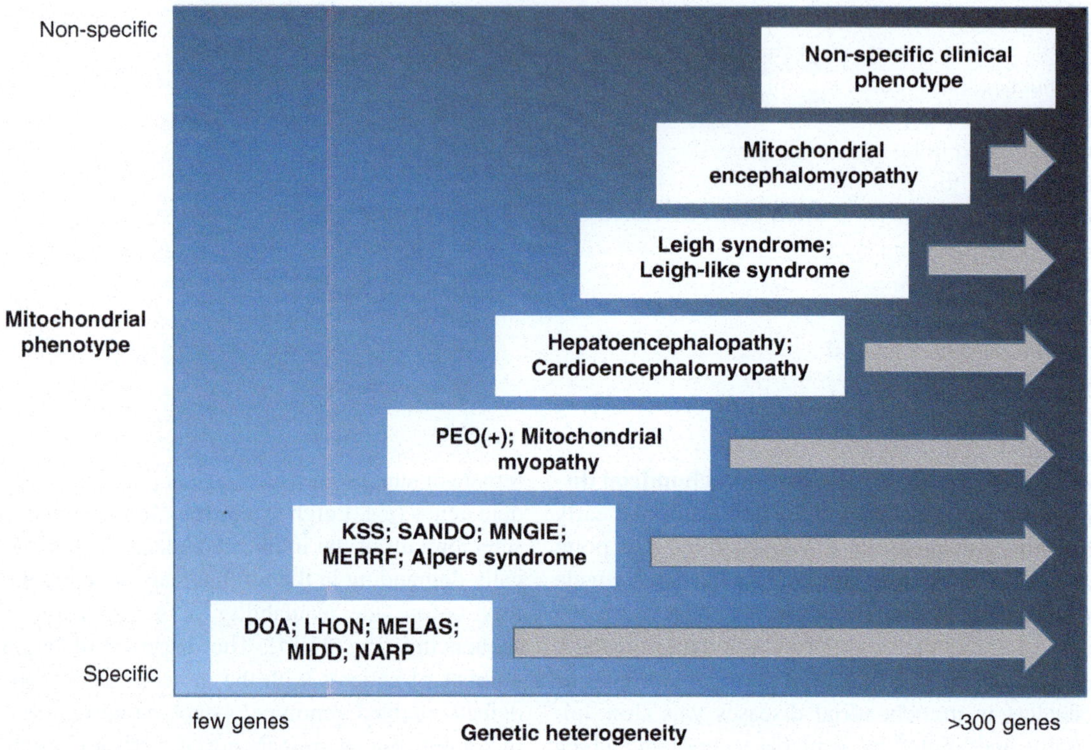

Fig. 1 Mitochondrial disease phenotypes are genetically heterogeneous and caused by mutations in an increasing number of genes. Some distinct phenotypes point towards specific genes or mutations of interest (bottom left), but many patients do not have a definite mitochondrial clinical syndrome (top right). In this instance, a large number of genes are implicated, which can only be screened effectively by next-generation sequencing approaches. Abbreviations: *DOA* dominant optic atrophy, *LHON* Leber hereditary optic neuropathy, *MELAS* mitochondrial encephalomyopathy, lactic acidosis, stroke-like episodes, *MIDD* maternally inherited diabetes and deafness, *NARP* neuropathy, ataxia, and retinitis pigmentosa, *KSS* Kearns-Sayre syndrome, *SANDO* sensory axonal neuropathy, dysarthria, and ophthalmoparesis, *MNGIE* mitochondrial neurogastrointestinal encephalopathy, *MERRF* myoclonus epilepsy with ragged red fibres, *PEO* progressive external ophthalmoparesis

muscle can provide evidence of mitochondrial pathology. The modified Gomori trichrome stain allows the detection of ragged-red fibres (RRFs) with abnormal sub-sarcolemmal proliferation of mitochondria, resulting from a compensatory response to a respiratory chain defect representing a characteristic histopathological feature of mitochondrial disorders. Although suggestive of mitochondrial disease, RRFs are not diagnostic because they are also seen with normal ageing and other muscle conditions [11]. Sequential cytochrome c oxidase (COX)/succinate dehydrogenase (SDH) histochemistry is the standard method used to assess the activities of the partially mtDNA-encoded complex IV (COX) and the fully nuclear-encoded complex II (SDH). By combining both reactions in a single slide (COX/SDH stain), fibres or cells with mitochondrial dysfunction are seen as a mosaic reduction of COX activity with preserved SDH activity (blue fibres), indicative of an underlying mtDNA-related abnormality [11]. The mtDNA abnormality can be the primary cause of the disease (e.g. m.8344A>G) or secondary to a nuclear gene defect which compromises mtDNA maintenance (e.g. multiple mtDNA deletions secondary to a nuclear gene mutation in *POLG*, which codes for the mtDNA polymerase). A quadruple immunofluorescent technique has been recently developed, enabling the quantification of key respiratory chain subunits of complexes I and IV, together with an indicator of mitochondrial mass and a cell membrane marker [12]. This assay allows an objective quantification of protein abundance in large numbers of individual muscle fibres, providing insight into the underlying molecular pathology [12]. However, the diagnostic utility of this approach has yet to be validated in multiple independent laboratories.

Biochemical measurement of respiratory chain (RC) enzyme activities has been widely used in the past 20 years to define the deficient enzyme and narrow down the number of potential candidate genes. Typically, RC defects are associated with mutations affecting the mitochondrial DNA (mtDNA) or nuclear genes coding for mitochondrial proteins. A defect of one or more RC enzymes provided the first laboratory diagnostic evidence for a mitochondrial disorder and guided subsequent DNA analysis (Sanger sequencing) of the mitochondrial DNA (mtDNA) and candidate nuclear genes encoding mitochondrial proteins [13, 14]. However, in a substantial proportion of cases with a RC defect, it has not been possible to reach a molecular diagnosis. It was assumed that most of these patients carry undetected mutations in genes coding for mitochondrial proteins; however, using unbiased genetic testing, it has been shown that several metabolic and neurodegenerative diseases may lead to secondary RC deficiency [15, 16], providing an alternative explanation. Moreover, defects in mitochondrial maintenance, fusion/fission or abnormalities in mitochondrial membrane integrity or transport have taught us that some of these disorders do not present always with significant oxidative phosphorylation (OXPHOS) complex deficiencies in the skeletal muscle biopsy [17]. On the other hand, the identification of new mutations often requires extensive research to prove its pathogenicity, which may include a muscle or skin biopsy [18]. It is also important to note that a muscle biopsy may help to identify other non-mitochondrial muscle disease which enters the differential diagnosis.

The introduction of massively parallel sequencing (MPS), a wide and rapid genetic screening with targeted panels, whole-exome sequencing (WES) or whole-genome sequencing (WGS), has become preferable to the laborious and costly sequential candidate gene sequencing [4, 13, 14, 19]. With the increased availability of next-generation sequencing (NGS), mainly whole-exome sequencing (WES) or targeted panels, most diagnostic centres have changed their diagnostic strategy in suspected mitochondrial disease [20, 21]. Currently, around 300 genes are known to be associated with mitochondrial disease [21], but this list is still growing rapidly, despite the predicted decline of novel gene discoveries in Mendelian disorders in the recent years post 2013 [22]. Over 1500 nuclear genes are thought to be important for mitochondrial biogenesis, implicating a further ~1200 genes as candidates for mitochondrial disease that have yet to be implicated in patients with established mitochondrial pathology [23].

In patients with a clinically diagnosed mitochondrial disease (compatible clinical signs and symptoms and/or a confirmed mitochondrial complex deficiency on skin fibroblasts or muscle biopsy), the first step is the exclusion of relevant common mtDNA mutations (m.3243A>G, LHON, single mtDNA deletion) and common nuclear variants known to cause mitochondrial diseases (*POLG, SPG7, OPA1*). The next step in the investigation algorithm is NGS, which has a variable success rate of between 16% and 60%, depending on patient selection, the genes covered and the informatics pipeline used [13, 14, 24–26]. Some mutations in known disease genes may still be missed for technical reasons (e.g. GC-rich regions in the first exon, which remain difficult to sequence) leading to the general consensus that currently known disease genes account for only ~60% of patients with suspected mitochondrial disease [22]. WES and WGS also capture mitochondrial DNA with a very high coverage due to the higher number of mtDNA molecules in all nucleated cells. This enables the detection of low heteroplasmy mtDNA variants at the same time as detecting relevant nuclear gene variants [27]. Based on these data, it is increasingly difficult to justify the use of an invasive procedure as a 'first-line' investigation, particularly in children (Fig. 2).

Mitochondrial disease criteria (MDC) have been developed to evaluate the probability of an underlying mitochondrial disease and the need for

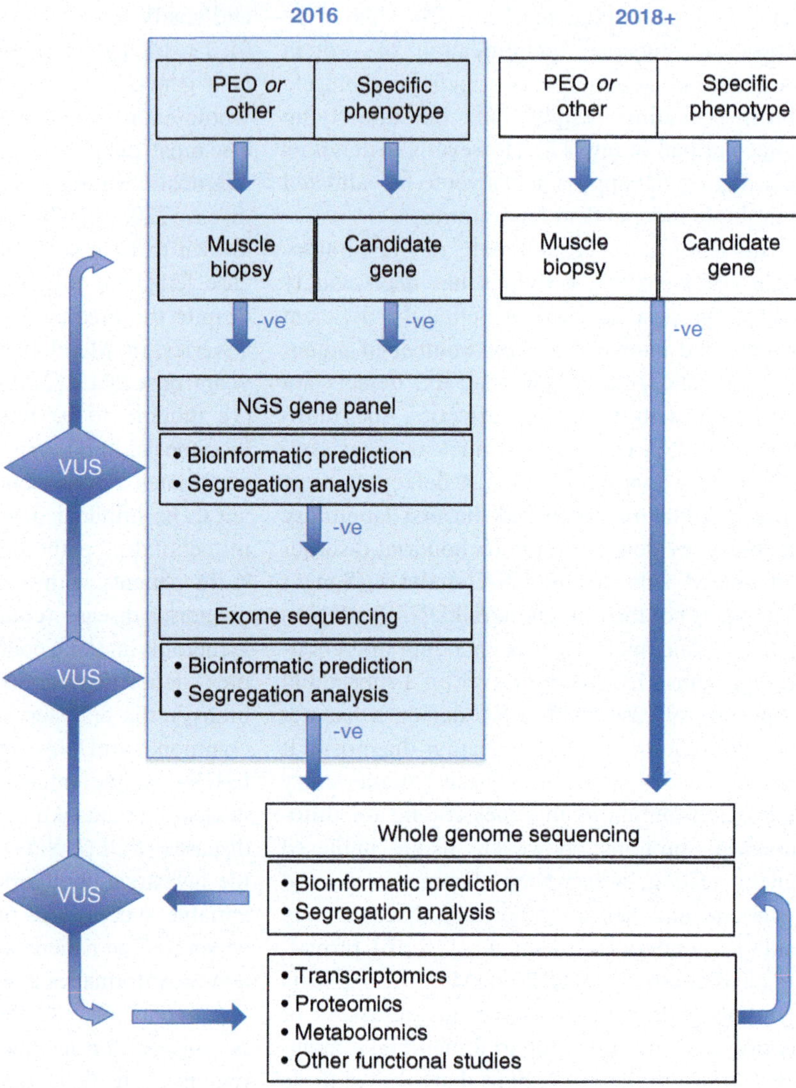

Fig. 2 Impact of NGS on the diagnosis of mitochondrial disease. Adapted from Horvath and Chinnery, 2017 [2]

a muscle biopsy [3]. Importantly, these criteria are tailored to the paediatric population and reflect the importance of monitoring natural history. This allows the evolution of new symptoms and signs to change the likelihood of a mitochondrial disorder and thus influence the decision to perform more extensive and invasive investigations to confirm the diagnosis [3]. The composite MDC score helps separate a mitochondrial aetiology from other multisystem diseases by quantifying the probability that a patient has an oxidative phosphorylation (OXPHOS) defect-related disease and weights the need to perform more invasive investigations such as a muscle biopsy. A recent study validated the diagnostic value of MDC and found that it remains very useful in the later phase of the clinical diagnosis of mitochondrial disease, including the interpretation of whole-exome sequencing results [28]. A new diagnostic algorithm has been recently suggested placing the muscle biopsy after the genetic investigations [28].

Based on current evidence, the following approach is proposed: if the MDC suggests 'probable' mitochondrial disease, and WES/WGS detected a pathogenic variant in a mitochondrial disease gene which segregates within the family and corresponds to the patient phenotype, the diagnosis is made and the muscle biopsy is not needed. Large control databases (ExAc) and better bioinformatics prediction programs support the filtering of variants of interest, and international sharing of genetic and phenotypic data enables matchmaking across centres, substantiating the diagnosis in many instances. A muscle (and/or liver) biopsy should only be performed when the diagnosis cannot be confirmed by first-line DNA testing [20, 24]. However, if there are questions on the pathogenicity of the mutation, or when other diseases affecting skeletal muscle enter the differential diagnosis, a muscle biopsy with OXPHOS measurements can assist with the interpretation of the clinical and genetic information. Therefore, many clinicians practising mitochondrial medicine question whether muscle biopsy is still the 'gold standard' as the first-line diagnostic test for mitochondrial disease [29].

New Technologies (RNAseq, Long-Read Sequencing, Proteomics, Metabolomics)

The decreasing cost of WES/WGS and their wide diagnostic role in inherited diseases places them in the frontline of the diagnosis of mitochondrial disease [29]. The diagnostic yield of genome-wide approaches can be further enhanced by the parallel use of other high-throughput, new omics technologies, such as RNAseq, long-read sequencing, proteomics and metabolomics further enhance the diagnostic yield of whole exome or genome sequencing. For example, a recent study in skin fibroblasts from patients with a clinical suspicion of mitochondrial disease showed that RNA sequencing identified the underlying defect in 10% (5 of 48) in patients where WES was unsuccessful in isolation. This approach identified altered gene expression, aberrant splicing events and mono-allelic expression of rare variants which are emerging as important molecular mechanisms [30]. Other new technologies are also becoming available in the research setting and are likely to contribute to routine diagnostics in the near future. These include long-read sequencing, which enables the better detection of rearrangements, and both proteomic and metabolomic platforms, which are currently used to underpin the pathomechanism of mitochondrial defects [31].

Final Remarks

Mitochondrial diseases are still difficult to diagnose because of their wide clinical and genetic heterogeneity. A more comprehensive phenotype characterization and clinical experience are still important in reaching the correct diagnosis as soon as possible. A recent survey suggested that patients with suspected mitochondrial disease still see more than eight clinicians on average (primary care physicians, neurologists, clinical geneticists, metabolic disease specialists, cardiologists, gastroenterologists, etc.) before they receive the final diagnosis of mitochondrial disease [32]. Faced with increasing numbers of disease causing genes and with more accessible sequencing techniques, the diagnosis of mitochondrial diseases has become less specialized. If the diagnosis is not straightforward on WES/WGS, the clinicians should consult with expert mitochondrial disease centres. The management of patients with mitochondrial disease has become more complex, and promising clinical trials are available in specialized centres; therefore, patients with mitochondrial disease should have the possibility to seek advice from a mitochondrial disease specialist linked to national and international networks of clinicians and researchers.

References

1. Gorman GS, Chinnery PF, DiMauro S, Hirano M, Koga Y, McFarland R, Suomalainen A, Thorburn DR, Zeviani M, Turnbull DM. Mitochondrial diseases. Nat Rev Dis Primers. 2016;2:16080.
2. Horvath R, Chinnery PF. The effect of neurological genomics and personalized mitochondrial medicine. JAMA Neurol. 2017;74(1):11–3.
3. Morava E, van den Heuvel L, Hol F, de Vries MC, Hogeveen M, Rodenburg RJ, Smeitink JA. Mitochondrial disease criteria: diagnostic applications in children. Neurology. 2006;67(10):1823–6.
4. Lake NJ, Compton AG, Rahman S, Thorburn DR. Leigh syndrome: one disorder, more than 75 monogenic causes. Ann Neurol. 2016;79(2):190–203.

5. Horvath R, Hudson G, Ferrari G, Fütterer N, Ahola S, Lamantea E, Prokisch H, Lochmüller H, McFarland R, Ramesh V, Klopstock T, Freisinger P, Salvi F, Mayr JA, Santer R, Tesarova M, Zeman J, Udd B, Taylor RW, Turnbull D, Hanna M, Fialho D, Suomalainen A, Zeviani M, Chinnery PF. Phenotypic spectrum associated with mutations of the mitochondrial polymerase gamma gene. Brain. 2006;129(Pt 7):1674–84.
6. Fratter C, Gorman GS, Stewart JD, Buddles M, Smith C, Evans J, Seller A, Poulton J, Roberts M, Hanna MG, Rahman S, Omer SE, Klopstock T, Schoser B, Kornblum C, Czermin B, Lecky B, Blakely EL, Craig K, Chinnery PF, Turnbull DM, Horvath R, Taylor RW. The clinical, histochemical, and molecular spectrum of PEO1 (Twinkle)-linked adPEO. Neurology. 2010;74(20):1619–26.
7. Pitceathly RD, Smith C, Fratter C, Alston CL, He L, Craig K, Blakely EL, Evans JC, Taylor J, Shabbir Z, Deschauer M, Pohl U, Roberts ME, Jackson MC, Halfpenny CA, Turnpenny PD, Lunt PW, Hanna MG, Schaefer AM, McFarland R, Horvath R, Chinnery PF, Turnbull DM, Poulton J, Taylor RW, Gorman GS. Adults with RRM2B-related mitochondrial disease have distinct clinical and molecular characteristics. Brain. 2012;135(Pt 11):3392–403.
8. Wedatilake Y, Brown RM, McFarland R, Yaplito-Lee J, Morris AA, Champion M, Jardine PE, Clarke A, Thorburn DR, Taylor RW, Land JM, Forrest K, Dobbie A, Simmons L, Aasheim ET, Ketteridge D, Hanrahan D, Chakrapani A, Brown GK, Rahman S. SURF1 deficiency: a multi-centre natural history study. Orphanet J Rare Dis. 2013;8:96.
9. Steele HE, Horvath R, Lyon JJ, Chinnery PF. Monitoring clinical progression with mitochondrial disease biomarkers. Brain. 2017;140(10): 2530–40.
10. de Beaurepaire I, Grévent D, Rio M, Desguerre I, de Lonlay P, Levy R, Dangouloff-Ros V, Bonnefont JP, Barcia G, Funalot B, Besmond C, Metodiev MD, Ruzzenente B, Assouline Z, Munnich A, Rötig A, Boddaert N. High predictive value of brain MRI imaging in primary mitochondrial respiratory chain deficiency. J Med Genet. 2018;55(6):378–83.
11. Alston CL, Rocha MC, Lax NZ, Turnbull DM, Taylor RW. The genetics and pathology of mitochondrial disease. J Pathol. 2017;241(2):236–50.
12. Rocha MC, Grady JP, Grünewald A, Vincent A, Dobson PF, Taylor RW, Turnbull DM, Rygiel KA. A novel immunofluorescent assay to investigate oxidative phosphorylation deficiency in mitochondrial myopathy: understanding mechanisms and improving diagnosis. Sci Rep. 2015;5:15037.
13. Taylor RW, Pyle A, Griffin H, et al. Use of whole-exome sequencing to determine the genetic basis of multiple mitochondrial respiratory chain complex deficiencies. JAMA. 2014;312(1):68–77.
14. Calvo SE, Compton AG, Hershman SG, et al. Molecular diagnosis of infantile mitochondrial disease with targeted next-generation sequencing. Sci Transl Med. 2012;4(118):118ra10.
15. Pyle A, Nightingale HJ, Griffin H, Abicht A, Kirschner J, Baric I, Cuk M, Douroudis K, Feder L, Kratz M, Czermin B, Kleinle S, Santibanez-Koref M, Karcagi V, Holinski-Feder E, Chinnery PF, Horvath R. Respiratory chain deficiency in nonmitochondrial disease. Neurol Genet. 2015;1(1):e6.
16. Stepien KM, Heaton R, Rankin S, Murphy A, Bentley J, Sexton D, Hargreaves IP Evidence of oxidative stress and secondary mitochondrial dysfunction in metabolic and non-metabolic disorders. J Clin Med. 2017;6(7). https://doi.org/10.3390/jcm6070071.
17. DiMauro S, Schon EA, Carelli V, Hirano M. The clinical maze of mitochondrial neurology. Nat Rev Neurol. 2013;9(8):429–44.
18. Saada A. Mitochondria: mitochondrial OXPHOS (dys) function ex vivo – the use of primary fibroblasts. Int J Biochem Cell Biol. 2014;48:60–5.
19. Plutino M, Chaussenot A, Rouzier C, Ait-El-Mkadem S, Fragaki K, Paquis-Flucklinger V, Bannwarth S. Targeted next generation sequencing with an extended gene panel does not impact variant detection in mitochondrial diseases. BMC Med Genet. 2018;19(1):57.
20. Parikh S, Goldstein A, Koenig MK, et al. Diagnosis and management of mitochondrial disease: a consensus statement from the Mitochondrial Medicine Society. Genet Med. 2015;17(9):689–701.
21. Craven L, Alston CL, Taylor RW, Turnbull DM. Recent advances in mitochondrial disease. Annu Rev Genomics Hum Genet. 2017;18:257–75.
22. Frazier AE, Thorburn DR, Compton AG. Mitochondrial energy generation disorders: genes, mechanisms and clues to pathology. J Biol Chem. 2017; https://doi.org/10.1074/jbc.R117.809194.
23. Vafai SB, Mootha VK. Mitochondrial disorders as windows into an ancient organelle. Nature. 2012;491(7424):374–83.
24. Morava E, Brown GK. Next generation mitochondrial disease: change in diagnostics with eyes on therapy. J Inherit Metab Dis. 2015;38(3):387–8.
25. Wortmann SB, Koolen DA, Smeitink JA, van den Heuvel L, Rodenburg RJ. Whole exome sequencing of suspected mitochondrial patients in clinical practice. J Inherit Metab Dis. 2015;38(3):437–43.
26. Kohda M, Tokuzawa Y, Kishita Y, Nyuzuki H, Moriyama Y, Mizuno Y, Hirata T, Yatsuka Y, Yamashita-Sugahara Y, Nakachi Y, Kato H, Okuda A, Tamaru S, Borna NN, Banshoya K, Aigaki T, Sato-Miyata Y, Ohnuma K, Suzuki T, Nagao A, Maehata H, Matsuda F, Higasa K, Nagasaki M, Yasuda J, Yamamoto M, Fushimi T, Shimura M, Kaiho-Ichimoto K, Harashima H, Yamazaki T, Mori M, Murayama K, Ohtake A, Okazaki Y. A comprehensive genomic analysis reveals the genetic landscape of mitochondrial respiratory chain complex deficiencies. PLoS Genet. 2016;12(1):e1005679.
27. Griffin HR, Pyle A, Blakely EL, Alston CL, Duff J, Hudson G, Horvath R, Wilson IJ, Santibanez-Koref M, Taylor RW, Chinnery PF. Accurate mitochondrial DNA sequencing using off-target reads provides a

single test to identify pathogenic point mutations. Genet Med. 2014;16(12):962–71.

28. Witters P, Saada A, Honzik T, Tesarova M, Kleinle S, Horvath R, Goldstein A, Morava E. Revisiting mitochondrial diagnostic criteria in the new era of genomics. Genet Med. 2018;20(4):444–51.
29. Raymond FL, Horvath R, Chinnery PF. First-line genomic diagnosis of mitochondrial disorders. Nat Rev Genet. 2018;19(7):399–400.
30. Kremer LS, Bader DM, Mertes C, Kopajtich R, Pichler G, Iuso A, Haack TB, Graf E, Schwarzmayr T, Terrile C, Koňaříková E, Repp B, Kastenmüller G, Adamski J, Lichtner P, Leonhardt C, Funalot B, Donati A, Tiranti V, Lombes A, Jardel C, Gläser D, Taylor RW, Ghezzi D, Mayr JA, Rötig A, Freisinger P, Distelmaier F, Strom TM, Meitinger T, Gagneur J, Prokisch H. Genetic diagnosis of Mendelian disorders via RNA sequencing. Nat Commun. 2017;8:15824.
31. Zhang Y, Avalos JL. Traditional and novel tools to probe the mitochondrial metabolism in health and disease. Wiley Interdiscip Rev Syst Biol Med. 2017;9(2). https://doi.org/10.1002/wsbm.1373.
32. Grier J, Hirano M, Karaa A, Shepard E, Thompson JLP. Diagnostic odyssey of patients with mitochondrial disease: results of a survey. Neurol Genet. 2018;4(2):e230.

Neuroimaging Findings in Primary Mitochondrial Cytopathies

César Augusto Pinheiro Ferreira Alves, Sara Reis Teixeira, Fabricio Guimaraes Goncalves, and Giulio Zuccoli

Abbreviations

AARS2	Alanyl-transfer RNA synthetase 2
ARS	Aminoacyl-transfer RNA synthetase
ATP	Adenosine triphosphate
CNS	Central nervous system
CoQ10	Coenzyme Q10
COX	Cytochrome oxidase
Cr	Creatine
CSF	Cerebrospinal fluid
CT	Computed tomography
DARS2	Aspartyl-tRNA synthetase 2
DNA	Deoxyribonucleic acid
DWI	Diffusion-weighted imaging
EARS2	Glutamyl-tRNA synthetase 2
GM	Gray matter
LBSL	Leukoencephalopathy with brainstem and spinal cord involvement and high lactate
LHON	Leber hereditary optic neuropathy
LS	Leigh syndrome
LTBL	Leukoencephalopathy with thalamus and brainstem involvement and high lactate
MELAS	Mitochondrial encephalomyopathy, lactic acidosis, and stroke-like episodes
MNGIE	Mitochondrial neurogastrointestinal encephalopathy
MPC	Mitochondrial pyruvate carrier
MRI	Magnetic resonance imaging
MRI	Magnetic resonance imaging
MRS	Magnetic resonance spectroscopy
mtDNA	Mitochondrial deoxyribonucleic acid
NAA	N-acetylaspartate
NADH	Reduced nicotinamide adenine dinucleotide
nuDNA	Nuclear deoxyribonucleic acid
OXPHOS	Oxidative phosphorylation
PCH	Pontocerebellar hypoplasia
PDHc	Pyruvate dehydrogenase complex
POLG	Polymerase gamma gene
POLGRD	Polymerase gamma gene-related disorders
RARS2	Arginyl-tRNA synthetase 2
TCA	Tricarboxylic acid
TP	Thymidine phosphorylase
tRNA	Transfer ribonucleic acid
WM	White matter

C. A. P. F. Alves · S. R. Teixeira · F. G. Goncalves
G. Zuccoli (✉)
Division of Neuroradiology, Department of Radiology, Children's Hospital of Philadelphia, Philadelphia, PA, USA
e-mail: zuccolig@email.chop.edu

Background

Mitochondrial cytopathies are genetic disorders resulting from either nuclear deoxyribonucleic acid (DNA) or mitochondrial DNA (mtDNA)

M. Mancuso, T. Klopstock (eds.), *Diagnosis and Management of Mitochondrial Disorders*,
https://doi.org/10.1007/978-3-030-05517-2_18

pathogenic variants, leading to decreased oxidative phosphorylation (OXPHOS) and, consequently, decreased cellular energy (adenosine triphosphate, ATP) production [1].

Mitochondrial cytopathies can manifest themselves as a single organ or as multisystem or multi-organ diseases resulting in severe metabolic and functional impairment of the targeted system and its metabolic turnover. The degree of involvement is relative to the bulk of mitochondria in a given system. Hence, the central nervous system (CNS) and the musculoskeletal system (MSK) are among the most commonly affected systems. Clinical onset shall occur at any age, yet particularly severe dysfunctions commonly affect newborns and young children [2].

In the last decades, the knowledge concerning the molecular, biochemical, and genetic background relative to mitochondrial cytopathies has substantially expanded. Significant development has also occurred on how those conditions are assessed by imaging, particularly in the field of magnetic resonance imaging (MRI). MRI is essential for mitochondrial cytopathies workup as it allows correlating imaging findings with some well-established imaging phenotypes. Moreover, it allows estimation of disease extension and severity [3]. Imaging pattern recognition approach to MD is a continually evolving field, and represents a diagnostic challenge for neuroradiologists.

As a general imaging rule, mitochondrial cytopathies are usually progressive. In the acute phase, CNS changes are characterized by symmetrical bilateral involvement of the supra- and infratentorial gray matter (GM) and white matter (WM), with restricted diffusion or vasogenic edema. It is appropriate to issue a caveat that substantial imaging and clinical findings have overlapping features among other metabolic disorders and mitochondrial cytopathies. Nevertheless, abnormalities in the deep GM nuclei or dorsal brainstem when associated with cerebellar atrophy, white matter disease, and increased lactate peak are likely expression of a mitochondrial cytopathy [4].

Mitochondrial DNA Syndromes

Mitochondrial Encephalomyopathy, Lactic Acidosis, and Stroke-Like Episodes

Mitochondrial encephalomyopathy, lactic acidosis, and stroke-like episodes (MELAS) is a condition related to the mitochondrial gene defect with transfer ribonucleic acid (tRNA) mutations, leading to the absence or deficit of subunits of the respiratory chain protein complexes. More than 80% of the cases of MELAS are linked to the m.3243A>G in the tRNALeu (UUR) (MTTL1) gene [5].

The disease onset occurs typically during childhood, with stroke-like episodes before 40 years old [6], and it is usually preceded by normal psychomotor development, although short stature and hearing loss may coexist in early childhood. Neurological symptoms can be highly variable. Acute unless epileptic seizure associated with stroke has been described [7].

Stroke-like brain imaging changes are the hallmark of the disorder. This can be explained by the presence of abnormal mitochondria in the endothelial and smooth muscle cells of blood vessels leading to an impairment of the autoregulatory vascular mechanisms [8]. These lesions are most often located in the posterior and lateral brain regions (occipital, parietal, or temporal lobes), corresponding to approximately 90% of the cases [9]. In MELAS, new stroke-like lesions usually do not overlap with older lesions.

In the acute stage, lesions are characterized by cytotoxic edema (i.e., restricted diffusion: high signal intensity on DWI and low signal intensity on ADC map) with sulci effacement. In the subacute-chronic phase, lesions usually portray vasogenic edema (i.e., facilitated diffusion: high signal intensity or iso intensity to normal parenchyma on DWI and high signal on ADC) [10]. Magnetic resonance spectroscopy (MRS) may be abnormal, which can demonstrate a lactate peak at 1.3 ppm in the affected area and also from the CSF inside the ventricle [11]. Additionally, a smaller lactate peak can be seen in the normal-appearing brain.

Cortical enhancement may be observed during the subacute phase, which can be explained by blood-brain barrier damage as a result of venous congestion or reperfusion-related damage [12, 13] (Fig. 1). The edematous lesions may sometimes evolve into cystic encephalomalacia [10, 14]. Scattered calcifications and cerebellar atrophy can also be identified; however, this is a finding observed in the late stages of the disease. MELAS imaging findings are summarized in Table 1.

Leber Hereditary Optic Neuropathy

Leber hereditary optic neuropathy (LHON) is a result of a homoplasmic (100%) mtDNA mutation (m.11778G>A, m.3460G>A, m.14484T>C), and all maternal offspring will inherit the mutation. Nevertheless, while 50% of males will be affected, only 10% of females will develop visual loss [15].

LHON is a predominantly organ-specific disease, considered to be one of the most common inherited optic neuropathies. The optic nerve retinal ganglion cells are the target of this condition. Once damaged, this ultimately leads to retinal ganglion cells degeneration, optic nerve atrophy, and central vision loss [16].

Visual loss frequently occurs between the ages of 20 and 40 years old, and it is more frequent in males. Unaffected LHON carriers are initially asymptomatic and may become symptomatic once exposed to specific triggers, such as cigarette smoke, alcohol, or specific antibiotics (i.e., macrolides, aminoglycosides, ethambutol, isoniazid, and linezolid) [17, 18].

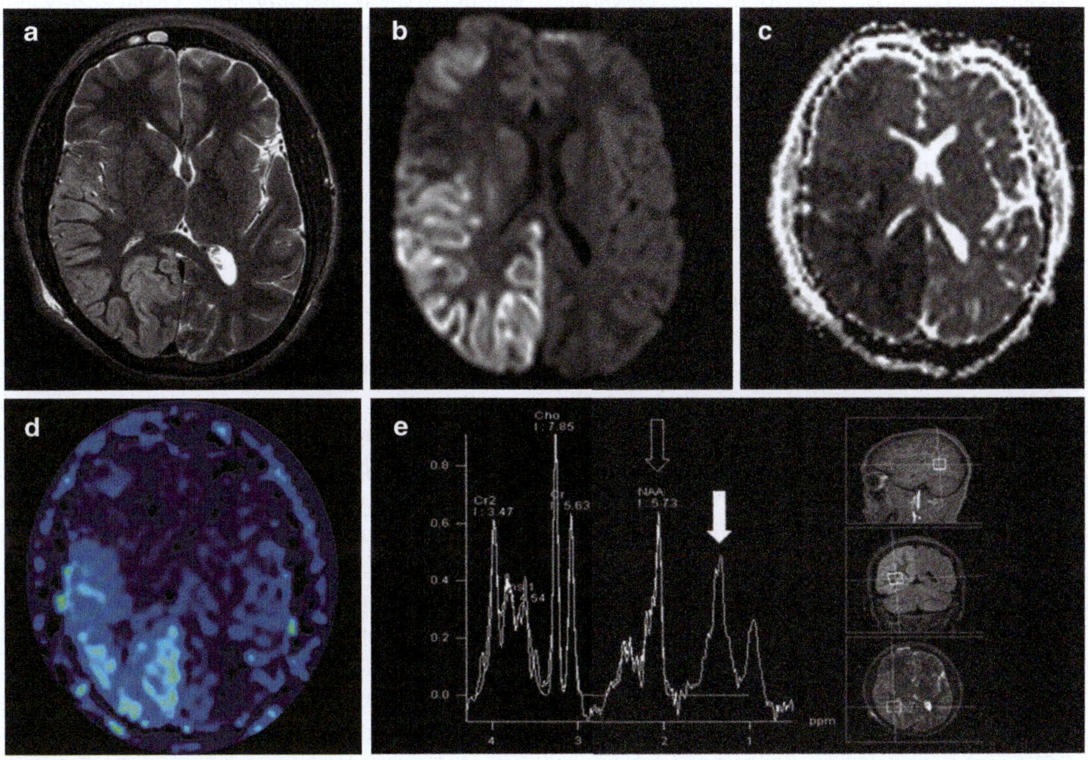

Fig. 1 A 10-year-old male with MELAS. Axial T2 and axial DWI show an abnormal hyperintensity and restricted diffusion in the right temporo-occipital gray matter (**a**, **b**) confirmed on the ADC map (**c**). Please note that T2 was not able to depict the metabolic impairment in the right frontal lobe seen on diffusion and ADC map (**b**, **c**). The axial ASL shows hyperperfusion in the right temporo-occipital gray mater (**d**). MRS (echo time 33 ms) with the voxel placed in the right occipital lobe demonstrates increased lactate (solid arrow, **e**) and decreased NAA (open arrow, **e**)

Table 1 MELAS

	Neuroimaging patterns	MRI			
		T1	T2	DWI	ASL perfusion
Acute-subacute	Migratory stroke-like lesions Occipital, parietal, and temporal lobes	Low signal Cortical enhancement	High signal	Restricted (high signal)	Increased flow
Chronic	Encephalomalacia Occipital, parietal, and temporal lobes Cerebellar atrophy	Low signal	High signal	Nonrestricted (low signal)	Decreased flow

LHON has a classic presentation of a subacute or acute, painless, central visual loss, typically unilateral with subsequent involvement of the contralateral eye within 2 months. Vision loss can be very severe, leading to blindness due to central scotoma in the majority of cases [19]. During the acute phase, the funduscopic examination show characteristic signs of pseudoedema of the peripapillary nerve fiber layer (optic disc elevation and hyperemia), retinal vascular tortuosity, and peripapillary telangiectatic microangiopathy [20]. At this stage, fluorescein angiography provides the distinction between the pseudoedema of LHON and true optic disc edema seen in other optic neuropathies.

Signs of idiopathic intracranial hypertension may be present before the acute phase of the disease and remains present during the disease onset [21]. Extraocular muscles atrophy and signal abnormalities can also be observed in selected patients [22]. Prompt diagnosis is essential, especially before the second eye becomes involved since idebenone-based therapy is available in Europe [23].

In affected patients, optical coherence tomography initially demonstrates thinning of the temporal and inferior peripapillary fibers, followed by thickening of the superior and ultimately of the nasal fibers, which are usually spared in the initial presentation [24].

As a general rule, the brain often appears normal in LHON patients. Nevertheless, lesions virtually indistinguishable from those seen in multiple sclerosis have been reported in patients with LHON, suggesting a link between mitochondrial dysfunction and neuroinflammation [25–27].

Atypical presentation of Leigh syndrome (LS) associated with LHON underling a primary mitochondrial DNA mutation has also been described in the literature [28]. In rare cases, MRI shows signal abnormalities in the visual pathways. Enlargement and enhancement of the optic chiasm may also occur in these patients [29, 30]. Chronic stages of LHON show reduced GM volume in the bilateral primary visual cortex and decreased WM volume in the optic chiasm, optic tracts, and bilateral optic radiations. These findings are more frequently observed in patients with LHON and WM abnormalities in comparison with isolated, "pure" LHON disease [31–33] (Fig. 2).

The imaging findings are summarized in Table 2.

Kearns-Sayre Syndrome

KSS is an uncommon sporadic multisystemic mitochondrial cytopathy caused by a single large-scale mtDNA de novo deletion which shows a marked heterogeneity with various types of inheritance already described [34].

The syndrome consists of a triad of progressive external ophthalmoplegia/ptosis, retinal pigmentary degeneration, and heart block requiring a prophylactic pacemaker, with onset age before 20 years [35]. Other clinical associations include low stature, with proximal myopathy, limb weakness, cardiomyopathy, sensorineural hearing loss, dementia, cerebellar ataxia, and endocrine dysfunction (diabetes, hypoparathyroidism, growth hormone deficiency) [36, 37].

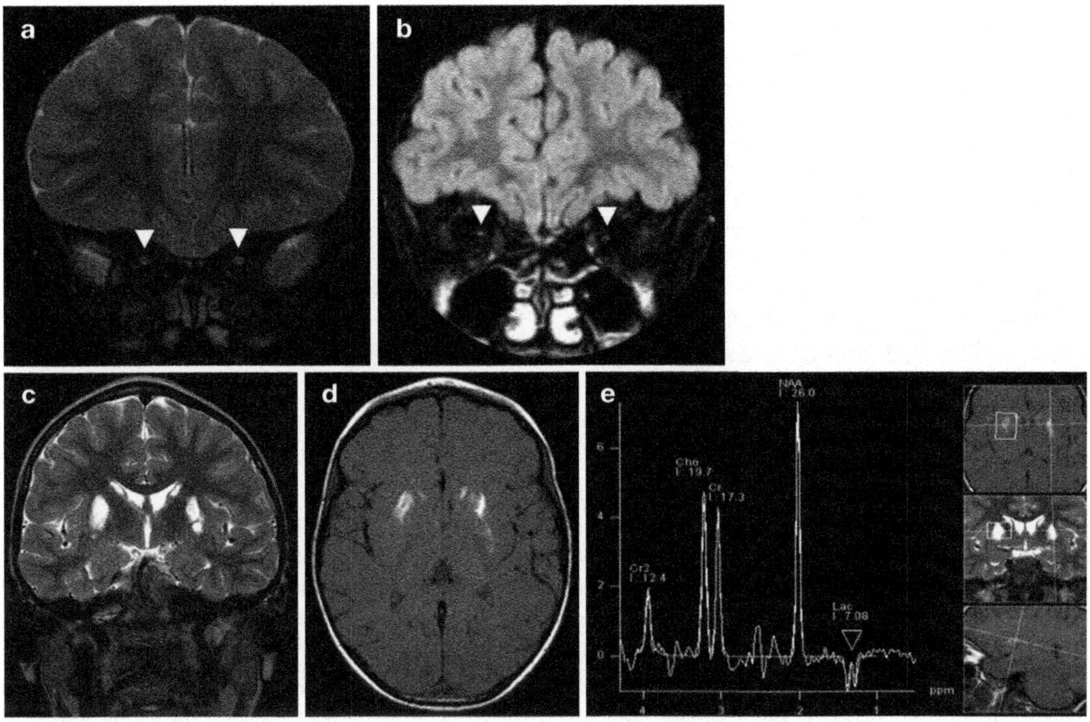

Fig. 2 An 8-year-old male with gradual bilateral visual loss and extrapyramidal symptoms with LHON "PLUS" diagnosis. Coronal T2 and FLAIR images show bilateral optic nerves hyperintensity and atrophy (arrowheads, **a**, **b**). Coronal T2 and axial T1 images show bilateral hyperintensities in the striatum (**c**, **d**) consistent with laminar necrosis. MRS (echo time 144 ms) with the voxel placed in the right striatum demonstrates mildly decreased NAA and increased lactate (open arrowhead, **e**)

Table 2 LHON

	Neuroimaging patterns	MRI			
		T1	T2	DWI	ASL perfusion
Acute-subacute	Optic pathway Enlargement of the optic chiasm	Low signal Optic chiasm enhancement	High signal	Restricted	N/A
Chronic	Reduced WM volume in the optic chiasm, optic tracts, and bilateral optic radiations Reduced GM volume in the bilateral primary visual cortex	Low signal	High signal	Nonrestricted	N/A

Note. *WM* white matter, *GM* gray matter

KSS patients may present with increased CSF proteins (>100 mg/dL). Diagnosis can be established by a combination of clinical, MRI, pathological, biochemical, and molecular findings. A muscle biopsy may be necessary to detect the mtDNA deletion, as it may not be found in the blood, also showing the characteristic histopathological findings of RRF with modified Gomori trichrome stain [38].

MRI findings range from an unremarkable examination to positive findings such as cerebral, cerebellar, and brainstem atrophy. Atrophic changes are commonly observed in the later stage of the disorder [39].

The most characteristic neuroimaging feature of KSS are T2 hyperintense lesions involving the subcortical U-fibers, with preservation of the periventricular WM [4]. Early involvement of the subcortical U-fibers is a typical imaging finding of KSS, which may aid in the differentiation from other entities such as lysosomal and peroxisomal disorders, in which the subcortical U-fibers are spared until the late stage of the disease [40].

Involvement of the mediodorsal thalamus, basal ganglia, and brainstem tegmentum is also commonly seen.

In the acute stage of the disease, brain lesions can show restricted diffusion. CT or MRI may show calcified deposits in the basal ganglia in the late stages. An unusual pattern of radially oriented T2 low signal intensity stripes within the abnormally myelinated WM has also been described [41] (Fig. 3).

KSS and L2-hydroxyglutaric aciduria may present with similar imaging features since the early subcortical U-fibers involvement and the basal ganglia lesions have been described in both disorders [42]. However, KSS may be differentiated from L2-hydroxyglutaric aciduria due to its peculiar involvement of the tegmentum of the brainstem and differences in clinical presentation.

The imaging findings are summarized in Table 3.

Nuclear DNA Syndromes

POLG-Related Disorders

POLG (polymerase gamma gene) is the unique DNA polymerase activated during the process of mtDNA transcription. Mutations in this nuclear gene can be autosomal dominant or autosomal recessive, both leading to a continuum of overlapping clinical phenotypes called POLG-related disorders (POLGRDs) [43, 44].

POLGRDs are often multisystemic diseases, and they may manifest over an extended period of time with a progressive intensification of symptoms over time. The onset of symptoms

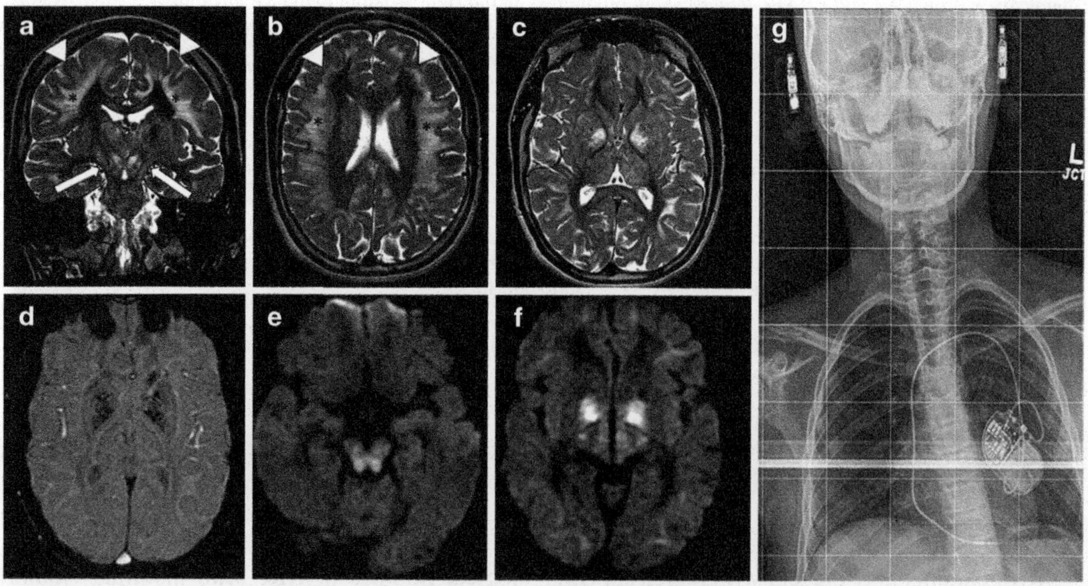

Fig. 3 An 8-year-old male with KSS diagnosis, with bilateral hearing loss and A-V block. Coronal and axial T2 images (**a**–**c**) show hyperintense corticospinal tracts (arrows, **a**), involvement of the subcortical U-fibers (arrowheads, **a**, **b**), radially oriented T2 low signal intensity stripes within the abnormal demyelinated WM (asterisks, **a**, **b**), and hyperintensities in the globus pallidum (**c**). Axial SW image shows multiple foci of hypointensities in the globus pallidum corresponding to calcifications (**d**). DW images show restricted diffusion in the dorsal segment of the mesencephalon and globus pallidum (**e**, **f**). Radiography of the thorax and head demonstrates cardiac pacemaker and auditive devices (**g**)

Table 3 Kearns-Sayre

	Neuroimaging patterns	MRI			
		T1	T2	DWI	ASL perfusion
Acute-subacute	Subcortical WM Basal ganglia Mediodorsal thalami Brainstem tegmentum	Low signal	High signal	Restricted[a]	N/A
Chronic	Subcortical WM Basal ganglia Mediodorsal thalami Brainstem tegmentum Cerebellar Atrophy	Low signal	High signal	Nonrestricted	N/A

Note: [a]Restricted diffusion in the thalami, basal ganglia, and brainstem

may occur at any age, from childhood to late adulthood, with some intrafamilial phenotypic constancy. There are many unsteady phenotypes associated to POLG mutations. One of them is known as the Alpers-Huttenlocher syndrome (AHS). This phenotype has a bimodal age distribution, with typical onset in toddlers or young adults.

The hallmark clinical features of AHS are intractable seizures, developmental regression, and liver dysfunction. Although liver involvement is a typical feature of AHS, it has a variable onset, and it may precede seizures in some patients, while in others, it only occurs at the late stages of the disease [45].

CT or MRI of the brain may be normal at the beginning of the course of AHS. As the disorder evolves, the cerebellum, basal ganglia, thalamus, and brainstem will sequentially become involved [46].

In patients presenting with lesions involving the dorsomedial thalamus, cerebellar white matter, and the inferior olivary nuclei, POLG should be included in the differential diagnoses [47].

Moreover, some patients with POLG1 mutation have been associated with a MELAS-like phenotype. However, due to clinical differences, it is unclear whether POLG1 mutation may either cause MELAS or represent a distinct pathological entity [48].

As a general rule, patients with POLGRD show progressive brain volume loss (basal ganglia > cortical) and ventriculomegaly.

In the acute phase, a characteristic of the disease is the asymmetrical brain involvement, with the classical restricted diffusion in the ipsilateral pulvinar thalamus and occipital lobe. Other nuclei of the thalamus may be also involved, also bilaterally. Atrophy and gliosis may affect the occipital lobes unilaterally or bilaterally (Fig. 4).

The cerebellum may be atrophic at the onset, or it may become progressively atrophic over the course of the disease. MRS may show reduced NAA, normal creatine, and a lactate peak [49].

The imaging findings are summarized on the Table 4.

Mitochondrial Neurogastrointestinal Encephalomyopathy

Mitochondrial neurogastrointestinal encephalopathy (MNGIE) is an autosomal recessive mitochondrial cytopathy associated with multiple deletions and depletion of mtDNA linked to TYMP gene mutations. This results in a loss of thymidine phosphorylase (TP) activity and consequently leading to nucleotide metabolism disorder. TP deficiency causes marked accumulation of systemic thymidine and deoxyuridine components, promoting a nucleotide pool imbalance with subsequent instability of mtDNA and impairment of the mitochondrial RC [50–52].

Clinically, MNGIE is characterized by the involvement of the digestive system and CNS, with onset in adolescence and young adulthood,

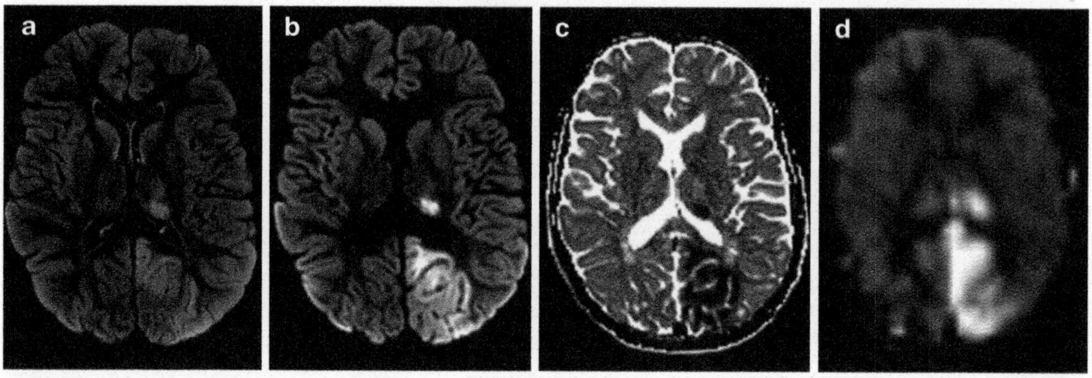

Fig. 4 A 6-year-old male with POLG disease. Axial FLAIR, DWI, ADC, and ASL show asymmetric cortical and subcortical hyperintensities, with restricted diffusion and hyperperfusion in the left occipital lobe and thalamus (**a**–**d**)

Table 4 POLGRD

	Neuroimaging patterns	MRI			
		T1	T2	DWI	ASL perfusion
Acute-subacute	Asymmetrical lesions distribution Cerebellum Basal ganglia Thalamus Brainstem (pulvinar and occipital lobe)	Low signal Cortical enhancement	High signal	Restricted	Increased flow
Chronic	Progressive cerebral volume loss (central > cortical) Ventriculomegaly Cerebellar atrophy	Low signal	High signal	Nonrestricted	Decreased flow

which progressively worsen over time. Patients with MNGIE usually present with gastrointestinal dysmotility and myopathy. Nevertheless, some MNGIE cases may have mild or no gastrointestinal or skeletal muscle involvement, despite mutations in the TYMP gene [53].

Cerebral and cerebellar WM involvement may be diffuse with increased signal intensity on T2/FLAIR sequences [54]. The corpus callosum, basal ganglia, and thalami can also be involved. MRS shows decreased N-acetylaspartate and choline in involved regions, without lactate peaks. In MINGIE brain lesions do not show restricted diffusion [55].

The imaging findings in MINGIE are summarized on the Table 5.

Coenzyme Q10 Deficiency

Coenzyme Q10 (CoQ10) is an essential cofactor of the mitochondrial electron transport chain, endogenously synthesized lipid responsible for carrier electrons from complexes I and II and the oxidation of fatty acids and branched-chain amino acids, via flavin-linked dehydrogenases, to complex III [56]. Coenzyme Q10 (CoQ10) is an essential cofactor of the mitochondrial electron transport chain. CoQ10 is an endogenously synthesized lipid responsible for carrier electrons from complexes I and II and the oxidation of fatty acids and branched-chain amino acids, via flavin-linked dehydrogenases, to complex III [57].

Table 5 MNGIE

	Neuroimaging patterns	MRI			
		T1	T2	DWI	ASL perfusion
Acute-subacute	Confluent and diffuse WM involvement Corpus callosum Basal ganglia Thalami	Low signal	High signal	Nonrestricted	N/A
Chronic	More evident lesions already observed in the acute phase	Low signal	High signal	Nonrestricted	N/A

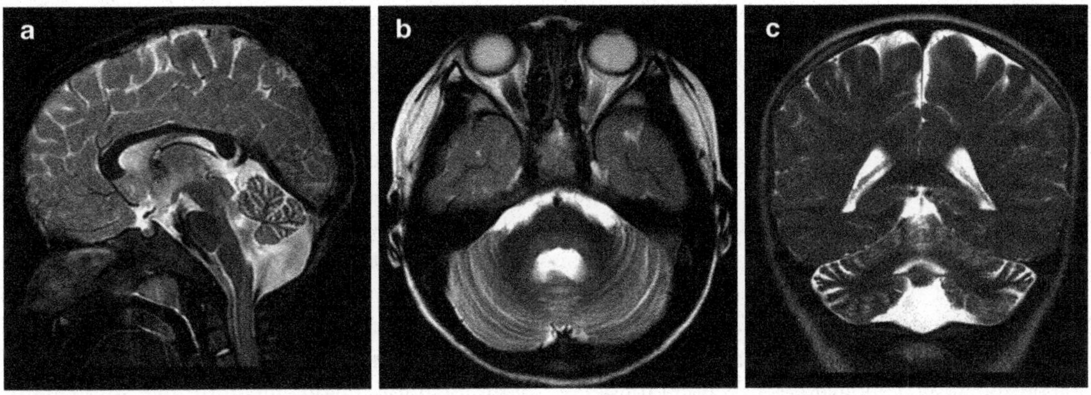

Fig. 5 A 4-year-old female with coenzyme Q10 deficiency. Sagittal, axial, and coronal T2 images show cerebellar atrophy with subtle hyperintense cortex (**a**–**c**)

The severity and age of onset of primary CoQ10 deficiency are variable. In the most critical patients, the disease manifests in childhood resulting in significant brain dysfunction and muscle weakness with other associations including, hypertrophic cardiomyopathy, optic atrophy, cataracts, sensorineural hearing loss, and nephropathy with focal and segmental glomerulosclerosis.

There are six significant phenotypes described in association with CoQ10 deficiency, characterized by seizures and ataxia: (1) severe and multisystem childhood form with encephalopathy, (2) cardiomyopathy and renal failure, (3) cerebellar form with ataxia and brain images with cerebellar atrophy, (4) Leigh syndrome, (5) isolated myopathic form, and (6) steroid-resistant nephrotic syndrome [58, 59].

MRI may demonstrate a broad spectrum of abnormalities from Leigh syndrome features to normal exam. The involvement of the cerebellum, commonly characterized by cerebellar atrophy [60], associated with T2 cortical hyperintensity known as "bright cerebellum" is typically observed in CoQ10 deficiency (Fig. 5).

The imaging findings of CoQ10 deficiency are summarized in Table 6.

Leigh Syndrome

Leigh syndrome (LS) or subacute necrotizing encephalomyelopathy is the most frequent mitochondrial cytopathy of infancy and childhood [61].

Causative genes of LS exist in both nuclear (nuDNA) and mtDNA genomes [62]. Up to now, more than 75 disease genes have been linked to LS, affecting the OXPHOS system, the pyruvate dehydrogenase complex (PDHc), and multiple other enzymes mostly related to OXPHOS system or a broader pathway of energy generation [63].

Table 6 CoQ10 deficiency

	Neuroimaging patterns	MRI			
		T1	T2	DWI	ASL perfusion
Acute-subacute	Cerebellum Basal ganglia and brainstem (Leigh pattern)	Low signal	High signal	Restricted[a]	N/A
Chronic	Cerebellum (atrophy) Basal ganglia and brainstem (Leigh pattern)	Low signal	High signal	Nonrestricted	N/A

Note: [a]In cases of LEIGH presentation, restricted diffusion may be observed in the basal ganglia, thalami, and brainstem

LS is characterized by a wide clinical, biochemical, and genetic variability. Despite its heterogeneity, LS is pathologically characterized by symmetric necrotic lesions, with demyelination, vascular proliferation, and gliosis, in the basal ganglia, diencephalon, brainstem, and spinal cord [64].

The age at onset among patients is variable, most often appears within the first years of life, followed by a progressive pattern; in most clinical presentation demonstrates psychomotor delay or regression, acute neurological or acidotic episodes, hypotonia, ataxia, spasticity, movement disorders, and the corresponding anomalies of the basal ganglia and brainstem on MRI [65].

Isolated complex I (NADH:ubiquinone oxidoreductase) deficiency is the most common biochemical defect observed in LS [66]. Other common defects are related to the disruption of complex IV or cytochrome oxidase (COX), within the OXPHOS pathway, more commonly linked with nuclear-encoded SURF1 mutated gene located on chromosome 9q34 [65], and abnormalities in the PDHc [67].

Due to the inconsistent nature of this disease and the distinct absence of a specific biochemical or molecular defect, the diagnosis is reached by consensus based on a combination of clinical, imaging findings and lactic acidosis [65].

The classical involvement of bilateral basal ganglia (putamen) with restricted diffusion has long been regarded as a consistent finding of LS on neuroimaging studies [67, 68] (Fig. 6). Other features include central tegmental tracts and substantia nigra, periaqueductal gray matter, and dentate nuclei involvement [11]. Lactate peak on MRS, a characteristic feature of mitochondrial cytopathies, may also be found in LS. Lesional hyperperfusion on ASL may also be observed in the acute stage of the disease [69].

LS can also affect the cervical cord and the white matter and the cerebral cortex [70, 71].

LS related to COX with *SURF1* gene mutation is a relatively homogeneous clinical entity with peculiar neuroimaging findings. The *SURF1* gene mutation has been described in association with bilateral involvement of the subthalamic nuclei [72]. Furthermore, it may affect the brainstem at different levels (medulla oblongata, pontine tegmentum, and periaqueductal area), despite a mild or even absent involvement of the basal ganglia (Fig. 7).

Other target areas include the interpeduncular nucleus and pallidum-cortical-nigro-cortical tracts [73, 74].

The imaging findings of LS are summarized in Table 7.

Pyruvate Metabolism Disorders

Pyruvate is the primary fuel for the mitochondria to produce energy, i.e., the ATP. It is derived from many sources within the cellular cytoplasm.

The PDHc is composed of four sub-complexes, each with subunits, and plays a core role in the cellular energy metabolism linking the glycolysis in the cytosol and the TCA cycle and OSPHOS in the mitochondria [75]. The acetyl-CoA, one of the molecules yielded from reactions generated by the PDHc upon the pyruvate, will drive the TCA cycle, and the net result will be high-energy

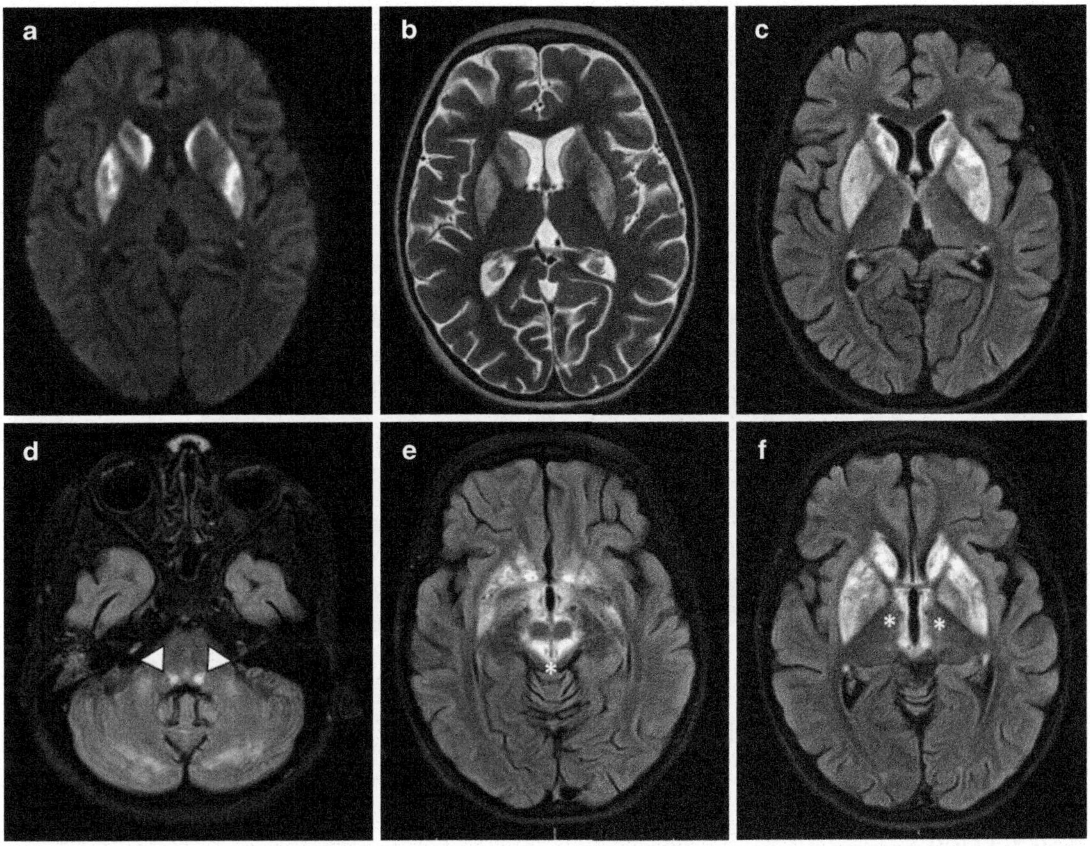

Fig. 6 A 5-year-old female with Leigh syndrome. Axial T2, FLAIR, and DW images show bilateral hyperintensity of the striatum (**a**, **b**) with restricted diffusion (**c**). Axial FLAIR images show symmetric hyperintensities in the cerebellar hemispheres and central tegmental tracts of the pons (arrowheads, **d**) and hyperintensity of the periaqueductal gray matter and medial portion of the thalami (asterisks, **e** and **f**)

molecules, such as ATP [75, 76]. Moreover, when the tissue demands more energy, such as muscle contraction during exercise, the enzyme pyruvate carboxylase (PC) will carboxylase the pyruvate and yield oxaloacetate, a reaction that will increase the capacity of the TCA cycle to metabolize acetyl-CoA [77]. Thus, PDHc and PC are of utmost importance to the metabolism of carbohydrate and energy production through the phosphorylation of the TCA cycle.

The main abnormalities of the pyruvate metabolism result from either impairment of one or a combination of the following: PDHc, lactate dehydrogenase, PC [77], pyruvate kinase, alanine aminotransferase, MPC [78], pyruvate dehydrogenase phosphatase, and pyruvate dehydrogenase kinase [79]. Neuroimaging abnormalities have been reported in patients with conditions associated to misregulations of the PDHc and PC [77, 79–81].

Brain energy depends upon carbohydrates metabolism. Impairments in any step of the pyruvate metabolism, TCA cycle, PDHc, or PC, to the genes that regulate their functions, may lead to neurological impairment [80, 82].

Pyruvate Dehydrogenase Complex

There are three major clinical presentations of PDHc deficiency [77, 80, 81], which were revised and proposed to be increased to four in the last decade [83]: (1) neonatal encephalopathy with lactic acidosis, (2) nonprogressive infantile

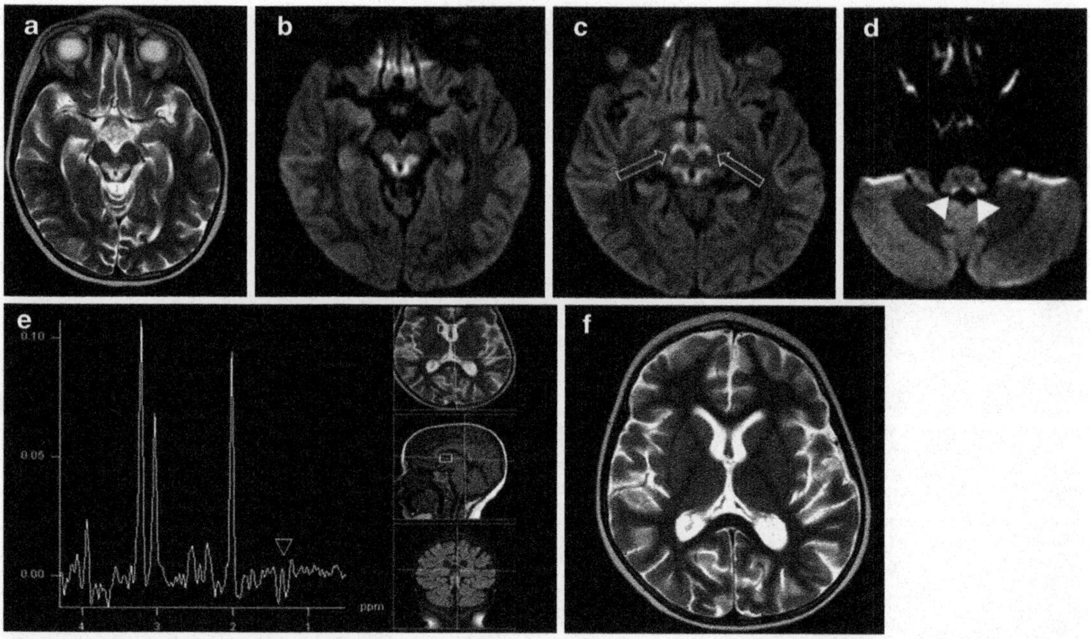

Fig. 7 A 4-year-old female with Leigh syndrome underlying SURF1 gene mutations. Axial T2 and DW images show hyperintensity and restricted diffusion of the periaqueductal gray matter (**a**, **b**) and selective restricted diffusion lesions in the substantia nigra (open arrows, **c**) and hypoglossal nucleus (arrowheads, **d**). MRS (echo time 144 ms) with voxel placed in the right lateral ventricle demonstrates increased lactate (open arrowhead, **e**). Axial T2 (**f**) shows the absence of basal ganglia abnormalities

Table 7 LEIGH syndrome

	Neuroimaging patterns	MRI			
		T1	T2	DWI	ASL perfusion
Acute-subacute	Basal ganglia (striatum) Brainstem (CTT, periaqueductal GM)	Low signal	High signal	Restricted	Increased flow
Chronic	Cerebral volume loss Basal ganglia (striatum) Cerebellar atrophy	Low signal	High signal	Nonrestricted	Decreased flow

Note: *CTT* central tegmental tracts

encephalopathy, (3) Leigh syndrome, and (4) relapsing ataxia. These clinical phenotypes differ semiologically and may respond to different treatments [83]. Males are more affected than females due to the predominantly maternal inheritance of mitochondria, though in women the disease is more severe [80, 83, 84]. However, there is neither correlation between the genotype and phenotype, and there is no correlation between neuroimaging findings and genotype [83–85].

Brain abnormalities related to PDHc deficiency may be either due to developmental anomalies or due to neurodegenerative changes [82, 86], though differences owing to these two pathological entities have not still elucidated jet [82, 86, 87]. It has been demonstrated that impairment of the activity of the PDHc will lead to abnormal migration and proliferation cells, a lower rate of cell differentiate into mature neurons, and decrease in the number of the Purkinje cells. Moreover, fatty acids in affected models are reduced due to the reduced de novo biosynthesis from acetyl-CoA via PDHc reactions [82].

Brain pathology and imaging studies will reflect these anomalies. Grossly, neuroimaging findings can be divided into two main patterns:

(1) perinatal, which is mainly found in females with lactic acidosis, hypotonia, and coma, eventually leading to precocious death, and (2) infancy or delayed pattern, which clinically mainly affects male patients with recurrent episodes of brainstem dysfunctions, dystonia and a past medical history of neonatal lactic acidosis, and ataxia or axonal neuropathy in previously normal children [83–85]. It is hypothesized that male fetuses need a significant enzyme residual activity to survive, and, therefore, they are more prone to present mild forms of the disease [83, 86, 88–91].

Asymmetrical supratentorial ventriculomegaly with a normal 4th ventricle; ventricular septations; parenchymal or subependymal pseudocysts; severe white matter volume loss, such as dysgenesis of the corpus callosum and hypoplasia of the pons and medullary pyramids; and migration anomalies, including periventricular heterotopia, polymicrogyria, and pachygyria, are the hallmark of the PDHc deficiency in females with severe lactic acidosis [83, 88–91] (Fig. 8). These findings may also be detected on prenatal imaging [86, 92–94].

A pattern resembling unilateral periventricular leukomalacia has also been described [95]. Neuropathology studies also showed microcalcifications and gliosis [86, 92–94] and marked vascular proliferation in the cerebrum and cerebellar white matter and in the basal ganglia [96], not yet demonstrated by neuroimaging.

In mild forms of the disease, MRI of the brain shows high-signal intensity on T2-weighted images in the basal ganglia [83, 88–91, 97], ranging from small punctate lesions to the classic pattern of Leigh syndrome with symmetrical lesions of the basal ganglia and brainstem and dentate nuclei [80, 83, 85, 88–91, 98, 99]. It is noteworthy to emphasize the importance of performing neuroimaging at clinical onset or disease relapse, as the characteristic imaging findings may be resolving with symptoms, which may delay diagnosis and treatment [85, 98]. Brain atrophy is the consequence of long-standing disease [85, 98].

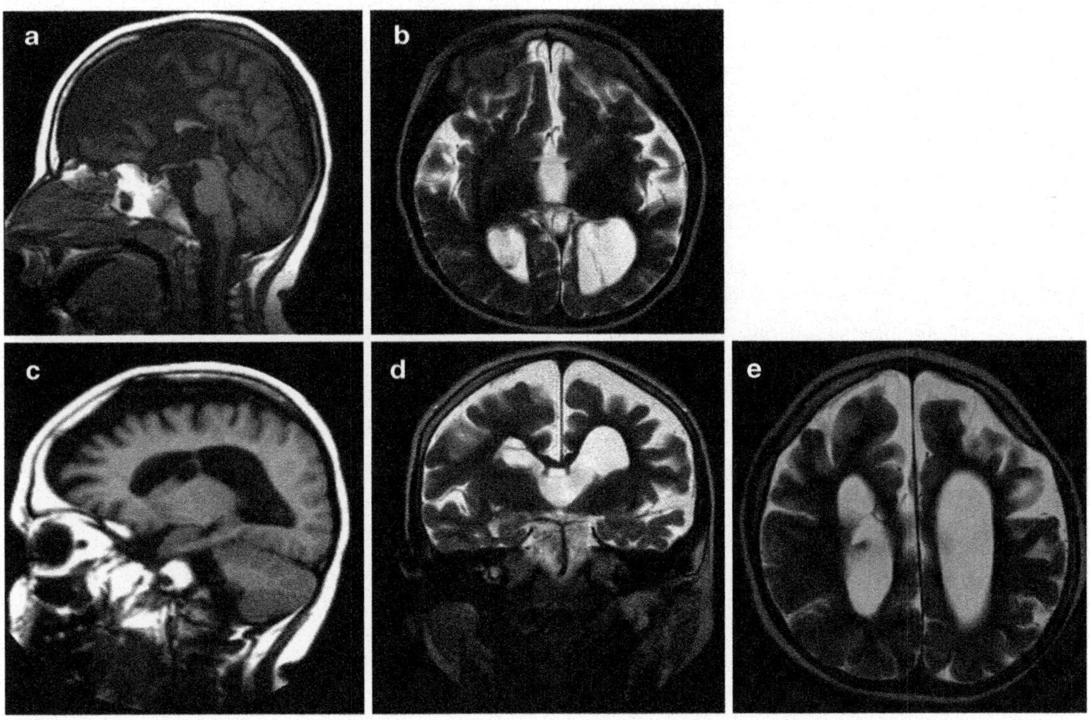

Fig. 8 A 4-year-old female with PDH deficiency. Sagittal T1 demonstrates a severe corpus callosum dysgenesis (**a**). Axial T2 demonstrates white matter reduction and asymmetrical ventriculomegaly (**b**). Sagittal T1 (**c**), coronal T2 (**d**), and axial T2 (**e**) show the presence of septations in the right lateral ventricle

MRS may add in the diagnosis of PDHc deficiency, aiding in the differential diagnosis, and can be used to monitor therapy [100]. Although not specific, in areas of signal intensity abnormalities, there is a lactate peak [80, 83, 85, 88–91, 98, 101, 102], and neuronal damage is expressed by decreasing the N-acetylaspartate/creatine (NAA/Cr) ratio [83, 88–91]. In addition, a pyruvate peak at 2.37 ppm can be depicted [83, 88–91] in severely affected children and should prompt the diagnosis toward PDH deficiency [102].

The imaging findings of pyruvate dehydrogenase complex are summarized in Table 8.

Pyruvate Carboxylase

The clinical phenotype of PC deficiency is classically divided into three types that may represent a continuum from the most severe form—the (B) neonatal or French form—the (A) infantile or North American form, to the less severe, (C) the benign form [77]. In type B PC deficiency, which is more common in France in patients with Arab descent, the affected neonate will typically present with hypotonia and tachypnea in the first 72 h that may come with additional signs, such as hepatomegaly, failure to thrive, abnormal limb and ocular movements, and sometimes generalized tonic-clonic seizures [103, 104]. Type A PC deficiency is more common among North American Indians with a typical age of onset of the disease of 2–5 months. Failure to thrive, hypotonia, nystagmus, seizures, and developmental delay are common clinical features of the disease. As there is no effective treatment, both types A and B have a poor prognosis expecting death by the first years and 3 months of life, respectively [77]. Type C is sporadic form with an age of onset of the disease in late infancy presenting with mild developmental delay and episodes of ketoacidosis and a longer expected survival rate [105].

Neuroimaging reports of types A and B describe similar features between PC and PDH deficiency, such as global white matter abnormalities and periventricular or subependymal pseudocysts [103, 104, 106], ventriculomegaly, and subcortical white matter hyperintensities on MRI [107, 108], which can be associated with brainstem signal intensities abnormalities [107, 108]. However, in contrast to what observed in PDH deficiency, patients with PC deficiency usually present with a more systemic disease which includes steatosis-related hepatomegaly and renal acidosis [77, 103]. Scarce literature is available regarding type C neuroimaging findings, though in one paper, no abnormalities on brain MRI were reported [105].

Table 8 Pyruvate dehydrogenase complex

	Neuroimaging patterns	MRI				
		T1	T2	DWI	ASL perfusion	MRS
Acute-subacute	Asymmetrical supratentorial ventriculomegaly Ventricular septations Subependymal pseudocysts Dysgenesis of the corpus callosum Hypoplasia of the pons and medullary pyramids Migration anomalies	Low signal	High signal	Restricted	N/A	Pyruvate peak (2.37 ppm)
Chronic	Same findings of acute stage, with cerebral volume loss	Low signal	High signal	Nonrestricted	N/A	Pyruvate peak (2.37 ppm)

Mitochondrial Translation

Protein translation is a critical step for the proper metabolism, survival of the cells, and propagation of information. The first step of translation requires the action of the aminoacyl-transfer RNA synthetase (ARS), which is an enzyme encoded by the nuclear DNA [109]. The ARSs can be classified as either cytoplasmic, mitochondrial, or bifunctional proteins, according to the location where they will facilitate translation [109]. Considering the many known mitochondrial translation related genes known, few mutations are known to give rise to human disease [109, 110].

EARS2-Leukoencephalopathy with Thalamus and Brainstem Involvement and High Lactate (LTBL)

Leukoencephalopathy with thalamus and brainstem involvement and high lactate (LTBL) is caused by glutamyl-tRNA synthetase 2 (EARS2) mutations [109]. LTBL has a severe and mild clinical phenotype [110]. The severe group includes newborns and infants with hypotonia and psychomotor developmental delay, which can be followed by seizures, spastic tetraparesis, and dystonia [110], with no further improvement [110, 111]. The milder clinical phenotype is patients with an overt onset of the disease after 6 months of age following a previously normal or mildly delayed development [110]. These patients improve after 2 years of age with attenuation of seizures, a disappearance of the spasticity, and regained milestones [110, 112]. Serum and cerebrospinal fluid lactate are elevated in both groups during the acute phase of the disease [110].

On MRI, the hallmark of the disease is diffuse T2 hyperintensity and T1 hypointensity of the deep white matter, sparing the periventricular white matter and abnormal signal intensity of the thalami, the striatum, and the brainstem [110–112]. In addition, abnormal signal may be present surrounding the dentate nuclei [113], and a peak of lactate may be depicted on MRS [110–112]. Following the clinical course of the disease, abnormal signal intensities detected on brain MRI may improve, reverse [110–113], or stabilize [110, 111]. In severely affected patients, thinning of the posterior part of the corpus callosum [110, 111] and absence of the thalami have been described, which may reflect early antenatal injuries [110, 111].

DARS2-Leukoencephalopathy with Brainstem and Spinal Cord Involvement and High Lactate (LBSL)

Leukoencephalopathy with brainstem and spinal cord involvement and high lactate (LBSL) is a rare hereditary disease with an autosomal recessive pattern caused by mutations of the aspartyl-tRNA synthetase 2 (DARS2) [109, 114]. The onset of the disease is during the childhood with 53% of the patients younger than 6 years old, though there are cases with an overt onset during the adolescence and adulthood, mainly in females [114]. Clinically, there is a slow progression of cerebellar ataxia, most of the patients requiring aid for walking after 18 years of age but not utterly dependent of a wheelchair, less severe manual ability, and 1/5 of them have an intellectual disability [114]. Patients with infantile onset of the disease are more severely affected than others, including rapid disease progression and a higher risk of death, though in general, LBSL patients have a normal life span [114].

The main neuroimaging findings have been described by van der Knaap more than a decade ago [115], and new diagnostic criteria have recently been published [116]. To fulfill the MRI criteria for this diagnosis, there should be at least abnormal signal intensity in all of the following brain structures, (1) the cerebral white matter with relative subcortical sparing, (2) the decussation of the medial lemniscus or pyramidal tract at the level of the medulla oblongata or both, and (3) the lateral corticospinal tracts and dorsal columns of the spinal cord, and one of the following minor signs, such as abnormalities of the cerebellum white matter, superior and inferior cerebellar peduncles, anterior spinocerebellar tracts in the medulla oblongata, trigeminal tracts

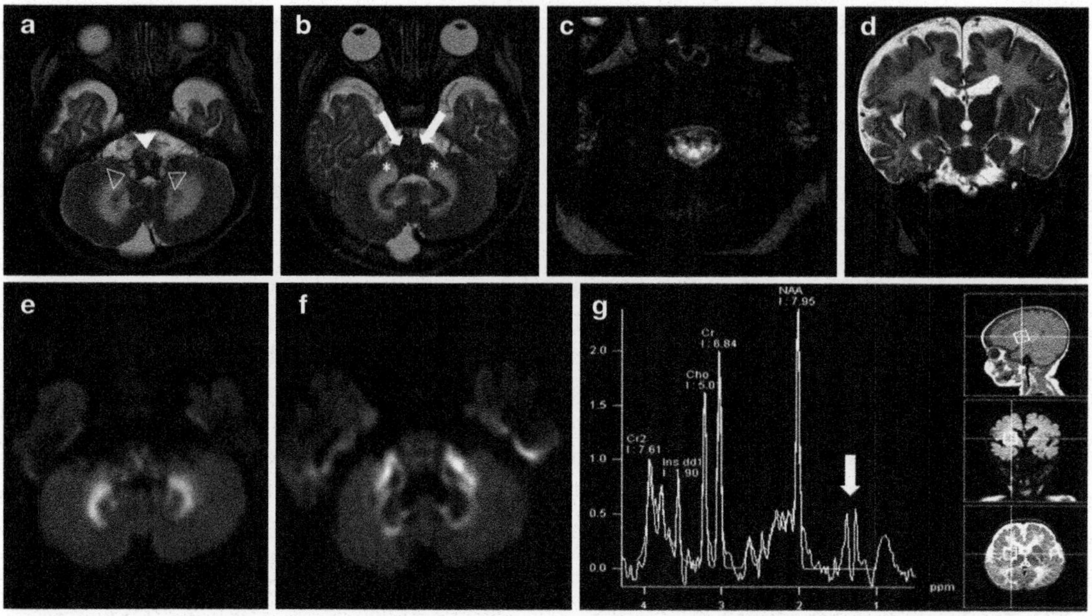

Fig. 9 A 1-year-old male with LBSL (DARS2). Brain and cervical spinal cord MRI studies. Axial T2 and DW images (**a**, **b** and **e**, **f**) show hyperintense lesions with restricted diffusion in the inferior cerebellar peduncles (open arrowheads, **a**) and pyramids (arrowhead, **a**). At the level of the pons, an abnormal signal in the pyramidal tracts (arrows, **b**), medial lemniscus, and mesencephalic trigeminal tracts (asterisks, **b**). Cervical spinal cord axial T2 image shows hyperintensities in the dorsal column and lateral corticospinal tracts (**c**). Coronal T2 image demonstrates cerebral periventricular WM hyperintensities also compromising the corticospinal tract (**d**). MRS (echo time 33 ms) with voxel placed in the right striatum demonstrates increased lactate (open arrowhead, **g**)

in the mesencephalon, intraparenchymal part of the trigeminal nerve, posterior limb of the internal capsule, and splenium of the corpus callosum [116]. DWI may show scattered areas of restricted diffusion in the white matter, a common feature in mitochondrial leukoencephalopathies, likely reflecting myelin vacuolization [117] (Fig. 9). No genotype-neuroimaging correlation has been described.

AARS2

Mutations of the alanyl-transfer RNA synthetase 2 (AARS2) have been related to a progressive adult-onset leukodystrophy, with ovarian involvement in females [118], and to infantile hypertrophic cardiomyopathy associated with brain disease and rapid progression to death [119, 120]. For the latter group, patterns of brain abnormalities have not been thoroughly explored, though cerebral atrophy and findings consistent with Leigh syndrome have been described in a few reports [120].

Knowledge of imaging findings in adult-onset leukodystrophy caused by AARS2 mutations has significantly improved [118]. In adult-onset leukodystrophy caused by AARS2 mutations, the characteristic neuroimaging findings are asymmetrical and heterogeneous abnormal signal intensity in the WM tracts, mainly involving the frontal and parietal lobes, sparing the subcortical WM. Typically, there is involvement of the corpus callosum and corticospinal tracts [118, 121, 122]. Patients presenting with prominent psychiatric symptoms and cognitive dysfunction show abnormalities in the frontopontine tract, while patients with a prominent motor dysfunction show pyramidal tract involvement [118, 121, 122]. In addition, mild infratentorial atrophy is more noticeable in the vermis, and scattered areas of restricted diffusion of the white matter can be seen on MRI [118].

RARS2

Mutations of the arginyl-tRNA synthetase 2 (RARS2) encoding gene have been related to pontocerebellar hypoplasia (PCH) type 6 [123–126]. However, this mutation is rare, accounting for only 2 out of 106 patients with genetically proven PCH, being one case PCH type 1-like with elevated CSF lactate [123–126]. There is a wide variability in its clinical phenotype; notwithstanding, neonatal and early infantile-onset encephalopathy represents the most common phenotype of the disease [127]. Patients present with hypotonia, a few hours or days after birth following an uneventful pregnancy, intractable seizures, progressive microcephaly, severe global development delay, and, in some cases, rapid progression to death [123–126]. Most patients have CSF, blood, or MRS elevated lactate [127].

Characteristic imaging findings of RARS2 mutations were initially described as PCH and harbored in the PCH type 6 group [123–126]. Nevertheless, most cases show progressive cerebral and cerebellar atrophy on serial images [123–127]. PCH is not as common as it was initially suspected. The initial MRI may show atrophy of the cerebellum with or without involvement of the vermis [127, 128], mild hypoplasia of the pons, and mild cerebral atrophy [127, 128]. Simplified gyral patterns [129] and subdural effusions [128, 130] are also imaging features described in cases of RARS2 mutations.

The main imaging findings of mitochondrial translation disorders are summarized in Table 9.

Table 9 Mitochondrial translation

Main mitochondrial translation disorders	Main neuroimaging patterns
EARS2 (LTBL)	Symmetric involvement of WM Diffuse: brainstem and thalami Cerebellar WM Dysgenesis of the CC Agenesis/hypoplasia of the thalamus
DARS2 (LBSL)	Symmetric involvement of WM (sparing subcortical WM) Lesions in mesencephalic trigeminal tract Inferior cerebellar peduncles Splenium of corpus callosum
AARS2	Symmetrical abnormal signal intensity of the WM tracts (corpus callosum and corticospinal tracts) Mainly in the periventricular WM of the frontal and parietal lobes
RARS2	Atrophy of the cerebellum including the vermis Hypoplasia of the pons Mild cerebral atrophy Simplified gyral pattern Subdural effusions

Note: All disorders can show MRI lesions with T1 hypointensity, T2/FLAIR hyperintensity, restrict diffusion in DWI sequence, and MRS with lactate peak in 1.3 ppm

Approaching the Respiratory Chain Subunit Defects

The respiratory chain (RC) in the mitochondria will eventually lead to the formation of ATP through OXPHOS, which relies upon the action of five protein complexes: complex I (NADH:ubiquinone oxidoreductase), complex II (succinate dehydrogenase), complex III (CoQH2-cytochrome C reductase), complex IV (cytochrome C oxidase), and complex V (ATP synthetase) [131, 132].

RC primary defects may be a challenging diagnosis for neurologists given its broad variability in clinical presentation. MRI may be a valuable tool in distinguishing primary RC deficiency from phenocopies and other etiologies, highlighting the detection of the brainstem and basal ganglia lesions, including common locations such as the pyramids of the medulla and the striatum [133]. Table 10 summarizes the neuroimaging features of disorders of the RC complexes.

Complex I Deficiency (NADH:Ubiquinone Oxidoreductase)

Mutations of the complex I components are the most frequent cause of respiratory chain disorders in childhood and encompass variable clinical

Table 10 Respiratory complex defects

RC main defect	Main neuroimaging findings
Complex I mtDNA	Bilateral basal ganglia Periaqueductal gray matter Brainstem Stroke-like lesions
Complex I nDNA	Necrotizing leukoencephalopathy cavitation Brainstem involvement
Complex II	Leukoencephalopathy Corticospinal tracts Pyramids of the medulla Transverse pontine fibers Middle cerebellar peduncles Spectroscopy: 2.4 ppm (succinate peak)
Complex III	Bilateral basal ganglia (putamen, caudate, and globus pallidum) Brainstem is *not* a consistent finding
CoQ10	Basal ganglia (bilateral putaminal) Periaqueductal gray matter Brainstem Cerebellar atrophy
COX (complex IV)	Diffuse leukoencephalopathy Basal ganglia Thalamus and subthalamic nucleus Brainstem Dentate nucleus
Complex V	Basal ganglia Cerebellar atrophy Stroke-like and WM lesions are *not* a consistent finding

Note: All disorders can show MRI lesions with restrict diffusion in DWI sequence (white matter or gray matter) and MRS with lactate peak in 1.3 ppm

presentations, among them LHON, Leigh syndrome, MELAS, and mitochondrial encephalomyopathy [134].

Bilateral signal intensity abnormalities in the striatum, centered in the putamen, and brainstem lesions are the neuroimaging hallmarks of patients suffering from complex I deficiency [135, 136]. Hence, the absence of brainstem involvement makes the diagnosis of complex I deficiency unlikely [135, 136].

There are, however, differences in neuroimaging findings between mutations of the proteins encoded by the mtDNA and the nuDNA [135, 136]. In up to 42% of the patients carrying mtDNA mutations, Lebre et al. [135, 136] described a pattern consistent with supratentorial stroke-like lesions without calcifications, which, coupled with brainstem involvement, is the key to differentiate complex I deficiency from MTTL1 mutations causing MELAS. Mitochondrial mutations leading to complex I deficiency may also cause corpus callosum edema and abnormal signal intensity of the cerebellum and then progressing to cerebellar atrophy in patients older than 5 years of age [135–137]. In contrast, patients with nuDNA mutations have a pattern consistent with necrotizing leukoencephalopathy [135, 136] (Fig. 10).

Complex II Deficiency (Succinate Dehydrogenase)

Complex II deficiencies have been associated with Leigh syndrome and with an increasing number of tumors, such as hereditary paragangliomas and renal neoplasms [138]. Leukoencephalopathy related to complex II deficiency is rare, and the most common mutations described are of the genes SDHA, SDHB, and SDHAF1. However, mutations in all of the genes encoding the complex II subunits or assembling proteins can potentially cause disease [138].

Characteristic brain MRI findings described are the involvement of the white matter of the frontal lobes, posterior regions of the temporal lobes, and parieto-occipital lobes sparing the U fibers, swollen appearance of the corpus callosum sparing its inner and outer blades, abnormal signal intensity of the corticospinal tracts including the pyramids of the medulla, and involvement of the dorsal regions of the cervical spinal cord [139, 140]. Helman et al. described these features in 73% up to 100% of the individuals in the early stage of the disease and all individuals at a late stage of the disease [139, 140]. Involvement of the lateral portions of the cerebellar peduncles and the transverse fibers of the pons are other imaging features that may be observed in patients with complex II [139, 140]. In early stage of the disease, restricted diffusion of the white matter is present. In late stage of the disease, the white matter involvement may progress to cystic degeneration. One specific

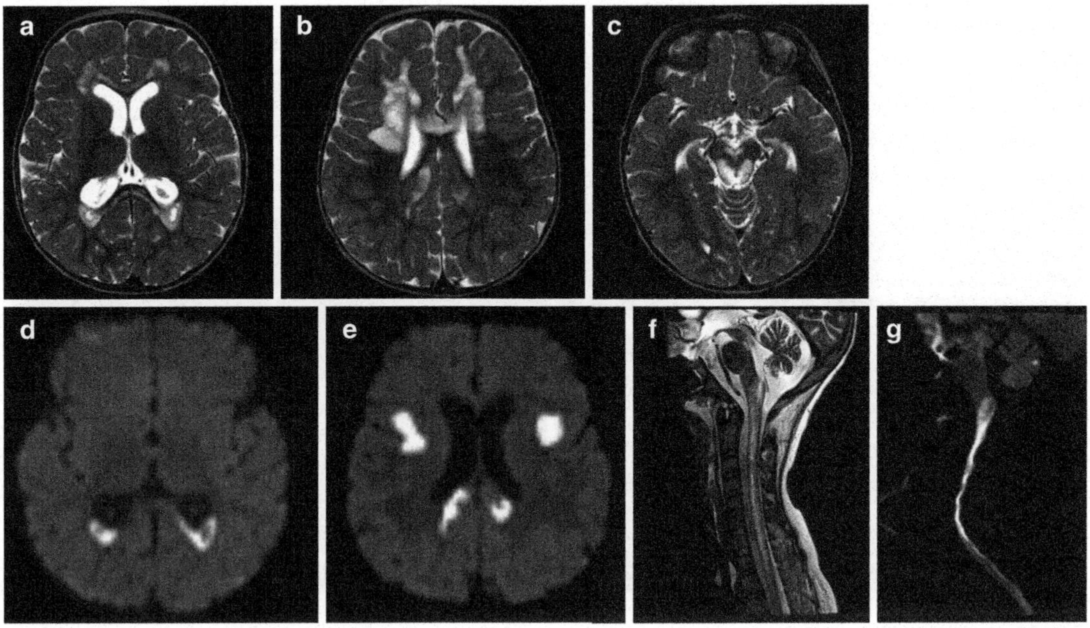

Fig. 10 Two different patients with complex I deficiency underlying the mutation of NDUFV1. A 6-year-old male (patient 1, **a–e**) axial T2 and DWI show tumefactive diffuse WM lesions with restricted diffusion (**a**, **b** and **d**, **e**). Axial T2 image at the level of the mesencephalon shows hyperintensities in the periaqueductal gray matter and mesial part of the cerebral peduncles (**c**). A 8-year-old male (patient 2, **f**, **g**) sagittal T2 and DW images of the cervical spinal cord show tumefactive diffuse hyperintense and restricted diffusion lesions (**f**, **g**)

finding of complex II deficiency is a peak at 2.4 ppm on MRS, which represents increased amounts of succinate [139, 140].

Complex III Deficiency (CoQH2-Cytochrome C Reductase)

Among all of the respiratory chain complex deficiencies causing encephalopathies, isolated complex III deficiency is the most uncommon. Mutations of the complex III have been related to a broad spectrum of clinical presentations and heterogeneous group of diseases in children and adults, encompassing exercise intolerance in mildly affected patients, liver failure, renal tubulopathy, GRACILE syndrome, and severe encephalopathy [141–144]. On neuroimaging, the pattern of Leigh syndrome has been described in few reports of patients with neurological symptoms due to complex III deficiency, though with no consistent involvement of the brainstem [141–146].

Complex IV Deficiency (Cytochrome C Oxidase)

The cytochrome C oxidase (COX) is encoded by both the mDNA and nDNA [147]. SURF1 deficiency is the most common cause of COX (complex IV) deficiency [148].

Clinically, patients present in the first year of age (75%) with poor feeding, vomiting, and reduced weight gain, followed by hypotonia, mostly after the neonatal period [148]. Clinical criteria for LS are met in the majority of patients with SURF1 mutations, though leukoencephalopathy and malabsorption syndrome have also been described [148]. MRI shows findings of LS but with the prominent involvement of the brainstem rather than the basal ganglia and constant bilateral involvement of the subthalamic nuclei [72]. Diffuse leukoencephalopathy and nearly normal brain imaging have also been described [148] (Fig. 11). Abnormal cerebral and cerebellar white matter may contain small cysts [72].

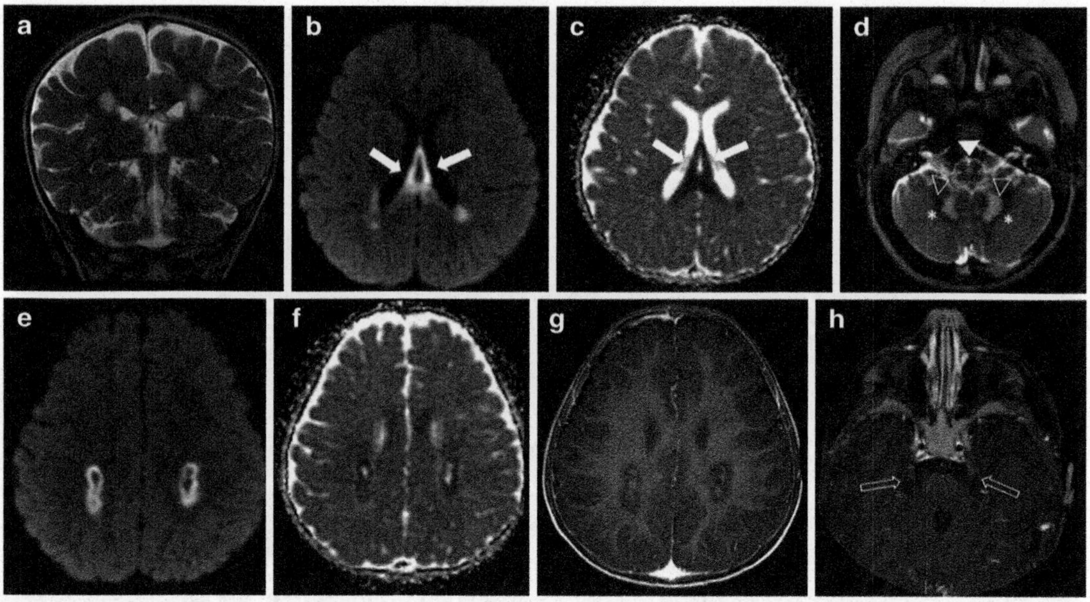

Fig. 11 A 9-year-old male with complex IV deficiency (W227x nonsense mutation in the Surf 1 gene). Coronal T2, axial DW, and ADC images (**a–c**, **e**, and **f**) show tumefactive hyperintense WM lesions with restricted diffusion, involving the fornices (arrows, **b** and **c**). Axial T2 image shows hyperintense lesions in the inferior cerebellar peduncles (open arrowheads, **d**), pyramids (arrowhead), and dentate nuclei (asterisks, **d**). Post-contrast T1 images show enhancing foci in the bilateral WM (**g**) and trigeminal nerves (open arrows, **h**)

Complex V Deficiency (Coupling with Oxidative Phosphorylation)

Clinical phenotypes of complex V deficiency may be severe, including neuropathy, ataxia, and retinitis pigmentosa (NARP), maternally inherited Leigh syndrome (MILS), neonatal mitochondrial encephalo(cardio)myopathy, and dysmorphic facial features [149]. Cerebellar hypoplasia is the most common imaging feature described in the few published series [150, 151].

Other brain imaging features described are white matter abnormalities, brainstem hypoplasia, and incomplete hippocampal inversion [150].

Differential Considerations

Hypoxic-Ischemic Encephalopathy

One of the main differential diagnoses of mitochondrial disorders in newborns and infants is hypoxic-ischemic encephalopathy (HIE). This is a frequent clinical challenge for clinicians and neuroradiologists.

Due to its higher incidence in the clinical practice compared to mitochondrial cytopathies and also due to many clinical and neuroimaging overlaps, HIE should be included in the differential considerations of primary mitochondrial disorders. An aggregate of careful history, neurological examination, can assist in differentiating HIE from mitochondrial cythopathies.

HIE and mitochondrial citopathies share common imaging findings. The central location of the lesions in the brain depends not only on the severity and duration of the hypoxic-ischemic event, but also the age of the patients [152, 153].

In severe preterms with low birth weight, the involvement of the cerebellar surface is a frequent finding [154]. It occurs as a result of the high metabolic rate in the cerebellar germinal matrix. Presence of hemorrhagic lesions compromising the cerebellar surface is a feature that can be better depicted by using susceptibility weighted imaging [155, 156].

In the later stage of the gestational age, either germinal matrix hemorrhages and/or supratentorial WM lesions, and the characteristic finding of periventricular leukomalacia with or without cystic cavitations are usually observed [154].

In HIE, WM lesions are characterized by hyperintense foci on T1WI [157] with or without restricthed diffision [158]. These imaging findings may overlap with of a mitochondrial cytopathy showing white matter cavitations.

HIE in term neonates with severe asphyxia tend to demonstrate injuries that compromise the deep GM, preferentially the ventrolateral thalami, putamen, dorsal brainstem, and occasionally perirolandic cortex. The presence of restricted diffusion is usually observed over the first 24 hours since the onset of the symptoms. However, less frequently, these lesions may appear only after 24 hours, as described in the literature [159, 160]. HIE may overlap image findings with some mitochondrial cytopathies, such as Leigh disease [161].

In patients with severe effects of HIE, apart from the age, impairment of the thalamus and cerebellum is a characteristic feature which can also be observed in some mitochondrial cytopathies, such as POLG and related disorders [162].

Infectious Diseases

Mitochondria play many functions in infected and noninfected cells, including energy generation, intracellular Ca^{2+} accumulation, innate immune signaling, and neuronal apoptosis [163]. Consequently, it is expected that primary mitochondrial cytopathies may share many similarities with infectious diseases.

Infectious diseases caused by different agents may demonstrate similar imaging features that are also seen in mitochondrial cytopathies. Particular attention must be paid to the involvement of the deep GM structures affected by viral agents [164].

Several viruses involve the basal ganglia [165]. Striatal and thalamic lesions may be included in the differential of infections caused by *Herpesviridae* family of viruses, some arbovirosis such as dengue, West Nile fever, Japanese encephalitis, and others. This pattern is also typical of bacteria and mycoplasma [166]. Involvement of the posterior brainstem, seen in mytochondrial disorders, has also been described in enteroviruses 68 and 71 infected patients [167, 168]. Basal ganglia and thalamic lesions can be observed in cases of acute necrotizing encephalitis (ANE), influenza A and B, novel influenza A (H1N1), parainfluenza, varicella, human herpesviruses 6 and 7 (HHV-6 and HHV-7), enterovirus, novel reovirus train (MRV2Tou05), rotavirus, herpes simplex virus, rubella, Coxsackie A9, measles, influenza virus and HHV-6 [169–177] (Fig. 12).

Other Neurometabolic Disorders

Biotin-Responsive Basal Ganglia Disease

Biotin-responsive basal ganglia disease (BBGD) is an autosomal recessive metabolic disorder caused by a mutation in the SLC19A3 gene which leads to a deficiency of a protein responsible for thiamin transporter [178, 179].

Clinical findings include recurrent subacute episodes of encephalopathy associated with dystonia, seizures, external ophthalmoplegia, and dysphagia, eventually leading to coma and even death [180].

This diagnosis must always be promptly considered, because it represents a treatable disorder and its outcome depends upon the quick recognition of the disease and the start of the appropriate treatment with biotin and thiamine.

BBGD can share some clinical and imaging features with mitochondrial cytopathies [181]. The presence of T2 hyperintense lesions associated with mass effect in the acute stage compromising the basal ganglia, thalamus, cortex, and cerebellum are typical findings. Cortical lesions are usually scattered in nature, both infra- and supra- tentorially [178, 182, 183].

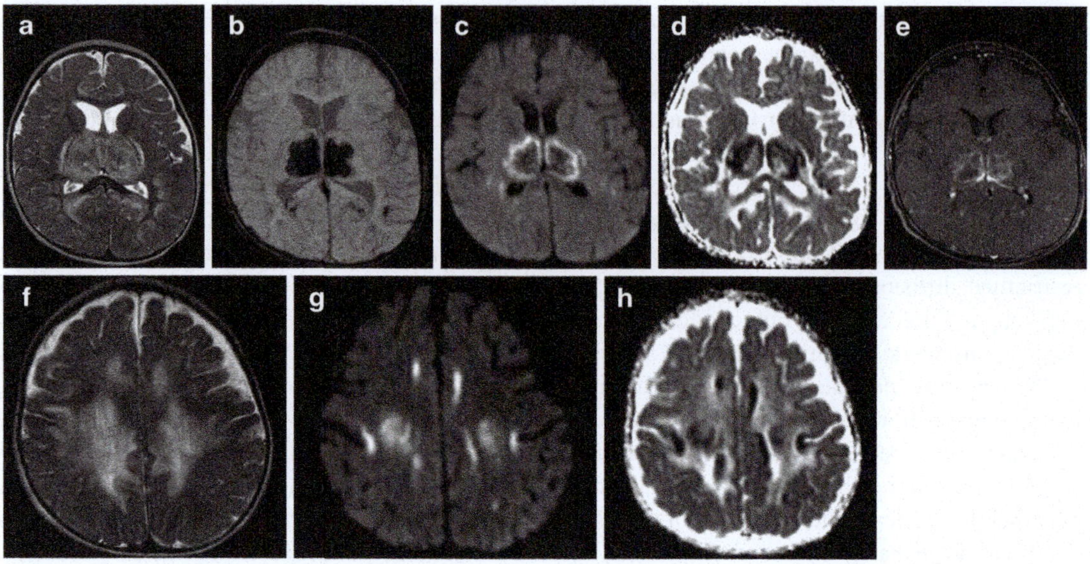

Fig. 12 A 1-year-old male with acute necrotizing encephalopathy (ANEC) and a recent history of enterovirus 71 infection. Axial T2, SWI, DWI, ADC, and enhanced T1 show symmetrical lesions in the thalami appearing hyperintense on T2 (**a**), very hypointense on SWI indicating an hemorrhagic component (**b**), and peripheral restricted diffusion confirmed on the ADC map (**c** and **d**) with heterogeneous enhancement (**e**). Axial T2, DWI, and ADC show also tumefactive hyperintense WM lesions (**f**) with restricted diffusion in the subcortical regions confirmed on the ADC map (**g**, **h**)

Ethylmalonic Encephalopathy

Ethylmalonic encephalopathy (EE) is a rare metabolic disorder, with an autosomal recessive inheritance caused by mutations in the ETHE1 gene, which codes a mitochondrial sulfur dioxygenase. EE is characterized by developmental delay, generalized microvascular damage, acrocyanosis, chronic diarrhea, and ethylmalonic, lactic, and methyl succinic aciduria. Neurologic deterioration accelerates following intercurrent infectious illness, and the majority of children die in the first decade [184]. Since there are therapeutic options for EE, differentiating between mitochondrial cytopathy and EE is important [185, 186].

Similar to mitochondrial cytopathies, in EE, brain MRI show T2 hyperintense lesions with a symmetrical pattern, involving the basal ganglia, brainstem, periventricular and subcortical WM, cerebellar WM, and dentate nuclei [187, 188]. On follow-up, brain MRI of patients with EE often show cortical atrophy and diffuse leukoencephalopathy [184, 189]. Congenital anomalies of the CNS, such as tethered cord and Chiari I malformation, have also been described in a few cases of EE [190].

References

1. Chinnery PF. Mitochondrial genetics. Br Med Bull. 2013;106:135–59.
2. Chi C-S. Diagnostic approach in infants and children with mitochondrial diseases. Pediatr Neonatol. 2015;56:7–18.
3. Gropman AL. Neuroimaging in mitochondrial disorders. Neurotherapeutics. 2012;10:273–85.
4. Saneto RP, Friedman SD, Shaw DWW. Neuroimaging of mitochondrial disease. Mitochondrion. 2008;8:396–413.
5. Kirby DM, et al. Mutations of the mitochondrial ND1 gene as a cause of MELAS. J Med Genet. 2004;41:784–9.
6. Hirano M, Pavlakis SG. Mitochondrial myopathy, encephalopathy, lactic acidosis, and strokelike episodes (MELAS): current concepts. J Child Neurol. 1994;9:4–13.

7. Robinson R. The wide phenotypic spectrum of the common MELAS-causing mutation. Neurol Today. 2007;7:26.
8. Busija DW, Katakam PV. Mitochondrial mechanisms in cerebral vascular control: shared signaling pathways with preconditioning. J Vasc Res. 2014;51:175–89.
9. Goto Y, et al. Mitochondrial myopathy, encephalopathy, lactic acidosis, and stroke-like episodes (MELAS): a correlative study of the clinical features and mitochondrial DNA mutation. Neurology. 1992;42:545–50.
10. Kim JH, et al. Diffusion and perfusion characteristics of MELAS (mitochondrial myopathy, encephalopathy, lactic acidosis, and stroke-like episode) in thirteen patients. Korean J Radiol. 2011;12:15.
11. Barkovich AJ, Good WV, Koch TK, Berg BO. Mitochondrial disorders: analysis of their clinical and imaging characteristics. AJNR Am J Neuroradiol. 1993;14:1119–37.
12. Kim IO, et al. Mitochondrial myopathy-encephalopathy-lactic acidosis-and strokelike episodes (MELAS) syndrome: CT and MR findings in seven children. Am J Roentgenol. 1996;166:641–5.
13. Hasuo K, et al. Computed tomography and angiography in MELAS (mitochondrial myopathy, encephalopathy, lactic acidosis and stroke-like episodes); report of 3 cases. Neuroradiology. 1987;29:393–7.
14. Yatsuga S, et al. MELAS: a nationwide prospective cohort study of 96 patients in Japan. Biochim Biophys Acta Gen Subj. 2012;1820:619–24.
15. Tuppen HAL, Blakely EL, Turnbull DM, Taylor RW. Mitochondrial DNA mutations and human disease. BBA-Bioenergetics. 2010;1797:113–28.
16. Newman NJ. Hereditary optic neuropathies: from the mitochondria to the optic nerve. Am J Ophthalmol. 2005;140:517.e1–9.
17. La Morgia C, Carbonelli M, Barboni P, Sadun AA, Carelli V. Medical management of hereditary optic neuropathies. Front Neurol. 2014;5:81.
18. Kirkman MA, et al. Gene–environment interactions in Leber hereditary optic neuropathy. Brain. 2009;132:2317–26.
19. Lee HK. Mitochondrial pathogenesis from genes and apoptosis to aging and disease. Overview. Ann N Y Acad Sci. 2004;1011:1–6.
20. Valentino ML, et al. Mitochondrial DNA nucleotide changes C14482G and C14482A in the ND6 gene are pathogenic for Leber's hereditary optic neuropathy. Ann Neurol. 2002;51:774–8.
21. Lamirel C, et al. Papilloedema and MRI enhancement of the prechiasmal optic nerve at the acute stage of Leber hereditary optic neuropathy. J Neurol Neurosurg Psychiatry. 2010;81:578–80.
22. Pitceathly RDS, et al. Extra-ocular muscle MRI in genetically-defined mitochondrial disease. Eur Radiol. 2015;26:130–7.
23. Lyseng-Williamson K, Idebenone A. A review in Leber's hereditary optic neuropathy. Drugs. 2016;76:805–13.
24. Barboni P, et al. Natural history of Leber's hereditary optic neuropathy: longitudinal analysis of the retinal nerve fiber layer by optical coherence tomography. Ophthalmology. 2010;117:623–7.
25. Küker W, Weir A, Quaghebeur G, Palace J. White matter changes in Leber's hereditary optic neuropathy: MRI findings. Eur J Neurol. 2007;14:591–3.
26. Parry-Jones AR, Mitchell JD, Gunarwardena WJ, Shaunak S. Leber's hereditary optic neuropathy associated with multiple sclerosis: Harding's syndrome. Pract Neurol. 2008;8:118–21.
27. Bargiela D, Chinnery PF. Mitochondria in neuroinflammation – multiple sclerosis (MS), leber hereditary optic neuropathy (LHON) and LHON-MS. Neurosci Lett. 2017. https://doi.org/10.1016/j.neulet.2017.06.051.
28. Fruhman G, et al. Atypical presentation of Leigh syndrome associated with a Leber hereditary optic neuropathy primary mitochondrial DNA mutation. Mol Genet Metab. 2011;103:153–60.
29. Blanc C, et al. MRI of the optic nerves and chiasm in patients with Leber hereditary optic neuropathy. J Neuroophthalmol. 2018;1. https://doi.org/10.1097/WNO.0000000000000621.
30. Phillips PH, Vaphiades M, Glasier CM, Gray LG, Lee AG. Chiasmal enlargement and optic nerve enhancement on magnetic resonance imaging in Leber hereditary optic neuropathy. Arch Ophthalmol. 2003;121:577–9.
31. Barcella V, et al. Evidence for retrochiasmatic tissue loss in Leber's hereditary optic neuropathy. Hum Brain Mapp. 2010;31:1900–6.
32. Rizzo G, et al. Secondary post-geniculate involvement in Leber's hereditary optic neuropathy. PLoS One. 2012;7:e50230.
33. Inglese M, et al. Magnetic resonance imaging, magnetisation transfer imaging, and diffusion weighted imaging correlates of optic nerve, brain, and cervical cord damage in Leber's hereditary optic neuropathy. J Neurol Neurosurg Psychiatry. 2001;70:444–9.
34. Zeviani M, et al. Deletions of mitochondrial DNA in Kearns-Sayre syndrome. Neurology. 1988;38:1339.
35. Kearns TP. Retinitis pigmentosa, external ophthalmoplegia, and complete heart block. AMA Arch Ophthalmol. 1958;60:280.
36. Harvey JN, Barnett D. Endocrine dysfunction in Kearns-Sayre syndrome. Clin Endocrinol. 1992;37:97–103.
37. Obara-Moszynska M, et al. A novel mitochondrial DNA deletion in a patient with Kearns-Sayre syndrome: a late-onset of the fatal cardiac conduction deficit and cardiomyopathy accompanying long-term rGH treatment. BMC Pediatr. 2013;13:117.

38. Becker LE. Lysosomes, peroxisomes and mitochondria: function and disorder. AJNR Am J Neuroradiol. 1992;13:609–20.
39. Wray SH, Provenzale JM, Johns DR, Thulborn KR. MR of the brain in mitochondrial myopathy. AJNR Am J Neuroradiol. 1995;16:1167–73.
40. Yu M, et al. Clinical and brain magnetic resonance imaging features in a cohort of Chinese patients with Kearns-Sayre syndrome. Chin Med J. 2016;129:1419–6.
41. Hourani R, Barada W, Al-Kutoubi A, Hourani M. Atypical MRI findings in Kearns-Sayre syndrome: T 2 radial stripes. Neuropediatrics. 2006;37:110–3.
42. Seijo-Martínez M, et al. L-2-hydroxyglutaric aciduria: clinical, neuroimaging, and neuropathological findings. Arch Neurol. 2005;62:666–70.
43. Horvath R. Phenotypic spectrum associated with mutations of the mitochondrial polymerase gene. Brain. 2006;129:1674–84.
44. Stumpf JD, Saneto RP, Copeland WC. Clinical and molecular features of POLG-related mitochondrial disease. Cold Spring Harb Perspect Biol. 2013;5:a011395.
45. Egger J, Harding BN, Boyd SG, Wilson J, Erdohazi M. Progressive neuronal degeneration of childhood (PNDC) with liver disease. Clin Pediatr (Phila). 2016;26:167–73.
46. Cohen BH, Naviaux RK. The clinical diagnosis of POLG disease and other mitochondrial DNA depletion disorders. Methods. 2010;51:364–73.
47. Henao AI, et al. Characteristic brain MRI findings in ataxia-neuropathy spectrum related to POLG mutation. Neuroradiol J. 2016;29:46–8.
48. Cheldi A, et al. POLG1 mutations and stroke like episodes: a distinct clinical entity rather than an atypical MELAS syndrome. BMC Neurol. 2013;13:8.
49. Wong L-JC, et al. Molecular and clinical genetics of mitochondrial diseases due to POLG mutations. Hum Mutat. 2008;29:E150–72.
50. Lara MC, Valentino ML, Torres-Torronteras J, Hirano M, Martí R. Mitochondrial neurogastrointestinal encephalomyopathy (MNGIE): biochemical features and therapeutic approaches. Biosci Rep. 2007;27:151–63.
51. Hirano M, Nishino I, Nishigaki Y, Martí R. Thymidine phosphorylase gene mutations cause mitochondrial neurogastrointestinal encephalomyopathy (MNGIE). Intern Med. 2006;45:1103.
52. Garone C, Tadesse S, Hirano M. Clinical and genetic spectrum of mitochondrial neurogastrointestinal encephalomyopathy. Brain. 2011;134:3326–32.
53. Martin MA, et al. Lack of gastrointestinal symptoms in a 60-year-old patient with MNGIE. Neurology. 2004;63:1536–7.
54. Millar WS, Lignelli A, Hirano M. MRI of five patients with mitochondrial neurogastrointestinal encephalomyopathy. Am J Roentgenol. 2004;182:1537–41.
55. Scarpelli M, et al. The role of brain MRI in mitochondrial neurogastrointestinal encephalomyopathy. Neuroradiol J. 2013;26:520–30.
56. Dallner G, Sindelar PJ. Regulation of ubiquinone metabolism. Free Radic Biol Med. 2000;29:285–94.
57. Mollet J, et al. Prenyldiphosphate synthase, subunit 1 (PDSS1) and OH-benzoate polyprenyltransferase (COQ2) mutations in ubiquinone deficiency and oxidative phosphorylation disorders. J Clin Invest. 2007;117:765–72.
58. Ogasahara S, Engel AG, Frens D, Mack D. Muscle coenzyme Q deficiency in familial mitochondrial encephalomyopathy. Proc Natl Acad Sci U S A. 1989;86:2379–82.
59. Goldstein AC, Bhatia P, Vento JM. Mitochondrial disease in childhood: nuclear encoded. Neurotherapeutics. 2013;10:212–26.
60. Musumeci O, et al. Familial cerebellar ataxia with muscle coenzyme Q10 deficiency. Neurology. 2001;56:849–55.
61. Zeviani M, Bertagnolio B, Uziel G. Neurological presentations of mitochondrial diseases. J Inherit Metab Dis. 1996;19:504–20.
62. Darin N, Oldfors A, Moslemi AR, Holme E, Tulinius M. The incidence of mitochondrial encephalomyopathies in childhood: clinical features and morphological, biochemical, and DNA abnormalities. Ann Neurol. 2001;49:377–83.
63. Lake NJ, Compton AG, Rahman S, Thorburn DR. Leigh syndrome: one disorder, more than 75 monogenic causes. Ann Neurol. 2015;79:190–203.
64. Leigh D. Subacute necrotizing encephalomyelopathy in an infant. J Neurol Neurosurg Psychiatry. 1951;14:216–21.
65. Saneto R, Ruhoy I. The genetics of Leigh syndrome and its implications for clinical practice and risk management. TACG. 2014;221. https://doi.org/10.2147/TACG.S46176.
66. Marin SE, et al. Leigh syndrome associated with mitochondrial complex I deficiency due to novel mutations In NDUFV1 and NDUFS2. Gene. 2013;516:162–7.
67. Medina L, Chi TL, DeVivo DC, Hilal SK. MR findings in patients with subacute necrotizing encephalomyelopathy (Leigh syndrome): correlation with biochemical defect. Am J Roentgenol. 1990;154:1269–74.
68. Sener RN. Diffusion magnetic resonance imaging patterns in metabolic and toxic brain disorders. Acta Radiol. 2004;45:561–70.
69. Whitehead MT, Lee B, Gropman A. Lesional perfusion abnormalities in Leigh disease demonstrated by arterial spin labeling correlate with disease activity. Pediatr Radiol. 2016;46:1309–16.
70. Arii J, Tanabe Y. Leigh syndrome: serial MR imaging and clinical follow-up. AJNR Am J Neuroradiol. 2000;21:1502–9.
71. Ng YS, et al. MT-ND5 mutation exhibits highly variable neurological manifestations at low mutant load. EBioMedicine. 2018;30:86–93.

72. Farina L, et al. MR findings in Leigh syndrome with COX deficiency and SURF-1 mutations. AJNR Am J Neuroradiol. 2002;23:1095–100.
73. Rossi A, et al. Leigh syndrome with COX deficiency and SURF1 gene mutations: MR imaging findings. AJNR Am J Neuroradiol. 2003;24:1188–91.
74. Savoiardo M, Zeviani M, Uziel G, Farina L. MRI in Leigh syndrome with SURF1 gene mutation. Ann Neurol. 2002;51:138–9.
75. Sugden MC, Holness MJ. Recent advances in mechanisms regulating glucose oxidation at the level of the pyruvate dehydrogenase complex by PDKs. Am J Physiol Endocrinol Metab. 2003;284:E855–62.
76. Harris RA, Bowker-Kinley MM, Huang B, Wu P. Regulation of the activity of the pyruvate dehydrogenase complex. Adv Enzym Regul. 2002;42:249–59.
77. Marin-Valencia I, Roe CR, Pascual JM. Pyruvate carboxylase deficiency: mechanisms, mimics and anaplerosis. Mol Genet Metab. 2010;101:9–17.
78. Brivet M. Impaired mitochondrial pyruvate importation in a patient and a fetus at risk. Mol Genet Metab. 2003;78:186–92.
79. Gray LR, Tompkins SC, Taylor EB. Regulation of pyruvate metabolism and human disease. Cell Mol Life Sci. 2013;71:2577–604.
80. Patel KP, O'Brien TW, Subramony SH, Shuster J, Stacpoole PW. The spectrum of pyruvate dehydrogenase complex deficiency: clinical, biochemical and genetic features in 371 patients. Mol Genet Metab. 2012;106:385–94.
81. Robinson BH. Cell culture studies on patients with mitochondrial diseases: molecular defects in pyruvate dehydrogenase. J Bioenerg Biomembr. 1988;20:313–23.
82. Pliss L, et al. Cerebral developmental abnormalities in a mouse with systemic pyruvate dehydrogenase deficiency. PLoS One. 2013;8:e67473.
83. Barnerias C, et al. Pyruvate dehydrogenase complex deficiency: four neurological phenotypes with differing pathogenesis. Dev Med Child Neurol. 2009;52:e1–9.
84. DeBrosse SD, et al. Spectrum of neurological and survival outcomes in pyruvate dehydrogenase complex (PDC) deficiency: lack of correlation with genotype. Mol Genet Metab. 2012;107:394–402.
85. Giribaldi G, et al. Intermittent-relapsing pyruvate dehydrogenase complex deficiency: a case with clinical, biochemical, and neuroradiological reversibility. Dev Med Child Neurol. 2012;54:472–6.
86. Pirot N, et al. Phenotypic and neuropathological characterization of fetal pyruvate dehydrogenase deficiency. J Neuropathol Exp Neurol. 2016;75:227–38.
87. Pliss L, Pentney RJ, Johnson MT, Patel MS. Biochemical and structural brain alterations in female mice with cerebral pyruvate dehydrogenase deficiency. J Neurochem. 2004;91:1082–91.
88. Soares-Fernandes JP, et al. Neonatal pyruvate dehydrogenase deficiency due to a R302H mutation in the PDHA1 gene: MRI findings. Pediatr Radiol. 2008;38:559–62.
89. Brown RM, Brown GK. Prenatal diagnosis of pyruvate dehydrogenase E1 alpha subunit deficiency. Prenat Diagn. 1994;14:435–41.
90. Shevell MI, et al. Cerebral dysgenesis and lactic acidemia: an MRI/MRS phenotype associated with pyruvate dehydrogenase deficiency. Pediatr Neurol. 1994;11:224–9.
91. Wada N, Matsuishi T, Nonaka M, Naito E, Yoshino M. Pyruvate dehydrogenase E1α subunit deficiency in a female patient: evidence of antenatal origin of brain damage and possible etiology of infantile spasms. Brain Dev. 2004;26:57–60.
92. Natarajan N, Tully HM, Chapman T. Prenatal presentation of pyruvate dehydrogenase complex deficiency. Pediatr Radiol. 2016;46:1354–7.
93. Robinson JN, et al. Prenatal diagnosis of pyruvate dehydrogenase deficiency using magnetic resonance imaging. Prenat Diagn. 2001;21:1053–6.
94. Tamaru S, et al. A case of pyruvate dehydrogenase E1α subunit deficiency with antenatal brain dysgenesis demonstrated by prenatal sonography and magnetic resonance imaging. J Clin Ultrasound. 2012;40:234–8.
95. Sharma R, Sharrard MJ, Connolly DJ, Mordekar SR. Unilateral periventricular leukomalacia in association with pyruvate dehydrogenase deficiency. Dev Med Child Neurol. 2012;54:469–71.
96. Michotte A, et al. Neuropathological findings of a patient with pyruvate dehydrogenase E1 alpha deficiency presenting as a cerebral lactic acidosis. Acta Neuropathol. 1993;85:674–8.
97. Head RA, et al. Clinical and genetic spectrum of pyruvate dehydrogenase deficiency: dihydrolipoamide acetyltransferase (E2) deficiency. Ann Neurol. 2005;58:234–41.
98. Mellick G, Price L, Boyle R. Late-onset presentation of pyruvate dehydrogenase deficiency. Mov Disord. 2004;19:727–9.
99. Brown GK, Otero LJ, LeGris M, Brown RM. Pyruvate dehydrogenase deficiency. J Med Genet. 1994;31:875–9.
100. Harada M, et al. Therapeutic efficacy of a case of pyruvate dehydrogenase complex deficiency monitored by localized proton magnetic resonance spectroscopy. Magn Reson Imaging. 1996;14:129–33.
101. Ah Mew N, et al. MRI features of 4 female patients with pyruvate dehydrogenase E1 alpha deficiency. Pediatr Neurol. 2011;45:57–9.
102. Zand DJ, et al. In vivo pyruvate detected by MR spectroscopy in neonatal pyruvate dehydrogenase deficiency. AJNR Am J Neuroradiol. 2003;24:1471–4.
103. García-Cazorla A, et al. Pyruvate carboxylase deficiency: metabolic characteristics and new neurological aspects. Ann Neurol. 2005;59:121–7.
104. Ortez C, et al. Infantile parkinsonism and gabaergic hypotransmission in a patient with pyruvate carboxylase deficiency. Gene. 2013;532:302–6.
105. Arnold GL, Griebel ML, Porterfield M, Brewster M. Pyruvate carboxylase deficiency. Report of a case

and additional evidence for the 'mild' phenotype. Clin Pediatr (Phila). 2001;40:519–21.

106. Brun N, et al. Pyruvate carboxylase deficiency: prenatal onset of ischemia-like brain lesions in two sibs with the acute neonatal form. Am J Med Genet. 1999;84:94–101.
107. Higgins JJ, Glasgow AM, Lusk M, Kerr DS. MRI, clinical, and biochemical features of partial pyruvate carboxylase deficiency. J Child Neurol. 1994;9:436–9.
108. Schiff M, et al. A case of pyruvate carboxylase deficiency with atypical clinical and neuroradiological presentation. Mol Genet Metab. 2006;87:175–7.
109. Antonellis A, Green ED. The role of aminoacyl-tRNA synthetases in genetic diseases. Annu Rev Genomics Hum Genet. 2008;9:87–107.
110. Steenweg ME, et al. Leukoencephalopathy with thalamus and brainstem involvement and high lactate 'LTBL' caused by EARS2 mutations. Brain. 2012;135:1387–94.
111. Kevelam SH, et al. Absent thalami caused by a homozygous EARS2 mutation: expanding disease spectrum of LTBL. Neuropediatrics. 2016;47:64–7.
112. Şahin S, et al. Leukoencephalopathy with thalamus and brainstem involvement and high lactate caused by novel mutations in the EARS2 gene in two siblings. J Neurol Sci. 2016;365:54–8.
113. Steenweg ME, et al. Novel hypomyelinating leukoencephalopathy affecting early myelinating structures. Arch Neurol. 2012;69:125–8.
114. van Berge L, et al. Leukoencephalopathy with brainstem and spinal cord involvement and lactate elevation: clinical and genetic characterization and target for therapy. Brain. 2014;137:1019–29.
115. van der Knaap MS, et al. A new leukoencephalopathy with brainstem and spinal cord involvement and high lactate. Ann Neurol. 2002;53:252–8.
116. Steenweg M, et al. Early-onset LBSL: how severe does it get? Neuropediatrics. 2012;43:332–8.
117. Steenweg ME, et al. Leucoencephalopathy with brainstem and spinal cord involvement and high lactate: quantitative magnetic resonance imaging. Brain. 2011;134:3333–41.
118. Dallabona C, et al. Novel (ovario) leukodystrophy related to AARS2 mutations. Neurology. 2014;82:2063–71.
119. Götz A, et al. Exome sequencing identifies mitochondrial Alanyl-tRNA synthetase mutations in infantile mitochondrial cardiomyopathy. Am J Hum Genet. 2011;88:635–42.
120. Kamps R, et al. Genetic defects in mtDNA-encoded protein translation cause pediatric, mitochondrial cardiomyopathy with early-onset brain disease. Eur J Hum Genet. 2018;108:206.
121. Szpisjak L, et al. Novel AARS2 gene mutation producing leukodystrophy: a case report. J Hum Genet. 2016;62:329–33.
122. Lakshmanan R, et al. Redefining the phenotype of ALSP and AARS2 mutation-related leukodystrophy. Neurol Genet. 2017;3:e135.
123. Edvardson S, et al. Deleterious mutation in the mitochondrial arginyl–transfer RNA synthetase gene is associated with pontocerebellar hypoplasia. Am J Hum Genet. 2007;81:857–62.
124. Namavar Y, et al. Clinical, neuroradiological and genetic findings in pontocerebellar hypoplasia. Brain. 2010;134:143–56.
125. Rankin J, et al. Pontocerebellar hypoplasia type 6: a British case with PEHO-like features. Am J Med Genet. 2010;152A:2079–84.
126. Cassandrini D, et al. Pontocerebellar hypoplasia type 6 caused by mutations in RARS2: definition of the clinical spectrum and molecular findings in five patients. J Inherit Metab Dis. 2012;36:43–53.
127. Nishri D, et al. RARS2 mutations cause early onset epileptic encephalopathy without ponto-cerebellar hypoplasia. Eur J Paediatr Neurol. 2016;20: 412–7.
128. Kastrissianakis K, et al. Subdural effusions and lack of early pontocerebellar hypoplasia in siblings with RARS2 mutations. Arch Dis Child. 2013;98:1004–7.
129. Joseph JT, et al. Neuropathologic features of pontocerebellar hypoplasia type 6. J Neuropathol Exp Neurol. 2014;73:1009–25.
130. van Dijk T, et al. JIMD reports, volume 33, vol. 33. Heidelberg: Springer; 2016. p. 87–92.
131. Hatefi Y. The mitochondrial electron transport and oxidative phosphorylation system. Annu Rev Biochem. 1985;54:1015–69.
132. CHANCE B, WILLIAMS GR. Respiratory enzymes in oxidative phosphorylation. I. Kinetics of oxygen utilization. J Biol Chem. 1955;217:383–93.
133. de Beaurepaire I, et al. High predictive value of brain MRI imaging in primary mitochondrial respiratory chain deficiency. J Med Genet. 2018;1807:378–83.
134. Loeffen JLCM, et al. Isolated complex I deficiency in children: clinical, biochemical and genetic aspects. Hum Mutat. 2000;15:123–34.
135. Lebre AS, et al. A common pattern of brain MRI imaging in mitochondrial diseases with complex I deficiency. J Med Genet. 2010;48:16–23.
136. Bricout M, et al. Brain imaging in mitochondrial respiratory chain deficiency: combination of brain MRI features as a useful tool for genotype/phenotype correlations. J Med Genet. 2014;51:429–35.
137. Kevelam SH, et al. NUBPL mutations in patients with complex I deficiency and a distinct MRI pattern. Neurology. 2013;80:1577–83.
138. Hoekstra AS, Bayley J-P. The role of complex II in disease. Biochim Biophys Acta. 2013;1827:543–51.
139. Helman G, et al. Magnetic resonance imaging spectrum of succinate dehydrogenase–related infantile leukoencephalopathy. Ann Neurol. 2016;79:379–86.
140. Grønborg S, et al. JIMD reports, volume 19, vol. 33. Heidelberg: Springer; 2016. p. 69–77.
141. Bénit P, Lebon S, Rustin P. Respiratory-chain diseases related to complex III deficiency. Biochim Biophys Acta. 2009;1793:181–5.

142. Jackson CB, et al. A novel mutation in BCS1L associated with deafness, tubulopathy, growth retardation and microcephaly. Eur J Pediatr. 2016;175:517–25.
143. Jiang J, Wang XL, Ma YY. Respiratory chain complex III deficiency in patients with tRNA-leu mutation. Genet Mol Res. 2015;14:18629–36.
144. Visapää I, et al. GRACILE syndrome, a lethal metabolic disorder with iron overload, is caused by a point mutation in BCS1L. Am J Hum Genet. 2002;71:863–76.
145. Barel O, et al. Mitochondrial complex III deficiency associated with a homozygous mutation in UQCRQ. Am J Hum Genet. 2008;82:1211–6.
146. Blázquez A, et al. Infantile mitochondrial encephalomyopathy with unusual phenotype caused by a novel BCS1L mutation in an isolated complex III-deficient patient. Neuromuscul Disord. 2009;19:143–6.
147. Sinkler CA, et al. Tissue- and condition-specific isoforms of mammalian cytochrome c oxidase subunits: from function to human disease. Oxidative Med Cell Longev. 2017;2017:1–19.
148. Wedatilake Y, et al. SURF1 deficiency: a multi-centre natural history study. Orphanet J Rare Dis. 2013;8:96.
149. Jonckheere AI, et al. Restoration of complex V deficiency caused by a novel deletion in the human TMEM70 gene normalizes mitochondrial morphology. Mitochondrion. 2011;11:954–63.
150. Diodato D, et al. JIMD reports, volume 19. Heidelberg: Springer; 2014. https://doi.org/10.1007/8904_2014_300.
151. De Meirleir L, et al. Respiratory chain complex V deficiency due to a mutation in the assembly gene ATP12. J Med Genet. 2004;41:120–4.
152. Ramenghi LA, Fumagalli M, Supramaniam V. Neonatology. Milano: Springer; 2012. p. 1067–78.
153. Huang BY, Castillo M. Hypoxic-ischemic brain injury: imaging findings from birth to adulthood. Radiographics. 2008;28:417–39.
154. Sannia A, et al. Different gestational ages and changing vulnerability of the premature brain. J Matern Fetal Neonatal Med. 2015;28:2268–72.
155. Steggerda SJ, et al. Cerebellar injury in preterm infants: incidence and findings on US and MR images. Radiology. 2009;252:190–9.
156. Volpe JJ. Cerebellum of the premature infant: rapidly developing, vulnerable, clinically important. J Child Neurol. 2009;24:1085–104.
157. Inder TE, Anderson NJ, Spencer C, Wells S, Volpe JJ. White matter injury in the premature infant: a comparison between serial cranial sonographic and MR findings at term. AJNR Am J Neuroradiol. 2003;24:805–9.
158. Martinez-Biarge M, et al. MRI based preterm white matter injury classification: the importance of sequential imaging in determining severity of injury. PLoS One. 2016;11:e0156245.
159. Robertson RL, et al. MR line-scan diffusion-weighted imaging of term neonates with perinatal brain ischemia. AJNR Am J Neuroradiol. 1999;20:1658–70.
160. Barkovich AJ, Westmark K, Partridge C, Sola A, Ferriero DM. Perinatal asphyxia: MR findings in the first 10 days. AJNR Am J Neuroradiol. 1995;16:427–38.
161. Gire C, et al. Clinical features and neuroradiological findings of mitochondrial pathology in six neonates. Childs Nerv Syst. 2002;18:621–8.
162. Henao AI, et al. Characteristic brain MRI findings in ataxia-neuropathy spectrum related to POLG mutation. Neuroradiol J. 2015;29:46–8.
163. Luethy LN, Pfeiffer JK. Viral infection brings mitochondrial traffic to a standstill. Cell Host Microbe. 2012;11:420–1.
164. Beattie GC, et al. Encephalitis with thalamic and basal ganglia abnormalities: etiologies, neuroimaging, and potential role of respiratory viruses. Clin Infect Dis. 2013;56:825–32.
165. Zuccoli G, Yannes MP, Nardone R, Bailey A, Goldstein A. Bilateral symmetrical basal ganglia and thalamic lesions in children: an update (2015). Neuroradiology. 2015;57:973–89.
166. El Hafidi N, Allouch B, Benbrahim F, Chellaoui M, El Mahraoui C. Encéphalite aiguë des noyaux gris centraux à Mycoplasma pneumoniae. Rev Neurol (Paris). 2012;168:49–52.
167. Chen F, Li J, Liu T, Wang L, Li Y. MRI characteristics of brainstem encephalitis in hand-foot-mouth disease induced by enterovirus type 71 – will different MRI manifestations be helpful for prognosis. Eur J Paediatr Neurol. 2013;17:486–91.
168. Maloney JA, et al. MRI findings in children with acute flaccid paralysis and cranial nerve dysfunction occurring during the 2014 enterovirus D68 outbreak. AJNR Am J Neuroradiol. 2015;36:245–50.
169. Okumura A, Abe S, Kidokoro H, Mizuguchi M. Acute necrotizing encephalopathy: a comparison between influenza and non-influenza cases. Microbiol Immunol. 2009;53:277–80.
170. Yadav S, Das CJ, Kumar V, Lodha R. Acute necrotizing encephalopathy. Indian J Pediatr. 2009;77:307–9.
171. Wang HS, Huang SC. Acute necrotizing encephalopathy of childhood. Chang Gung Med J. 2001;24:1–10.
172. Bassuk AG, Burrowes DM, McRae W. Acute necrotizing encephalopathy of childhood with radiographic progression over 10 hours. Neurology. 2003;60:1552–3.
173. Ouattara LA, et al. Novel human reovirus isolated from children with acute necrotizing encephalopathy. Emerg Infect Dis. 2011;17:1436–44.
174. Seo H-E, et al. Clinical spectrum and prognostic factors of acute necrotizing encephalopathy in children. J Korean Med Sci. 2010;25:449.
175. Kim Y-N, You SJ. A case of acute necrotizing encephalopathy associated with parainfluenza virus infection. Korean J Pediatr. 2012;55:147.
176. Martin A, Reade EP. Acute necrotizing encephalopathy progressing to brain death in a pediatric patient with novel influenza A (H1N1) infection. Clin Infect Dis. 2010;50:e50–2.
177. Kubo T, et al. A case of HHV-6 associated acute necrotizing encephalopathy with increase

of CD56bright NKcells. Scand J Infect Dis. 2009;38:1122–5.

178. Ozand PT, et al. Biotin-responsive basal ganglia disease: a novel entity. Brain. 1998;121(Pt 7):1267–79.
179. Zeng W-Q, et al. Biotin-responsive basal ganglia disease maps to 2q36.3 and is due to mutations in SLC19A3. Am J Hum Genet. 2005;77:16–26.
180. Tabarki B, et al. Biotin-responsive basal ganglia disease revisited: clinical, radiologic, and genetic findings. Neurology. 2013;80:261–7.
181. Distelmaier F, et al. JIMD reports, volume 19, vol. 13. Heidelberg: Springer; 2013. p. 53–7.
182. Yamada K, et al. A wide spectrum of clinical and brain MRI findings in patients with SLC19A3 mutations. BMC Med Genet. 2010;11:171.
183. Kassem H, Wafaie A, Alsuhibani S, Farid T. Biotin-responsive basal ganglia disease: neuroimaging features before and after treatment. AJNR Am J Neuroradiol. 2014;35:1990–5.
184. Grosso S, et al. Ethylmalonic encephalopathy. J Neurol. 2002;249:1446–50.
185. Dionisi-Vici C, et al. Liver transplant in ethylmalonic encephalopathy: a new treatment for an otherwise fatal disease. Brain. 2016;139:1045–51.
186. Boyer M, et al. Response to medical and a novel dietary treatment in newborn screen identified patients with ethylmalonic encephalopathy. Mol Genet Metab. 2018;124:57–63.
187. Pigeon N, Campeau PM, Cyr D, Lemieux B, Clarke JTR. Clinical heterogeneity in ethylmalonic encephalopathy. J Child Neurol. 2009;24:991–6.
188. Cavusoglu D, et al. An unusual cause of cavitating leukoencephalopathy: ethylmalonic encephalopathy. Acta Neurol Belg. 2018;118:309–12.
189. Heberle LC, Al Tawari AA, Ramadan DG, Ibrahim JK. Ethylmalonic encephalopathy—report of two cases. Brain Dev. 2006;28:329–31.
190. Nowaczyk MJ, Blaser SI, Clarke JT. Central nervous system malformations in ethylmalonic encephalopathy. Am J Med Genet. 1998;75:292–6.

Outcome Measures and Quality of Life in Mitochondrial Diseases

S. Koene, C. Jimenez-Moreno, and G. S. Gorman

Introduction

Mitochondrial diseases are an important group of inherited neurometabolic disorders that invariably exhibit multi-organ involvement and are relentlessly progressive, resulting in significant morbidity and mortality. While pharmacological agents are emerging for mitochondrial disease, there is a paucity of effective therapies [1, 2]. Hence there is a significant, unmet clinical need for the development of new therapeutic strategies. To be specific and sensitive enough to detect the effectiveness of new therapies, well-designed clinical studies need to be executed. Previously, a Cochrane review on treatment studies in patients with mitochondrial disease stated that the quality of many of the previously performed studies is low [3]. One of the main problems arising in these low-quality studies includes the heterogeneity of the, often small-numbered, study population and the lack of sufficiently sensitive patient-centred outcome measures and endpoints.

Recently, significant efforts have been made to identify appropriate instruments to measure clinically relevant aspects of health and quality of life in children and adults with mitochondrial disease [4, 5]. These instruments are commonly referred to as outcome measures, and while there is not yet an 'ideal' outcome measure or set of outcome measures to assess all patients with mitochondrial disease, there are certainly instruments currently available that are relevant and with proven psychometric properties applicable within the population. However, further research in the field is needed to improve their use.

In this chapter, you will find a description of some of the most frequently used outcome measures in mitochondrial diseases and provide guidance on choosing robust and clinically meaningful outcomes. Stakeholders interested in assessing this population of patients must be confident that the measure used is adequate enough to measure the intended outcome and in their interpretability. But perhaps most importantly, it considers the phenotypic heterogeneity of mitochondrial disease when selecting an outcome and defining the endpoint for a clinical trial, since the results of validation studies may not be generalizable to all (if any) forms of mitochondrial disease.

Outcome Measures in Mitochondrial Disease

In medical terms, outcome measures are defined as instruments providing information about cer-

S. Koene
Radboud Center for Mitochondrial Medicine, Nijmegen, The Netherlands

C. Jimenez-Moreno · G. S. Gorman (✉)
Wellcome Centre for Mitochondrial Research, Institute of Neuroscience, Newcastle University, Newcastle Upon Tyne, UK
e-mail: Grainne.Gorman@newcastle.ac.uk

M. Mancuso, T. Klopstock (eds.), *Diagnosis and Management of Mitochondrial Disorders*,
https://doi.org/10.1007/978-3-030-05517-2_19

tain disease aspects, such as disease severity, response to therapy or remission of the disease [6]. Outcome measures help define endpoints (i.e. objectively measured events in time to determine whether an intervention is effective or safe). However, if these outcome measures have been poorly validated in the disease in question, the established endpoint may be unrealistic or simply not adequate (or feasible) to measure the desired outcome. The FDA defines clinically meaningful endpoints as those that directly measure how a patient feels, functions or survives [7]. It is said that 'Clinical trials are only as credible as their endpoints' [8], as only endpoints assessed with valid instruments (i.e. outcomes) provide meaningful data. Hence, the selection of a robust instrument for the targeted population can only lead to the enhanced quality of trials. We will elaborate on the strategy and efforts invested to date to identify outcomes appropriate for clinical trials in patients with mitochondrial disease but also those deemed relevant for the patients.

Appropriately designing a clinical study to prove treatments are efficacious in patients, and especially children, with mitochondrial disorders is challenging for many reasons (Table 1). Mitochondrial disorders are rare, heterogeneous diseases involving multiple organs, and the clinical disease course is unpredictable, variable and often oscillating. Although the variability in affected organs and degree of disability may warrant grouping of patients into homogeneous clinical cohorts, both the external validation of the results of the trial and the potential to detect clinical benefit for a small group of patients with specific biochemical or genetic abnormalities are hampered when setting very strict inclusion criteria. Lastly, the unpredictable disease course requires such large cohorts that patient recruitment will be impossible despite the participation of multiple centres. However, the emergence of adaptive trial design may help mitigate some of these difficulties in conducting reliable and valid trials in such patient groups exhibiting marked genotypic and phenotypic heterogeneity, in addition to low patient numbers. Pre-specification of the adaptation schedule and processes relating to modification of sample size, based on data analysis of the primary outcome, can serve to improve efficiency, increase the likelihood of success and improve understanding of the therapeutic effects of the therapy or molecule under interrogation.

Table 1 Hurdles in proving treatment effects in patients with mitochondrial disease

Rare disorders
Clinically, biochemically and genetically heterogeneous disorders
Clinical heterogeneity within one genetic entity, both in mitochondrial DNA and nuclear DNA mutations
Unpredictable, variable and sometimes oscillating natural disease course
Multi-system disease with variable involvement of organs
Patients may be very disabled and unable to perform functional tests
Abilities of patients vary widely

Selection of Outcome Measures

According to the World Health Organization (WHO), health is a multidimensional construct: 'a state of complete physical, mental and social well-being and not merely the absence of disease or infirmity'. Forty-six years after the rather non-specific but holistic definition of health, the WHO developed a framework for thinking about health in chronic conditions, taking into account the bio psychosocial aspect of human functioning [9]. This framework, the International Classification of Functioning, Disability and Health (ICF, Fig. 1), comprises four dimensions: (1) body functions, (2) body structure, (3) activities and participation, and (4) environmental factors. These dimensions clarify and expand on the different disease parameters that can potentially be measured, either as part of a combined assessment or by themselves.

In the ICF model, the severity of the experienced disability is seen as a dynamic and interactive process among the interconnected components of functioning [10]. For example, an increase in muscle strength may not necessarily correlate with an improvement in daily functioning [11] and may be irrelevant to a patient not able to adequately coordinate movements.

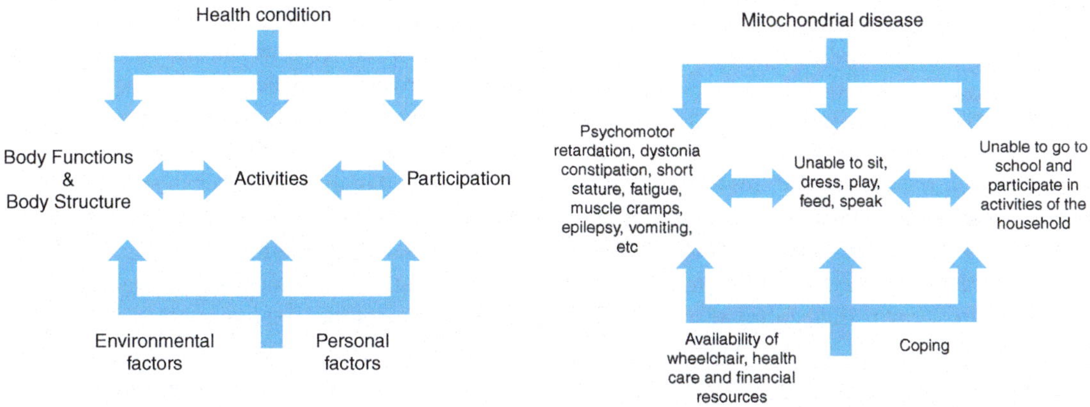

Fig. 1 The International Classification of Functioning, Disability and Health (ICF) framework. The structure of the ICF (left) filled out as an example for the symptoms, limitations and disabilities that can be observed in patients with mitochondrial disease (right). Note the interplay between the health condition on physical function, activity and participation on one side and the influence of environmental and personal factors on the other

Surely, any improvement in health and disability after the intended treatment should be experienced by and relevant to the patient. This is endorsed by regulatory authorities such as the US Food and Drug Administration (FDA) and the European Medicines Agency (EMA), preferring the inclusion of clinically meaningful outcomes in clinical trials. To systematically identify the chief complaints and limitations relevant to all, or at least a large majority of patients with mitochondrial disease, the framework provided by the ICF may be of major assistance and has already been adapted by other forms of neuromuscular disease [12].

The selection of appropriate outcome measures for a clinical trial starts with detailed knowledge of the clinical spectrum of phenotype(s) to be included in the study. This inventory should preferably follow the framework of the ICF, in which not only medical complaints but also the activities and social participation in which the patient is facing limitations are included. When the relevant aspects of the disease are known, instruments measuring functional and structural consequences of it can be identified. These instruments should be indicative of the parameter of disease severity aimed to be measured (i.e. validity) and should detect change with any disease progression or regression (i.e. responsiveness) to be applicable as an outcome measure in clinical trials [13]. Additionally, in the case of mitochondrial diseases, the level of reliability (i.e. the degree to which the measurement is free from measurement error) should be as high as possible to allow for small sample sizes and heterogeneous phenotypes.

The selected outcome measure should correspond closely to the parameter of the health condition to be measured. The selection of an outcome measure to define the (primary) endpoint depends on many factors including the research goal, the type of intervention and the inclusion criteria (including age and mental capacities and functional abilities of the intended patient group) [14]. While early proof-of-principle studies would prefer to study a more narrowly defined population using highly detailed endpoints, larger trials require a larger population and thus more generally applicable outcome measures as not to render recruitment a challenge [15]. Still, neither of these should negatively impact on validity and should present evidence relevant and specific for this population. Unfortunately, the outcome measures that have been used to date in clinical trials of patients with mitochondrial disease have rarely been disease-specific and validated and do not always measure symptoms and complaints experienced by or relevant to the patient.

Outcome Measures in Mitochondrial Diseases

In blockbuster disease clinical trials, in, for example, cardiovascular diseases or cancer, time-to-event (i.e. relapse, stroke, myocardial infarction or death), histological results or radiological results are often used as endpoints [16–18]. Since at this time no markers for mitochondrial dysfunction are known that correlate with disease progression nor applicable to the whole population [19–23], identifying quantifiable tools that can support the definition of disease-specific endpoints is essential to move forward into clinical trials.

However, mitochondrial diseases face specific difficulties as any other rare disease when it comes to the selection of outcome measures [24]. Since the number of patients to be included in a clinical trial (sample size) depends on the expected effect of the intervention, there needs to be either a large treatment effect to be easily detected or a very precise (i.e. sensitive) outcome measure that will identify minimal differences, if any, even in a small number of patients. Given therapies are currently expected to slow disease progression rather than reverse morbidity by targeting the underlying biochemical defect [25, 26], there is a huge challenge to identify instruments able to reliably quantify more subtle changes in, for example, strength, gait and endurance.

When including a clinically heterogeneous group of mitochondrial diseases in a clinical trial, a non-categorical approach, like addressing limitations in daily functioning seen as common manifestations of impaired health rather than specific to particular aetiologies, maybe more suitable. Such a 'one-size-fits-all' approach increases the number of patients for which the instrument is relevant [11]. On the other hand, when assessing a more homogeneous cohort, more disease-specific instruments can be used. An example of a clinically homogeneous mitochondrial disorder is Leber's hereditary optic neuropathy (LHON), a disease largely limited to a single organ, the eye. In a randomised, placebo-controlled trial of idebenone, a collaboration of several mitochondrial expert centres in which a symptom-specific secondary outcome (i.e. visual acuity; discordant vision) allowed the detection of effectiveness of the treatment to allow its subsequent prescription by specialists in LHON [27]. However, in order to detect subtle but meaningful changes in heterogeneous populations with a more generic instrument, either large numbers of participants or disease-specific outcomes responsive for all the different phenotypes are required.

For the purposes of this chapter, we present a series of examples classified according to the Food and Drug Administration (FDA)'s clinical outcome assessments (COA) classification. The COA classification is part of the Drug Development Tool Qualification Program, a guidance for FDA submitters towards the inclusion of well-defined, specific and reliable outcomes. Including COA in a clinical trial design allows not only the assessment of a treatment's effectiveness but also to define its safeness. There are four types of COA, all referring to measures of the effects of a disease or condition on how the patient functions or feels. All these COA may be influenced by human choices, judgement or motivation. Other surrogate measures reflecting more biological processes often referred to as biomarkers are considered independently.

Clinician-Observed Outcomes

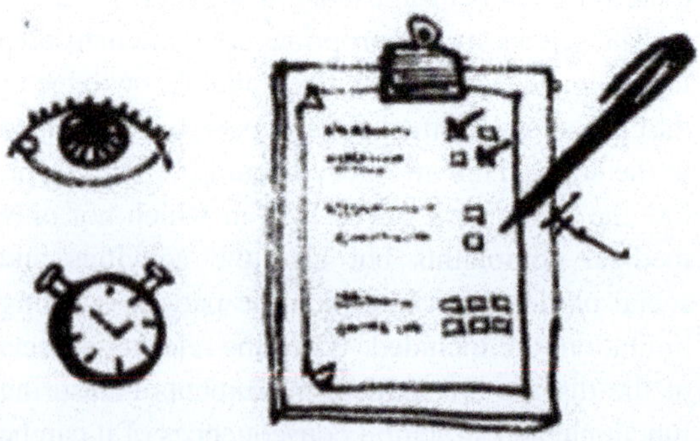

These outcomes are based on reports from a trained health-care professional and their interpretation of a patient's health condition or status. Clinician-observed examples suitable for mitochondrial diseases include:

(a) Sections II and III of the Newcastle Mitochondrial Disease Scale for Adults (NMDAS [28]), a semi-quantitative rating scale specifically developed for mitochondrial disorders and that allows a longitudinal follow-up of patients with mitochondrial disease. This scale comes with an assessment manual to improve inter-rater reliability. This scale includes two sections that are not clinician-observed based but are scored according to the patient's judgement of their health status (section I) and quality of life (section IV). Notably, section I may reflect the clinician's perspective as this section is completed following an interview with the patient or the caregiver and a score is assigned by the assessor based on their responses to each enquiry. There is the parallel version of this scale specific for the paediatric population with different forms for each age range group (the Newcastle Paediatric Mitochondrial Disease Scale; NPMDS [29]). This has recently been translated and validated for use in Brazil [30]. It was first used in a clinical trial testing a variant of CoEnzyme Q10 (EPI-743, also known as Vincerinone). This study showed minimal differences for sections I to III of the NPMDS but improvement in section IV (quality of life) in 10 out of the 12 patients completing the study [31]. A lack of change in the clinician-observed outcomes of these scales, may not necessarily relate to a lack of treatment efficacy. These data may be difficult to interpret due to the phenotype and genotype heterogeneity of the sample or due to the broadness of the questionnaire and the innate properties of the scales to assess parameters over a more protracted timeframe. As these scales assess a variety of parameters that may be affected by the disease but not specifically those that may benefit from the treatment, the specific points responding to the treatment may be hidden among the rest. This example highlights the importance of selecting an outcome measure not only valid for the target disease but also specific for the outcome expected to respond to the intervention. However, this is not as easy as it sounds as with new treatment options offering solutions at early stages in the pathophysiological chain, it is difficult to predict where the real impact will be realised.

(b) The International Paediatric Mitochondrial Disease Scale (IPMDS [32]) is an evolution of the NPMDS and the Paediatric Evaluation of Disability Inventory (PEDI). It has been devised by the implementation of a Delphi-based process including patients, parents and mitochondrial disease experts in the decision-making, making it suitable for international use. Section II of IPMDS corresponds to the physical examination assessing factors like growth, visual performance and muscle tone, among others. As the NMDAS, this is a global scale and its interpretation carries a note of caution, as within the same patient it may be reliable to assess overall disease progression but any changes as a global scale may not translate with the same significance from patient to patient.

(c) A physician/investigator's global assessment (PGA) is usually a 5- or 6-point Likert scoring system or a 10-cm visual analogue scale used broadly to assess disease severity or disease activity. This tool has not been developed specifically for mitochondrial disease, and there is not yet a standardised version for it. However, it is a scale that allows symptom specificity, and it has been used in other disease states such as arthritis and cerebral palsy to support FDA approval. Overall severity can also be rated on a seven-point scale in the Clinical Global Impression of Improvement or Severity of Illness (CGI-I and CGI-S [33]). These scales provide an overall clinician-determined overview of disease severity and change (if any) from the initiation of any treatment. Both are self-explanatory and quick to complete. Although the original version of this scale was developed for psychiatric disorders, its rationale has been implemented in other diseases as it allows to address independently any changes on the disease per se or a symptom in specific from the overall disease status; ideally, improvements in one scale should follow the other. However, this is based purely on the physician's judgement and may not translate to what the patient or caregiver may perceive. The choice of either the PGA or the CGI scales is dependent on the rated symptom, patient characteristics and the aimed precision of the measurement (continuous versus dichotomous).

Patient-Reported Outcomes

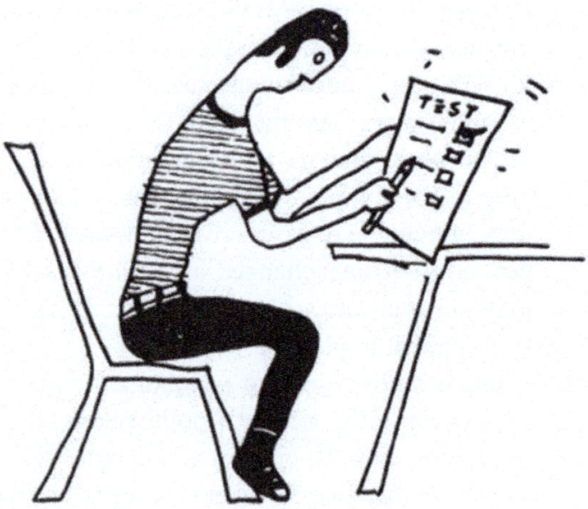

These measures are derived from the patient's self-reports about their health condition or its impact on daily life performance and satisfaction. This should *not* incorporate clinicians nor anyone else's point of view, except that of the patient. Both the FDA and the World Health Organization (WHO) support the inclusion of patient-reported outcomes to describe the patient's perspective on the effectiveness of the drug [7, 34].

Health-Related Quality of Life

Advances in drug development have led to an increased understanding and appreciation from stakeholders (including researchers and regulatory agencies) of the importance of quality of life as a dimension to be measured in clinical trials. Indeed, it is important to better consider patient perceptions when selecting outcome measures and those patient-centred outcomes that best reflect quality-of-life status.

Health-related quality of life (HRQOL), either generic or disease-specific [35], is the most frequently used patient-reported outcome measure. HRQOL is known to be only weakly to moderately correlated to physiological and functional parameters [36–38], suggesting both that HRQOL instruments provide a unique perspective on the outcome of treatment and that universally applicable QOL questionnaires are influenced by other factors than simply disease severity alone. Although measuring HRQOL may appear more like an art than a science compared to more robust parameters such as measuring blood pressure, it is interesting to note that most HRQOL questionnaires show better precision than diastolic blood pressure measurement [39]. Patient-reported outcomes specifically developed for mitochondrial patients are IPMDS (section I), section IV of NMDAS which corresponds to an age-specific quality-of-life questionnaire and the Newcastle Mitochondrial Quality of life measure (NMQ) [40]. This latter can be considered a disease-specific patient-centred HRQOL tool, but its applicability in clinical trials has yet to be investigated.

However, HRQOL is not the only relevant patient-reported outcome. There is an extensive list of symptoms that can be assessed in this way including pain (numerical pain rating scale or visual analogue scale, VAS), mood (such as Hospital Anxiety and Depression Scale [41], Beck Depression Inventory [42, 43]) and perceived fatigue or physical exertion (such as Fatigue Impact Scale, FIS [44]; Fatigue Severity Scale, FSS [45]; Checklist Individual Strength, CIS [46]; and the Borg Rating of Perceived Exertion Scale [47]). A recent phase 2 cross-over study with KH176 in patients with mitochondrial disease was able to detect statistically significant differences in questionnaires measuring mood on treatment versus placebo [48]. This suggests that these questionnaires, although not specific for mitochondrial disease, maybe sensitive to small changes in patient-experienced health.

Other outcome measures allow a picture of patients' perceived performance in daily life activities and their level of social participation and identify barriers probably underestimated by standard clinical assessments. Two examples possibly relevant for this population would include (1) the international physical activity questionnaire (IPAQ [49]), assessing type, frequency and intensity of the respondent's physical activity, and (2) the Patient-Reported Outcomes Measurement Information System (PROMIS [50]) social function measures that assess participation in social roles and level of satisfaction.

Of course, the main questions for subjects included in a clinical trial are 'In your opinion, does your treatment (or placebo) work? And how do you feel different?' Although very easily asked, these questions are rarely included in a clinical trial due to the criticisms of quantifying qualitative data. However, this information may prove invaluable to inform future trial design and execution and are currently under further evaluation.

Observer-Reported Outcomes

Observer-reported outcomes are based on the observation and reports about the patient's health from someone other than the patient and health professional (e.g. caregivers, parents) [51]. These type of outcomes may not be as commonly used as the two outlined above; however, in clinical trials where the final care decision relies on a third person (e.g. in the cases of children, adults who lack cognitive capacity, emergency/life-death scenarios), the voice of the 'observers' may be as relevant and valid as the clinicians or even the patient, depending on the specific circumstances. In patients with cognitive or functional impairment that rely highly on caregivers for daily living activities, observer-reported outcomes may provide secondary endpoints of significance and the opportunity to assess treatment effects otherwise possibly undetermined. An example here would be Leigh syndrome: a population with a disease status that can vary from day to day and in which patients are commonly unable to communicate their symptoms to the health-care practitioners, either because of impaired communication skills or young age. These type of outcomes can also be useful in these type of diseases in which cooperation to perform functional tests may vary significantly from visit to visit.

An observer-reported outcome can be an ideal secondary outcome for a clinical trial, and it could fill the unmet need for at-home disease status reporting. The ideal observer-reported outcome must be able to be reliably detected by a sense or senses of the 'observer' (i.e. see, heard, smelled or touch) and either quantified or categorised [52]. Section I of the IPMDS and the initial four questions of this scale regarding the disease status and happiness levels over the previous 2 days, and the parent-reported quality-of-life questionnaire (section IV of the NPMDS), are good examples of observer-reported outcomes suitable for paediatric mitochondrial patients. However, we should also consider these type of outcomes when assessing adults also, as these may be a relevant source of data in trials assessing daily life physical activity or behaviours.

Performance Outcome Measures

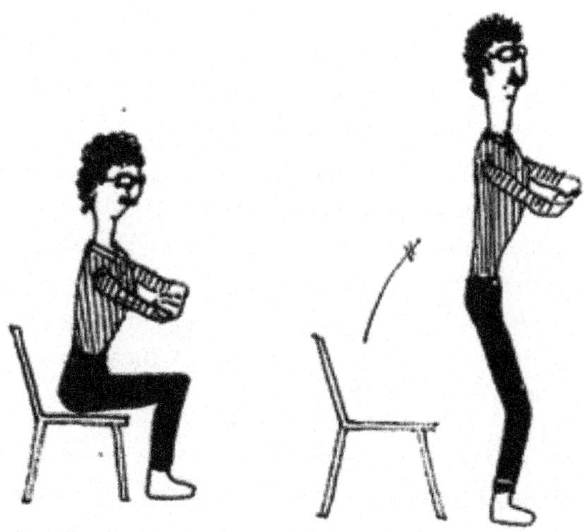

These may be the most commonly known and used type of outcomes. Performance outcome measures are based on specific task(s) performed by the patient under the guidance and scoring of a health-care professional. These outcomes usually imply cooperation and motivation from the participant and a specific methodology of implementation.

Examples of these outcomes currently in use or previously reported in mitochondrial disease trials include the following: 6-min walking test

(6MWT), 10-m walk test, Time up and Go (TUG), gait assessment, activity monitors (accelerometers), usual gait speed (UGS) and the short physical performance battery (SPPB), visual acuity and VO2 kinetics.

When choosing an instrument assessing functionality (either as a reported outcome or as an objective assessment like the performance outcome measures), it is important to distinguish between instruments measuring ((sub)maximal) capacity and those measuring real-world performance in daily life. Capacity is the ability to perform a certain task in an 'ideal' environment (e.g. on a level floor, assessor's support and encouragement, hospital facilities), while performance describes what an individual can do and does in his own environment on a daily basis (with both barriers and available aids and help) [53]. Both constructs have their own advantages and disadvantages. For example, a laboratory situation in which a patient is encouraged to make a single maximum effort in a clinical environment by a relative stranger may allow assessments with less confounding factors but is likely not to fully reflect the disabilities experienced in daily life. On the other hand, motor performance levels only partly reflect the motor capacities of the patient [53], and contextual (physical, environmental) and personal factors (anxiety, motivation) are likely to play a significant role. The development of accelerometer-based wearable technology may help circumvent these limitations in future clinical trials.

Biomarkers

Since all functional outcome measures are to some extent subjective instruments, either to the patient, to their relatives or to the investigator, one may feel a demand for more objective outcome measures that can be assessed using more reliable and unbiased assays or devices. These so-called surrogate endpoints are easy to measure variables that give an indirect indication of the toxicity or therapeutic benefit of a compound. Although surrogate endpoints have many advantages, such as a reduction of sample size and the possibility to indicate changes in biochemical processes that would be unethical to measure otherwise, drawbacks are numerous.

First and foremost, a change in a surrogate endpoint does not necessarily reflect a clinically meaningful effect of the treatment to the patient [54, 55]. Moreover, technical problems, fluctuations due to seasonal variation, physiological maturation and development, diurnal rhythm, hormonal cycle, food intake, exercise and local laboratory variations (measurement variability, storage and timing) add to the complexity of using it as an endpoint in a clinical trial. The current view is that functional outcome measures are only good indicators of the aspects of function that reflect everyday activities [15].

Making a diagnosis of mitochondrial disease can be challenging and remains heavily dependent on the clinical acumen of the examining physician. Non-specific biomarkers indicative of defective oxidative phosphorylation have traditionally been used in clinical practice to support physicians in making a diagnosis of mitochondrial disease. These conventionally have included lactate, pyruvate, lactate/pyruvate ratio, alanine and creatine kinase. Other laboratory tests may include acylcarnitine and organic acids. Urinary organic acid can be very useful for the detection of childhood-onset mitochondrial diseases such as methylmalonic aciduria in *SUCLA2 and SUCLG1* [56–60] or 3-methylglutaconic aciduria in *TAZ, TMEM70* and *SERAC1* mutations [61–66]. While certain biomarkers are extremely useful for making specific diagnosis, e.g. thymidine and deoxyuridine levels in mitochondrial neurogastrointestinal encephalopathy (MNGIE) syndrome, however, the majority of these parameters are recognised to exhibit poor sensitivity and specificity.

Recently, there has potentially been the identification of more useful mitochondrial disease biomarkers that appear to exhibit greater sensitivity and sensitivity indicative of oxidative phosphorylation dysfunction. These include levels of fibroblast growth factor (FGF21) and growth/differentiation factor 15 (GDF15). FGF21 was first reported as a potential useful biomarker of muscle manifesting mitochondrial disease in 2011

[67]. While recognised to be elevated in other metabolic disorders, its sensitivity and specificity (>90%) has far exceeded other traditional biomarkers to date. Subsequently, serum GDF15 has been shown to also be increased in mitochondrial disease and exhibits excellent sensitivity (98%) and good specificity (86%) [68–70].

However, both FGF21 and GDF15 have demonstrated only moderate correlation to disease severity [20, 21], which may suggest these markers cannot be used as surrogate markers for mitochondrial disease severity in general. There may be a role as a more specific (disease severity) biomarker for mtDNA maintenance and translational disorders [71]. So, although surrogate outcome measures may serve as reliable and unbiased indications of proof of concept, their reflection of the final goal of the treatment, namely, to improve the functional abilities or survival of the patient, should be established before using it in efficacy studies [72]. Only sensitive and responsive biomarkers, closely related to a valid clinical endpoint, treatment response and the pathophysiology of the disease may suit as a surrogate endpoint [73]. Moreover, changes in surrogate endpoints should always be supported by changes in clinically relevant parameters.

Selecting the Most Appropriate Outcome for Clinical Trials in Patients with Mitochondrial Disease

Since different tools will provide unique and relevant information, it is expected that the inclusion of more instruments in a trial will be needed to gather sufficient information on the clinical condition of the patient. Naturally, the size of the set of outcome measures and the sequence of the tests should be adapted to the abilities and energy level of the patient. One should also realise that many tests are confronting to patients and their parents and therefore 'less is more'.

Selecting COA for a clinical trial must take into consideration the stakeholders involved and the final aim of the study results as the type and robustness of the COA may vary from one stakeholder to the other. The COA selected for a two-time point natural history study will most likely differ from those chosen to assess the effectiveness of a drug that will target muscle power. In a clinical trial, the outcome most relevant for a physiotherapist may differ from the one relevant to the pathologist, and these two may differ from those expected by the FDA for drug approval or that patient organisations will like to see changing.

Agreement on Which Outcome Measures to Use

Because of the nature of the mitochondrial diseases as rare diseases, we should assume that for future clinical trials and natural history studies, multicentre collaboration will be required, most likely multinational. Hence, international feasibility and applicability (translation and cross-cultural adaptation) should be considered when selecting an outcome measure. When executing such an international trial, differences between sites should be minimised [51, 74]. As first instance, the way of delivery and interpretation of any of these outcomes should be standardised. This will provide reliable information for both, interpreting clinical trials as for communicating the prognosis in relevant terms to patients and families. Special care should be taken to guarantee training for all raters and to test and diminish inter-rater reliability. If patients are too scattered around the world, one might think of relocating patients and their families to the study site or of a combination of centralised pre- and post-treatment evaluations in combination with assessments which can be performed using telemedicine or devices to quantify functional abilities [75].

Several initiatives have tried to get international agreement on which COA to use [4, 5], although the lack of validation studies or clinical trials using these outcomes impairs the interpretability of these recommendations. The International Society for Pharmacoeconomics and Outcomes Research Task Force has developed a consensus compendium highlighting current challenges associated with the selection and use of COAs in rare disease clinical trials [51, 76] and presents potential solutions to these.

Selection of Outcome Measures for Trials in Children with Mitochondrial Disease

Selecting an appropriate outcome measure for clinical trials in children with mitochondrial disease is challenging for many more reasons (Table 2). Not only are children developing and growing (requiring age-specific tests and the use of age- and size-matched reference values), but also their understanding and enthusiasm for and cooperation during the test may highly influence the test results. The feasibility of measuring disease progression in severely mentally impaired children, whom are sometimes not even able to communicate effectively with their environment, let alone respond to an instruction, is limited. Since virtually all functional tests require the child to show the best (s)he can do, even children having milder mental impairments might not show consistent results because of attention deficit and difficulties understanding the relevance of the tests. The measured results are therefore not only dependent on the stage of disease or grade of disability but also on age, gender, intellectual functions and environment and personal factors.

Table 2 Child-specific challenges when selecting outcome measures for trials in children

Children are in constant change (i.e. developing and growing)
Outcome measures for children mostly have a limited age range for which they were created or validated
Might present communication barriers
Might have a shorter attention span and are less likely to follow the instructions completely requiring specific considerations for assessments
The cooperation required for some tests is highly dependent on the level of enthusiasm for the test and the mental abilities of the child
High reliance on parents, caregivers and/or assessor's experience to perform assessments properly

Patient Preferences in the Selection of Outcome Measures and Clinical Endpoints

Between 2013 and 2017, a series of meetings have been convening as part of the patient-focused drug development initiative (established in 2012) by the FDA to incorporate patient perspective into the drug development decision-making process. The relevance of patient perspective has now been recognised when trying to fully understand the context for the assessment of benefits and risks of an intervention. One of the priority questions is always about which health effect of the disease (i.e. sign, symptom, problem) is most challenging for the patient (either responded by patients themselves or by caregivers). In heterogeneous diseases like mitochondrial diseases, this response may vary not only from patient to patient but within the patients themselves along the natural progression of their disease. This variability may frame the results of certain outcomes, as targeting specific symptoms may impact more on quality of life of those affected the most by it. However, it is essential to identify, document and measure the priority symptoms as established by the patients or their caregivers as this would support the FDA decision-making process when pushing for the approval of a new treatment. Likewise, the health technology assessment (HTA) has criticised the presumed effectiveness of some orphan drugs due to their lack of achievement in outcomes known to be clinically relevant to patients.

Not only identifying patient's chief concerns but also the level of relevance of how to measure the symptom(s) and how to interpret the results is important. Do the results provided by the selected COA really measure something meaningful for the population? How much change in this COA reflects a significant change in a patient's life? Including patients' preferences (i.e. what it is important to them) into the decision-making process for outcomes and endpoints when designing a clinical trial may provide invaluable insight into the impact of the disease and treatment on patients. The International Rare Diseases Research Consortium (IRDiRC) presented in

2016 the patient-centred outcome measures (PCOM). This initiative in the field of rare diseases proposes to systematically incorporate patient perspectives to measure the outcomes that really matter the most to patients [52, 77]. By following a systematic approach like this, we can expect a better informed outcome measure selection that places patients and their family and carers at the heart of the decisions concerning their health assessment and attention.

Conclusion

The field of clinical trials in mitochondrial medicine has been gaining momentum in the past decade. It is now widely accepted that patients should not be exposed to low-quality studies. The responsibility of the international expert centres is now to set guidelines for high-quality studies and to facilitate improvements in trial design, e.g. by harmonising outcome measures. Naturally, the decision on which outcome measures to use for natural history studies and clinical trials should be guided by the research question and taken by an expert panel and based on data obtained from experiments in the population intended to be included in the clinical trial.

References

1. Koopman WJ, et al. Mitochondrial disorders in children: toward development of small-molecule treatment strategies. EMBO Mol Med. 2016;8(4):311–27.
2. Gorman GS, et al. Mitochondrial diseases. Nat Rev Dis Primers. 2016;2:16080.
3. Pfeffer G, et al. New treatments for mitochondrial disease-no time to drop our standards. Nat Rev Neurol. 2013;9(8):474–81.
4. Mancuso M, et al. International Workshop:: Outcome measures and clinical trial readiness in primary mitochondrial myopathies in children and adults. Consensus recommendations. 16–18 November 2016, Rome, Italy. Neuromuscul Disord. 2017;27(12):1126–37.
5. Koene S, et al. Outcome measures for children with mitochondrial disease: consensus recommendations for future studies from a Delphi-based international workshop. J Inherit Metab Dis. 2018;41(6):1267–73. https://doi.org/10.1007/s10545-018-0229-5.
6. Brunner HI, Ravelli A. Developing outcome measures for paediatric rheumatic diseases. Best Pract Res Clin Rheumatol. 2009;23(5):609–24.
7. Adminstration, F.F.a.D. Guidance for Industry: Patient-Reported Outcome Measures: Use in Medical Product Development to Support Labeling Claims. U.S. Department of Health and Human Services. 2009.
8. Tugwell P, Boers M. OMERACT conference on outcome measures in rheumatoid arthritis clinical trials: introduction. J Rheumatol. 1993;20(3):528–30.
9. Organisation, W.W.H. International Classification of Functioning, Disability and Health. World Health Organization Press. 2001.
10. Ronen GM, Fayed N, Rosenbaum PL. Outcomes in pediatric neurology: a review of conceptual issues and recommendations. The 2010 Ronnie Mac Keith Lecture. Dev Med Child Neurol. 2011;53(4):305–12.
11. Merlini L, et al. Motor function-muscle strength relationship in spinal muscular atrophy. Muscle Nerve. 2004;29(4):548–52.
12. Kierkegaard M, et al. Perceived functioning and disability in adults with myotonic dystrophy type 1: a survey according to the International Classification of Functioning, Disability and Health. J Rehabil Med. 2009;41(7):512–20.
13. Mokkink LB, et al. The COSMIN study reached international consensus on taxonomy, terminology, and definitions of measurement properties for health-related patient-reported outcomes. J Clin Epidemiol. 2010;63(7):737–45.
14. Schiariti V, et al. Comparing contents of outcome measures in cerebral palsy using the international classification of functioning (ICF-CY): a systematic review. Eur J Paediatr Neurol. 2014;18(1):1–12.
15. Mercuri E, Mazzone E. Choosing the right clinical outcome measure: from the patient to the statistician and back. Neuromuscul Disord. 2011;21(1):16–9.
16. Etzioni R, Gulati R, Lin DW. Measures of survival benefit in cancer drug development and their limitations. Urol Oncol. 2015;33(3):122–7.
17. Fernandez-Martos C. Clinically relevant study end points in rectal cancer. Eur J Cancer. 2012;48:S1.
18. Preiss D, Sattar N, McMurray JJ. A systematic review of event rates in clinical trials in diabetes mellitus: the importance of quantifying baseline cardiovascular disease history and proteinuria and implications for clinical trial design. Am Heart J. 2011;161(1):210–219.e1.
19. Lee SK, et al. Initial experiences with proton MR spectroscopy in treatment monitoring of mitochondrial encephalopathy. Yonsei Med J. 2010;51(5):672–5.
20. Koene S, et al. Serum FGF21 levels in adult m.3243A>G carriers: clinical implications. Neurology. 2014;83(2):125–33.
21. Koene S, et al. Serum GDF15 levels correlate to mitochondrial disease severity and myocardial strain, but not to disease progression in adult m.3243A>G carriers. JIMD Rep. 2015;24:69–81.

22. Koene S, et al. Natural disease course and genotype-phenotype correlations in complex I deficiency caused by nuclear gene defects: what we learned from 130 cases. J Inherit Metab Dis. 2012;35(5):737–47.
23. Koene S, et al. Is 2D speckle tracking echocardiography useful for detecting and monitoring myocardial dysfunction in adult m.3243A>G carriers? - a retrospective pilot study. J Inherit Metab Dis. 2017;40(2):247–59.
24. Augustine EF, Adams HR, Mink JW. Clinical trials in rare disease: challenges and opportunities. J Child Neurol. 2013;28(9):1142–50.
25. Kang PB. Beyond the Gowers sign: measuring outcomes in Duchenne muscular dystrophy. Muscle Nerve. 2013;48(3):315–7.
26. Friedman LS, et al. Measuring the rate of progression in Friedreich ataxia: implications for clinical trial design. Mov Disord. 2010;25(4):426–32.
27. Klopstock T, et al. A randomized placebo-controlled trial of idebenone in Leber's hereditary optic neuropathy. Brain. 2011;134(Pt 9):2677–86.
28. Schaefer AM, et al. Mitochondrial disease in adults: a scale to monitor progression and treatment. Neurology. 2006;66(12):1932–4.
29. Phoenix C, et al. A scale to monitor progression and treatment of mitochondrial disease in children. Neuromuscul Disord. 2006;16(12):814–20.
30. Campolina-Sampaio GP, et al. The Newcastle pediatric mitochondrial disease scale: translation and cultural adaptation for use in Brazil. Arq Neuropsiquiatr. 2016;74(11):909–13.
31. Enns GM, et al. Initial experience in the treatment of inherited mitochondrial disease with EPI-743. Mol Genet Metab. 2012;105(1):91–102.
32. Koene S, et al. International paediatric mitochondrial disease scale. J Inherit Metab Dis. 2016;39(5):705–12.
33. Busner J, Targum SD. The clinical global impressions scale: applying a research tool in clinical practice. Psychiatry (Edgmont). 2007;4(7):28–37.
34. Bonnemann CG, et al. 173rd ENMC International Workshop: congenital muscular dystrophy outcome measures 5-7 March 2010, Naarden, The Netherlands. Neuromuscul Disord. 2011;21(7):513–22.
35. Patrick DL, Deyo RA. Generic and disease-specific measures in assessing health status and quality of life. Med Care. 1989;27(3 Suppl):S217–32.
36. Houwen-van Opstal SL, et al. Health-related quality of life and its relation to disease severity in boys with Duchenne muscular dystrophy: satisfied boys, worrying parents—a case-control study. J Child Neurol. 2014;29(11):1486–95.
37. Juniper EF, et al. Clinically important improvements in asthma-specific quality of life, but no difference in conventional clinical indexes in patients changed from conventional beclomethasone dipropionate to approximately half the dose of extrafine beclomethasone dipropionate. Chest. 2002;121(6):1824–32.
38. Davis SE, et al. The PedsQL in pediatric patients with Duchenne muscular dystrophy: feasibility, reliability, and validity of the pediatric quality of life inventory neuromuscular module and generic core scales. J Clin Neuromuscul Dis. 2010;11(3):97–109.
39. Hahn EA, et al. Precision of health-related quality-of-life data compared with other clinical measures. Mayo Clin Proc. 2007;82(10):1244–54.
40. Elson JL, et al. Initial development and validation of a mitochondrial disease quality of life scale. Neuromuscul Disord. 2013;23(4):324–9.
41. Barczak P, et al. Patterns of psychiatric morbidity in a genitourinary clinic - a validation of the hospital anxiety depression scale (HAD). Br J Psychiatry. 1988;152:698–700.
42. Emslie GJ, et al. Depressive symptoms by self-report in adolescence: phase I of the development of a questionnaire for depression by self-report. J Child Neurol. 1990;5(2):114–21.
43. Beck AT, et al. An inventory for measuring depression. Arch Gen Psychiatry. 1961;4(6):561–71.
44. Fisk JD, et al. Measuring the functional impact of fatigue: initial validation of the fatigue impact scale. Clin Infect Dis. 1994;18(Suppl 1):S79–83.
45. Krupp LB, et al. The fatigue severity scale. Application to patients with multiple sclerosis and systemic lupus erythematosus. Arch Neurol. 1989;46(10):1121–3.
46. Vercoulen JH, et al. Dimensional assessment of chronic fatigue syndrome. J Psychosom Res. 1994;38(5):383–92.
47. Borg G. Psychophysical scaling with applications in physical work and the perception of exertion. Scand J Work Environ Health. 1990;16(Suppl 1):55–8.
48. Janssen MCH, et al. The KHENERGY study: safety and efficacy of KH176 in mitochondrial m.3243A>G spectrum disorders. Clin Pharmacol Ther. 2019;105(1):101–11.
49. Hagstromer M, Oja P, Sjostrom M. The international physical activity questionnaire (IPAQ): a study of concurrent and construct validity. Public Health Nutr. 2006;9(6):755–62.
50. Cella D, et al. The patient-reported outcomes measurement information system (PROMIS): progress of an NIH roadmap cooperative group during its first two years. Med Care. 2007;45(5 Suppl 1):S3–S11.
51. Benjamin K, et al. Patient-reported outcome and observer-reported outcome assessment in rare disease clinical trials: an ISPOR COA emerging good practices task force report. Value Health. 2017;20(7):838–55.
52. International Rare Diseases Research Consortium (IRDiRC). Patient-Centered Outcome Measures Initiatives in the Field of Rare Diseases. 2016.
53. Holsbeeke L, et al. Capacity, capability, and performance: different constructs or three of a kind? Arch Phys Med Rehabil. 2009;90(5):849–55.
54. Beenakker EA, et al. Functional ability and muscle force in healthy children and ambulant Duchenne muscular dystrophy patients. Eur J Paediatr Neurol. 2005;9(6):387–93.
55. Parreira SL, et al. Comparison of motor strength and function in patients with Duchenne muscular dystrophy with or without steroid therapy. Arq Neuropsiquiatr. 2010;68(5):683–8.

56. Liu Y, et al. [Heterogeneous phenotypes, genotypes, treatment and prevention of 1 003 patients with methylmalonic acidemia in the mainland of China]. Zhonghua Er Ke Za Zhi. 2018;56(6):414-420.
57. Maalej M, et al. Clinical, molecular, and computational analysis in two cases with mitochondrial encephalomyopathy associated with SUCLG1 mutation in a consanguineous family. Biochem Biophys Res Commun. 2018;495(2):1730–7.
58. El-Hattab AW, Scaglia F. SUCLA2-Related Mitochondrial DNA Depletion Syndrome, Encephalomyopathic Form with Methylmalonic Aciduria. In: Adam MP, et al., editors. GeneReviews((R)). Seattle, WA: University of Washington, Seattle; 1993.
59. Carrozzo R, et al. Succinate-CoA ligase deficiency due to mutations in SUCLA2 and SUCLG1: phenotype and genotype correlations in 71 patients. J Inherit Metab Dis. 2016;39(2):243–52.
60. Carrozzo R, et al. SUCLA2 mutations are associated with mild methylmalonic aciduria, Leigh-like encephalomyopathy, dystonia and deafness. Brain. 2007;130(Pt 3):862–74.
61. Tort F, et al. Exome sequencing identifies a new mutation in SERAC1 in a patient with 3-methylglutaconic aciduria. Mol Genet Metab. 2013;110(1-2):73–7.
62. Wortmann SB, et al. 3-Methylglutaconic aciduria—lessons from 50 genes and 977 patients. J Inherit Metab Dis. 2013;36(6):913–21.
63. Barth PG, Wanders RJ, Vreken P. X-linked cardioskeletal myopathy and neutropenia (Barth syndrome)-MIM 302060. J Pediatr. 1999;135(3):273–6.
64. Stojanovic V, Doronjski A. Mild form of 3-methylglutaconic aciduria type IV and mutation in the TMEM70 genes. J Pediatr Endocrinol Metab. 2013;26(1-2):151–4.
65. Tort F, et al. Screening for nuclear genetic defects in the ATP synthase-associated genes TMEM70, ATP12 and ATP5E in patients with 3-methylglutaconic aciduria. Clin Genet. 2011;80(3):297–300.
66. Shchelochkov OA, et al. Milder clinical course of type IV 3-methylglutaconic aciduria due to a novel mutation in TMEM70. Mol Genet Metab. 2010;101(2-3):282–5.
67. Suomalainen A, et al. FGF-21 as a biomarker for muscle-manifesting mitochondrial respiratory chain deficiencies: a diagnostic study. Lancet Neurol. 2011;10(9):806–18.
68. Ji X, et al. Growth differentiation factor 15 is a novel diagnostic biomarker of mitochondrial diseases. Mol Neurobiol. 2017;54(10):8110–6.
69. Suomalainen A. Fibroblast growth factor 21: a novel biomarker for human muscle-manifesting mitochondrial disorders. Expert Opin Med Diagn. 2013;7(4):313–7.
70. Davis RL, Liang C, Sue CM. A comparison of current serum biomarkers as diagnostic indicators of mitochondrial diseases. Neurology. 2016;86(21):2010–5.
71. Lehtonen JM, et al. FGF21 is a biomarker for mitochondrial translation and mtDNA maintenance disorders. Neurology. 2016;87(22):2290–9.
72. Tukey JW. Some thoughts on clinical trials, especially problems of multiplicity. Science. 1977;198(4318):679–84.
73. Schuller Y, et al. Factors contributing to the efficacy-effectiveness gap in the case of orphan drugs for metabolic diseases. Drugs. 2017;77(13):1461–72.
74. Mayhew JE, et al. Reliable surrogate outcome measures in multicenter clinical trials of Duchenne muscular dystrophy. Muscle Nerve. 2007;35(1):36–42.
75. Filipovic Pierucci A, et al. Quantifiable evaluation of cerebellar signs in children. Neurology. 2015;84(12):1225–32.
76. ISPOR Good Practices for Outcomes Research Index. 2018. https://www.ispor.org/workpaper/practices_index.asp.
77. Morel T, Cano SJ. Measuring what matters to rare disease patients - reflections on the work by the IRDiRC taskforce on patient-centered outcome measures. Orphanet J Rare Dis. 2017;12(1):171.

The Pathophysiology of Exercise and Effect of Training in Mitochondrial Myopathies

Tina Dysgaard Jeppesen and John Vissing

The Pathophysiological Response to Exercise in Mitochondrial Myopathies

Mitochondrial myopathy is most often associated with a multisystem disease [1–3], but muscle symptoms are typically prominent. In skeletal muscle, mtDNA mutation load is often high in mitochondrial myopathies [4–6]. This coupled with an unprecedented high oxidative demand of skeletal muscle, with up to 100-fold increases in oxygen consumption from rest to peak exercise in healthy persons [7, 8], makes exercise intolerance the most common symptom in patients with mtDNA mutations [9–12]. In a clinical setting, the degree of exercise intolerance is difficult to grade and distinguish from limited physical fitness due to sedentary lifestyle or cardiopulmonary diseases. Exercise limitations in patients with mitochondrial myopathy can be assessed with provocative exercise tests. In the following paragraph, we describe oxygen uptake, delivery, and extraction and fuel utilization during exercise in patients with mitochondrial myopathies. As exercise tests can reveal pathophysiologic consequences of mitochondrial impairment, we also present the potential diagnostic strength of the different physiological parameters.

Maximal Oxygen Uptake

Since transfer of oxygen from air to muscle was first described in 1923 [13], maximal oxygen uptake (VO_{2max}) has been an omnipresent parameter in exercise studies used to evaluate exercise capacity in healthy persons [14–16] and patients with a variety of diseases [11, 17–19]. Maximal oxygen uptake (VO_{2max}) is the maximal rate of oxygen used for energy (ATP) production of working muscle. Maximal oxygen uptake depends on three factors: (1) the ability to deliver oxygen from air to blood (lung conductance), (2) the circulatory capacity to deliver oxygen to working muscle, and (3) mitochondrial capacity to extract oxygen and produce ATP [20, 21] (Fig. 1).

The range of VO_{2max} in patients with mtDNA mutations ranges from normal to as low as 10 mL/kg/min, which is less than that required for slow walking [4, 6]. In healthy individuals, cardiac output is rate-limiting for VO_{2max} [20, 22, 23], while VO_{2max} is limited by mitochondrial capacity in patients with mitochondrial myopathy [11, 12]. As a consequence of this, there is an inverse correlation between VO_{2max} and mtDNA mutation load in exercising muscle of patients with mitochondrial myopathy [4, 6, 24]. The

T. D. Jeppesen (✉) · J. Vissing
Department of Neurology, Copenhagen Neuromuscular Center at Rigshospitalet, University of Copenhagen, Copenhagen, Denmark
e-mail: tina.dysgaard.jeppesen.03@regionh.dk

M. Mancuso, T. Klopstock (eds.), *Diagnosis and Management of Mitochondrial Disorders*,
https://doi.org/10.1007/978-3-030-05517-2_20

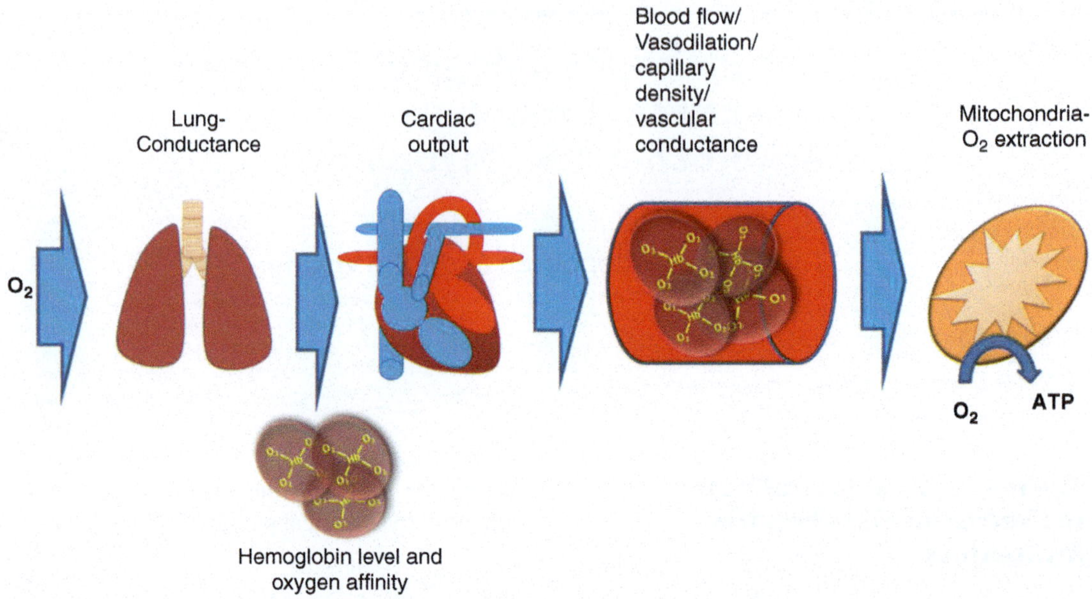

Fig. 1 Oxygen delivery from air to mitochondria. Oxygen uptake from mitochondria depends on lung conductance, hemoglobin level and affinity for oxygen, cardiac output capacity, blood delivery that is dependent on flow, vasodilation, capillary density and vascular conductance, and finally, the content and function of mitochondria

mutation threshold in muscle, at which oxidative capacity becomes impaired, has been shown to be around 85% in in vitro studies [25, 26], but in vivo, this threshold appears to be closer to 65% in patients with point mutations and 50% in patients with single, large-scale deletions of mtDNA [4, 6, 24].

Findings of correlation between VO_{2max} and mtDNA mutation load in exercising muscle [4, 6, 24] indicate that VO_{2max} is a good marker of the severity of a mitochondrial myopathy. However, low VO_{2max} is not specific for low oxidative capacity due to primary mitochondrial disease. Besides mitochondrial function, VO_{2max} depends on many factors including cardiac [27] and pulmonary capacity [28]. Additionally, most patients with primary muscle disease with exercise intolerance will have low VO_{2max} due to muscle weakness [29, 30] (Fig. 2). Additionally, patients with metabolic myopathies also have low oxidative capacity due to fuel limitations [10, 11, 31, 32]. Thus, measurement of VO_{2max} is important in characterization of mitochondrial dysfunction and oxidative impairment when examining mitochondrial myopathy but cannot be used for diagnostic purposes for mitochondrial disease.

Ventilatory Response

The rate of pulmonary ventilation (respiratory frequency, VE) increases linearly with exercise intensity until the VE threshold is reached [33–35]. From this point, VE exceeds oxygen uptake and lactate is accumulated [36]. VE is tightly regulated by areas in the central nervous system, by feedback from chemo-, mechano- and thermoreceptors in the peripheral nervous system, and by negative feedback from carbon dioxide tension [37, 38]. There is also a direct feedback from muscle prompted by a decrease in the ATP/ADP ratio [36]. Patients with mitochondrial myopathy have an excessive ventilator response during exercise [6, 10, 11, 39, 40], and the level correlates with mtDNA mutation load in contracting muscle [6, 41]. The mechanisms inducing excessive VE are unknown but likely relate to increased motor unit recruitment and excessive buildup of

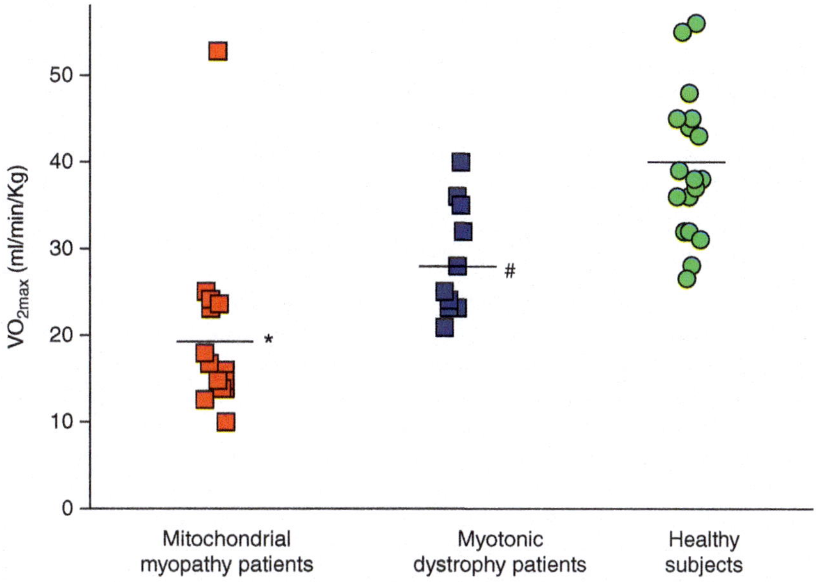

Fig. 2 Maximal oxygen uptake in 15 patients with mitochondrial myopathy compared with 2 control groups, 10 patients with myotonic dystrophy, and 10 healthy subjects. *, different from myotonic dystrophy patients and healthy subjects ($p < 0.05$). #, different from healthy subjects ($p < 0.05$)

ADP, lactate, and other metabolites in exercising muscle. Hyperventilation during exercise occurs in other diseases, including metabolic myopathies [11, 31, 42, 43]. Thus, ventilation rate is a good indicator of oxidative capacity but cannot be used as a diagnostic parameter for mitochondrial myopathy.

Oxygen Extraction

Maximal oxygen uptake is limited by the mitochondrial capacity to extract oxygen from blood in patients with mitochondrial myopathy. Larsson and Linderholm were the first to demonstrate arterialization of venous blood from contracting muscle during cycle exercise in patients with mitochondrial myopathy [44]. Since then, several studies have confirmed this paradox physiologic response to exercise via indices of reduced oxygen extraction using near-infrared spectroscopy technique during forearm and/or treadmill exercise [45–49], measurement of oxygen saturation in venous blood from exercising muscle [49, 50], and calculation of arterial-venous oxygen (a-vO_2) differences from cardiac output measured via acetylene rebreathing technique [6, 49, 51]. One study investigated oxygen extraction capacity and related mechanisms by direct methods (ultrasound Doppler and a-vO_2 tension differences over exercising skeletal muscle) [52] in patients with high levels of mtDNA mutation in skeletal muscle. The study showed that patients with mitochondrial myopathy had a normal oxygen extraction at rest but were unable to increase extraction levels during exercise.

Two studies have shown that limitation in oxygen extraction can be used for diagnostic purposes for mitochondrial myopathy. Thus, the studies found that measurement of oxygen saturation in blood from contracting forearm muscle at exercise intensity of 40–50% is diagnostically sensitive and quite specific for mitochondrial myopathy [49, 50] (Fig. 3).

Cardiac Output

A central feature of circulatory regulation in exercise is a strict relationship between oxygen delivery (cardiac output) and utilization, which in healthy persons is 5 L blood for every 1 L VO_2 irrespective of age, gender, or physical conditioning [7, 22]. In healthy persons, the regulation of cardiac output relates to multiple different factors, including stimuli from muscle (local vasomotor effect), increased venous return (systemic vasoconstriction and respiratory pump),

Fig. 3 Exercise induced change in venous oxygen saturation. Individual peak changes in cubital venous oxygen saturation during handgrip exercise in 12 patients with mutation of mtDNA, 10 patients with muscular dystrophy, and 12 age- and gender-matched healthy subjects. *, different from both control groups ($p < 0.05$)

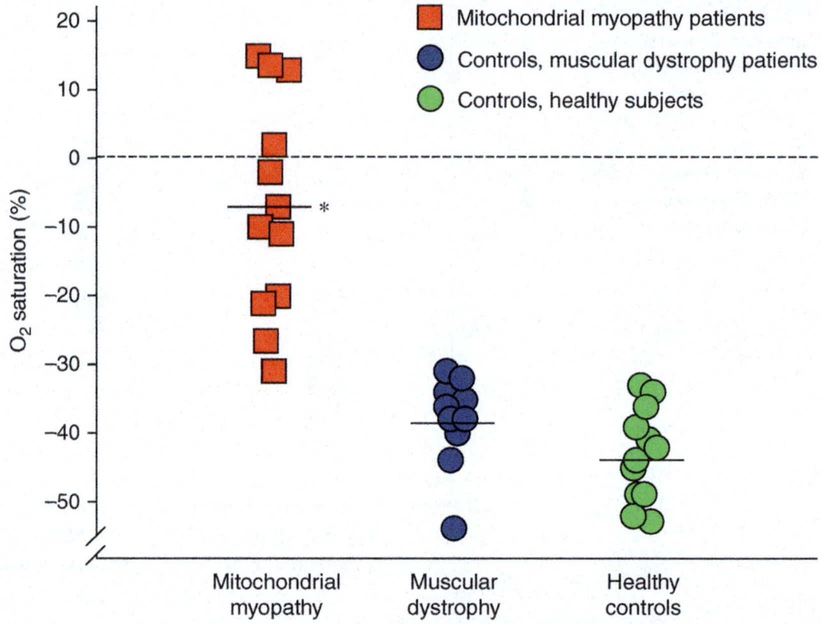

reduced afterload (systemic vasodilatation), CNS stimuli of heart rate and contractility, and redistribution of blood from non-active muscle cells. The limited oxygen extraction in patients with mitochondrial myopathy occurs along with a hyperkinetic circulatory response [6, 39, 44–47, 49, 50]. Two studies found a close relationship between the cardiac output relative to maximal workload and oxygen utilization during whole body exercise, irrespective of age, gender, or conditioning level [6, 49], indicating that the degree of impaired mitochondrial function determines the level of exaggerated cardiac output in patients with mitochondrial myopathy. Interestingly, other metabolic myopathies like myophosphorylase and PFK deficiency also exhibit this hyperkinetic circulatory response during exercise, which indicates that this paradox response to exercise is not linked to primary mitochondrial dysfunction but merely impaired oxidative capacity due to any dysfunction in extracting oxygen from blood [11, 31].

The skewed relationship between oxygen extraction and delivery in mitochondrial myopathy indicates that skeletal muscle receives excessive blood during contraction. This has been substantiated by findings of workload-adjusted maximal exercise leg hyperemia up to ~twofold (mean 65%) higher in skeletal muscle in patients with mtDNA mutation [52]. The hyperemic response was not a result of endothelial dysfunction in lower leg, which has previously been suggested [53–56]. Instead, the increased blood flow was apparently induced by ATP that was found to be elevated during exercise in patients with mitochondrial myopathy [52]. ATP is released from red blood cells in response to offloading of oxygen and deformation, and ATP is a potent vasodilator [57, 58] (Fig. 4). In order to preserve blood pressure and to redirect blood from inactive to active muscle during exercise, norepinephrine is released. In contracting muscle, blood flow has to be sustained by vasodilation and thus overrule the vasoconstrictive effect of norepinephrine, a phenomenon coined functional sympatholysis [59]. Studies have found that patients with mitochondrial myopathy have an increased level of norepinephrine during exercise [6, 9, 32, 60–62], which together with increased blood flow indicates that functional sympatholysis is highly exaggerated in this condition. The factors driving this paradox physiologic phenomenon are unknown, but since ATP has been shown to effectively overrule vasoconstrictive effects of norepinephrine [63, 64], it is likely that the increased ATP found in mitochon-

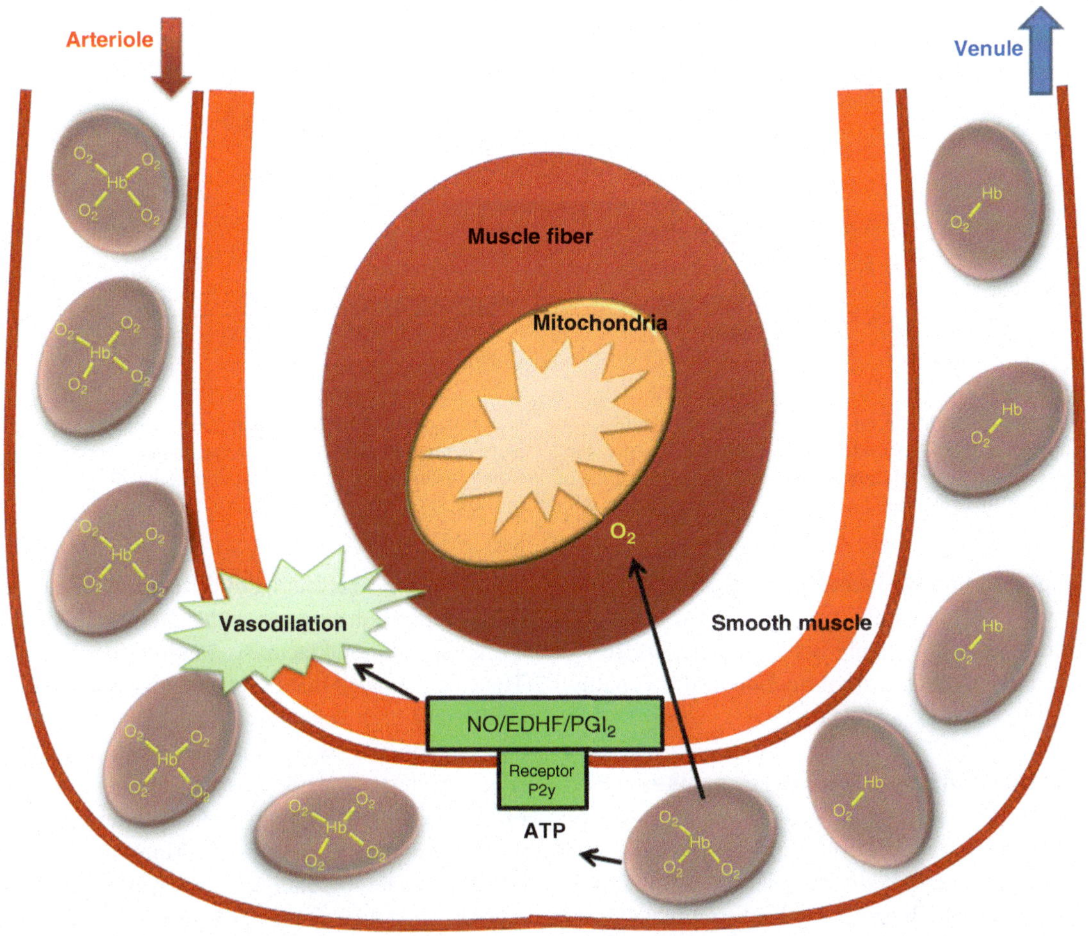

Fig. 4 Vasodilatory effect of ATP udloaded by red blood cells. The figure shows that when circulating red blood cells unload oxygen, they simultaneously unload ATP. ATP acts through P2y receptor that activates release of nitric oxide (NO), nonprostaglandin-mediated endothelium-dependent vasodilation (EDHF), and prostacyclin (PGI2), resulting in vasodilation through action on smooth muscle of arterioles

drial myopathy during exercise is responsible for the exaggerated functional sympatholysis in this condition [52].

Fuel Metabolism During Exercise in Mitochondrial Myopathy

The relative contribution of carbohydrate and fat for energy (ATP) synthesis during exercise varies with duration and intensity of exercise [65, 66]. At rest, the principle substrate for ATP production is free fatty acids (FFA). During exercise, FFA is the primary source to ATP generation until exercise intensity reaches 50% of VO_{2max}, after which the contribution of carbohydrates increase [66–68]. FFA and carbohydrate oxidation reach maximal rates at exercise intensities of 65% and 85% of VO_{2max}, respectively. At exercise intensities beyond 85% of VO_{2max}, anaerobic metabolism becomes increasingly important until peak VO_2 [69]. Since oxidation of glucose releases more ATP per molecule O_2 used compared to oxidation of FFA, it could be speculated that carbohydrate is a preferred substrate in favor of FFA during exercise in patients with mitochondrial myopathy. However, two studies have shown that this is not the case [60, 61], and FFA oxidation is similar in patients with mitochondrial myopathy compared to healthy subjects

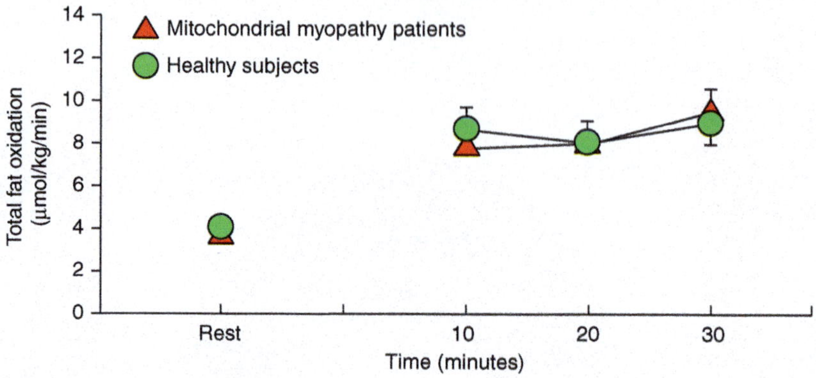

Fig. 5 Whole body fat oxidation during exercise in patients with mitochondrial myopathy vs. healthy subjects. Total fat oxidation at rest and during 30 min of exercise at a workload of 70 Watt in 10 patients with mutation of mtDNA (red triangles) vs. ten healthy subjects (green circles). All exercise values were significantly different from rest in patients and healthy subjects ($p < 0.05$)

(Fig. 5). For the same reason, changing diet toward carbohydrate or pre-exercise carbohydrate load would likely not increase exercise tolerance in patients with mitochondrial myopathy.

Lactate Turnover During Exercise

In the initial phase of exercise, there is a net release of lactate from healthy muscle. After a few minutes, oxygen delivery is restored so it matches the oxygen demand for oxidation of glucose and FFA for ATP production to contracting healthy skeletal muscle. Until exercise intensity reaches 60% of VO_{2max}, there is no release of lactate to the circulation although there is an ongoing lactate production in contracting muscle fibers. The produced lactate is taken up and oxidized in adjacent muscle fibers [69]. Only when exercise intensity exceeds 60% of VO_{2max}, there is a net release of lactate, but even at high exercise intensities, lactate is continuously taken up by muscle fibers and oxidized [69, 70]. In patients with mitochondrial myopathy, resting plasma lactate levels correlates with mtDNA mutation load in skeletal muscle, which has prompted the idea that the net lactate release from skeletal muscle in these patients depends on oxidative capacity in skeletal muscle [24]. However, a study investigating lactate metabolism showed that lactate oxidation capacity even in skeletal muscle with high level of mtDNA mutation is not limited. Instead, the increased levels of lactate seem to be related to differences in lactate release/uptake during rest and exercise rather than a limitation in total lactate oxidation [61] (Fig. 6). The study showed that during exercise there was a continuous high lactate oxidation in skeletal muscle of patients with mitochondrial myopathy (Fig. 6b) that matched the absolute rate and level of that found in healthy age- and gender-matched healthy subjects [61] (Fig. 6c). Along with a substantial lactate oxidation, there was still a net release of lactate from contracting muscle. The constant release of lactate from muscle together with a substantial uptake in patients with mitochondrial myopathy could relate to a different mitochondrial function among muscle fibers. In healthy muscle, mitochondrial function varies between type I and II fibers, but the mitochondrial capacity within each fiber type is rather uniformly distributed. In patients with mtDNA mutations, however, mtDNA mutation load varies among fibers, even among the same type of muscle fiber [71–73] (Fig. 7). Thus, in fibers with high mtDNA mutation load, ATP production rely solely on anaerobic glycolysis resulting in lactate production while adjacent muscle fibers with low or no mtDNA mutations are able to oxidize lactate (Fig. 8). In total, this structural composition can in theory induce the higher lactate production from some fibers along with a simultaneous efficient lactate oxidation in other muscle fibers.

The premature fatigue that is often seen in patients with mitochondrial myopathy has been

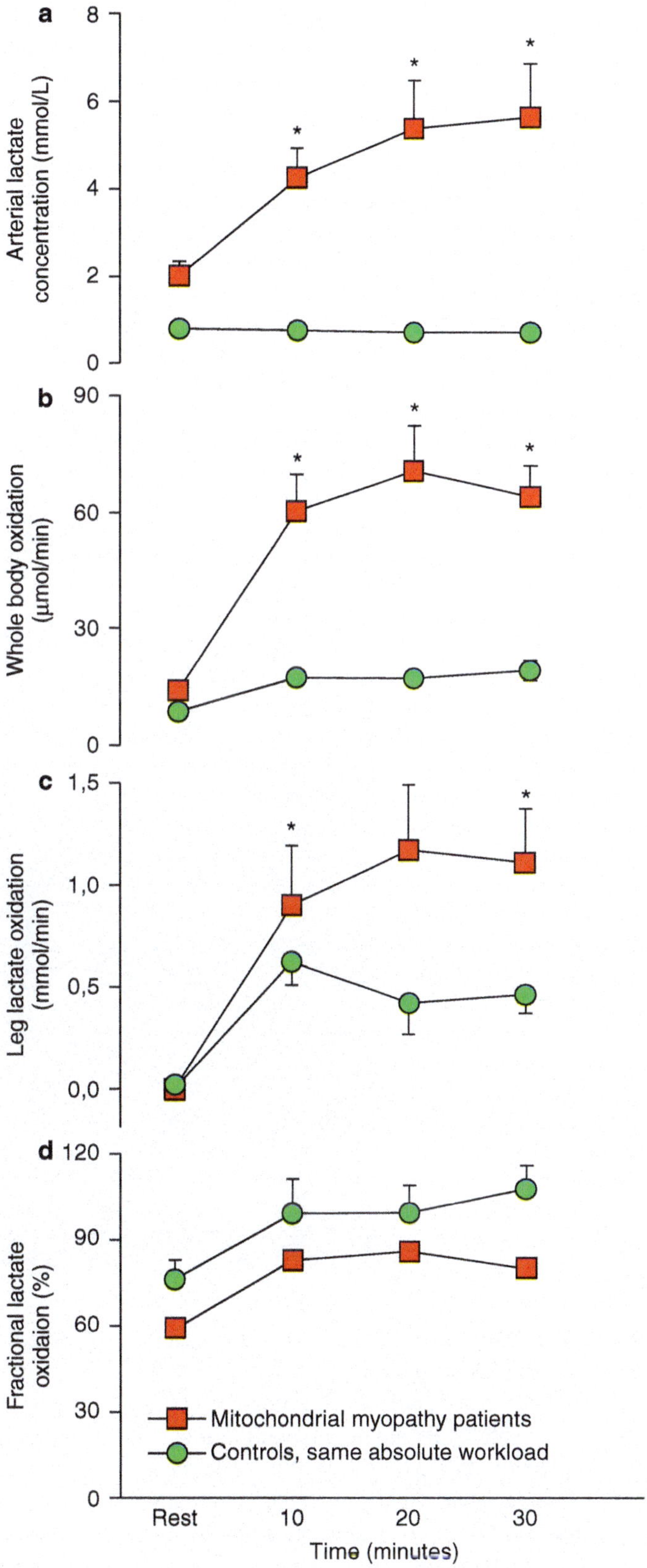

Fig. 6 Limb lactate kinetics under resting and exercising conditions in ten patients with mitochondrial myopathy and ten healthy subjects. (**a**) Arterial lactate concentration; (**b**) Whole ody lactate oxidation; (**c**) lactate oxidation across the leg and (**d**) lactate oxidation as a percentage of the unidirectional lactate uptake. *, $p < 0.05$ vs. healthy subjects. §, $p < 0.05$ vs. rest

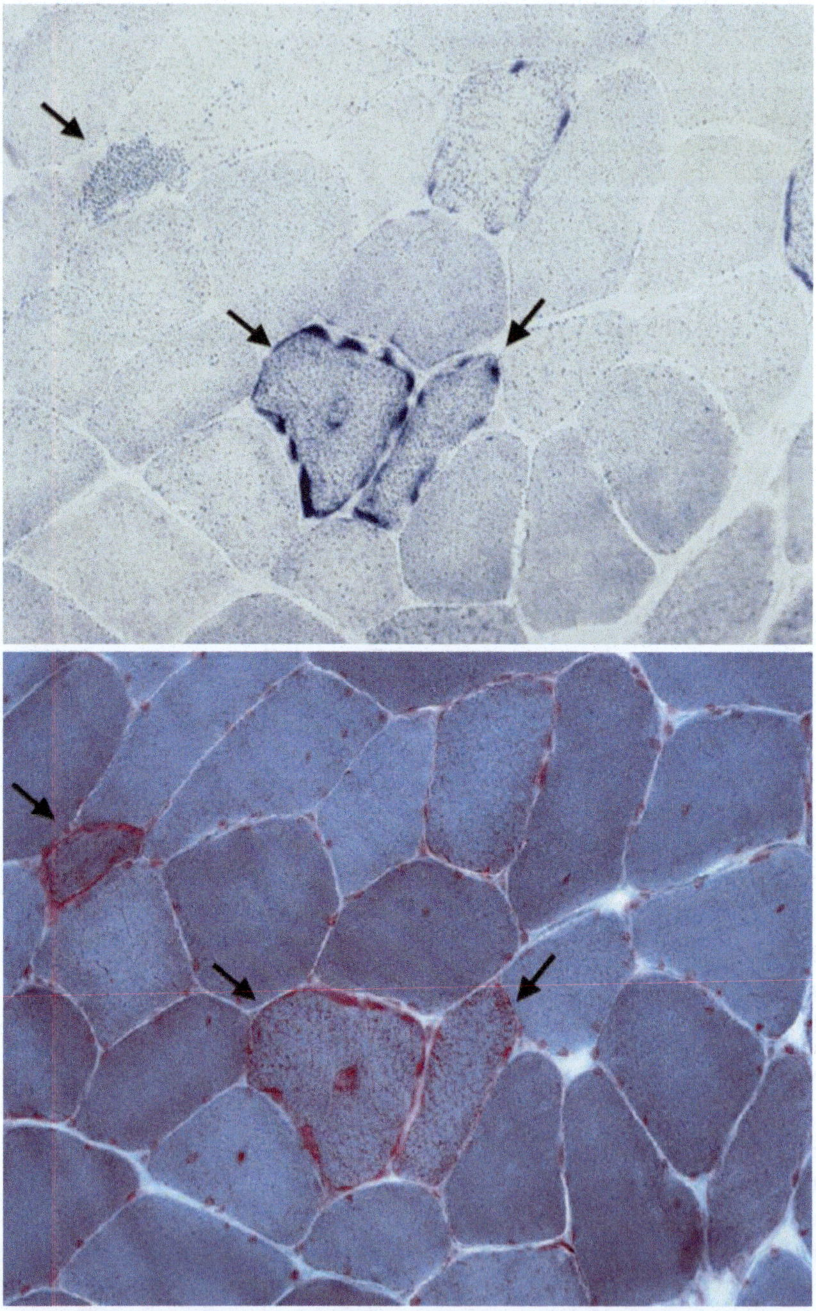

Fig. 7 Muscle biopsy of a patient with mutation of mtDNA mutation. Skeletal muscle biopsy obtained from a patient with a single, large-scale deletion of mtDNA stained with succinate dehydrogenase (upper) and trichrome (lower) staining. The arrow points to fibers with upregulated content of mitochondria as a sign of mitochondrial defect/ disease

linked to the excessive buildup of lactate due to impaired oxidative capacity [74, 75]. However, an additional factor could relate to higher recruitment of muscle fibers in patients with mitochondrial myopathy compared to healthy. This is so, since muscle fibers with high mtDNA mutation load that rely heavily on anaerobic glycolysis are prone for depleting glycogen storage fast, which inevitably result in recruitment of additional muscle fibers for contraction. The higher recruitment of muscle fibers in skeletal muscle of patients with mitochondrial myopathy will result in premature fatigue compared to healthy subjects exercising at the same relative workload [67].

Lactate is associated with anaerobic metabolism, and thus exercise test with measurement of lactate level as a primary endpoint potentially could be diagnostic for patients with oxidative

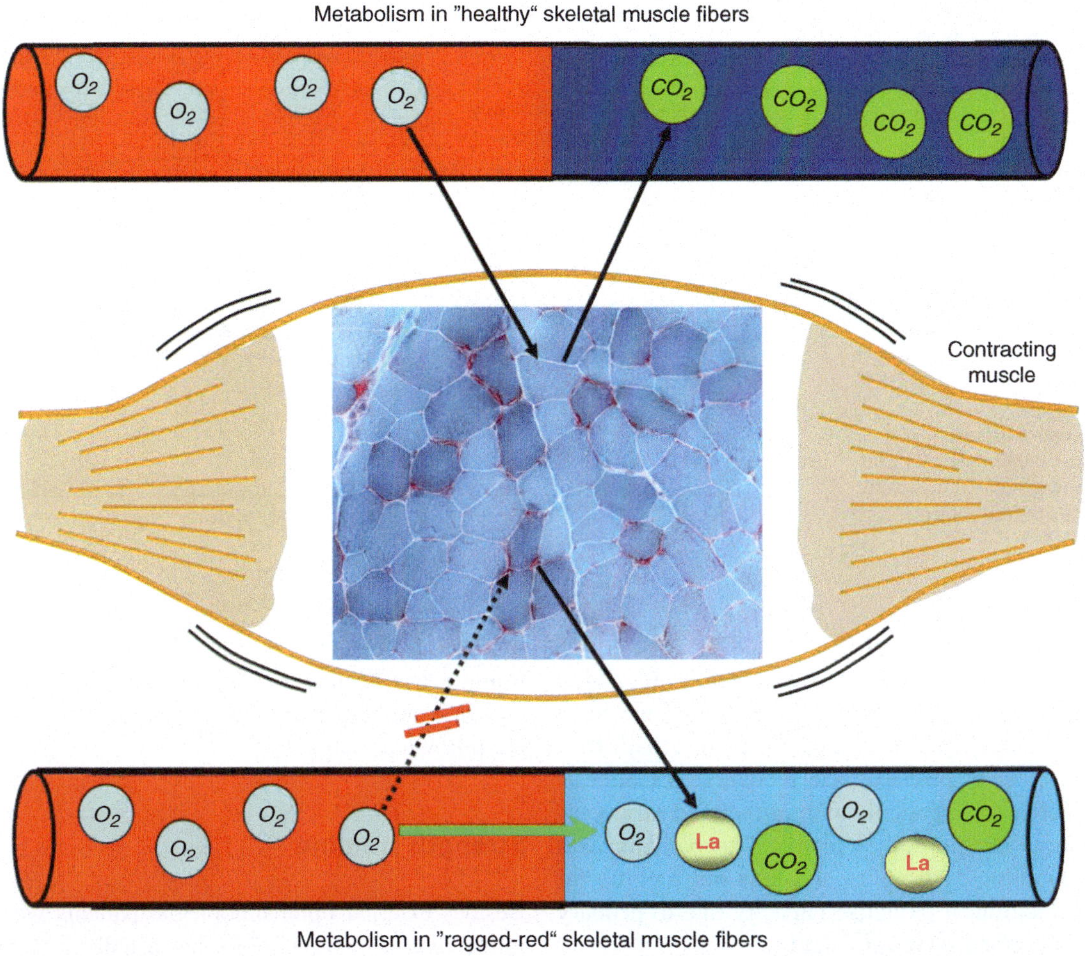

Fig. 8 Differential lactate metabolism in muscle fibers with low and high mutation loads. The figure illustrates how lactate in one muscle fiber can be efficiently oxidized (in muscle fiber with low mtDNA mutations and thus intact oxidative capacity), while lactate is released from fibers with high mtDNA mutation load, explaining a simultaneous high lactate release in muscle fibers with high mtDNA mutation burden vs. high lactate oxidation capacity in fibers with low mutation loads

impairment [75–78]. Exercise-induced peak lactate level depends on duration of exercise above anaerobic threshold, which depends on training status, pain threshold, and physiologic factors. Thus, even though patients with mitochondrial myopathy theoretically should reach higher levels of plasma lactate relative to workload performed compared to healthy subjects, healthy well-trained subjects often reach higher levels of plasma lactate at peak exercise [79]. This is so, since patients with mitochondrial myopathy may often stop exercising at pre-peak levels, which is substantiated by findings of lower maximal heart rates in this condition. Moreover, increased lactate levels at peak exercise are also found in patients with congestive heart failure, obstructive pulmonary disease, and anemia. Thus, peak exercise lactate is not diagnostically sensitive or specific for mitochondrial myopathy [79]. At constant workload exercise, the relationship between workload and lactate production is well-controlled, and psychological factors (the will to continue above lactate threshold) can be disregarded. Lactate threshold is lower in patients with mitochondrial myopathy, and thus exercise tests at a fixed or same relative (55–65% of VO_{2max}) workload have been proposed as diagnostic for mitochondrial myopathy [74, 76, 80–82]. However, even though lactate measured during a constant workload test may seem indicative of mitochondrial myopathy (Fig. 9), the diagnostic sensitivity and specificity is not different from simple testing of

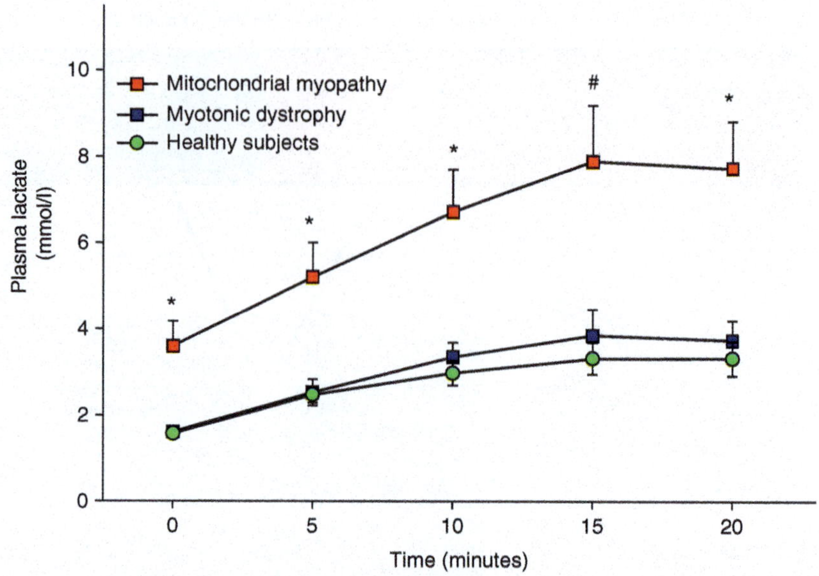

Fig. 9 Plasma lactate during a steady-state cycle exercise test at 65% of VO_{2max}. Plasma lactate level at rest and during 20 min of steady-state exercise at 65% of VO_{2max} in 15 patients with mitochondrial myopathy, 9 patients with myotonic dystrophy, and 18 healthy control subjects. *, $p < 0.05$ in patients with mitochondrial myopathy vs. both control groups. $^\#$, $p < 0.05$ in patients with mitochondrial myopathy vs. healthy subjects

resting lactate level (Fig. 10). Thus, cycle testing with measurement of lactate does not add to the diagnostic work-up of a patients suspected for mitochondrial myopathy. In line with this, the rate of post exercise recovery of lactate is increased in patients with mitochondrial myopathy, but the rate is identical to patients with myotonic dystrophies and thus not specific for limitation of oxidative capacity due to primary mitochondrial disease [79].

Exercise Training in Patients with Mitochondrial Myopathy

Exercise can improve and even prevent conditions like obesity [83], diabetes [84], and hypertension [85]. Muscle is a highly adaptable tissue, and even a single bout of exercise can change mRNA levels of multiple genes [86–88]. With long-term aerobic training, mitochondrial concentration, aerobic threshold, and functional work capacity are increased in skeletal muscle in both healthy subjects [89, 90] and patients with chronic diseases [29, 30, 91]. The exercise intolerance seen in patients with mitochondrial myopathy is enhanced by a sedentary lifestyle that not only worsens the already impaired exercise capacity but also increases their susceptibility for contracting diabetes and cardiovascular diseases. In order to enhance exercise tolerance, exercise training has been tested in patients with mitochondrial myopathy which will be described in the following sections.

Strength Training

Besides external ophthalmoplegia, patients with mitochondrial myopathy are not usually associated with muscle weakness or muscle atrophy. Nevertheless, patients with large-scale deletions often have mild to moderate proximal weakness with significant progression over time [92]. In line with this, muscle histology often shows increased connective tissue [93], and MRI shows increased muscle fat fractions [94]. Thus, it has been speculated if strength training could be used to counteract the myopathy found in this genotype [95]. Besides increased motor unit recruitment and increased glycolysis capacity, the increase in force is maintained by activation of skeletal muscle stem cell that through activation and additional divisions fuses with the adult myofiber [96].

Only a few studies have investigated the effect of strength training in patients with mitochondrial myopathy [62, 97, 98]. The overall conclusion from those studies is that resistance training increases strength without adverse effects in patients with mitochondrial myopathy. Additionally, resistance

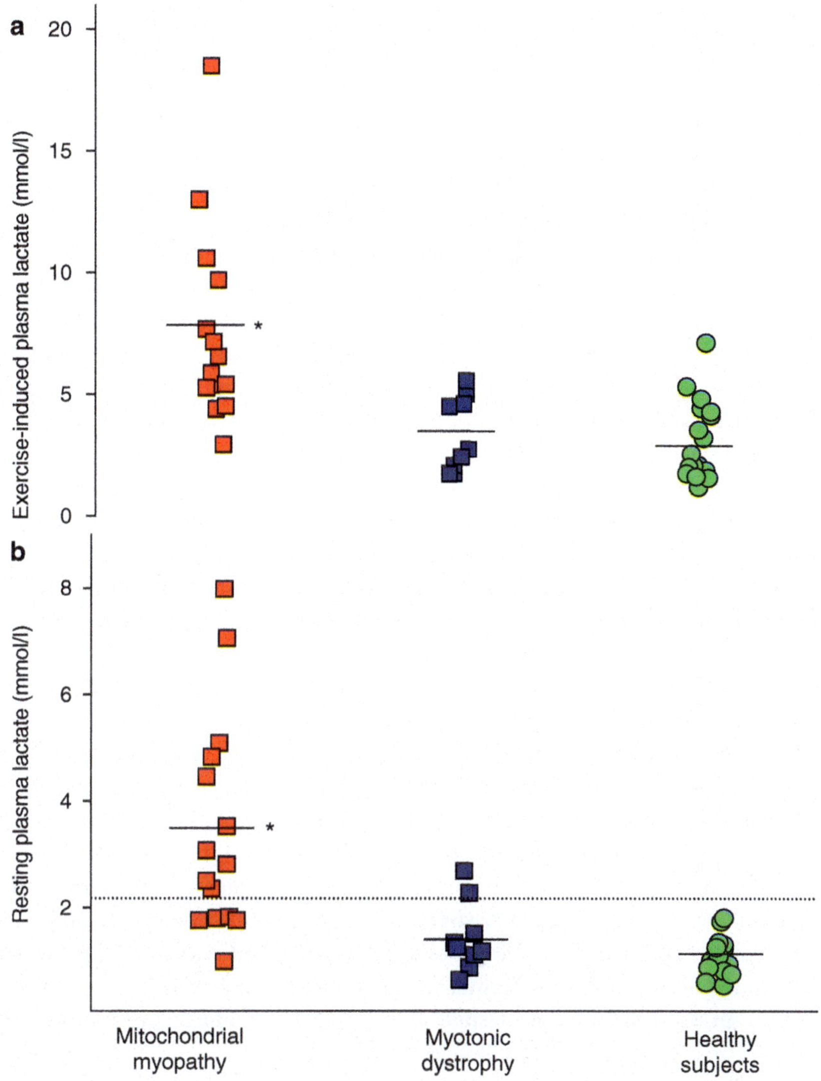

Fig. 10 Plasma lactate during a steady-state cycle exercise test at 65% of VO_{2max} (**a**) and resting plasma lactate levels (**b**). Individual lactate levels in the 20th minute of steady-state cycle exercise at 65% of VO_{2max} (**a**) and resting plasma lactate levels (**b**) in 14 patients with mitochondrial myopathy, 9 patients with myotonic dystrophy, and 18 healthy control subjects. The findings show that the levels of lactate concentration show the same pattern among groups at rest and during exercise). *, $p < 0.05$ in patients with mitochondrial myopathy vs. both control groups. #, $p < 0.05$ in patients with mitochondrial myopathy vs. healthy subjects. #, $p < 0.05$ in patients with mtDNA mutations vs. healthy subjects

training has been used for genetic shift in mtDNA mutation load [97–100]. A case study indicated that satellite cells of patients with sporadic mutations of mtDNA harbor very little if no mtDNA mutation [71], which indicated that induction of myotrauma and thus satellite cell activation and fusion with existing myofiber would result in decrease in mtDNA mutation load. Studies, such as inducing myotrauma artificially by myotoxic agent [100] and muscle biopsies [99] in patients with mitochondrial myopathy, found a substantial upregulation of wild-type mtDNA in regenerated muscle fibers. However, even though a case study indicated that resistance training might be able to induce physiological adaptations in muscle resulting in mtDNA mutation decrease [97], a follow-up study performed in eight patients with single, large-scale deletions showed that 12 weeks of resistance training improved strength, but despite significant myotrauma in trained muscle, there was no significant change in mtDNA mutation load [98]. More recent data on satellite cells of patients with sporadic mtDNA mutations has also questioned previous findings of reluctant mtDNA mutation load in satellite cells, since this study found that satellite cells may, after all, contain the same amount of mutated mtDNA copies, than that of mature muscle cells [101], which for the same reason questions the rationale for gene shifting through myotrauma in skeletal muscle of patients with mitochondrial myopathy.

Endurance Training

Aerobic training induces multiple adaptations which together improve exercise capacity. Among many, some of the important physiologic adaptations include increased oxygen delivery through increased cardiac output, increased vascular tone through induction of vascular conductance, and increased oxygen delivery to contracting muscle through increased number of capillaries in muscle fibers [7, 67]. On muscle fiber level, the level of type I and type IIa fibers is increased [102] due to the increased oxidative demand. Fuel turnover changes from carbohydrate to increased fatty acid oxidation [66, 103], which is met by substantial increase in mitochondrial biogenesis, including increased respiratory chain enzyme levels [7, 89, 104]. The rate and slope of these changes depend on pre-training status, duration, and intensity of training.

Since endurance training obviously increases mitochondrial function, studies have investigated endurance training as potential treatment for impaired oxidative capacity in patients with mitochondrial myopathy [51, 62, 105–112]. These studies have investigated the effect 8–14 weeks of aerobic training (bicycle or treadmill) at workloads of 60–85% of VO_{2max}. The studies found that the change in mitochondrial biogenesis and related lowering of relative level of plasma lactate production from exercised muscle despite high mtDNA mutation load was similar to that found in healthy control subjects. However, finding of increased mtDNA mutation load in 6 of 9 patients after 14 weeks of cycle exercise questioned the safety of aerobic training in patients with mtDNA mutations [51]. Mitochondria are very dynamic organelles and increase in size and number with training and decrease with deconditioning [113]. It is assumed that mtDNA content replicates when mitochondrial number is increased [106, 114–116]. The potential mechanism behind an increase in mutated mtDNA could be that shorter (mutated) mtDNA copies have a replicative advantage over longer (wild-type) copies [71–73, 117, 118], resulting in training-induced increase in mtDNA mutation load when size and number of mitochondria increases [51]. In order to investigate this further, additionally three studies were conducted, investigating the effect of short-term endurance training (12–14 weeks) followed by deconditioning (8–14 weeks) [108, 109] and long-term training (24 months) [112] on mitochondrial biogenesis, i.e., oxygen uptake, mitochondrial respiratory enzyme activity, citrate synthase level, and mtDNA mutation load and copy number. The studies did not find any change in mtDNA mutation load despite a substantial up- and downregulation of mitochondrial capacity with training and deconditioning in the patients with mitochondrial myopathy (Fig. 11). Along with unchanged pathologic findings on muscle biopsy, the studies indicated

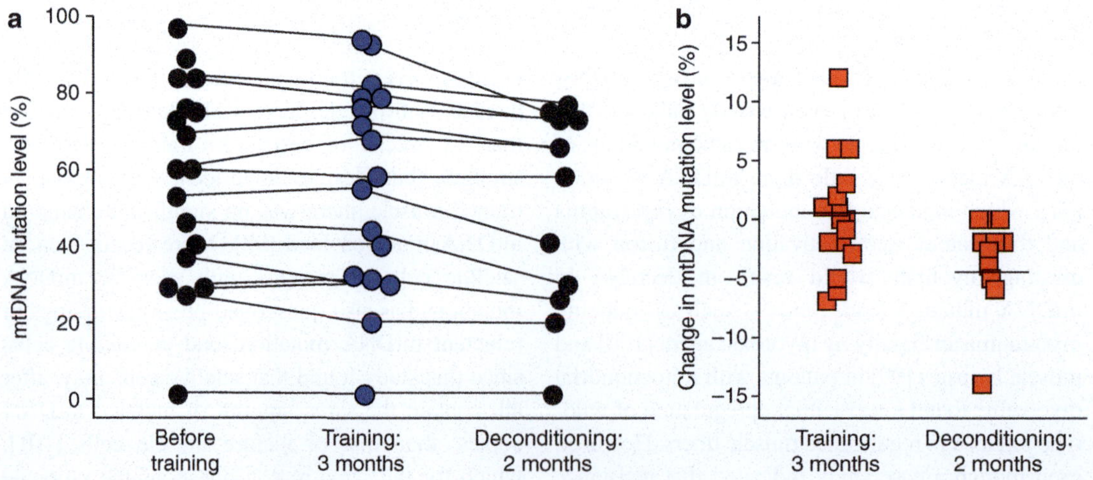

Fig. 11 Training and deconditioning effects on mtDNA mutation load level in skeletal muscle. Individual absolute levels (**a**) and changes (**b**) in mtDNA mutation load level before and after 3 months of training and after 2 months of deconditioning in 20 patients with a wide range of mtDNA mutation load in skeletal muscle (2–99%)

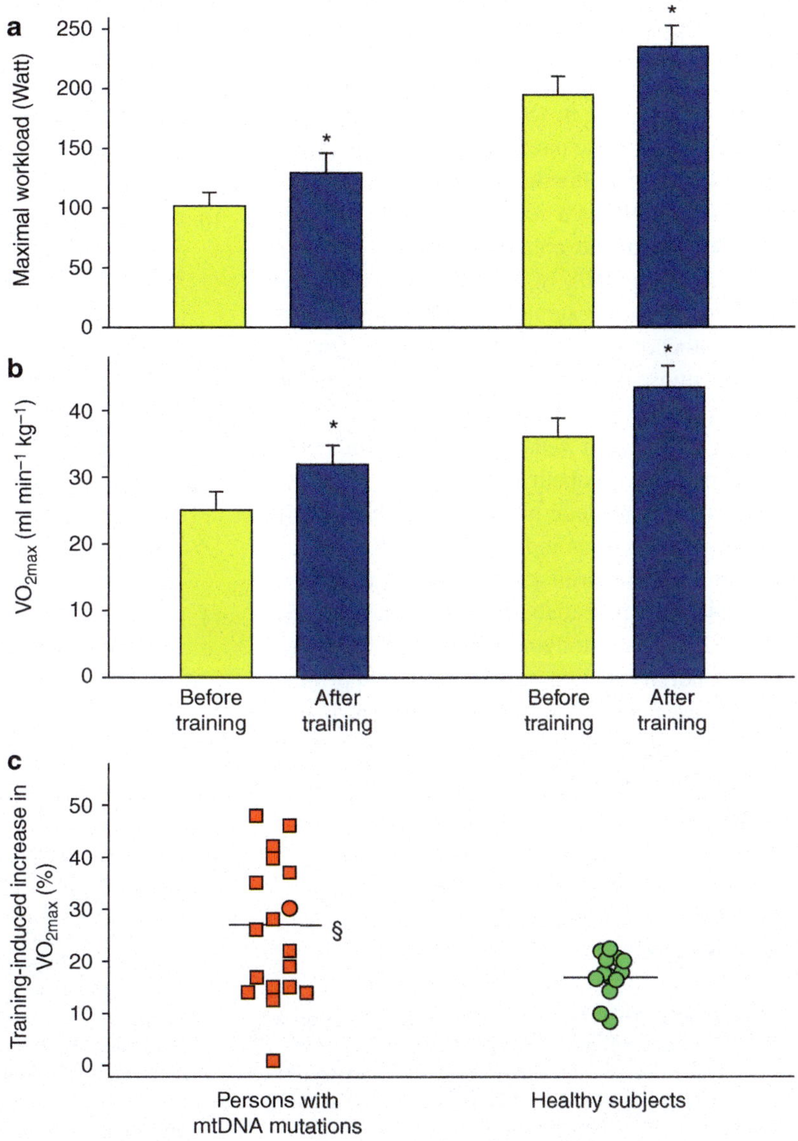

Fig. 12 Training effect on maximal workload capacity and maximal oxygen uptake in patient with mtDNA mutation vs. healthy subjects. Maximal workload (**a**) and oxygen uptake (**b**) before and after 12 weeks of training and training-induced increases in VO_{2max} (**c**) in 20 subjects with mutations of mtDNA (left) and in 13 healthy subjects (open circles). Each symbol in **c** represents a subject. *, $p < 0.05$ compared to before training. §, $p < 0.05$ vs. healthy subjects

that mtDNA mutation may not be selectively replicated over wild type. Thus, endurance training seems to be an efficient and safe method to enhance exercise tolerance in patients with mitochondrial myopathy (Fig. 12).

It is a general concern that patients with mtDNA mutation, due to uncoupling of complexes in the respiratory chain, have an increased level of reactive oxygen species (ROS), which potentially could increase mtDNA mutation burden with time [111, 119–122]. ROS can induce mitochondrial permeability pore, and additionally dysfunctional mitochondria may be even more susceptible to this damage than wild-type mitochondria [119, 121]. Considering this, studies have questioned the safety of long-term training [111, 123]. However, one study investigating the effect after 24 months of endurance training did not find indices of adverse effects of endurance training including an unchanged level of pathological fibers on muscle biopsy, indicating that a potential increased ROS production over 24 months was not able to induce functional deleterious effect on skeletal muscle [112].

Due to the multiorgan affection, patients with mitochondrial myopathy are likely to have both primary (due to beta cell affection in pancreas) and secondary (due to sedentary lifestyle) insulin insensitivity/glucose intolerance. In line with this, patients with mitochondrial insulin resistance and deafness (MIDD) is a common phenotype found in patients with the common 3243A > G point mutation of mtDNA [4, 5, 124]. Thus, another important factor in exercise intolerance in patients with mitochondrial myopathy may be insulin resistance/insensitivity. To our knowledge, no study to date has investigated the influence of training on insulin sensitivity in patients with mitochondrial myopathy. Since mitochondrial dysfunction in skeletal muscle is associated with insulin resistance, as indicated by a 30% reduction in mitochondrial content and function in patients with type 2 diabetes compared to healthy [125, 126]. Thus, studying insulin sensitivity and mitochondrial function in patients with a primary dysfunctional mitochondria would provide insight into the mechanisms behind insulin insensitivity vand exercise intolerance and the influence of mitochondrial dysfunction.

References

1. Fine PE. Mitochondrial inheritance and disease. Lancet Lond Engl. 1978;2(8091):659–62.
2. Leonard JV, Schapira AH. Mitochondrial respiratory chain disorders I: mitochondrial DNA defects. Lancet. 2000;355(9200):299–304.
3. Leonard JV, Schapira AH. Mitochondrial respiratory chain disorders II: neurodegenerative disorders and nuclear gene defects. Lancet. 2000;355(9201):389–94.
4. Jeppesen TD, Schwartz M, Frederiksen AL, Wibrand F, Olsen DB, Vissing J. Muscle phenotype and mutation load in 51 persons with the 3243A>G mitochondrial DNA mutation. Arch Neurol. 2006;63(12):1701–6.
5. Frederiksen AL, Andersen PH, Kyvik KO, Jeppesen TD, Vissing J, Schwartz M. Tissue specific distribution of the 3243A->G mtDNA mutation. J Med Genet. 2006;43(8):671–7.
6. Taivassalo T, Jensen TD, Kennaway N, DiMauro S, Vissing J, Haller RG. The spectrum of exercise tolerance in mitochondrial myopathies: a study of 40 patients. Brain J Neurol. 2003;126(Pt 2):413–23.
7. Andersen P, Saltin B. Maximal perfusion of skeletal muscle in man. J Physiol. 1985;366(1):233–49.
8. Bassett DR Jr, Howley ET. Limiting factors for maximum oxygen uptake and determinants of endurance performance. Med Sci Sports Exerc. 2000;32(1):70–84.
9. Vissing J, Galbo H, Haller RG. Exercise fuel mobilization in mitochondrial myopathy: a metabolic dilemma. Ann Neurol. 1996;40(4):655–62.
10. Haller RG, Lewis SF, Estabrook RW, DiMauro S, Servidei S, Foster DW. Exercise intolerance, lactic acidosis, and abnormal cardiopulmonary regulation in exercise associated with adult skeletal muscle cytochrome c oxidase deficiency. J Clin Invest. 1989;84(1):155–61.
11. Haller RG, Lewis SF. Pathophysiology of exercise performance in muscle disease. Med Sci Sports Exerc. 1984;16(5):456–9.
12. Haller RG, Mukherjee A, Gaffney FA, Blomquist CG. Mitochondrial myopathy presenting as exercise intolerance. Trans Am Neurol Assoc. 1978;103:6–10.
13. Hill AV, Lupton H. Muscular exercise, lactic acid, and the supply and utilization of oxygen. QJM Int J Med. 1923;os-16(62):135–71.
14. Hoppeler H, Weibel ER. Limits for oxygen and substrate transport in mammals. J Exp Biol. 1998;201(Pt 8):1051–64.
15. di Prampero PE. Factors limiting maximal performance in humans. Eur J Appl Physiol. 2003;90(3–4):420–9.
16. Mitchell JH, Sproule BJ, Chapman CB. The physiological meaning of the maximal oxygen intake test. J Clin Invest. 1958;37(4):538–47.
17. Abbott JA, Hirschfeld DS, Kunkel FW, Scheinman MM, Modin G. Graded exercise testing in patients with sinus node dysfunction. Am J Med. 1977;62(3):330–8.
18. Grimby G. Peripheral limiting factors during exercise in chronic lung diseases. Bull Eur Physiopathol Respir. 1977;13(3):381–6.
19. Ørngreen MC, Olsen DB, Vissing J. Exercise tolerance in carnitine palmitoyltransferase II deficiency with IV and oral glucose. Neurology. 2002;59(7):1046–51.
20. Saltin B. Physiological adaptation to physical conditioning. Old problems revisited. Acta Med Scand Suppl. 1986;711:11–24.
21. Bangsbo J, Krustrup P, González-Alonso J, Boushel R, Saltin B. Muscle oxygen kinetics at onset of intense dynamic exercise in humans. Am J Physiol Regul Integr Comp Physiol. 2000;279(3): R899–906.
22. Saltin B, Strange S. Maximal oxygen uptake: "old" and "new" arguments for a cardiovascular limitation. Med Sci Sports Exerc. 1992;24(1):30–7.
23. Berglund B, Ekblom B. Effect of recombinant human erythropoietin treatment on blood pressure and some haematological parameters in healthy men. J Intern Med. 1991;229(2):125–30.
24. Jeppesen TD, Schwartz M, Olsen DB, Vissing J. Oxidative capacity correlates with muscle muta-

tion load in mitochondrial myopathy. Ann Neurol. 2003;54(1):86–92.
25. Chomyn A, Martinuzzi A, Yoneda M, Daga A, Hurko O, Johns D, et al. MELAS mutation in mtDNA binding site for transcription termination factor causes defects in protein synthesis and in respiration but no change in levels of upstream and downstream mature transcripts. Proc Natl Acad Sci U S A. 1992;89(10):4221–5.
26. Boulet L, Karpati G, Shoubridge EA. Distribution and threshold expression of the tRNA(Lys) mutation in skeletal muscle of patients with myoclonic epilepsy and ragged-red fibers (MERRF). Am J Hum Genet. 1992;51(6):1187–200.
27. Charlton GA, Crawford MH. Physiologic consequences of training. Cardiol Clin. 1997;15(3):345–54.
28. Lindstedt SL, Conley KE. Human aerobic performance: too much ado about limits to V(O(2)). J Exp Biol. 2001;204(Pt 18):3195–9.
29. Sveen ML, Jeppesen TD, Hauerslev S, Køber L, Krag TO, Vissing J. Endurance training improves fitness and strength in patients with Becker muscular dystrophy. Brain J Neurol. 2008;131(Pt 11):2824–31.
30. Sveen M-L, Jeppesen TD, Hauerslev S, Krag TO, Vissing J. Endurance training: an effective and safe treatment for patients with LGMD2I. Neurology. 2007;68(1):59–61.
31. Haller RG, Vissing J. Spontaneous "second wind" and glucose-induced second "second wind" in McArdle disease: oxidative mechanisms. Arch Neurol. 2002;59(9):1395–402.
32. Vissing J, Vissing SF, MacLean DA, Saltin B, Quistorff B, Haller RG. Sympathetic activation in exercise is not dependent on muscle acidosis. Direct evidence from studies in metabolic myopathies. J Clin Invest. 1998;101(8):1654–60.
33. Davis JA, Whipp BJ, Lamarra N, Huntsman DJ, Frank MH, Wasserman K. Effect of ramp slope on determination of aerobic parameters from the ramp exercise test. Med Sci Sports Exerc. 1982;14(5):339–43.
34. Martin BJ, Weil JV. CO2 and exercise tidal volume. J Appl Physiol. 1979;46(2):322–5.
35. Goldstein I, Goldstein S, Urbanetti JA, Anthonisen NR. Effects of expiratory threshold loading during steady-state exercise. J Appl Physiol. 1975;39(5):697–701.
36. Davis HA, Bassett J, Hughes P, Gass GC. Anaerobic threshold and lactate turnpoint. Eur J Appl Physiol. 1983;50(3):383–92.
37. Dempsey JA, Vidruk EH, Mitchell GS. Pulmonary control systems in exercise: update. Fed Proc. 1985;44(7):2260–70.
38. Forster HV, Pan LG. Breathing during exercise: demands, regulation, limitations. Adv Exp Med Biol. 1988;227:257–76.
39. Flaherty KR, Wald J, Weisman IM, Zeballos RJ, Schork MA, Blaivas M, et al. Unexplained exertional limitation: characterization of patients with a mitochondrial myopathy. Am J Respir Crit Care Med. 2001;164(3):425–32.
40. Heinicke K, Taivassalo T, Wyrick P, Wood H, Babb TG, Haller RG. Exertional dyspnea in mitochondrial myopathy: clinical features and physiological mechanisms. Am J Physiol Regul Integr Comp Physiol. 2011;301(4):R873–84.
41. Taivassalo T, Haller RG. Exercise and training in mitochondrial myopathies. Med Sci Sports Exerc. 2005;37(12):2094–101.
42. Lykidis CK, Kumar P, Balanos GM. The respiratory responses to the combined activation of the muscle metaboreflex and the ventilatory chemoreflex. Adv Exp Med Biol. 2009;648:281–7.
43. Ørngreen MC, Vissing J, Laforét P. No effect of bezafibrate in patients with CPTII and VLCAD deficiencies. J Inherit Metab Dis. 2015;38(2):373–4.
44. Larsson LE, Linderholm H, Mueller R, Ringqvist T, Soernaes R. Hereditary metabolic myopathy with paroxysmal myoglobinuria due to abnormal glycolysis. J Neurol Neurosurg Psychiatry. 1964;27:361–80.
45. Abe K, Matsuo Y, Kadekawa J, Inoue S, Yanagihara T. Measurement of tissue oxygen consumption in patients with mitochondrial myopathy by noninvasive tissue oximetry. Neurology. 1997;49(3):837–41.
46. Bank W, Chance B. An oxidative defect in metabolic myopathies: diagnosis by noninvasive tissue oximetry. Ann Neurol. 1994;36(6):830–7.
47. Bank W, Chance B. Diagnosis of defects in oxidative muscle metabolism by non-invasive tissue oximetry. Mol Cell Biochem. 1997;174(1–2):7–10.
48. Ozawa T, Sahashi K, Nakase Y, Chance B. Extensive tissue oxygenation associated with mitochondrial DNA mutations. Biochem Biophys Res Commun. 1995;213(2):432–8.
49. Taivassalo T, Abbott A, Wyrick P, Haller RG. Venous oxygen levels during aerobic forearm exercise: an index of impaired oxidative metabolism in mitochondrial myopathy. Ann Neurol. 2002;51(1):38–44.
50. Jensen TD, Kazemi-Esfarjani P, Skomorowska E, Vissing J. A forearm exercise screening test for mitochondrial myopathy. Neurology. 2002;58(10):1533–8.
51. Taivassalo T, Shoubridge EA, Chen J, Kennaway NG, DiMauro S, Arnold DL, et al. Aerobic conditioning in patients with mitochondrial myopathies: physiological, biochemical, and genetic effects. Ann Neurol. 2001;50(2):133–41.
52. Jeppesen TD, Vissing J, González-Alonso J. Influence of erythrocyte oxygenation and intravascular ATP on resting and exercising skeletal muscle blood flow in humans with mitochondrial myopathy. Mitochondrion. 2012;12(3):414–22.
53. Fujii T, Okuno T, Ito M, Hattori H, Mutoh K, Go T, et al. 123I-IMP SPECT findings in mitochondrial encephalomyopathies. Brain Dev. 1995;17(2):89–94.
54. Gropen TI, Prohovnik I, Tatemichi TK, Hirano M. Cerebral hyperemia in MELAS. Stroke. 1994;25(9):1873–6.

55. Ohama E, Ohara S, Ikuta F, Tanaka K, Nishizawa M, Miyatake T. Mitochondrial angiopathy in cerebral blood vessels of mitochondrial encephalomyopathy. Acta Neuropathol (Berl). 1987;74(3):226–33.
56. Nishioka J, Akita Y, Yatsuga S, Katayama K, Matsuishi T, Ishibashi M, et al. Inappropriate intracranial hemodynamics in the natural course of MELAS. Brain Dev. 2008;30(2):100–5.
57. González-Alonso J, Olsen DB, Saltin B. Erythrocyte and the regulation of human skeletal muscle blood flow and oxygen delivery: role of circulating ATP. Circ Res. 2002;91(11):1046–55.
58. González-Alonso J, Mortensen SP, Jeppesen TD, Ali L, Barker H, Damsgaard R, et al. Haemodynamic responses to exercise, ATP infusion and thigh compression in humans: insight into the role of muscle mechanisms on cardiovascular function. J Physiol. 2008;586(9):2405–17.
59. Saltin B. Exercise hyperaemia: magnitude and aspects on regulation in humans. J Physiol. 2007;583(Pt 3):819–23.
60. Jeppesen TD, Orngreen MC, van Hall G, Haller RG, Vissing J. Fat metabolism during exercise in patients with mitochondrial disease. Arch Neurol. 2009;66(3):365–70.
61. Jeppesen TD, Orngreen MC, Van Hall G, Vissing J. Lactate metabolism during exercise in patients with mitochondrial myopathy. Neuromuscul Disord. 2013;23(8):629–36.
62. Cejudo P, Bautista J, Montemayor T, Villagómez R, Jiménez L, Ortega F, et al. Exercise training in mitochondrial myopathy: a randomized controlled trial. Muscle Nerve. 2005;32(3):342–50.
63. Rosenmeier JB, Yegutkin GG, González-Alonso J. Activation of ATP/UTP-selective receptors increases blood flow and blunts sympathetic vasoconstriction in human skeletal muscle. J Physiol. 2008;586(Pt 20):4993–5002.
64. Rosenmeier JB, Hansen J, González-Alonso J. Circulating ATP-induced vasodilatation overrides sympathetic vasoconstrictor activity in human skeletal muscle. J Physiol. 2004;558(Pt 1):351–65.
65. Hawley JA, Burke LM, Phillips SM, Spriet LL. Nutritional modulation of training-induced skeletal muscle adaptations. J Appl Physiol (1985). 2011;110(3):834–45.
66. Saltin B, Astrand PO. Free fatty acids and exercise. Am J Clin Nutr. 1993;57(5 Suppl):752S–7S; discussion 757S-758S
67. Saltin B. Muscle fibre recruitment and metabolism in prolonged exhaustive dynamic exercise. Ciba Found Symp. 1981;82:41–58.
68. Gollnick PD, Piehl K, Saltin B. Selective glycogen depletion pattern in human muscle fibres after exercise of varying intensity and at varying pedalling rates. J Physiol. 1974;241(1):45–57.
69. Van Hall G, Jensen-Urstad M, Rosdahl H, Holmberg H-C, Saltin B, Calbet JAL. Leg and arm lactate and substrate kinetics during exercise. Am J Physiol Endocrinol Metab. 2003;284(1):E193–205.
70. van Hall G. Lactate kinetics in human tissues at rest and during exercise. Acta Physiol (Oxf). 2010;199(4):499–508.
71. Fu K, Hartlen R, Johns T, Genge A, Karpati G, Shoubridge EA. A novel heteroplasmic tRNAleu(CUN) mtDNA point mutation in a sporadic patient with mitochondrial encephalomyopathy segregates rapidly in skeletal muscle and suggests an approach to therapy. Hum Mol Genet. 1996;5(11): 1835–40.
72. Moraes CT, DiMauro S, Zeviani M, Lombes A, Shanske S, Miranda AF, et al. Mitochondrial DNA deletions in progressive external ophthalmoplegia and Kearns-Sayre syndrome. N Engl J Med. 1989;320(20):1293–9.
73. Weber K, Wilson JN, Taylor L, Brierley E, Johnson MA, Turnbull DM, et al. A new mtDNA mutation showing accumulation with time and restriction to skeletal muscle. Am J Hum Genet. 1997;60(2):373–80.
74. Finsterer J, Shorny S, Capek J, Cerny-Zacharias C, Pelzl B, Messner R, et al. Lactate stress test in the diagnosis of mitochondrial myopathy. J Neurol Sci. 1998;159(2):176–80.
75. Dengler R, Wohlfarth K, Zierz S, Jobges M, Schubert M. Muscle fatigue, lactate, and pyruvate in mitochondrial myopathy with progressive external ophthalmoplegia. Muscle Nerve. 1996;19(4):456–62.
76. Siciliano G, Rossi B, Manca L, Angelini C, Tessa A, Vergani L, et al. Residual muscle cytochrome c oxidase activity accounts for submaximal exercise lactate threshold in chronic progressive external ophthalmoplegia. Muscle Nerve. 1996;19(3):342–9.
77. Chan A, Reichmann H, Kögel A, Beck A, Gold R. Metabolic changes in patients with mitochondrial myopathies and effects of coenzyme Q10 therapy. J Neurol. 1998;245(10):681–5.
78. Elliot DL, Buist NR, Goldberg L, Kennaway NG, Powell BR, Kuehl KS. Metabolic myopathies: evaluation by graded exercise testing. Medicine (Baltimore). 1989;68(3):163–72.
79. Jeppesen TD, Olsen D, Vissing J. Cycle ergometry is not a sensitive diagnostic test for mitochondrial myopathy. J Neurol. 2003;250(3):293–9.
80. Finsterer J, Milvay E. Lactate stress testing in 155 patients with mitochondriopathy. Can J Neurol Sci. 2002;29(1):49–53.
81. Finsterer J. Lactate stress testing by bedside lactate determination. Metab Brain Dis. 2003;18(4):265–72.
82. Dandurand RJ, Matthews PM, Arnold DL, Eidelman DH. Mitochondrial disease. Pulmonary function, exercise performance, and blood lactate levels. Chest. 1995;108(1):182–9.
83. Di Meo S, Iossa S, Venditti P. Improvement of obesity-linked skeletal muscle insulin resistance by strength and endurance training. J Endocrinol. 2017;234(3):R159–81.
84. Bruce CR, Hawley JA. Improvements in insulin resistance with aerobic exercise training: a

lipocentric approach. Med Sci Sports Exerc. 2004;36(7):1196–201.
85. Cornelissen VA, Buys R, Smart NA. Endurance exercise beneficially affects ambulatory blood pressure: a systematic review and meta-analysis. J Hypertens. 2013;31(4):639–48.
86. Babij P, Booth FW. Sculpturing new muscle phenotypes. News Physiol Sci. 1988;3:100–2.
87. Booth FW, Watson PA. Control of adaptations in protein levels in response to exercise. Fed Proc. 1985;44(7):2293–300.
88. Hargreaves M, Cameron-Smith D. Exercise, diet, and skeletal muscle gene expression. Med Sci Sports Exerc. 2002;34(9):1505–8.
89. Hoppeler H, Fluck M. Plasticity of skeletal muscle mitochondria: structure and function. Med Sci Sports Exerc. 2003;35(1):95–104.
90. Hood DA. Invited Review: contractile activity-induced mitochondrial biogenesis in skeletal muscle. J Appl Physiol (1985). 2001;90(3):1137–57.
91. Puente-Maestu L, Lázaro A, Tejedor A, Camaño S, Fuentes M, Cuervo M, et al. Effects of exercise on mitochondrial DNA content in skeletal muscle of patients with COPD. Thorax. 2011;66(2):121–7.
92. Grady JP, Campbell G, Ratnaike T, Blakely EL, Falkous G, Nesbitt V, et al. Disease progression in patients with single, large-scale mitochondrial DNA deletions. Brain J Neurol. 2014;137(Pt 2):323–34.
93. Krag TO, Hauerslev S, Jeppesen TD, Duno M, Vissing J. Muscle regeneration in mitochondrial myopathies. Mitochondrion. 2013;13(2):63–70.
94. Hedermann G, Dahlqvist JR, Løkken N, Vissing CR, Knak KL, Andersen LK, et al. Progressive fat replacement of muscle contributes to the disease mechanism of patients with single, large-scale deletions of mitochondrial DNA. Neuromuscul Disord. 2018;28(5):408–13.
95. Phillips BA, Mastaglia FL. Exercise therapy in patients with myopathy. Curr Opin Neurol. 2000;13(5):547–52.
96. Schultz E. Satellite cell behavior during skeletal muscle growth and regeneration. Med Sci Sports Exerc. 1989;21(5 Suppl):S181–6.
97. Taivassalo T, Fu K, Johns T, Arnold D, Karpati G, Shoubridge EA. Gene shifting: a novel therapy for mitochondrial myopathy. Hum Mol Genet. 1999;8(6):1047–52.
98. Murphy JL, Blakely EL, Schaefer AM, He L, Wyrick P, Haller RG, et al. Resistance training in patients with single, large-scale deletions of mitochondrial DNA. Brain J Neurol. 2008;131(Pt 11):2832–40.
99. Shoubridge EA, Johns T, Karpati G. Complete restoration of a wild-type mtDNA genotype in regenerating muscle fibres in a patient with a tRNA point mutation and mitochondrial encephalomyopathy. Hum Mol Genet. 1997;6(13):2239–42.
100. Clark KM, Bindoff LA, Lightowlers RN, Andrews RM, Griffiths PG, Johnson MA, et al. Reversal of a mitochondrial DNA defect in human skeletal muscle. Nat Genet. 1997;16(3):222–4.
101. Spendiff S, Reza M, Murphy JL, Gorman G, Blakely EL, Taylor RW, et al. Mitochondrial DNA deletions in muscle satellite cells: implications for therapies. Hum Mol Genet. 2013;22(23):4739–47.
102. McDermott JC, Bonen A. The regulation of myosin gene transcription in skeletal muscle: effects of altered functional demand. Can J Sport Sci. 1991;16(3):210–22.
103. Bylund AC, Bjurö T, Cederblad G, Holm J, Lundholm K, Sjöstroöm M, et al. Physical training in man. Skeletal muscle metabolism in relation to muscle morphology and running ability. Eur J Appl Physiol. 1977;36(3):151–69.
104. Holloszy JO. Adaptation of skeletal muscle to endurance exercise. Med Sci Sports. 1975;7(3):155–64.
105. Siciliano G, Manca ML, Renna M, Prontera C, Mercuri A, Murri L. Effects of aerobic training on lactate and catecholaminergic exercise responses in mitochondrial myopathies. Neuromuscul Disord. 2000;10(1):40–5.
106. Taivassalo T, De Stefano N, Chen J, Karpati G, Arnold DL, Argov Z. Short-term aerobic training response in chronic myopathies. Muscle Nerve. 1999;22(9):1239–43.
107. Taivassalo T, Matthews PM, De Stefano N, Sripathi N, Genge A, Karpati G, et al. Combined aerobic training and dichloroacetate improve exercise capacity and indices of aerobic metabolism in muscle cytochrome oxidase deficiency. Neurology. 1996;47(2):529–34.
108. Taivassalo T, Gardner JL, Taylor RW, Schaefer AM, Newman J, Barron MJ, et al. Endurance training and detraining in mitochondrial myopathies due to single large-scale mtDNA deletions. Brain J Neurol. 2006;129(Pt 12):3391–401.
109. Jeppesen TD, Schwartz M, Olsen DB, Wibrand F, Krag T, Dunø M, et al. Aerobic training is safe and improves exercise capacity in patients with mitochondrial myopathy. Brain J Neurol. 2006;129(Pt 12):3402–12.
110. Taivassalo T, De Stefano N, Argov Z, Matthews PM, Chen J, Genge A, et al. Effects of aerobic training in patients with mitochondrial myopathies. Neurology. 1998;50(4):1055–60.
111. Siciliano G, Simoncini C, Lo Gerfo A, Orsucci D, Ricci G, Mancuso M. Effects of aerobic training on exercise-related oxidative stress in mitochondrial myopathies. Neuromuscul Disord. 2012;22(Suppl 3):S172–7.
112. Jeppesen TD, Dunø M, Schwartz M, Krag T, Rafiq J, Wibrand F, et al. Short- and long-term effects of endurance training in patients with mitochondrial myopathy. Eur J Neurol. 2009;16(12):1336–9.
113. Neufer PD. The effect of detraining and reduced training on the physiological adaptations to aerobic exercise training. Sports Med. 1989;8(5):302–20.
114. Zoladz JA, Grassi B, Majerczak J, Szkutnik Z, Korostyński M, Karasiński J, et al. Training-induced acceleration of O(2) uptake on-kinetics precedes muscle mitochondrial biogenesis in humans. Exp Physiol. 2013;98(4):883–98.

115. Menshikova EV, Ritov VB, Fairfull L, Ferrell RE, Kelley DE, Goodpaster BH. Effects of exercise on mitochondrial content and function in aging human skeletal muscle. J Gerontol A Biol Sci Med Sci. 2006;61(6):534–40.
116. Lyons CN, Mathieu-Costello O, Moyes CD. Regulation of skeletal muscle mitochondrial content during aging. J Gerontol A Biol Sci Med Sci. 2006;61(1):3–13.
117. Chinnery PF, Samuels DC. Relaxed replication of mtDNA: a model with implications for the expression of disease. Am J Hum Genet. 1999;64(4):1158–65.
118. Larsson NG, Holme E, Kristiansson B, Oldfors A, Tulinius M. Progressive increase of the mutated mitochondrial DNA fraction in Kearns-Sayre syndrome. Pediatr Res. 1990;28(2):131–6.
119. Wu S-B, Ma Y-S, Wu Y-T, Chen Y-C, Wei Y-H. Mitochondrial DNA mutation-elicited oxidative stress, oxidative damage, and altered gene expression in cultured cells of patients with MERRF syndrome. Mol Neurobiol. 2010;41(2–3):256–66.
120. Ikawa M, Okazawa H, Arakawa K, Kudo T, Kimura H, Fujibayashi Y, et al. PET imaging of redox and energy states in stroke-like episodes of MELAS. Mitochondrion. 2009;9(2):144–8.
121. Liu C-Y, Lee C-F, Wei Y-H. Activation of PKCdelta and ERK1/2 in the sensitivity to UV-induced apoptosis of human cells harboring 4977 bp deletion of mitochondrial DNA. Biochim Biophys Acta. 2009;1792(8):783–90.
122. Lu C-Y, Wang EK, Lee H-C, Tsay H-J, Wei Y-H. Increased expression of manganese-superoxide dismutase in fibroblasts of patients with CPEO syndrome. Mol Genet Metab. 2003;80(3):321–9.
123. Adhihetty PJ, Taivassalo T, Haller RG, Walkinshaw DR, Hood DA. The effect of training on the expression of mitochondrial biogenesis- and apoptosis-related proteins in skeletal muscle of patients with mtDNA defects. Am J Physiol Endocrinol Metab. 2007;293(3):E672–80.
124. Frederiksen AL, Jeppesen TD, Vissing J, Schwartz M, Kyvik KO, Schmitz O, et al. High prevalence of impaired glucose homeostasis and myopathy in asymptomatic and oligosymptomatic 3243A>G mitochondrial DNA mutation-positive subjects. J Clin Endocrinol Metab. 2009;94(8):2872–9.
125. Hesselink MKC, Schrauwen-Hinderling V, Schrauwen P. Skeletal muscle mitochondria as a target to prevent or treat type 2 diabetes mellitus. Nat Rev Endocrinol. 2016;12(11):633–45.
126. Hallan S, Sharma K. The role of mitochondria in diabetic kidney disease. Curr Diab Rep. 2016;16(7):61.

Mitochondrial Symptomatic Treatments

Felix Distelmaier and Thomas Klopstock

Introduction

Mitochondrial diseases comprise a heterogeneous group of disorders that can affect any organ system and manifest at any age. The diseases cause a wide range of clinical symptoms including neurodevelopmental regression, movement disorders, muscle weakness, fatigue, epilepsy, depression, neuropathic pain, and progressive multiple-organ dysfunction. Accordingly, mitochondrial diseases impose a severe burden upon patients and their caregivers.

During the last years, researchers have made significant progress in elucidating the genetic and biochemical processes underlying mitochondrial diseases. In view of this knowledge, innovative approaches to treating affected individuals are eagerly awaited. Currently, several studies try to establish causal treatment strategies for specific mitochondrial disease subgroups [1]. However, so far no clinical breakthrough is in sight.

Therefore, management of patients suffering from mitochondrial diseases still mainly relies on symptomatic treatments. Although these approaches do not act on the evolution of the disease, they may improve quality of life and lengthen survival. In the following, we will provide an overview of the symptomatic treatment options for the most relevant clinical problems in mitochondrial disease patients.

Treatment of Epilepsy in Mitochondrial Diseases

High energy demands of the brain make this tissue specifically vulnerable to mitochondrial dysfunction. Clinical features of brain pathology include developmental delay, epilepsy, and movement disorders. Epileptic seizures are a frequently encountered problem in patients with mitochondrial diseases. Most prominent examples are nuclear-encoded defects in *POLG* as well as the mitochondrial DNA-encoded MELAS mutation m.3243A>G or MERRF mutation m.8344A>G [2]. Also patients with pyruvate dehydrogenase complex (PDHc) deficiency typically develop epilepsy during the disease course. In addition, there are numerous other mitochondrial diseases that can manifest with seizures.

F. Distelmaier (✉)
Medical Faculty, Department of General Pediatrics, Neonatology and Pediatric Cardiology, University Children's Hospital, Heinrich-Heine-University, Düsseldorf, Germany
e-mail: Felix.distelmaier@med.uni-duesseldorf.de

T. Klopstock
Department of Neurology, Friedrich-Baur-Institute, Ludwig-Maximilians-University of Munich, Munich, Germany

German Center for Neurodegenerative Diseases (DZNE), Munich, Germany

Munich Cluster for Systems Neurology (SyNergy), Munich, Germany
e-mail: Thomas.Klopstock@med.uni-muenchen.de

M. Mancuso, T. Klopstock (eds.), *Diagnosis and Management of Mitochondrial Disorders*,
https://doi.org/10.1007/978-3-030-05517-2_21

Clinicians involved in the care of these patients frequently feel insecure about antiepileptic drug treatment because of potential side effects on mitochondrial function. This problem is best known for valproate toxicity with liver failure in patients with *POLG* mutations. The mechanism behind this phenomenon appears to be the activation of mitochondrial-dependent apoptosis by permeability transition pore opening [3]. Apart from valproate, also other antiepileptic drugs were discussed to exert negative effects on mitochondrial function. These include carbamazepine, phenytoin, and phenobarbital [4]. However, information on antiepileptic drug mitochondrial toxicity mainly relates to in vitro studies, and clinical reports are limited to single cases. Therefore, it is difficult to provide general recommendations regarding the use of these antiepileptic drugs in mitochondrial disease patients.

For most antiepileptic drugs, information on their interference with mitochondrial energy metabolism is scarce. In clinical practice, antiepileptic drug monotherapy using substances with favorable drug profiles (e.g., levetiracetam, lamotrigine, etc.) is the preferred initial management approach for mitochondrial disease patients. However, for treatment of severe drug-resistant epilepsy, also other antiepileptic drugs and combination of antiepileptic drugs may be considered (also including phenobarbital). In this context, also cannabidiol, a non-psychotropic component of *Cannabis sativa*, might be of interest since it was reported to exhibit beneficial effects on mitochondrial functions in vitro and proved to be beneficial as adjuvant treatment in pediatric-onset drug-resistant epilepsy [5, 6].

Of note, certain mitochondrial defects may specifically improve with ketogenic diet. This treatment option consists of high-fat and low-carbohydrate nutrition, leading to increased formation of ketone bodies, which can be used as alternative substrates for cellular energy metabolism. Especially patients with PDHc deficiency appear to benefit from this strategy [7]. In addition, ketogenic diet was reported to be beneficial in patients with LHON-, MELAS-, or POLG-related mitochondrial diseases. Before starting ketogenic diet, the biochemical and/or genetic defect should be clearly established, and contraindications like fatty acid oxidation disorders, pyruvate carboxylase deficiency, gluconeogenesis disorders, or defects of ketone body synthesis/utilization should be ruled out.

Treatment of Movement Disorders in Mitochondrial Diseases

CNS manifestations of mitochondrial diseases are variable and include symmetric brain stem and basal ganglia lesions (Leigh/Leigh-like disease) as well as leukoencephalopathy or structural abnormalities like dysgenesis of corpus callosum or cerebellar hypoplasia/atrophy. Accordingly, movement disorders are a frequent feature of mitochondrial diseases. Depending on the underlying CNS pathology, patients may suffer from spasticity, dystonia, or ataxia.

Early start of physiotherapy and exercise training as well as adequate supply with mobility aids and orthotic devices are important to improve or preserve motoric functions in mitochondrial disease patients. The use of special seating systems in children with muscular hypotonia facilitates an upright sitting posture for better visual interaction with the environment. Pressure suits are applied in patients with ataxia to increase postural stability.

Drug treatment includes baclofen for treatment of spasticity. Moreover, botulinum toxin injections might be considered. Anticholinergic agents (trihexyphenidyl, biperiden), gabapentin, and/or benzodiazepines are used in patients suffering from dystonia (for overview, see Koy et al. 2016 [8]). Interestingly, certain mitochondrial defects (*MT-ATP6* mutations) can manifest with episodic muscle weakness, mimicking periodic paralysis due to channelopathies [9]. Affected individuals may improve with acetazolamide treatment.

Invasive treatment options such as deep brain stimulation or intrathecal baclofen pump can be considered in severely affected patients. However, in view of the progressive disease course and the risk of metabolic decompensation during an operation, indication for such approaches should be critically discussed. In cases of severe spasticity with joint contractures or painful hip dislocation, orthopedic surgery might be required.

Of note, despite severe movement disorders, cognitive function in many mitochondrial disease patients may be preserved. Therefore, computer-assisted communication devices should be considered.

Management of Nutrition, Feeding Problems, and Metabolic Acidosis

Adequate caloric supply and avoidance of catabolism are the mainstay for many inborn errors of metabolism. This also holds true for patients with mitochondrial diseases. In most cases, no specific diet is required (exceptions are ketogenic diet for PDHc patients, etc.). Of note, patients suffering from mitochondrial diseases may develop feeding problems due to swallowing difficulties, and placement of a nasogastric tube or a percutaneous endoscopic gastrostomy is frequently required.

Importantly, during febrile infections, episodes with vomiting or diarrhea, as well as during fasting periods for diagnostic procedures or operations, infusion therapy should be administered. Intravenous glucose can be started at a rate of 6–8 mg/kg body weight/min and further increased depending on how well infusion therapy is tolerated (e.g., monitoring of lactate and glucose; see below). Intravenous fat can be supplied with around 2–4 g/kg body weight/day [10]. Of note, in some cases rapid intravenous administration of glucose may lead to a parallel increase of blood lactate as well as blood sugar, indicating a problem with cellular glucose metabolism. In such cases, glucose administration rate should be lowered, and caloric supply can be counterbalanced with increased supplementation of fat. Importantly, some mitochondrial defects are also associated with hyperammonemia (e.g., *TMEM70* or *ATP5F1D* mutations), which requires additional detoxification therapy with drugs like L-arginine and sodium benzoate during episodes of metabolic decompensation.

In general, mitochondrial disease patients appear to be at nutritional risk with depletion of muscle mass and a higher incidence of food intolerances [11]. Therefore, regular weight control and nutrition counseling are important for the management of patients with mitochondrial diseases. Of note, failure to thrive and problems gaining weight are variable features, which are of specific relevance in certain disease subgroups. For example, children with *TMEM70* defects typically present with poor weight despite adequate caloric supply. Moreover, patients with mitochondrial neurogastrointestinal encephalopathy (MNGIE) suffer from severe weight loss and vomiting, which can mimic anorexia nervosa or inflammatory bowel disease.

Besides feeding problems, also chronic metabolic acidosis may cause weight loss and failure to thrive. Therefore, oral buffering therapy using sodium bicarbonate or sodium citrate might be considered in some patients. During episodes with severe lactic acidosis during metabolic decompensation, intravenous buffering should be applied (for details, see Danhauser et al., 2015 [10]).

Dietary Supplements

There exist numerous ideas and theories about supplementary treatments with vitamins and cofactors for patients with mitochondrial diseases. These dietary supplements are also known as "nutraceuticals," suggesting that they are food-derived compounds with comparable properties as regular pharmaceuticals. The main hypotheses about these therapeutic strategies include improvement of respiratory chain function, reduction of oxidative stress, and augmentation of cellular energy pools.

Typical examples of nutraceuticals include vitamins with cofactor properties like thiamine (vitamin B1), riboflavin (vitamin B2), and biotin (vitamin B7), as well as the non-vitamin cofactor coenzyme Q_{10} (and its derivatives). In addition, antioxidants like alpha lipoic acid, γ-tocopherol (vitamin E), and ascorbic acid (vitamin C) are frequently used in the context of mitochondrial disorders. Finally, energy substrates such as carnitine or creatine are often part of such "mito-cocktails."

In most patients, these strategies are not evidence-based and therapeutic effects were only described for individual cases. Therefore, clear recommendations regarding dosage and combination of these compounds are difficult to provide. Nevertheless, it should be appreciated that certain patients may benefit from dietary supplements and it is important to discuss these options openly with affected families. Of note, it is recommended to establish baseline parameters for monitoring the treatment course (e.g., physical exam and laboratory parameters before and during supplementation therapy, etc.).

Importantly, there are several disorders among the large group of mitochondrial diseases that specifically benefit from vitamin or cofactor administration [12]. The most important example is thiamine deficiency disorders caused by defects in transporter proteins (e.g., *SLC19A3* mutations, etc.). Children typically present with acute episodes with encephalopathy, dystonia, seizures, and Leigh-like basal ganglia changes on brain MRI. Administration of thiamine (20–40 mg/kg body weight/day) and biotin (15 mg/kg body weight/day) greatly improves the clinical condition in these patients and prevents further episodes with metabolic decompensation. Therefore, in children with unclear basal ganglia lesions, a therapeutic trial with thiamine is recommended.

Apart from thiamine, riboflavin is an important cofactor that plays a role in the assembly of mitochondrial complex I. Accordingly, riboflavin treatment (around 10 mg/kg body weight/day) can be tried in patients with mitochondrial complex I deficiency. Especially some of the patients with *ACAD9* mutations appear to benefit from this strategy.

Supplementation of coenzyme Q_{10} is the treatment of choice in coenzyme Q_{10} biosynthesis defects (around 30 mg/kg body weight/day). However, clinical response to treatment is variable, and especially early-onset diseases with severe CNS involvement have a poor prognosis despite coenzyme Q_{10} therapy. The main problem with oral coenzyme Q_{10} supplementation is the low bioavailability. Different coenzyme Q_{10} formulations try to solve this problem. However, clinical studies investigating the efficiency of such approaches are lacking. In theory, therapies using CoQ precursor compounds targeting the specific genetic defect might offer a future treatment perspective [13].

Finally, patients with mitochondrial disease may develop secondary carnitine deficiency, and supplementation of L-carnitine (50–100 mg/kg/day) should be performed in case of abnormal acylcarnitine profile analysis [14].

Management of Headaches and Metabolic Strokes in Mitochondrial Diseases

Migraine as well as migraine-like headaches is an important feature of different mitochondrial diseases including MELAS and MERRF. The reason for this phenomenon is still unclear. In MELAS patients, there seems to be a smooth transition between migraine-like headaches and metabolic strokes, suggesting a problem with vascular energy metabolism and autoregulation (see below). However, in the general mitochondrial disease population, tension-type headache seems to be the most frequent headache phenotype [15]. The underlying pathophysiology of tension-type headache is multifactorial and includes peripheral mechanisms (myofascial nociception) as well as central mechanisms (inadequate endogenous pain control [16]).

Therapy of headaches in mitochondrial diseases usually does not differ compared to headaches caused by other conditions [17]. There are no general contraindications known regarding frequently used drugs like metamizole, nonsteroidal anti-inflammatory drugs, triptans, benzodiazepines, or steroids.

As discussed above, migraine-like headaches may herald metabolic strokes. These are characteristic complications of the common MELAS m.3243A>G mutation. However, they can also occur in a variety of other mitochondrial diseases [18]. The underlying pathophysiology involves disturbed energy metabolism in cerebral endothelial smooth muscle cells and reduced circulating nitric oxide levels in specific brain regions [19]. Of note, stroke-like lesions do not follow a typical vascular territory pattern like thrombotic strokes.

In 2005, Koga et al. reported that L-arginine ameliorates the clinical course of MELAS patients during stroke-like episodes [20]. In the following, several clinical studies further supported this concept. Moreover, it was shown that also mitochondrial diseases other than MELAS might benefit from this strategy [18]. During acute stroke-like episodes, it is suggested giving L-arginine 500 mg/kg body weight as an intravenous bolus over 1–3 h. This approach can be repeated every 24 h in case of insufficient response to initial therapy [18]. Oral L-arginine maintenance therapy comprises 100–300 mg/kg body weight/day.

Apart from L-arginine, also intravenous corticosteroids were described as effective by several authors during the acute management of stroke-like episodes [21]. Moreover, treatment of epileptic seizures during stroke-like episodes appears to be most important to avoid further neuronal damage. Other substances like dichloroacetate, coenzyme Q_{10}, or idebenone are of no proven value in stroke-like episodes.

Extracerebral Organ Manifestations in Mitochondrial Diseases

Mitochondrial diseases can affect multiple organ systems outside of the CNS including the skeletal and heart muscle, liver, pancreas, kidneys, thyroid, as well as bone marrow. The involvement of these organ systems varies greatly among the different disease subgroups and may be characteristic for specific genetic defects in some patients. Accordingly, a detailed interdisciplinary workup of affected individuals is important for identifying specific clinical problems that need to be addressed.

A typical example of mitochondrial diseases with gastrointestinal problems is mitochondrial neurogastrointestinal encephalopathy (MNGIE). The disease is characterized by progressive gastrointestinal dysmotility and cachexia in combination with ophthalmoparesis, leukoencephalopathy, and peripheral neuropathy [22]. Patients suffer from nausea, dysphagia, abdominal pain, and diarrhea. Management comprises antiemetic drugs, parenteral feeding, and antibiotics for intestinal bacterial overgrowth, hemodialysis for detoxification with removal of thymidine and deoxyuridine, as well as bone marrow transplantation [23].

Another example is Pearson syndrome, a disorder caused by mtDNA deletions leading to exocrine pancreatic insufficiency, bone marrow failure, and variable CNS involvement. Supportive therapy includes pancreatic enzyme replacement, blood transfusions, as well as granulocyte-colony-stimulating factor application [24].

In addition, there are several mitochondrial diseases that manifest with liver failure (e.g., defects in *DGUOK*, *MPV17*, *SUCLG1*, *POLG1*, etc.). Supportive management includes supplementation of vitamin K, administration of fresh frozen plasma, and treatment of hypoglycemia. Of note, among the mitochondrial diseases with liver failure, defects in *TRMU* play a special role as they cause transient hepatic problems, which resolve spontaneously after the first year of life. In view of the favorable long-term prognosis without neurological impairment, liver transplantation is a therapeutic option in *TRMU* patients with severe liver failure.

Endocrine dysfunction is a variable feature of different mitochondrial diseases and comprises diabetes mellitus, growth hormone deficiency, adrenal dysfunction, hypogonadism, and hypoparathyroidism as well as thyroid dysfunction [25]. The most prominent examples of mitochondrial diseases with multiple endocrinopathies are MELAS (especially for the m.3243A>G mutation) and Kearns-Sayre syndrome [26]. MELAS patients frequently develop diabetes mellitus. Moreover, growth hormone deficiency and hypogonadism are recognized disease features. Patients with Kearns-Sayre syndrome may suffer from hypoparathyroidism, thyroid dysfunction, hypogonadism, and growth hormone deficiency. Primary testicular or ovarian failure was reported in patients with *POLG* mutations as well as in patients with MNGIE. In general, endocrine laboratory workup should be performed on a regular basis in mitochondrial disease patients, and manifest hormone deficiencies should be treated with replacement therapies.

Renal involvement in mitochondrial diseases ranges from tubulopathy with loss of electrolytes to steroid-resistant nephrotic syndrome and renal failure [27]. Again, patients with MELAS have to be mentioned in this context as many affected individuals develop focal segmental glomerular sclerosis and proteinuria. Steroid-resistant nephrotic syndrome is a characteristic feature of several coenzyme Q_{10} biosynthesis defects. Especially mutations in *COQ2* appear to cause this problem. Of note coenzyme Q_{10} biosynthesis defects might benefit from coenzyme Q_{10} substitution (see above). However, response to treatment mostly appears to be unsatisfactory. Regarding *COQ2* defects, 4-hydroxybenzoic acid might be a promising compound for future trials [28]. Renal tubulopathy is a variable feature observed in many different mitochondrial diseases [29]. Clinical features range from asymptomatic patients to cases with severe electrolyte imbalance requiring substitution therapies. In cases with renal failure, peritoneal dialysis might be required.

Sensorineural hearing loss can be a feature of a variety of mitochondrial diseases including MELAS, MERRF, and Kearns-Sayre syndrome, *POLG*-related disorders, CoQ_{10} biosynthesis defects, etc. [30]. Onset of symptoms can be slowly progressive or sudden (e.g., during episodes with stress, trauma, and metabolic decompensation). In some mitochondrial diseases, there is an increased susceptibility to aminoglycoside-induced ototoxicity. This is especially the case in m.1555A>G and the m.1494C>T mutations, affecting the mitochondrial 12S rRNA. Diagnosis of hearing loss is essential to avoid problems with speech development in young children. Application of hearing aids as well as cochlear implants should be considered.

Apart from skeletal muscle, cardiac muscle as well as the cardiac conduction system is affected in many mitochondrial diseases. The prevalence of cardiac affection in children with mitochondrial disease was estimated as high as 20–40% [31]. Hypertrophic cardiomyopathy is the most common form and constitutes a characteristic disease feature in a broad range of genetic defects including *TMEM70*, *ACAD9*, *NDUFS4*, *SUCLG1*, *SDHA*, *COX10*, *COX14*, *COX15*, etc. However, also other types of cardiomyopathies were reported in literature (e.g., dilated, restrictive, or non-compaction cardiomyopathy). Heart failure, arrhythmias, and sudden cardiac death might be the consequence. Therefore, regular monitoring of cardiac function is important in mitochondrial disease patients (especially in genetic defects with known cardiac involvement). Symptomatic treatments include drug therapy (e.g., propranolol, diuretics), cardiac pacing, as well as defibrillator placement [32].

Ophthalmic manifestations of mitochondrial disease comprise progressive external ophthalmoplegia, pigmentary retinopathy, and optic neuropathy [33]. The most important examples of mitochondrial diseases with optic neuropathy are LHON and autosomal dominant as well as autosomal recessive optic atrophy. Pigmentary retinopathy is a typical complication in the course of NARP (neurogenic muscle weakness, ataxia, and retinitis pigmentosa), MELAS, MERRF, and Kearns-Sayre syndrome. In the case of LHON, administration of idebenone is the most important approach for treating visual impairment. For other mitochondrial diseases with ocular involvement, supportive treatment consisting of visual aids/special glasses or suspension surgery for severe ptosis is still the mainstay of therapy.

Treatment of Psychiatric Conditions in Mitochondrial Diseases

Neuropsychiatric conditions in mitochondrial diseases range from depression and anxiety to attention-deficit hyperactivity disorders or autism spectrum disorders. Especially depressive disorders constitute an important problem in adolescents and adults suffering from mitochondrial diseases [34]. Diagnosis of a chronic disorder with unfavorable prognosis as well as progressive organ dysfunction (e.g., visual impairment, hearing problems, stroke-like episodes, etc.) leads to a disruption of everyday life, affecting work and school as well as social and family contexts. Accordingly, physicians should screen mitochondrial disease patients for distress, and psychiatrists, psychologists, and social workers should be involved in the care of patients with mood disorders. Psychotherapy as well as antidepressant medication might be required.

Some children with mitochondrial diseases may present with severe behavioral problems (e.g., hyperactivity, aggression, etc.), and application of antipsychotic (e.g., risperidone, dipiperon) is a therapeutic option. In cases with sleep disturbances, melatonin can be a safe and effective treatment option [35]. Chloral hydrate as well as clobazam might be administered in children for the acute management of severe irritability.

Palliative Care in Mitochondrial Diseases

Progressive multi-organ affection in mitochondrial diseases may cause a broad range of clinical problems including abnormal breathing patterns, respiratory insufficiency, swallowing difficulties, central fever, dystonia, or spasticity. Accordingly, mitochondrial diseases constitute a high burden for patients and primary caregivers. Moreover, frequent hospitalizations may impair quality of life for affected individuals. Given the lack of therapeutic options, palliative care should be considered in the management of these patients. This especially holds true for infants and young children with severe, early-onset mitochondrial diseases (e.g., infantile Leigh syndrome, etc.). Specialized palliative care teams may provide a support system for affected families, including management of distressing symptoms, social and practical help, as well as psychological support. Thereby, the rate of hospitalizations can be reduced and patients may spend more of their remaining time in a familiar environment. Although the clinical course of severe mitochondrial diseases is difficult to predict, communicating the prognosis and end-of-life issues is an important part of patient care. Ideally, these discussions should take place in a non-acute setting. The aim is to agree on clear directives regarding the patient's/parent's wishes about the extent of medical care at the end of life (e.g., to limit life-sustaining treatments, etc.).

References

1. Koopman WJ, Beyrath J, Fung CW, Koene S, Rodenburg RJ, Willems PH, Smeitink JA. Mitochondrial disorders in children: toward development of small-molecule treatment strategies. EMBO Mol Med. 2016;8:311–27.
2. Whittaker RG, Devine HE, Gorman GS, Schaefer AM, Horvath R, Ng Y, Nesbitt V, Lax NZ, McFarland R, Cunningham MO, Taylor RW, Turnbull DM. Epilepsy in adults with mitochondrial disease: a cohort study. Ann Neurol. 2015;78:949–57.
3. Li S, Guo J, Ying Z, Chen S, Yang L, Chen K, Long Q, Qin D, Pei D, Liu X. Valproic acid-induced hepatotoxicity in Alpers syndrome is associated with mitochondrial permeability transition pore opening-dependent apoptotic sensitivity in an induced pluripotent stem cell model. Hepatology. 2015;61:1730–9.
4. Finsterer J, Zarrouk Mahjoub S. Epilepsy in mitochondrial disorders. Seizure. 2012;21:316–21.
5. Finsterer J, Scorza FA. Effects of antiepileptic drugs on mitochondrial functions, morphology, kinetics, biogenesis, and survival. Epilepsy Res. 2017;136:5–11.
6. Stockings E, Zagic D, Campbell G, Weier M, Hall WD, Nielsen S, Herkes GK, Farrell M, Degenhardt L. Evidence for cannabis and cannabinoids for epilepsy: a systematic review of controlled and observational evidence. J Neurol Neurosurg Psychiatry. 2018;89(7):741–53. https://doi.org/10.1136/jnnp-2017-317168.
7. Scholl-Bürgi S, Höller A, Pichler K, Michel M, Haberlandt E, Karall D. Ketogenic diets in patients with inherited metabolic disorders. J Inherit Metab Dis. 2015;38:765–73.
8. Koy A, Lin JP, Sanger TD, Marks WA, Mink JW, Timmermann L. Advances in management of movement disorders in children. Lancet Neurol. 2016;15:719–35.
9. Auré K, Dubourg O, Jardel C, Clarysse L, Sternberg D, Fournier E, Laforêt P, Streichenberger N, Petiot P, Gervais-Bernard H, Vial C, Bedat-Millet AL, Drouin-Garraud V, Bouillaud F, Vandier C, Fontaine B, Lombès A. Episodic weakness due to mitochondrial DNA MT-ATP6/8 mutations. Neurology. 2013;81:1810–8.
10. Danhauser K, Smeitink JA, Freisinger P, Sperl W, Sabir H, Hadzik B, Mayatepek E, Morava E, Distelmaier F. Treatment options for lactic acidosis and metabolic crisis in children with mitochondrial disease. J Inherit Metab Dis. 2015;38:467–75.
11. Aubry E, Aeberhard C, Bally L, Nuoffer JM, Risch L, Mühlebach S, Burgunder JM, Stanga Z. Are patients affected by mitochondrial disorders at nutritional risk? Nutrition. 2018;47:56–62.
12. Distelmaier F, Haack TB, Wortmann SB, Mayr JA, Prokisch H. Treatable mitochondrial diseases: cofactor metabolism and beyond. Brain. 2017;140:e11.

13. Herebian D, López LC, Distelmaier F. Bypassing human CoQ10 deficiency. Mol Genet Metab. 2018;123:289–91.
14. Infante JP, Huszagh VA. Secondary carnitine deficiency and impaired docosahexaenoic (22:6n-3) acid synthesis: a common denominator in the pathophysiology of diseases of oxidative phosphorylation and beta-oxidation. FEBS Lett. 2000;468:1–5.
15. Kraya T, Deschauer M, Joshi PR, Zierz S, Gaul C. Prevalence of headache in patients with mitochondrial disease: a cross-sectional study. Headache. 2018;58:45–52.
16. Fumal A, Schoenen J. Tension-type headache: current research and clinical management. Lancet Neurol. 2008;7:70–83.
17. Finsterer J, Zarrouk-Mahjoub S. Headache in mitochondrial disorders. Clin Neurol Neurosurg. 2018;166:44–9.
18. Ganetzky RD, Falk MJ. 8-year retrospective analysis of intravenous arginine therapy for acute metabolic strokes in pediatric mitochondrial disease. Mol Genet Metab. 2018;123:301–8.
19. Koenig MK, Emrick L, Karaa A, Korson M, Scaglia F, Parikh S, Goldstein A. Recommendations for the management of strokelike episodes in patients with mitochondrial encephalomyopathy, lactic acidosis, and strokelike episodes. JAMA Neurol. 2016;73:591–4.
20. Koga Y, Akita Y, Nishioka J, Yatsuga S, Povalko N, Tanabe Y, Fujimoto S, Matsuishi T. L-arginine improves the symptoms of strokelike episodes in MELAS. Neurology. 2005;64:710–2.
21. Fryer RH, Bain JM, De Vivo DC. Mitochondrial encephalomyopathy lactic acidosis and stroke-like episodes (MELAS): a case report and critical reappraisal of treatment options. Pediatr Neurol. 2016;56:59–61.
22. Hirano M. Mitochondrial neurogastrointestinal encephalopathy disease. In: Adam MP, Ardinger HH, Pagon RA, Wallace SE, Bean LJH, Stephens K, Amemiya A, editors. GeneReviews® [Internet]. Seattle, WA: University of Washington, Seattle; 1993–2018; 2005. [updated 2016 Jan 14]
23. Halter J, Schüpbach W, Casali C, Elhasid R, Fay K, Hammans S, Illa I, Kappeler L, Krähenbühl S, Lehmann T, Mandel H, Marti R, Mattle H, Orchard K, Savage D, Sue CM, Valcarcel D, Gratwohl A, Hirano M. Allogeneic hematopoietic SCT as treatment option for patients with mitochondrial neurogastrointestinal encephalomyopathy (MNGIE): a consensus conference proposal for a standardized approach. Bone Marrow Transplant. 2011;46:330–7.
24. Baertling F, Meissner T, Troeger A, Pillekamp F, Mayatepek E, Laws HJ, Distelmaier F. Granulocyte colony stimulating factor for treatment of neutropenia-associated infection in Pearson syndrome. Klin Padiatr. 2014;226:190–1.
25. Chow J, Rahman J, Achermann JC, Dattani MT, Rahman S. Mitochondrial disease and endocrine dysfunction. Nat Rev Endocrinol. 2017;13:92–104.
26. Schaefer AM, Walker M, Turnbull DM, Taylor RW. Endocrine disorders in mitochondrial disease. Mol Cell Endocrinol. 2013;379:2–11.
27. Emma F, Salviati L. Mitochondrial cytopathies and the kidney. Nephrol Ther. 2017;13(Suppl 1):S23–8.
28. Herebian D, Seibt A, Smits SHJ, Rodenburg RJ, Mayatepek E, Distelmaier F. 4-Hydroxybenzoic acid restores CoQ10 biosynthesis in human COQ2 deficiency. Ann Clin Transl Neurol. 2017;4:902–8.
29. Martín-Hernández E, García-Silva MT, Vara J, Campos Y, Cabello A, Muley R, Del Hoyo P, Martín MA, Arenas J. Renal pathology in children with mitochondrial diseases. Pediatr Nephrol. 2005;20:1299–305.
30. Yelverton JC, Arnos K, Xia XJ, Nance WE, Pandya A, Dodson KM. The clinical and audiologic features of hearing loss due to mitochondrial mutations. Otolaryngol Head Neck Surg. 2013;148:1017–22.
31. El-Hattab AW, Scaglia F. Mitochondrial cardiomyopathies. Front Cardiovasc Med. 2016;3:25.
32. Lee TM, Hsu DT, Kantor P, Towbin JA, Ware SM, Colan SD, Chung WK, Jefferies JL, Rossano JW, Castleberry CD, Addonizio LJ, Lal AK, Lamour JM, Miller EM, Thrush PT, Czachor JD, Razoky H, Hill A, Lipshultz SE. Pediatric cardiomyopathies. Circ Res. 2017;121:855–73.
33. Finsterer J, Mancuso M, Pareyson D, Burgunder JM, Klopstock T. Mitochondrial disorders of the retinal ganglion cells and the optic nerve. Mitochondrion. 2018;42:1–10. https://doi.org/10.1016/j.mito.2017.10.003.
34. Morava E, Gardeitchik T, Kozicz T, de Boer L, Koene S, de Vries MC, McFarland R, Roobol T, Rodenburg RJ, Verhaak CM. Depressive behaviour in children diagnosed with a mitochondrial disorder. Mitochondrion. 2010;10:528–33.
35. Ayyash HF, Preece P, Morton R, Cortese S. Melatonin for sleep disturbance in children with neurodevelopmental disorders: prospective observational naturalistic study. Expert Rev Neurother. 2015;15:711–7.

Experimental Therapies

Carlo Viscomi and Massimo Zeviani

Introduction

Experimental Therapeutic Strategies

Remarkable progress has been made in recent years on understanding both the fundamental pathogenic processes underlying mitochondrial disease and the mechanisms of mitochondrial biogenesis and signalling. Building on this wealth of knowledge, a number of therapeutic strategies have recently been proposed to combat mitochondrial disorders, for which experimental evidence is accumulating in cellular and animal models. These can be broadly divided in approaches that could in principle be applied to a wide spectrum of different disease conditions and strategies tailored to a single disease (Table 1). The first group of strategies includes (1) activation of mitochondrial biogenesis; (2) regulation/activation of mitochondrial stress response pathways; (3) inhibition of apoptosis; (4) scavenging of toxic compounds; (5) bypass of electron transfer chain defects; and (6) nuclear transfer. The second group includes (1) scavenging of specific toxic compounds in specific diseases, (2) supplementation of nucleotides, and (3) gene and cell replacement therapies. Each of these strategies can be implemented by several approaches, such as pharmacological treatments, gene transfer which replaces the missing gene or expresses a therapeutic protein, and stem cell/organ transplantation. This chapter will focus on emerging experimental (i.e. preclinical) therapies for mitochondrial disease.

C. Viscomi · M. Zeviani (✉)
MRC-Mitochondrial Biology Unit, University of Cambridge, Cambridge, UK
e-mail: mdz21@mrc-mbu.cam.ac.uk

Pharmacological and Metabolic Interventions

Increasing Mitochondrial Biogenesis

Mitochondrial diseases are hallmarked by bioenergetics defects, ultimately leading to decreased ATP synthesis. Thus, therapeutic interventions aimed at increasing the ATP levels available to cells may be beneficial. Importantly, mitochondrial disease become manifest when the residual activity of the defective gene product, either mitochondrial or nuclear encoded, falls below a critical threshold, suggesting that even partial restoration of the activity may be sufficient to rescue or at least ameliorate the phenotype. The idea that mitochondrial biogenesis is critical to determine the phenotypic outcome of disease has been boosted by the recent observation that increased mitochondrial content protects non-manifesting carriers of the LHON mutations. This can partly explain the incomplete penetrance of the disease and opens the possibility to stimulate mitochondrial biogenesis as a therapeutic strategy for LHON [1].

M. Mancuso, T. Klopstock (eds.), *Diagnosis and Management of Mitochondrial Disorders*,
https://doi.org/10.1007/978-3-030-05517-2_22

Increased mitochondrial biogenesis is a physiological response to stress conditions (e.g. cold, exercise, nutritional status), which is activated to meet the energetic requirements of tissues [2].

The best characterized pathways controlling mitochondrial biogenesis (Fig. 1) are centred on the actions of the peroxisome proliferator-activated receptor gamma (PPARγ) coactivators 1α and β (the PGC family). PGC proteins interact with and activate several transcription factors, including the nuclear respiratory factors (NRF1 and NRF2) and the peroxisome proliferator-activated receptors (PPAR α, β, and γ), among others. NRFs and PPARs in turn increase the transcription of genes related to oxidative phosphorylation (OXPHOS) and fatty acid oxidation (FAO) pathways, respectively. PGC-1α is the best characterized PGC protein. Its activity is inhibited by acetylation, which in turn is controlled by the acetylase GCN5 and deacetylase SIRT1, and is increased by phosphorylation, which depends on the activities of several kinases, including AMP-dependent kinase (AMPK) [3, 4]. Importantly, as AMPK and SIRT1 are druggable enzymes, they have been exploited in several preclinical experiments to activate PGC-1α and induce mitochondrial biogenesis.

Table 1 Experimental therapies for mitochondrial diseases

	Strategy
Generalist	• Activation of mitochondrial biogenesis • Modulation of autophagy • Inhibition of apoptosis • Scavenging of ROS
	• Endurance training • Dietary manipulation
	• Bypassing RC block • ZFNs or TALENs to shift heteroplasmy • Overexpressing aaRSs to stabilize mutated mt-tRNA • Somatic nuclear transfer
Disease-tailored	• Scavenging of toxic compounds • Supplementation of nucleotides
	• Replacement of the missing gene

Several compounds have been proposed to stimulate mitochondrial biogenesis, including bezafibrate [4], a pan-PPAR agonist widely used to treat metabolic syndrome and diabetes; AICAR, an agonist of the AMP-dependent kinase (AMPK); and nicotinamide riboside, a precursor of NAD^+. Bezafibrate was shown to improve the defective activities of the respiratory chain complexes, dependent on the induction of PGC-1α activity in cellular models carrying mutations in genes encoding complex I subunits and in cybrids harbouring pathological tRNA mutations [5] and complex IV in *SCO2*-mutant fibroblasts [6]. Bastin et al. [7]

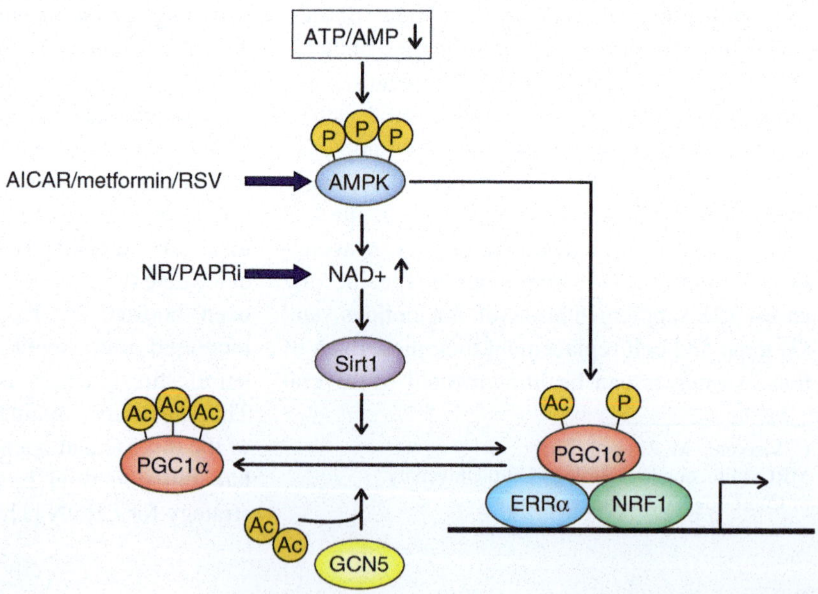

Fig. 1 PGC1α-dependent mitochondriogenic pathway and its pharmacological modulation (From [117] with permission)

reported an increase of OXPHOS markers in bezafibrate-treated CPT2-mutant patients, but no evidence of clinical efficacy in mitochondrial disease patients has so far been reported.

By using the AMPK agonist AICAR, Viscomi et al. obtained robust induction of OXPHOS-related gene transcription and increase of respiratory chain complex activities in three models of COX deficiency, namely, a *Surf1* constitutive knockout mouse (*Surf1*$^{-/-}$), a *Sco2* knockout/knockin (*Sco2*^{KOKI}) mouse, and a muscle-specific *Cox15* (*ACTA-Cox15*$^{-/-}$) mouse [8]. The increase in the respiratory chain activities resulted in striking improvement of motor endurance in the *Sco2*^{KOKI}, but not in *ACTA-Cox15*$^{-/-}$ mice, possibly because of the more severe clinical phenotype of the *ACTA-Cox15*$^{-/-}$ mouse model. Interestingly, Peralta and coworkers showed that AICAR improves muscle function by promoting fibre regeneration and that the effect on mitochondrial biogenesis is part of this reparative process [9].

A further strategy to activate PGC-1α is to promote its deacetylation via Sirtuin 1 (Sirt1). Sirt1 is a nuclear deacetylase that utilizes the NAD^+ moiety to deacetylate acetyl-lysine residues of proteins. Notably, NAD^+ exerts a substrate-dependent activation of Sirt1, which plays a homeostatic role by setting up mitochondrial biogenesis to NAD^+ availability. We showed that the NAD^+ pool can be increased by diet supplementation with its natural precursor nicotinamide riboside (NR) or by genetic or pharmacological inhibition of poly(ADP) ribosyl-polymerase 1 (Parp1), a NAD^+ consumer and Sirt1 competitor. These treatments lead to activation of Sirt1 (and other sirtuins) and boost mitochondrial respiration by inducing OXPHOS genes via the PGC-1α axis [10]. As a result, *Sco2*^{KOKI} mice showed improved motor performance up to normal values. NR was also effective in delaying the disease progression of the *deletor* mouse, another model of mitochondrial myopathy due to expression of a mutant variant of Twinkle, the mtDNA helicase [11].

More work is warranted to transfer these strategies to the patients. For instance, pharmacokinetics data in a nonrandomized, open-label healthy volunteers have been reported and showed that NR (1000 mg bid) was well-tolerated, had a half-life of 2.7 h, and led to an increase in NAD^+ concentration up to about 100%, which was stable for 9 days [12].

Endurance Training

Endurance training has also been exploited to trigger mitochondrial biogenesis and shown to delay the effects of ageing in mice [5, 13]. In addition to PGC-1α activation, endurance training seems to activate PGC-1β, as well as AMPK, p38γ MAPK, and the hypoxia inducible factors (HIFs) [14]. Irrespective of the molecular mechanism, endurance exercise has been reported as beneficial and safe in patients affected by mitochondrial myopathy [15–17], in muscle-specific *Cox10* knockout mice [18], and in the mtDNA *mutator* mice, where it appears to rescue progeroid ageing [13]. Importantly, these beneficial effects were not limited to skeletal muscle but also involved other organs, including the brain.

Scavenging Toxic Compounds

Pharmacological interventions have been used to modify the course of specific mitochondrial diseases characterized by metabolic blocks in mitochondria, which lead to accumulation of toxic substances. A first example is the use of N-acetylcysteine (NAC) and metronidazole to dump high levels of hydrogen sulphide (H_2S) characteristic of ethylmalonic encephalopathy (EE) [19]. EE is a devastating, multisystem disease of infancy due to mutations in *ETHE1*, a gene encoding a mitochondrial sulphur dioxygenase (SDO) involved in the disposal of H_2S. H_2S is produced by the catabolism of sulfurated amino acids in tissues and by the anaerobic bacterial flora in the large intestine. In concentrations above nanomolar, H_2S is highly toxic, leading to profound inhibition of fatty acids beta-oxidation and, more importantly, COX, as well as direct damage to endothelial lining of small vessels [20]. Accumulation of H_2S then causes a generalized microvasculopathy and COX deficiency, with multiple organ damage, including the brain, skin (with petechial purpura and orthostatic acrocyanosis), skeletal muscle, and large intestine. NAC is a cell-permeable precursor of GSH, which can act as an intracellular H_2S buffer. Metronidazole is an antibiotic specifically active against H_2S-producing anaerobic bacteria and protozoa. Administration of NAC and metronidazole significantly prolonged the lifespan and clinical conditions of an *Ethe1*$^{-/-}$ mouse model, when administered singly or, more effectively, in combination [19]. The same compounds were also effective in a cohort of EE patients, ameliorating some of the clinical hallmarks of the disease, including chronic diarrhoea and diffuse microvasculopathy with acrocyanosis. Some signs of CNS involvement were also improved, leading to increased alertness and wakefulness, and decreased number and duration of epileptic seizures [19].

A second important class of toxic compounds accumulating in mitochondrial dysfunction are the reactive oxygen species (ROS). ROS are generated at various sites along the respiratory chain and may lead to damage of cellular structures, including proteins, lipids, and nucleic acids, but can also play important role as signalling molecules in a number of pathways including adaptation to hypoxia, regulation of autophagy, control of immunological responses, promotion of cell differentiation, and set-up of longevity [21, 22]. These observations constitute the rational basis for the use of antioxidants in the therapy of mitochondrial diseases. Cocktails of antioxidant compounds, including lipoic acid, vitamins C and E, CoQ, etc., have extensively been used in the therapy of mitochondrial diseases for a long time, but no quantitative studies have been carried out in animal models to validate their use. Likewise, randomized double blind trials are still missing to support their efficacy in patients [23, 24]. In addition, although a transgenic mouse overexpressing a mitochondrially targeted catalase shows increased lifespan and resistance to oxidative damage [25], the efficacy of antioxidants in cellular and/or animal models of OXPHOS defects is still controversial.

Interestingly, Mootha and colleagues recently showed that chronic hypoxia leads to a marked improvement in survival, body weight, body temperature, behaviour, neuropathology, and disease biomarkers in a genetic mouse model of Leigh syndrome [26, 27]. Future work is anyway warranted to explore the molecular mechanism of this striking effect.

Supplementation of Nucleotides

Supplementation of deoxyribonucleotides can effectively correct mtDNA depletion in patients' fibroblasts carrying mutations in enzymes involved in the control of the mitochondrial nucleotide and deoxynucleotide pools (e.g. deoxyguanosine kinase, dGK, and thymidine phosphorylase, TP, encoded by the *DGUOK* and *TYMP* genes, respectively). Likewise, mtDNA depletion has also been corrected in vivo, by treating a *Tymp* knockout mouse model with either dCtd or tetrahydrouridine, an inhibitor of nucleotide catabolism [28–31].

Mutations in human *TYMP1*, encoding TP, are responsible of mitochondrial neurogastrointestinal encephalomyopathy, MNGIE [32]. MNGIE is a severe, autosomal recessive mitochondrial disorder of early adulthood, characterized by painful gastrointestinal dysmotility causing chronic diarrhoea and leading to cachexia, progressive external ophthalmoplegia with mitochondrial myopathy, and severe sensory-motor peripheral neuropathy. Patients usually die of complications due to their critical nutritional status, with an average age at death of 37 years [33]. TP is a cytosolic enzyme catalysing the first step of thymidine (dThd) and deoxyuridine (dUrd) catabolism. As a consequence of TP dysfunction, MNGIE patients accumulate dThd and dUrd systemically, which ultimately results in imbalances of the mitochondrial pool of deoxyribonucleoside triphosphates (dNTPs) [34]. This dNTP imbalance is mutagenic for mitochondrial DNA (mtDNA), resulting in depletion, multiple deletions, and point mutations accumulating in post-mitotic organs, notably intestinal smooth muscle, skeletal muscle, and the nervous system, and causes progressive mitochondrial deficiency and organ failure. Although the mouse model has hardly any clinical sign, it is clearly characterized by markedly abnormal dNTP pools, similar to MNGIE patients. The use of nucleotides is thus aimed at correcting the imbalance in the dNTP pools.

Similarly, positive results were also obtained in a thymidine kinase 2 (*Tk2*) H126N knockin mouse reproducing a pathological mutation found in patients. *Tk2* encodes the gene for the mitochondrial thymidine kinase, which phosphorylates thymidine and deoxycytidine pyrimidine nucleosides to generate deoxythymidine monophosphate (dTMP) and deoxycytidine monophosphate (dCMP). Absence of *Tk2* determines an imbalance of dNTP pools leading to mtDNA instability and depletion with early-onset fatal encephalomyopathy due to mtDNA depletion and multiple RC defects. Treatment with dTMP+dCMP (200 or 400 mg/Kg/day) leads to increased dNTP concentrations and mtDNA content, rescuing the RC defects, and significantly prolonging lifespan in H126N knockin mouse from 13 to 34 days [35]. Promising results were also obtained by administering the nucleosides deoxythymidine (dT) and deoxycytidine (dC) to the same mouse model, while co-administration of the deaminase inhibitor, tetrahydrouridine (THU), with dTMP+dCMP reduced the lifespan compared to dTMP+dCMP alone [36].

Rapamycin

Rapamycin is the first described inhibitor of mTORC1, a cytosolic serine-threonine kinase targeting a large number of proteins and regulating important pathways including autophagy, translation, and lipid and nucleotide synthesis. Administration of rapamycin led to a remarkable prolongation of the lifespan, delay of the neurological derangement, and reduction of neuroinflammation in *Ndufs4*$^{-/-}$ mice, a model of severe complex I deficiency [37].

Post-onset oral administration of rapamycin at the same dose previously used ip (8 mg/Kg), which is higher than the corresponding dose used in humans to prevent organ rejection, delayed the development of the encephalopathy in the *Ndufs4*$^{-/-}$ mouse [38].

Encouraging results using rapamycin were also obtained in neurons derived from induced pluripotent stem cells (iPSCs) from a patient with maternally inherited Leigh syndrome (MILS), carrying a mutation in the MT-ATP6 gene [39], in a thymidine kinase 2 (Tk2) knockin mouse [40], and in the deletor mouse [41]. However, the mechanisms for these positive results remain only partially understood.

Dietary Manipulations

Several approaches based on dietary measures have been attempted, with controversial results [42]. Ketogenic diet (KD), i.e. a high-fat, low-carbohydrate diet, has been proposed to stimulate mitochondrial beta-oxidation and provide ketones, which constitute an alternative energy source for the brain, heart, and skeletal muscle. Ketone bodies are metabolized to acetyl-CoA, which enters the Krebs cycle and is oxidized to feed the RC and ultimately generate ATP via OXPHOS. This pathway partially bypasses complex I via increased synthesis of succinate, which donates electrons to the respiratory chain via complex II. KD reduced the mutation load of a heteroplasmic mtDNA deletion in a cybrid cell lines from a Kearns-Sayre syndrome patient [43], was shown to increase the expression levels of uncoupling proteins and mitochondrial biogenesis in the hippocampus of mice and rats [44, 45], and increased mitochondrial GSH levels [46] in rat brain. In a preclinical trial on the *deletor* mouse, KD slowed the progression of mitochondrial myopathy [47]. However, other reports showed that KD can have the opposite effect and worsens the mitochondrial defect in vivo, for instance, in the *Mterf2*$^{-/-}$ [48]or the *Mpv17*$^{-/-}$ mouse models [49].

The administration of a ketogenic (high-fat, low-carbohydrate) modified Atkins diet (mAD) to five patients with PEO and exercise intolerance caused by single or multiple mitochondrial DNA (mtDNA) deletions induced acute muscle damage with burning sensation and muscle pain spreading from their lower limbs to the back, with elevated creatine kinase (CK), transaminases, and myoglobin levels within days from initiating the mAD regimen, unlike their age- and sex-matched controls. These findings were accompanied by selective necrotic degeneration of ragged-red fibres (RRF) in PEO patients. All the symptoms quickly reverted after cessation of the diet regimen. However, after 2.5 years muscle strength had mildly improved in three out of four patients [50, 51]. These results suggest that reparative processes triggered by acute damage could lead, in the long term, to an amelioration of the myopathic phenotype in these patients.

Molecular Approaches to Treat Mitochondrial Diseases

Targeted Re-expression of the Mutated Gene

Correction of a mutation by expressing the wild-type gene in critical organs has for long been envisaged as the definitive cure for genetic diseases. Although we are still far from having achieved a general strategy for gene replacement in the whole body, large-size organs (e.g. skeletal muscle), or impermeable organs (e.g. brain), several successes have been reported in the last years for a number of genetic diseases, in both preclinical models and patients. In fact, while expression of therapeutic genes through the whole body is still unachievable, and quantitative targeting of skeletal muscle is only feasible in small rodents but not in humans, smaller organs can be targeted by exploiting currently available technologies. In particular the introduction of adeno-associated viral (AAVs) vectors has given new stamina to gene therapy. AAVs belong to the parvoviridae family, which are not associated with any disease in humans or animals, and remain episomic in the cells for prolonged time, thus reducing the risk of insertional mutagenesis [52]. In addition, several serotypes with different cellular specificities have been selected, allowing specific targeting of several organs and tissues [53] (Fig. 2).

We reported that a recombinant construct expressing *Ethe1*^{wt} could be targeted to the liver using a hepatotropic AAV2/8 serotype. When titres >10^{12} viral genomes/Kg were injected in 3-week old *Ethe1*$^{-/-}$ mice, Ethe1-associated SDO activity was completely recovered in the liver [20], leading to efficient clearance of H_2S from the bloodstream. This treatment was associated with significant rescue of the profound COX deficiency due to the inhibitory effect of H_2S, correction of the other biomarkers of the disease (e.g. high plasma and urine levels of ethylmalonate, lactate, and thiosulfate), remarkable clinical improvement, and marked prolongation of the lifespan, from a few weeks in untreated animals to over 8 months in AAV-treated littermates [54].

The same liver-specific AAV2/8 vector has been exploited to treat a mouse model for MNGIE [55]. Although the *Tymp*$^{-/-}$ mouse displays hardly any clinical sign, it is characterized by markedly abnormal dNTP pools, similar to MNGIE patients. Intravenous injection of AAV2/8 particles expressing human wt *TYMP* (10^{12}–10^{13} viral DNA/kg) normalized dCTP and dTTP levels in plasma and tissues for up to 8 months of age. In addition, the effects of an AAV containing the TYMP coding sequence transcriptionally targeted to the liver persisted for at least 21 months at a dose of 2×10^{12} vg/kg in mice [56].

The encouraging proof-of-principle results on EE and MNGIE models support the transferability of the AAV2/8 treatment to the patients. However, the possibility of improving the clinical phenotype using the liver as an organ suitable to scavenge toxic compounds prompted the use of liver transplant for these diseases in a few patients, with promising preliminary results [57, 58].

The current standard treatment for MNGIE relies on bone marrow transplantation [59, 60], which is anyway burdened by a >50% post-graft mortality due to poor clinical conditions of the recipient patients. A noninvasive and safe procedure like systemic administration of suitably engineered AAV vectors is clearly more acceptable and can lead to substantial improvement of the otherwise ominous prognosis of this extremely invalidating disorder.

AAV2/9 vector carrying the human *NDUFS4* coding sequence (*hNDUFS4*) has been administered by intravenous (IV) and/or intracerebroventricular (ICV) routes to either newborn or young Ndufs4$^{-/-}$ mice. IV administration alone was only able to correct the cI deficiency in peripheral organs, whereas ICV administration partially corrected the deficiency in the brain. However, both treatments failed to improve the clinical phenotype or to prolong the lifespan of *Ndufs4*$^{-/-}$ mice. In contrast, combined IV and ICV treatments resulted, along with increased cI activity, in the amelioration of the rotarod performance and in a significant prolongation of the lifespan [61].

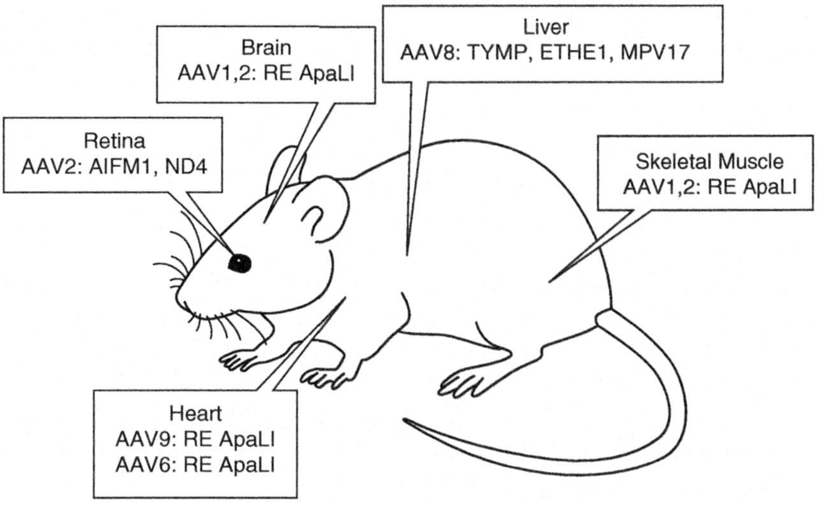

Fig. 2 AAV-based gene therapies in mouse models of mitochondrial diseases (From [117] with permission)

A number of issues will need to be addressed in the coming years, including the development of suitable strategies to effectively target extrahepatic, critical organs such as the skeletal muscle, heart, and brain.

A strategy repeatedly proposed to correcting mtDNA mutations in protein-encoding genes is based on allotopic expression. In this approach, the recoded wild-type gene, transfected to the nucleus, expresses a recombinant protein containing a mitochondrial targeting sequence (MTS), to address it to mitochondria. A 3′-UTR signal is usually added that in yeast serves to target transcripts of mitochondrial proteins to the organelle surface. These transcripts are then translated by a local pool of ribosomes into proteins, which can promptly be imported into the organelle. This approach has been attempted in fibroblasts carrying mutations in ND1, ND4, and ATP6 genes [62–64] and in a rat model of LHON [65]. These results are very controversial, as conflicting data have been obtained by different groups on the ability of recoded mitochondrially targeted mtDNA gene products that can effectively been imported and correctly inserted within the respiratory chain complexes [66]. Nevertheless, open-label clinical trials based on AAV-mediated allotopic expression of mtDNA genes for LHON are currently recruiting patients (https//clinicaltrial.gov).

The multiploidy organization of mtDNA, its confinement within an almost impermeable double-membrane barrier, and the virtual absence of homologous recombination are formidable hurdles against the direct, controlled manipulation of this genome for therapeutic intervention. Nevertheless, several approaches have been proposed to this aim, and some are giving promising results. A first strategy was based on the use of protein nucleic acids (PNAs) as an "antigenomic" device [67, 68]. PNAs are synthetic DNA-like molecules in which the pyrimidine and purine residues are linked to an aminoethyl (pseudopeptide) backbone. Since these molecules are not charged at physiological pH, a PNA binds its complementary DNA with greater affinity than natural nucleic acids, so that PNA-DNA hybrids are more stable than DNA-DNA hybrids. PNAs complementary to either the mtDNA stretch containing the 8344A>G MERRF mutation in mt-tRNA^{Lys} [69] or the breakpoint junction associated with the mtDNA common deletion were shown to be imported into mitochondria, where they inhibited the replication of mutant but not wild-type mtDNA, but no such effect was demonstrated in cell lines [70].

An alternative approach had been used to target allotopically expressed tRNAs and mRNAs to the mitochondria, taking advantage from the observation that RNase P, a ribonucleoprotein deemed to be involved in the processing of mitochondrial transcripts, is imported into mitochondria through a supposedly specialized system (PNPase) that specifically recognizes its RNA component (H1 RNA). By fusing the gene of interest with a 20-ribonucleotide stem-loop sequence from the H1 RNA, some evidence was provided in support of correction of mt-tRNA and COII gene mutations in cell lines [71, 72]. However, the human mtRNase P was shown specifically not to contain any *trans*-acting RNA [73], so these results should be taken cautiously.

Manipulating mtDNA Heteroplasmy

As pathogenic mutations of mtDNA are often heteroplasmic and behave as "recessive-like" mutations, suitable therapeutic intervention can be envisaged, aimed at eliminating or reducing the amount of mutated DNA below the threshold at which the disease manifests. This result has been achieved in cellular models by targeting to mitochondria recombinant restriction endonucleases [74–76], zinc finger endonucleases [77], or TALENs [78].

While the strategy based on restriction enzymes can be used therapeutically only if a unique restriction site is created by an mtDNA mutation, as in the case of the 8993T>G NARP, an exceptionally rare event. The recent development of zinc finger nuclease and TALEN technologies can offset this limitation. Zinc finger nucleases (ZFNs) are chimeric enzymes in which the modular Cys_2His_2 zinc finger DNA-binding domains present in numerous transcription factors are conjugated to the C-terminal catalytic subunit of the type II restriction enzyme *Fok*I [79, 80]. Each zinc finger domain recognizes three nucleotides, so that appropriate arrangements of the zinc finger modules permit to target virtually any DNA sequence for nucleolytic cleavage. ZFN can be targeted to mitochondria by adding a suitable MTS at the N-terminus. Likewise, transcription activator-like effectors nucleases (TALEN) exploit DNA-binding domains of the *Xanthomonas* bacteria composed of 33–35 amino acid repeats, each recognizing a single base pair, fused with the *Fok*I nuclease. Again, TALENs can be targeted to mitochondria via an N-terminal MTS (MitoTALENs).

MitoTALENs [78] have been proven to eliminate heteroplasmic mutant mtDNA in cybrid cells carrying either the m.8483_13459del4977 common mtDNA deletion [81–83] or the m.14459G>A LHON/dystonia mutation in the MT-ND6 gene [84]. In both cases, a transient decrease in total mtDNA levels occurred, followed by repopulation with wild-type mtDNA up to normal values.

Likewise, mitochondrially targeted ZFNs (mtZFNs) were successfully used in heteroplasmic cybrids to cleave mtDNA harbouring either the heteroplasmic m.8993T>G NARP mutation [85] or the common deletion. As for TALENS and restriction enzymes, mtZFNs led to a reduction in mutant mtDNA haplotype load and subsequent repopulation of wild-type mtDNA, associated with restoration of mitochondrial respiration [77].

Stabilizing Mutant mt-tRNA

More than 50% of the mtDNA mutations are localized in tRNA genes, leading to a wide range of syndromes, such as MELAS or MERRF. Aminoacyl-tRNA synthetases (aaRSs) are ubiquitously expressed, essential enzymes performing the attachment of amino acids to their cognate tRNA molecules as the first step of protein synthesis [86]. Several lines of evidence in yeast and human cell lines indicate that overexpressing cognate mt-aaRS can attenuate the detrimental effects of mt-tRNA point mutations [87–90]. For instance, overexpression of mt-leucyl-tRNA synthetase (mt-LeuRS) corrects the respiratory chain deficiency of transmitochondrial cybrids harbouring the MELAS mutation in the mt-$tRNA^{Leu(UUR)}$ gene (*MTTL1*) [86, 89]. Likewise, overexpressing the cognate mt-valyl-tRNA synthetase (mt-ValRS) restored, at least in part, steady-state levels of mutated mt-$tRNA^{Val}$ in cybrid cell lines [90]. Finally, constitutive high levels of mt-isoleucyl-tRNA synthetase (mt-IleRS) were shown to be associated with reduced penetrance of the homoplasmic m.4277T>C mt-$tRNA^{Ile}$ mutation, which causes hypertrophic cardiomyopathy [91]. In addition, experiments in yeast and human cells have shown that the overexpression of either human mt-LeuRS or mt-ValRS was able of rescuing the pathological phenotype associated with mutations in both the cognate and the non-cognate mt-tRNA. A region in the carboxy-terminal domain of mt-LeuRS was found necessary and sufficient to determine this phenomenon, probably via a chaperone-like stabilizing effect [92, 93].

An alternative approach to the same issue was based on the observation that in yeast some tRNAs were encoded in the nuclear genome and imported into the mitochondria. So, tRNA mutations in mtDNA may in principle be complemented by expressing a xenotopic nDNA-encoded yeast mitochondrial tRNA from the mammalian nucleus [72, 94, 95]. However, there results are highly controversial because of the lack of convincing evidence that RNAs can be imported into mitochondria.

Targeting Fission and Fusion

Mitochondria are highly dynamic organelles whose shape and mass are finely tuned by the activity of pro-fusion proteins, such as mitofusin 1 (MFN1), MFN2, and optic atrophy protein 1 (OPA1), and pro-fission proteins, such as dynamin-related protein 1 (DRP1) and mitochondrial fission 1 protein (FIS1) [96, 97]. Alterations in the genes encoding these complex machineries lead to disease in humans. For instance, mutations in *OPA1* are associated with autosomal dominant optic atrophy [98], and mutations in *MFN2* cause Charcot-Marie-Tooth disease type 2A [99]. In addition, disruption of *Mfn1* and *Mfn2* in the skeletal muscle of the *POLG*^{D257A} *mutator* mouse leads to striking worsening of the phenotype, due to accumulation of mtDNA mutations, suggesting that the physiological balance between fission and fusion protects the integrity of mtDNA through continuous mixing of mtDNA pools [100]. Two additional observations are relevant in this context. First, overexpression of *Opa1*, a multitasking GTPase involved in shaping mitochondrial cristae and promoting fusion of the inner mitochondrial membrane, has been shown to increase respiratory efficiency by stabilizing the respiratory chain supercomplexes [101] and to increase survival and improve clinical conditions of *Ndufs4*$^{-/-}$ and *ACTA-Cox15*$^{-/-}$ mouse models [102]. In addition, overexpression of Opa1 also ameliorated the outcome of a number of insults with mitochondrial involvement, including ischemia-reperfusion, denervation-induced muscle atrophy, and hepatocellular apoptosis [103]. Second, some compounds affecting fission and fusion have been identified, such as the Drp1 inhibitor MDIVI-1 and M1-hydrazone that probably promotes fusion by acting on Mfn or Opa1. However, the therapeutic potential of these compounds for mitochondrial diseases has still to be proved.

Bypassing the Block of the Respiratory Chain

An emerging concept in mitochondrial medicine is the possibility to bypass the block of OXPHOS due to mutations affecting the RC complexes by using the “alternative” enzymes NADH dehydrogenase/CoQ reductase (Ndi1) and CoQ/O2 alternative oxidase (AOX).

These are single-peptide enzymes, located in the mitochondrial inner membrane, which transfer electrons to (Ndi1) and from (AOX) CoQ, without pumping protons across the membrane. Ndi1 substitutes complex I in yeast mitochondria. AOX is an alternative electron transport system present in lower eukaryotes, plants, and several invertebrates that bypasses the complex III + IV segment of the respiratory chain. Expression of these proteins is well-tolerated in mammalian cells [104], flies, and mice [105] and has successfully been exploited to bypass complex I or complex III/IV defects in human cells [106, 107] and *Drosophila* models [108–110]. The therapeutic mechanism is based on the capacity of these enzymes to restore the electron flow through the quinone pool, thus preventing accumulation of reduced intermediates and oxidative damage [111]. However, this is not accompanied by restoration of proton translocation across the inner mitochondrial membrane and does not directly increase ATP production. Nevertheless, the restoration of the electron flow can reactivate the unaffected RC complexes, thus indirectly promoting the rebuilding of the proton gradient and the reactivation of OXPHOS. AOX-expressing mice have recently been created and shown to be viable and fertile [105], thus opening the possibility to test whether this approach is amenable in a mammalian organism, using suitable mouse models of complex III or IV deficiency.

Somatic Nuclear Transfer

Given the difficulty of manipulating mtDNA and the uncertainties of genetic counselling for mtDNA mutations, prenatal or preimplantation genetic diagnosis is nowadays the best option available to women carrying pathogenic mtDNA mutations. However, these techniques can only be applied to subjects with low levels of mtDNA mutations in oocytes and are technically challenging. Recent technical improvements in nonhuman primates [112] and nonviable human embryos [113, 114] have paved the way to replace the mutated maternal mtDNA with that obtained from a healthy woman, by transferring either the spindle-chromosomal complex of mature oocytes before fertilization or the pronuclei during the prezygotic stage of fertilized egg [115]. Both techniques have been refined in order to minimize the amount of mutant mtDNA carried over into the recipient ooplasm, whose consequences are largely unknown [115, 116]. A child born by these procedures will carry the nuclear genes of the affected mother (and healthy father) but the healthy mitochondrial genes of the donor.

Conclusions

Mitochondrial diseases are amazingly complex and its biology has so far prevented the development of effective therapy for most of them. Nevertheless, the last few years witnessed numerous attempts to significantly modify the phenotype in cellular and animal models by using either disease-specific or wide-spectrum strategies applicable to several disorders. The wealth of knowledge accumulated in over 25 years of intensive studies aimed at elucidating the genetic causes and the pathogenic mechanisms of mitochondrial diseases has driven these first "proof of concept" successes that now need to be translated and tested on patients. In addition, mitochondrial dysfunction is nowadays acknowledged as central in several diseases, including diabetes and neurodegenerative diseases, and advances in these fields will very likely affect the research on primary mitochondrial disease and vice versa.

Acknowledgments This work was supported by the MRC-QQR Grant 2015-2020 (to MBU), ERC Advanced Grant ERC FP7-322424, and NRJ-Institute de France (to M.Z.).

References

1. Giordano C, Iommarini L, Giordano L, Maresca A, Pisano A, Valentino ML, et al. Efficient mitochondrial biogenesis drives incomplete penetrance in Leber's hereditary optic neuropathy. Brain J Neurol. 2014;137(Pt 2):335–53.
2. Scarpulla RC. Transcriptional paradigms in mammalian mitochondrial biogenesis and function. Physiol Rev. 2008;88(2):611–38.
3. Fernandez-Marcos PJ, Auwerx J. Regulation of PGC-1alpha, a nodal regulator of mitochondrial biogenesis. Am J Clin Nutr. 2011;93(4):884S–90.
4. Bastin J, Aubey F, Rotig A, Munnich A, Djouadi F. Activation of peroxisome proliferator-activated receptor pathway stimulates the mitochondrial respiratory chain and can correct deficiencies in patients' cells lacking its components. J Clin Endocrinol Metab. 2008;93(4):1433–41.
5. Wenz T, Wang X, Marini M, Moraes CT. A metabolic shift induced by a PPAR panagonist markedly reduces the effects of pathogenic mitochondrial tRNA mutations. J Cell Mol Med. 2011;15(11):2317–25.
6. Casarin A, Giorgi G, Pertegato V, Siviero R, Cerqua C, Doimo M, et al. Copper and bezafibrate cooperate to rescue cytochrome c oxidase deficiency in cells of patients with SCO2 mutations. Orphanet J Rare Dis. 2012;7:21.
7. Djouadi F, Bastin J. Species differences in the effects of bezafibrate as a potential treatment of mitochondrial disorders. Cell Metab. 2011;14(6):715–6; author reply 7
8. Viscomi C, Bottani E, Civiletto G, Cerutti R, Moggio M, Fagiolari G, et al. In vivo correction of COX deficiency by activation of the AMPK/PGC-1alpha axis. Cell Metab. 2011;14(1):80–90.
9. Peralta S, Garcia S, Yin HY, Arguello T, Diaz F, Moraes CT. Sustained AMPK activation improves muscle function in a mitochondrial myopathy mouse model by promoting muscle fiber regeneration. Hum Mol Genet. 2016;25(15):3178–91.
10. Cerutti R, Pirinen E, Lamperti C, Marchet S, Sauve AA, Li W, et al. NAD(+)-dependent activation of Sirt1 corrects the phenotype in a mouse

model of mitochondrial disease. Cell Metab. 2014;19(6):1042–9.
11. Khan NA, Auranen M, Paetau I, Pirinen E, Euro L, Forsstrom S, et al. Effective treatment of mitochondrial myopathy by nicotinamide riboside, a vitamin B3. EMBO Mol Med. 2014;6(6):721–31.
12. Airhart SE, Shireman LM, Risler LJ, Anderson GD, Nagana Gowda GA, Raftery D, et al. An open-label, non-randomized study of the pharmacokinetics of the nutritional supplement nicotinamide riboside (NR) and its effects on blood NAD+ levels in healthy volunteers. PLoS One. 2017;12(12):e0186459.
13. Safdar A, Bourgeois JM, Ogborn DI, Little JP, Hettinga BP, Akhtar M, et al. Endurance exercise rescues progeroid aging and induces systemic mitochondrial rejuvenation in mtDNA mutator mice. Proc Natl Acad Sci U S A. 2011;108(10):4135–40.
14. Rowe GC, El-Khoury R, Patten IS, Rustin P, Arany Z. PGC-1alpha is dispensable for exercise-induced mitochondrial biogenesis in skeletal muscle. PLoS One. 2012;7(7):e41817.
15. Jeppesen TD, Schwartz M, Olsen DB, Wibrand F, Krag T, Duno M, et al. Aerobic training is safe and improves exercise capacity in patients with mitochondrial myopathy. Brain J Neurol. 2006;129(Pt 12):3402–12.
16. Zeviani M. Train, train, train! No pain, just gain. Brain J Neurol. 2008;131(Pt 11):2809–11.
17. Murphy JL, Blakely EL, Schaefer AM, He L, Wyrick P, Haller RG, et al. Resistance training in patients with single, large-scale deletions of mitochondrial DNA. Brain J Neurol. 2008;131(Pt 11):2832–40.
18. Wenz T, Diaz F, Hernandez D, Moraes CT. Endurance exercise is protective for mice with mitochondrial myopathy. J Appl Physiol. 2009;106(5):1712–9.
19. Viscomi C, Burlina AB, Dweikat I, Savoiardo M, Lamperti C, Hildebrandt T, et al. Combined treatment with oral metronidazole and N-acetylcysteine is effective in ethylmalonic encephalopathy. Nat Med. 2010;16(8):869–71.
20. Tiranti V, Viscomi C, Hildebrandt T, Di Meo I, Mineri R, Tiveron C, et al. Loss of ETHE1, a mitochondrial dioxygenase, causes fatal sulfide toxicity in ethylmalonic encephalopathy. Nat Med. 2009;15(2):200–5.
21. Raimundo N. Mitochondrial pathology: stress signals from the energy factory. Trends Mol Med. 2014;20(5):282–92.
22. Sena LA, Chandel NS. Physiological roles of mitochondrial reactive oxygen species. Mol Cell. 2012;48(2):158–67.
23. Kanabus M, Heales SJ, Rahman S. Development of pharmacological strategies for mitochondrial disorders. Br J Pharmacol. 2014;171(8):1798–817.
24. Wallace DC, Fan W, Procaccio V. Mitochondrial energetics and therapeutics. Annu Rev Pathol. 2010;5:297–348.
25. Schriner SE, Linford NJ, Martin GM, Treuting P, Ogburn CE, Emond M, et al. Extension of murine life span by overexpression of catalase targeted to mitochondria. Science. 2005;308(5730):1909–11.
26. Ferrari M, Jain IH, Goldberger O, Rezoagli E, Thoonen R, Cheng KH, et al. Hypoxia treatment reverses neurodegenerative disease in a mouse model of Leigh syndrome. Proc Natl Acad Sci U S A. 2017;114(21):E4241–E50.
27. Jain IH, Zazzeron L, Goli R, Alexa K, Schatzman-Bone S, Dhillon H, et al. Hypoxia as a therapy for mitochondrial disease. Science. 2016;352(6281):54–61.
28. Taanman JW, Muddle JR, Muntau AC. Mitochondrial DNA depletion can be prevented by dGMP and dAMP supplementation in a resting culture of deoxyguanosine kinase-deficient fibroblasts. Hum Mol Genet. 2003;12(15):1839–45.
29. Bulst S, Abicht A, Holinski-Feder E, Muller-Ziermann S, Koehler U, Thirion C, et al. In vitro supplementation with dAMP/dGMP leads to partial restoration of mtDNA levels in mitochondrial depletion syndromes. Hum Mol Genet. 2009;18(9):1590–9.
30. Bulst S, Holinski-Feder E, Payne B, Abicht A, Krause S, Lochmuller H, et al. In vitro supplementation with deoxynucleoside monophosphates rescues mitochondrial DNA depletion. Mol Genet Metab. 2012;107(1–2):95–103.
31. Camara Y, Gonzalez-Vioque E, Scarpelli M, Torres-Torronteras J, Caballero A, Hirano M, et al. Administration of deoxyribonucleosides or inhibition of their catabolism as a pharmacological approach for mitochondrial DNA depletion syndrome. Hum Mol Genet. 2014;23(9):2459–67.
32. Nishino I, Spinazzola A, Hirano M. Thymidine phosphorylase gene mutations in MNGIE, a human mitochondrial disorder. Science. 1999;283(5402):689–92.
33. Nishino I, Spinazzola A, Hirano M. MNGIE: from nuclear DNA to mitochondrial DNA. Neuromuscul Disord. 2001;11(1):7–10.
34. Spinazzola A, Marti R, Nishino I, Andreu AL, Naini A, Tadesse S, et al. Altered thymidine metabolism due to defects of thymidine phosphorylase. J Biol Chem. 2002;277(6):4128–33.
35. Garone C, Garcia-Diaz B, Emmanuele V, Lopez LC, Tadesse S, Akman HO, et al. Deoxypyrimidine monophosphate bypass therapy for thymidine kinase 2 deficiency. EMBO Mol Med. 2014;6(8):1016–27.
36. Lopez-Gomez C, Levy RJ, Sanchez-Quintero MJ, Juanola-Falgarona M, Barca E, Garcia-Diaz B, et al. Deoxycytidine and deoxythymidine treatment for thymidine kinase 2 deficiency. Ann Neurol. 2017;81(5):641–52.
37. Johnson SC, Yanos ME, Kayser EB, Quintana A, Sangesland M, Castanza A, et al. mTOR inhibition alleviates mitochondrial disease in a mouse model of Leigh syndrome. Science. 2013;342(6165):1524–8.
38. Felici R, Buonvicino D, Muzzi M, Cavone L, Guasti D, Lapucci A, et al. Post onset, oral rapamycin treatment delays development of mitochondrial encephalopathy only at supramaximal doses. Neuropharmacology. 2017;117:74–84.

39. Zheng X, Boyer L, Jin M, Kim Y, Fan W, Bardy C, et al. Alleviation of neuronal energy deficiency by mTOR inhibition as a treatment for mitochondria-related neurodegeneration. Elife. 2016;5
40. Siegmund SE, Yang H, Sharma R, Javors M, Skinner O, Mootha V, et al. Low-dose rapamycin extends lifespan in a mouse model of mtDNA depletion syndrome. Hum Mol Genet. 2017;26(23):4588–605.
41. Khan NA, Nikkanen J, Yatsuga S, Jackson C, Wang L, Pradhan S, et al. mTORC1 regulates mitochondrial integrated stress response and mitochondrial myopathy progression. Cell Metab. 2017;26(2):419–28 e5.
42. Kuszak AJ, Espey MG, Falk MJ, Holmbeck MA, Manfredi G, Shadel GS, et al. Nutritional interventions for mitochondrial OXPHOS deficiencies: mechanisms and model systems. Annu Rev Pathol. 2018;13:163–91.
43. Santra S, Gilkerson RW, Davidson M, Schon EA. Ketogenic treatment reduces deleted mitochondrial DNAs in cultured human cells. Ann Neurol. 2004;56(5):662–9.
44. Sullivan PG, Rippy NA, Dorenbos K, Concepcion RC, Agarwal AK, Rho JM. The ketogenic diet increases mitochondrial uncoupling protein levels and activity. Ann Neurol. 2004;55(4):576–80.
45. Bough KJ, Wetherington J, Hassel B, Pare JF, Gawryluk JW, Greene JG, et al. Mitochondrial biogenesis in the anticonvulsant mechanism of the ketogenic diet. Ann Neurol. 2006;60(2):223–35.
46. Jarrett SG, Milder JB, Liang LP, Patel M. The ketogenic diet increases mitochondrial glutathione levels. J Neurochem. 2008;106(3):1044–51.
47. Ahola-Erkkila S, Carroll CJ, Peltola-Mjosund K, Tulkki V, Mattila I, Seppanen-Laakso T, et al. Ketogenic diet slows down mitochondrial myopathy progression in mice. Hum Mol Genet. 2010;19(10):1974–84.
48. Wenz T, Luca C, Torraco A, Moraes CT. mTERF2 regulates oxidative phosphorylation by modulating mtDNA transcription. Cell Metab. 2009;9(6):499–511.
49. Bottani E, Giordano C, Civiletto G, Di Meo I, Auricchio A, Ciusani E, et al. AAV-mediated liver-specific MPV17 expression restores mtDNA levels and prevents diet-induced liver failure. Mol Ther. 2014;22(1):10–7.
50. Ahola S, Auranen M, Isohanni P, Niemisalo S, Urho N, Buzkova J, et al. Modified Atkins diet induces subacute selective ragged-red-fiber lysis in mitochondrial myopathy patients. EMBO Mol Med. 2016;8(11):1234–47.
51. Pitceathly RD, Viscomi C. Effects of ketosis in mitochondrial myopathy: potential benefits of a mitotoxic diet. EMBO Mol Med. 2016;8(11):1231–3.
52. Mingozzi F, High KA. Therapeutic in vivo gene transfer for genetic disease using AAV: progress and challenges. Nat Rev Genet. 2011;12(5):341–55.
53. Gao GP, Alvira MR, Wang L, Calcedo R, Johnston J, Wilson JM. Novel adeno-associated viruses from rhesus monkeys as vectors for human gene therapy. Proc Natl Acad Sci U S A. 2002;99(18):11854–9.
54. Di Meo I, Auricchio A, Lamperti C, Burlina A, Viscomi C, Zeviani M. Effective AAV-mediated gene therapy in a mouse model of ethylmalonic encephalopathy. EMBO Mol Med. 2012;4(9):1008–14.
55. Torres-Torronteras J, Viscomi C, Cabrera-Perez R, Camara Y, Di Meo I, Barquinero J, et al. Gene therapy using a liver-targeted AAV vector restores nucleoside and nucleotide homeostasis in a murine model of MNGIE. Mol Ther. 2014;22(5):901–7.
56. Torres-Torronteras J, Cabrera-Perez R, Vila-Julia F, Viscomi C, Camara Y, Hirano M, et al. Long-term sustained effect of liver-targeted Adeno-associated virus gene therapy for mitochondrial Neurogastrointestinal Encephalomyopathy. Hum Gene Ther. 2018;29(6):708–18.
57. De Giorgio R, Pironi L, Rinaldi R, Boschetti E, Caporali L, Capristo M, et al. Liver transplantation for mitochondrial neurogastrointestinal encephalomyopathy. Ann Neurol. 2016;80(3):448–55.
58. Dionisi-Vici C, Diodato D, Torre G, Picca S, Pariante R, Giuseppe Picardo S, et al. Liver transplant in ethylmalonic encephalopathy: a new treatment for an otherwise fatal disease. Brain J Neurol. 2016;139(Pt 4):1045–51.
59. Hirano M, Marti R, Casali C, Tadesse S, Uldrick T, Fine B, et al. Allogeneic stem cell transplantation corrects biochemical derangements in MNGIE. Neurology. 2006;67(8):1458–60.
60. Rahman S, Hargreaves IP. Allogeneic stem cell transplantation corrects biochemical derangements in MNGIE. Neurology. 2007;68(21):1872; author reply; discussion-3
61. Di Meo I, Marchet S, Lamperti C, Zeviani M, Viscomi C. AAV9-based gene therapy partially ameliorates the clinical phenotype of a mouse model of Leigh syndrome. Gene Ther. 2017;24(10):661–7.
62. Bonnet C, Kaltimbacher V, Ellouze S, Augustin S, Benit P, Forster V, et al. Allotopic mRNA localization to the mitochondrial surface rescues respiratory chain defects in fibroblasts harboring mitochondrial DNA mutations affecting complex I or v subunits. Rejuvenation Res. 2007;10(2):127–44.
63. Kaltimbacher V, Bonnet C, Lecoeuvre G, Forster V, Sahel JA, Corral-Debrinski M. mRNA localization to the mitochondrial surface allows the efficient translocation inside the organelle of a nuclear recoded ATP6 protein. RNA. 2006;12(7):1408–17.
64. Bonnet C, Augustin S, Ellouze S, Benit P, Bouaita A, Rustin P, et al. The optimized allotopic expression of ND1 or ND4 genes restores respiratory chain complex I activity in fibroblasts harboring mutations in these genes. Biochim Biophys Acta. 2008;1783(10):1707–17.
65. Ellouze S, Augustin S, Bouaita A, Bonnet C, Simonutti M, Forster V, et al. Optimized allotopic expression of the human mitochondrial ND4 prevents blindness in a rat model of mitochondrial dysfunction. Am J Hum Genet. 2008;83(3):373–87.

66. Perales-Clemente E, Fernandez-Silva P, Acin-Perez R, Perez-Martos A, Enriquez JA. Allotopic expression of mitochondrial-encoded genes in mammals: achieved goal, undemonstrated mechanism or impossible task? Nucleic Acids Res. 2011;39(1):225–34.
67. Taylor RW, Chinnery PF, Turnbull DM, Lightowlers RN. Selective inhibition of mutant human mitochondrial DNA replication in vitro by peptide nucleic acids. Nat Genet. 1997;15(2):212–5.
68. Chinnery PF, Taylor RW, Diekert K, Lill R, Turnbull DM, Lightowlers RN. Peptide nucleic acid delivery to human mitochondria. Gene Ther. 1999;6(12):1919–28.
69. Shoffner JM, Lott MT, Lezza AM, Seibel P, Ballinger SW, Wallace DC. Myoclonic epilepsy and ragged-red fiber disease (MERRF) is associated with a mitochondrial DNA tRNA(Lys) mutation. Cell. 1990;61(6):931–7.
70. Muratovska A, Lightowlers RN, Taylor RW, Turnbull DM, Smith RA, Wilce JA, et al. Targeting peptide nucleic acid (PNA) oligomers to mitochondria within cells by conjugation to lipophilic cations: implications for mitochondrial DNA replication, expression and disease. Nucleic Acids Res. 2001;29(9):1852–63.
71. Wang G, Chen HW, Oktay Y, Zhang J, Allen EL, Smith GM, et al. PNPASE regulates RNA import into mitochondria. Cell. 2010;142(3):456–67.
72. Wang G, Shimada E, Zhang J, Hong JS, Smith GM, Teitell MA, et al. Correcting human mitochondrial mutations with targeted RNA import. Proc Natl Acad Sci U S A. 2012;109(13):4840–5.
73. Gammage PA, Moraes CT, Minczuk M. Mitochondrial genome engineering: the revolution may not be CRISPR-Ized. Trends Genet. 2018;34(2):101–10.
74. Bacman SR, Williams SL, Hernandez D, Moraes CT. Modulating mtDNA heteroplasmy by mitochondria-targeted restriction endonucleases in a 'differential multiple cleavage-site' model. Gene Ther. 2007;14(18):1309–18.
75. Bacman SR, Williams SL, Duan D, Moraes CT. Manipulation of mtDNA heteroplasmy in all striated muscles of newborn mice by AAV9-mediated delivery of a mitochondria-targeted restriction endonuclease. Gene Ther. 2012;19(11):1101–6.
76. Srivastava S, Moraes CT. Manipulating mitochondrial DNA heteroplasmy by a mitochondrially targeted restriction endonuclease. Hum Mol Genet. 2001;10(26):3093–9.
77. Gammage PA, Rorbach J, Vincent AI, Rebar EJ, Minczuk M. Mitochondrially targeted ZFNs for selective degradation of pathogenic mitochondrial genomes bearing large-scale deletions or point mutations. EMBO Mol Med. 2014;6(4):458–66.
78. Bacman SR, Williams SL, Pinto M, Peralta S, Moraes CT. Specific elimination of mutant mitochondrial genomes in patient-derived cells by mitoTALENs. Nat Med. 2013;19(9):1111–3.
79. Kim YG, Cha J, Chandrasegaran S. Hybrid restriction enzymes: zinc finger fusions to Fok I cleavage domain. Proc Natl Acad Sci U S A. 1996;93(3):1156–60.
80. Smith J, Bibikova M, Whitby FG, Reddy AR, Chandrasegaran S, Carroll D. Requirements for double-strand cleavage by chimeric restriction enzymes with zinc finger DNA-recognition domains. Nucleic Acids Res. 2000;28(17):3361–9.
81. Schon EA, Rizzuto R, Moraes CT, Nakase H, Zeviani M, DiMauro S. A direct repeat is a hotspot for large-scale deletion of human mitochondrial DNA. Science. 1989;244(4902):346–9.
82. Corral-Debrinski M, Horton T, Lott MT, Shoffner JM, Beal MF, Wallace DC. Mitochondrial DNA deletions in human brain: regional variability and increase with advanced age. Nat Genet. 1992;2(4):324–9.
83. Soong NW, Hinton DR, Cortopassi G, Arnheim N. Mosaicism for a specific somatic mitochondrial DNA mutation in adult human brain. Nat Genet. 1992;2(4):318–23.
84. Jun AS, Trounce IA, Brown MD, Shoffner JM, Wallace DC. Use of transmitochondrial cybrids to assign a complex I defect to the mitochondrial DNA-encoded NADH dehydrogenase subunit 6 gene mutation at nucleotide pair 14459 that causes Leber hereditary optic neuropathy and dystonia. Mol Cell Biol. 1996;16(3):771–7.
85. Holt IJ, Harding AE, Petty RK, Morgan-Hughes JA. A new mitochondrial disease associated with mitochondrial DNA heteroplasmy. Am J Hum Genet. 1990;46(3):428–33.
86. Park SG, Schimmel P, Kim S. Aminoacyl tRNA synthetases and their connections to disease. Proc Natl Acad Sci U S A. 2008;105(32):11043–9.
87. De Luca C, Besagni C, Frontali L, Bolotin-Fukuhara M, Francisci S. Mutations in yeast mt tRNAs: specific and general suppression by nuclear encoded tRNA interactors. Gene. 2006;377:169–76.
88. De Luca C, Zhou Y, Montanari A, Morea V, Oliva R, Besagni C, et al. Can yeast be used to study mitochondrial diseases? Biolistic tRNA mutants for the analysis of mechanisms and suppressors. Mitochondrion. 2009;9(6):408–17.
89. Li R, Guan MX. Human mitochondrial leucyl-tRNA synthetase corrects mitochondrial dysfunctions due to the tRNALeu(UUR) A3243G mutation, associated with mitochondrial encephalomyopathy, lactic acidosis, and stroke-like symptoms and diabetes. Mol Cell Biol. 2010;30(9):2147–54.
90. Rorbach J, Yusoff AA, Tuppen H, Abg-Kamaludin DP, Chrzanowska-Lightowlers ZM, Taylor RW, et al. Overexpression of human mitochondrial valyl tRNA synthetase can partially restore levels of cognate mt-tRNAVal carrying the pathogenic C25U mutation. Nucleic Acids Res. 2008;36(9):3065–74.
91. Perli E, Giordano C, Tuppen HA, Montopoli M, Montanari A, Orlandi M, et al. Isoleucyl-tRNA synthetase levels modulate the penetrance of a homoplasmic m.4277T>C mitochondrial tRNA(Ile)

mutation causing hypertrophic cardiomyopathy. Hum Mol Genet. 2012;21(1):85–100.
92. Hornig-Do HT, Montanari A, Rozanska A, Tuppen HA, Almalki AA, Abg-Kamaludin DP, et al. Human mitochondrial leucyl tRNA synthetase can suppress non cognate pathogenic mt-tRNA mutations. EMBO Mol Med. 2014;6(2):183–93.
93. Perli E, Giordano C, Pisano A, Montanari A, Campese AF, Reyes A, et al. The isolated carboxy-terminal domain of human mitochondrial leucyl-tRNA synthetase rescues the pathological phenotype of mitochondrial tRNA mutations in human cells. EMBO Mol Med. 2014;6(2):169–82.
94. Kolesnikova OA, Entelis NS, Jacquin-Becker C, Goltzene F, Chrzanowska-Lightowlers ZM, Lightowlers RN, et al. Nuclear DNA-encoded tRNAs targeted into mitochondria can rescue a mitochondrial DNA mutation associated with the MERRF syndrome in cultured human cells. Hum Mol Genet. 2004;13(20):2519–34.
95. Comte C, Tonin Y, Heckel-Mager AM, Boucheham A, Smirnov A, Aure K, et al. Mitochondrial targeting of recombinant RNAs modulates the level of a heteroplasmic mutation in human mitochondrial DNA associated with Kearns Sayre Syndrome. Nucleic Acids Res. 2013;41(1):418–33.
96. Friedman JR, Nunnari J. Mitochondrial form and function. Nature. 2014;505(7483):335–43.
97. Mishra P, Chan DC. Mitochondrial dynamics and inheritance during cell division, development and disease. Nat Rev Mol Cell Biol. 2014;15(10):634–46.
98. Alexander C, Votruba M, Pesch UE, Thiselton DL, Mayer S, Moore A, et al. OPA1, encoding a dynamin-related GTPase, is mutated in autosomal dominant optic atrophy linked to chromosome 3q28. Nat Genet. 2000;26(2):211–5.
99. Zuchner S, Mersiyanova IV, Muglia M, Bissar-Tadmouri N, Rochelle J, Dadali EL, et al. Mutations in the mitochondrial GTPase mitofusin 2 cause Charcot-Marie-Tooth neuropathy type 2A. Nat Genet. 2004;36(5):449–51.
100. Chen H, Vermulst M, Wang YE, Chomyn A, Prolla TA, McCaffery JM, et al. Mitochondrial fusion is required for mtDNA stability in skeletal muscle and tolerance of mtDNA mutations. Cell. 2010;141(2):280–9.
101. Cogliati S, Frezza C, Soriano ME, Varanita T, Quintana-Cabrera R, Corrado M, et al. Mitochondrial cristae shape determines respiratory chain supercomplexes assembly and respiratory efficiency. Cell. 2013;155(1):160–71.
102. Chin RM, Panavas T, Brown JM, Johnson KK. Optimized mitochondrial targeting of proteins encoded by modified mRNAs rescues cells harboring mutations in mtATP6. Cell Rep. 2018;22(11):2818–26.
103. Varanita T, Soriano ME, Romanello V, Zaglia T, Quintana-Cabrera R, Semenzato M, et al. The OPA1-dependent mitochondrial cristae remodeling pathway controls atrophic, apoptotic, and ischemic tissue damage. Cell Metab. 2015;21(6):834–44.
104. Hakkaart GA, Dassa EP, Jacobs HT, Rustin P. Allotopic expression of a mitochondrial alternative oxidase confers cyanide resistance to human cell respiration. EMBO Rep. 2006;7(3):341–5.
105. El-Khoury R, Dufour E, Rak M, Ramanantsoa N, Grandchamp N, Csaba Z, et al. Alternative oxidase expression in the mouse enables bypassing cytochrome c oxidase blockade and limits mitochondrial ROS overproduction. PLoS Genet. 2013;9(1):e1003182.
106. Perales-Clemente E, Bayona-Bafaluy MP, Perez-Martos A, Barrientos A, Fernandez-Silva P, Enriquez JA. Restoration of electron transport without proton pumping in mammalian mitochondria. Proc Natl Acad Sci U S A. 2008;105(48):18735–9.
107. Dassa EP, Dufour E, Goncalves S, Paupe V, Hakkaart GA, Jacobs HT, et al. Expression of the alternative oxidase complements cytochrome c oxidase deficiency in human cells. EMBO Mol Med. 2009;1(1):30–6.
108. Fernandez-Ayala DJ, Sanz A, Vartiainen S, Kemppainen KK, Babusiak M, Mustalahti E, et al. Expression of the Ciona intestinalis alternative oxidase (AOX) in Drosophila complements defects in mitochondrial oxidative phosphorylation. Cell Metab. 2009;9(5):449–60.
109. Sanz A, Soikkeli M, Portero-Otin M, Wilson A, Kemppainen E, McIlroy G, et al. Expression of the yeast NADH dehydrogenase Ndi1 in Drosophila confers increased lifespan independently of dietary restriction. Proc Natl Acad Sci U S A. 2010;107(20):9105–10.
110. Kemppainen KK, Rinne J, Sriram A, Lakanmaa M, Zeb A, Tuomela T, et al. Expression of alternative oxidase in Drosophila ameliorates diverse phenotypes due to cytochrome oxidase deficiency. Hum Mol Genet. 2014;23(8):2078–93.
111. Rustin P, Jacobs HT. Respiratory chain alternative enzymes as tools to better understand and counteract respiratory chain deficiencies in human cells and animals. Physiol Plant. 2009;137(4):362–70.
112. Tachibana M, Sparman M, Sritanaudomchai H, Ma H, Clepper L, Woodward J, et al. Mitochondrial gene replacement in primate offspring and embryonic stem cells. Nature. 2009;461(7262):367–72.
113. Tachibana M, Amato P, Sparman M, Woodward J, Sanchis DM, Ma H, et al. Towards germline gene therapy of inherited mitochondrial diseases. Nature. 2013;493(7434):627–31.
114. Craven L, Tuppen HA, Greggains GD, Harbottle SJ, Murphy JL, Cree LM, et al. Pronuclear transfer in human embryos to prevent transmission of mitochondrial DNA disease. Nature. 2010;465(7294):82–5.
115. Herbert M, Turnbull D. Progress in mitochondrial replacement therapies. Nat Rev Mol Cell Biol. 2018;19(2):71–2.
116. Yamada M, Emmanuele V, Sanchez-Quintero MJ, Sun B, Lallos G, Paull D, et al. Genetic drift can compromise mitochondrial replacement by nuclear transfer in human oocytes. Cell Stem Cell. 2016;18(6):749–54.
117. Viscomi C, Bottani E, Zeviani M. Emerging concepts in the therapy of mitochondrial disease. Biochim Biophys Acta. 2015;1847(6–7):544–57.

Reproductive Options for Women with Mitochondrial Disease

Lyndsey Craven and Doug M. Turnbull

Introduction

Mitochondrial disease is the collective term for a group of genetic disorders characterised by defects in oxidative phosphorylation. These diseases lead to a wide range of clinical symptoms involving any organ or body system but particularly those with high energy demands [1]. Mitochondrial disease is often progressive and can be associated with high morbidity and mortality in both children and adults. The mutations that cause mitochondrial disease are found in the nuclear DNA (nDNA) or mitochondrial DNA (mtDNA), reflecting the dual genetic control of mitochondrial function. This genetic heterogeneity can make diagnosis difficult and is exacerbated by the fact that >290 genetic defects have been identified in patients with mitochondrial disease [2]. The advent of next generation sequencing has resulted in an increasing number of pathogenic mutations being reported, which has led to a dramatic improvement in the diagnostic rate over recent years [3].

The significance of a genetic diagnosis in patients with mitochondrial disease is that it enables genetic counselling and allows for calculations of recurrence risk, which will depend entirely on the causative mutation. For inherited nuclear DNA mutations, the recurrence risk can be determined in much the same way as other nuclear genetic diseases and will depend on the pattern of inheritance, which can include autosomal dominant, autosomal recessive and X-linked. The difficulty arises when trying to calculate recurrence risk for inherited mtDNA mutations, which are only transmitted by female carriers due to the strict maternal inheritance of mtDNA.

Features of Mitochondrial Genetics

The challenge in providing accurate genetic advice to women affected by mitochondrial DNA disease is partly explained by the complex and unique features of mitochondrial genetics, including the multicopy nature of the mitochondrial genome. This is exemplified by human gametes, with individual sperm estimated to contain ~100 copies of mtDNA compared to mature oocytes that can contain >100,000 mtDNA copies. In some patients with a pathogenic mtDNA mutation, all copies of the mitochondrial genome will be identical, and only mutant mtDNA presents within cells, which is termed homoplasmy. In most patients, however, there is a combination of both wild-type and mutant mtDNA, which is termed heteroplasmy. When heteroplasmy exists, it is the ratio of wild-type to mutant mtDNA that

L. Craven (✉) · D. M. Turnbull
Wellcome Centre for Mitochondrial Research, Institute of Neuroscience, Newcastle University, Newcastle Upon Tyne, UK
e-mail: Lyndsey.Butterworth@ncl.ac.uk; Doug.Turnbull@ncl.ac.uk

M. Mancuso, T. Klopstock (eds.), *Diagnosis and Management of Mitochondrial Disorders*, https://doi.org/10.1007/978-3-030-05517-2_23

is important for the clinical presentation of disease, with higher levels of mutant mtDNA (and lower levels of wild-type mtDNA) often associated with more severe symptoms. This is known as the threshold effect, which denotes the level of mutant mtDNA that must be reached within a cell for a biochemical defect to become apparent. This level can differ depending on the precise mtDNA mutation and cell type but can also vary considerably between patients, with ongoing research beginning to elucidate other factors that could influence clinical expression of disease [4]. It is also well documented that heteroplasmy levels can shift dramatically both within and between generations due to a phenomenon known as the mitochondrial genetic bottleneck. This is an event thought to occur during early development of the female germ line that restricts the number of mtDNA molecules transmitted to the next generation and can result in offspring with divergent levels of heteroplasmy. The presence of this genetic bottleneck makes it difficult to predict the severity of disease in any children born, and consequently, genetic counselling is a challenge.

Reproductive Options for Mitochondrial Disease

In much the same way that genetic counselling for mitochondrial disease is governed by the genetic diagnosis, the reproductive options that are available to at-risk couples will also depend on the causative mutation. Most of these options are not exclusive to those affected by mitochondrial disease but may be considered by any individual who wishes to prevent transmission of an inherited genetic disease. These include voluntary childlessness and adoption, which are both options that will stop a disease recurring within a family. For carriers of nuclear DNA mutations, another reproductive option that can be considered is egg or sperm donation (depending on which parent is the carrier of the mutation), which will remove the risk of the disease gene being transmitted from the affected parent. For those couples who both wish to contribute genetically to their offspring, options include prenatal testing and preimplantation genetic diagnosis (PGD), which can be used to determine the carrier status of the resulting child. Although there can be exceptions, counselling couples on the outcome of these tests is relatively straightforward, with the presence or absence of the nuclear DNA mutation used to establish if the child will be affected or unaffected.

The reproductive options available to women who carry mtDNA mutations are similar, but the complex features of mitochondrial genetics mean that the results may be difficult to interpret and may not always guarantee prevention of mitochondrial DNA disease. Furthermore, not all the options will be suitable for every woman affected by mitochondrial DNA disease, highlighting the importance of mitochondrial specialists in providing advice that will help couples to make informed reproductive choices. Egg donation is one option that will prevent the maternal inheritance of an mtDNA mutation and will completely eradicate any risk of mitochondrial DNA disease (Fig. 1). For those women who wish to be genetically related to the child, prenatal testing and PGD can be used to determine the heteroplasmy level in the offspring and reduce the risk of having a severely affected child (Fig. 1). Both techniques have been available for several years and have resulted in the birth of healthy children, confirming their value for some affected families [5].

Prenatal Testing for mtDNA Mutations

Prenatal testing to prevent transmission of mitochondrial DNA disease is a reproductive option available to some women at risk of transmitting an mtDNA mutation to their offspring. The major drawback is that it involves determining the heteroplasmy level in foetal cells removed from an early pregnancy and so couples may need to consider a termination based on the prenatal result. The heteroplasmy level determined in the prenatal sample is reflective of the heteroplasmy level in the developing foetus [6–8] and allows the risk of mitochondrial disease in the resulting child to

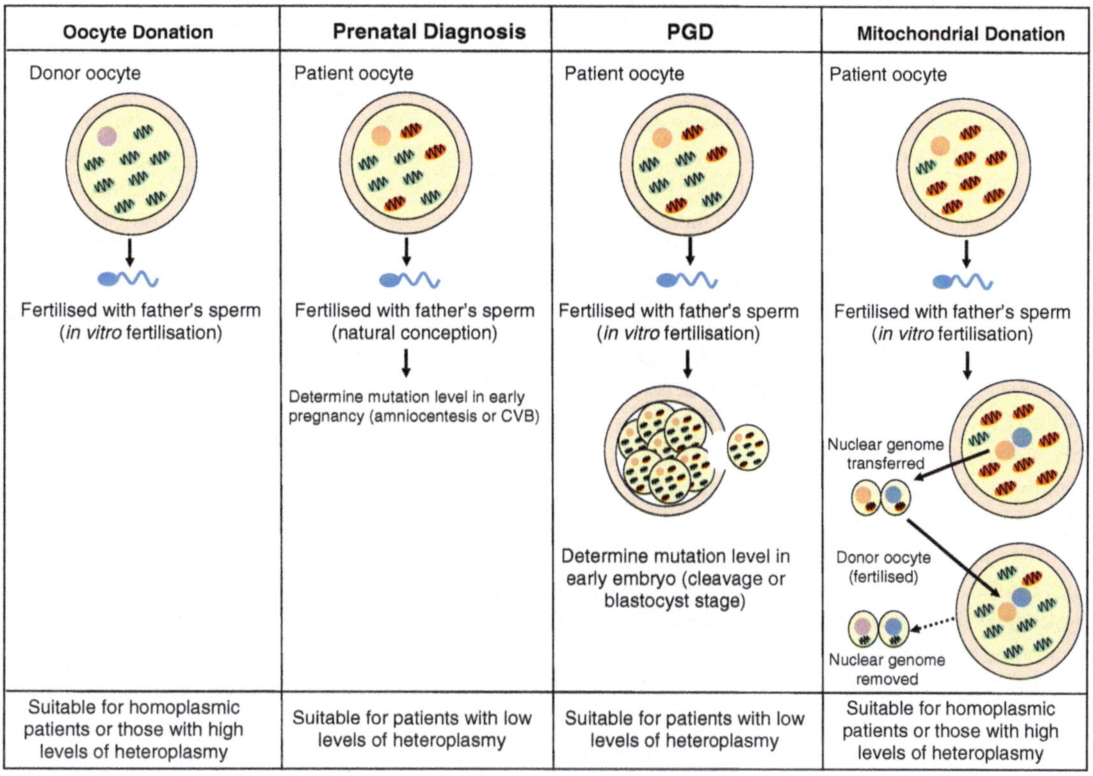

Fig. 1 Reproductive options for women with pathogenic mtDNA mutations [52]

be estimated. The outcome is easy to predict if undetectable or low levels of heteroplasmy are detected in the foetal sample, providing reassurance for parents that the risk of mitochondrial DNA disease in their child will be low. If high levels of heteroplasmy are detected, the outcome is also relatively easy to predict but will be accompanied by parents having to make the difficult choice to terminate the pregnancy knowing there is a high risk of the child being severely affected by mitochondrial DNA disease. This is even more challenging if intermediate heteroplasmy levels are reported, with some parents having to consider terminating an established pregnancy based on a theoretical disease risk. Despite this, prenatal testing is a reproductive option that has been successfully used for many different mtDNA mutations, with demand increasing among families affected by mitochondrial disease [9]. It may also be useful for providing reassurance to those couples who have had a previously affected child but a low recurrence risk [10]. For prenatal testing to be a suitable option that will reduce the risk of mitochondrial DNA disease, however, women who carry mtDNA mutations must produce oocytes with low heteroplasmy levels to prevent transmission of the disease.

Preimplantation Genetic Diagnosis (PGD) for mtDNA Mutations

PGD for mitochondrial DNA disease is another reproductive option that may be available for some women at risk of transmitting mtDNA mutations to their offspring. This technique involves determining the heteroplasmy level in cell(s) removed from early embryos produced during an in vitro fertilisation cycle and allows embryo(s) with a reduced risk of mitochondrial disease to be selected for implantation or cryopreserved for future use. PGD is being offered for an increasing number of mtDNA mutations and has successfully identified suitable embryos with undetectable or low levels of the mtDNA mutation for transfer to the uterus [11–16]. The majority of reported PGD cases have involved testing one or two blastomeres removed from cleavage-stage embryos, with the heteroplasmy level in the biopsied cell(s) indicative of the heteroplasmy level within the remaining embryo [17]. This assumes that the mtDNA mutation segregates uniformly during embryo cleavage, which appears to be the case for the majority of mtDNA mutations [12, 14, 16] although exceptions can occur [14, 18]. Alternatively, PGD can involve testing a small number of trophectoderm cells removed from blastocyst-stage embryos, which appears to reduce the impact of the biopsy on subsequent embryo development [19]. For this to be reliable, it requires that the heteroplasmy level is evenly distributed throughout the trophectoderm and that it corresponds to the heteroplasmy level in the inner cell mass, with limited data suggesting this is the case for human embryos [16]. There are currently few reports of blastocyst biopsy for mtDNA mutations [11, 16], with some inconsistency in the outcomes [20]. Despite this, PGD to reduce the transmission of mtDNA mutations has resulted in the birth of healthy children with a lower risk of mitochondrial DNA disease and so provides a promising option for some affected families. For this approach to be successful, however, women who carry mtDNA mutations must produce embryos with a heteroplasmy level below the critical threshold for disease expression. A level of 18% has been proposed as the threshold [21], although this varies between clinics and will depend on the precise mtDNA mutation. This highlights that PGD will not be suitable for all women who carry an mtDNA mutation, especially those who are homoplasmic or produce only oocytes with high levels of heteroplasmy.

Mitochondrial Donation Techniques

The development of mitochondrial donation techniques, also known as mitochondrial replacement, provides an alternative reproductive option that may give some women who carry an mtDNA mutation the opportunity to have a genetically related child whilst reducing the risk of mitochondrial DNA disease [22]. This option may be appropriate for a select group of patients when PGD is unlikely to succeed and could benefit ~150 women each year in the UK [23]. Importantly, before the development of this novel IVF treatment, no other reproductive option was available that would allow these women to contribute genetically to their offspring without a high risk of having a child severely affected by mitochondrial DNA disease. The procedure involves 'replacing' mutated mtDNA in human oocytes or zygotes by transferring the nuclear DNA to a donated oocyte or zygote with wild-type mtDNA from which the nuclear DNA has been removed. The reconstituted oocyte or zygote will contain the nuclear DNA from the intending parents with the majority of mtDNA provided by the donor oocyte or zygote, and as such, the risk of severe mitochondrial DNA disease will be dramatically reduced. Interestingly, it is this genetic contribution from three different people that led to the now infamous term 'three-parent baby' which was coined by journalists over a decade ago but has since appeared in nearly all media coverage of mitochondrial donation.

The transfer of nuclear DNA required for mitochondrial donation can be performed at various stages of oocyte development using unfertilised oocytes and techniques known as polar body transfer (PBT) and maternal spindle transfer (MST) or can be performed using fertilised oocytes (zygotes) and a technique known as pronuclear transfer (PNT) (Fig. 2). The basic principle is the same, but subtle differences between each technique mean there are advantages and disadvantages that need to be considered when investigating the safest and most effective method to reduce the risk of mitochondrial DNA disease. The most detailed preclinical study to date investigated the use of PNT to reduce the risk of mtDNA disease [24], but similar studies have been published for MST [25–27] and, to a lesser extent, PBT [28]. Importantly, there are currently more scientific data to support the clinical application of MST and PNT, with no evidence to

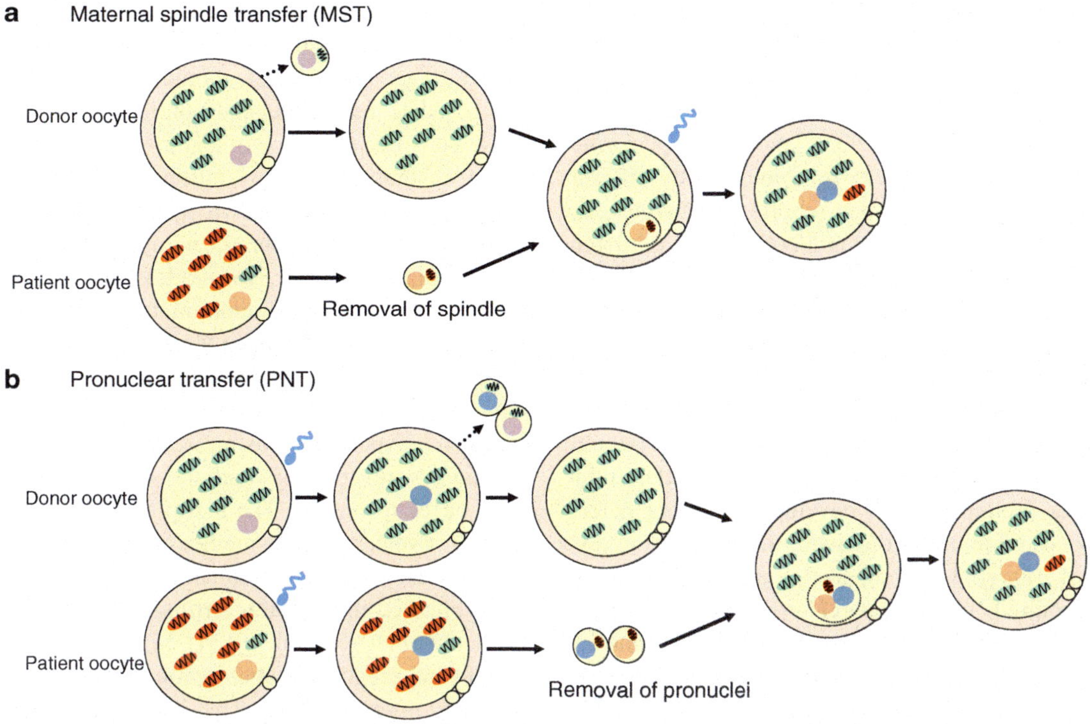

Fig. 2 Mitochondrial donation techniques. Mitochondrial donation involves removing the nuclear DNA from an oocyte/zygote carrying a pathogenic mtDNA mutation and transferring it to an enucleated donor oocyte/zygote with wild-type mtDNA. The reconstituted embryo contains predominantly wild-type mtDNA associated with a reduced risk of mitochondrial DNA disease. The transfer of nuclear DNA can be done between unfertilised oocytes using (**a**) maternal spindle transfer (MST) or between fertilised zygotes using (**b**) pronuclear transfer (PNT) [52]

suggest that one technique is preferable over the other (http://www.hfea.gov.uk/docs/Fourth_scientific_review_mitochondria_2016.PDF). This is reflected in the current UK legislation, with the Human Fertilisation and Embryology (Mitochondrial Donation) Regulations 2015 permitting MST and PNT for clinical use. The choice of technique will mostly depend on the expertise of the fertility centre offering mitochondrial donation but may also be influenced by the ethical, religious or cultural beliefs of the intending parents [29].

Pronuclear Transfer

PNT involves the transfer of nuclear DNA within two structures that become visible in the zygote following normal fertilisation. These structures, known as the pronuclei, have a well-defined membrane and contain the nuclear DNA from both parents. A method to efficiently transfer the pronuclei was initially developed using mouse zygotes [30] and involved removing the pronuclei in the presence of cytoskeletal inhibitors, which resulted in their removal within a membrane-bound karyoplast surrounded by a small volume of cytoplasm. Importantly, this allowed the pronuclei to be removed without disruption to the surrounding membrane, which dramatically improved zygote survival following the manipulation. Following removal, the pronuclear karyoplasts were exposed to a cell fusion protein called HVJ-E (haemagglutinating virus of Japan envelope) and transferred to an enucleated zygote to allow fusion to occur. Subsequent culture of these reconstituted zygotes revealed that they could develop efficiently to the blastocyst stage and resulted in live offspring when transferred to foster females [30]. This experimental strategy went on to form the basis of all subsequent PNT research, including several studies that assessed the level of mtDNA transferred to the donor zygote within the pronuclear karyoplast during the PNT procedure. One such study performed PNT using zygotes from mice with different mtDNA genotypes and reported a mean level of karyoplast-associated mtDNA of 19%, whilst the level within tissues of the offspring produced from these reconstituted zygotes varied from 0% to 69% [31, 32]. This level of 'mtDNA carryover' is important and must be minimal if mitochondrial donation is to reduce the risk of mitochondrial disease. The overall aim of this early study was to investigate the segregation of mtDNA during preimplantation development using heteroplasmic mice, and as such, minimising the level of karyoplast-associated mtDNA was not required. This is apparent when the mtDNA carryover levels are compared to a recent publication that reported much lower levels of karyoplast-associated mtDNA following PNT between mouse zygotes, with an average level of 0.29% [33]. Another study described the use of PNT to reduce transmission of a large-scale mtDNA deletion responsible for respiration defects in a mouse model of mitochondrial disease [34]. This demonstrated the feasibility of PNT to reduce transmission of an mtDNA mutation, with PNT mice displaying increased survival compared to controls.

The first study to evaluate the potential of PNT to prevent transmission of mitochondrial disease in humans used abnormally fertilised human zygotes consented to research by couples undergoing IVF treatments [35]. This revealed that the approach developed to perform PNT between mouse zygotes could not be directly applied to human zygotes and modifications were required to account for the many differences between mouse and human zygotes. Following optimisation of the procedure, the study revealed that PNT could successfully reduce levels of mtDNA carryover to <2% on average, with most reconstituted zygotes containing undetectable levels of karyoplast-associated mtDNA. The study also demonstrated that reconstituted zygotes were capable of development to the blastocyst stage, although at a reduced rate when compared to unmanipulated controls. This was most likely due to the use of abnormally fertilised zygotes which often arrest during embryo development and could lack a paternal/maternal genome or have an incorrect number of centrosomes following PNT. Nonetheless, this proof-of-concept study was important to confirm the potential of PNT to reduce the risk of mitochondrial DNA disease. Before clinical application could be considered, however, it was vital to repeat the experiments using normally fertilised human zygotes to assess both the safety and efficacy of the technique. The first preclinical study of PNT revealed that the methodology developed for abnormally fertilised human zygotes was not well tolerated in normally fertilised zygotes and needed further refinement [24], highlighting the benefit of creating human embryos for some research purposes [29]. The key modification involved changing the timing of PNT, with the transfer being performed immediately after formation of the pronuclei (~8 h post-fertilisation) rather than just before onset of mitosis (~16 h post-fertilisation). This modified technique, referred to as 'early PNT' (ePNT), improved survival of the reconstituted zygotes, leading to improved development of good quality blastocysts. Several other safety issues were investigated in this study, with analysis of aneuploidy and global gene expression revealing no significant differences between ePNT blastocysts and unmanipulated controls. The mtDNA carryover was <2% in the majority of ePNT blastocysts, but when these blastocysts were used to derive human embryonic stem cells, a limited number of hESC lines revealed that the level of karyoplast-associated mtDNA progressively increased during continued culture despite low levels at the blastocyst stage [24]. This led the authors to conclude that PNT has the potential to reduce the risk of mitochondrial DNA disease but may not guarantee prevention and, as such, should be considered in combination with prenatal testing.

Maternal Spindle Transfer

MST involves the transfer of nuclear DNA as a spindle-chromosome complex, also known as the maternal spindle, present in mature oocytes arrested at the metaphase II (MII) stage. The ability to visualise this microtubular structure using polarised microscopy, and importantly without the use of nuclear stains that can indirectly damage DNA, marked a significant advance in the development of MST and is fundamental to the possible clinical application of the technique. An efficient method to perform MST was first reported in non-human primates (*Macaca mulatta*) and involved removing the maternal spindle surrounded by a small volume of cytoplasm within a karyoplast in the presence of cytoskeletal inhibitor [36]. The karyoplast was exposed to HVJ-E and transferred to an enucleated MII recipient oocyte, followed by intracytoplasmic sperm injection (ICSI) to fertilise the reconstituted oocytes. The study reported comparable fertilisation and blastocyst rates to unmanipulated control oocytes and revealed that ESC lines derived from MST blastocysts had normal euploid karyotypes and minimal mtDNA carryover (lower detection limit of 3%). Moreover, the transfer of MST embryos to foster females resulted in the birth of healthy offspring with undetectable levels of mtDNA carryover in all tissues tested [26, 36]. The same technique has also been performed between mouse oocytes, confirming efficient blastocyst formation and an average mtDNA carryover of <1% [33]. Taken together, these animal studies confirm the potential of MST to prevent transmission of mitochondrial DNA disease.

The first study to perform MST in human oocytes confirmed the feasibility of the technique but also reported a high rate of abnormally fertilised MST zygotes following ICSI [26]. It was proposed that this could be due to either premature oocyte activation or spindle damage during the procedure. Despite this, the blastocyst rate in normally fertilised MST oocytes was comparable to controls, whilst the level of karyoplast-associated mtDNA in MST embryos was <1% and remained low in hESCs derived from MST blastocysts. Another study performed MST between human oocytes but used parthenogenetic activation of MST oocytes rather than ICSI and demonstrated that premature oocyte activation could be avoided by reducing the temperature or cryopreserving the oocytes before MST to partially depolymerise the spindle [37]. The study confirmed low levels of mtDNA carryover in reconstructed MST embryos, with undetectable levels reported in hESCs derived from MST blastocysts. Similar findings were published in recent MST studies, with low or undetectable levels of karyoplast-associated mtDNA in the majority of hESC lines derived from MST blastocysts [25, 27]. This was not a consistent finding, however, with a limited number of hESC lines showing an increase in the level of karyoplast-associated mtDNA after each passage. This phenomenon was also observed in the first research study to use human oocytes carrying a pathogenic mtDNA mutation to evaluate the potential of MST to prevent mitochondrial disease [25]. The data confirmed that MST could reduce the transmission of an mtDNA mutation to <1% but that this could undergo complete reversion to the karyoplast-associated mtDNA genotype in a limited number of hESC lines. Taken together with the data from the preclinical PNT study [24], this suggests that low levels of mtDNA carryover could increase to levels above the critical threshold and so mitochondrial donation may not prevent mitochondrial DNA disease irrespective of the technique used. The results must be interpreted with some caution, however, as the behaviour of mtDNA in hESCs could be very different from the situation that occurs during embryonic or foetal development [38].

In addition to the preclinical research investigating the potential of MST to reduce the risk of mitochondrial DNA disease, there is currently one case study describing the clinical application of MST to prevent transmission of a pathogenic mtDNA mutation [39]. The procedure was performed in Mexico due to pending approval in the

USA and resulted in the first live birth of an apparently healthy baby boy. The case involved a 36-year-old woman who suffered four miscarriages and had two children who died due to high levels of a maternally inherited mtDNA mutation (>95%) that causes Leigh syndrome (m.8993T>G). Following MST, the average level of the mtDNA mutation in the only euploid MST blastocyst selected for embryo transfer was 5.73%, whilst the level within several tissues tested after birth ranged from 2.36% to 9.23% [39]. This confirms that MST is compatible with a viable pregnancy leading to a live birth and that MST can reduce transmission of a pathogenic mtDNA mutation. However, the level of mtDNA carryover determined in the MST blastocyst was higher than previously reported in other studies and highlights the importance of long-term follow-up of any children born following MST or PNT to confirm the safety of this IVF treatment while still at the research stage.

Towards Clinical Application of Mitochondrial Donation

The research studies using both animal models and human oocytes have provided scientific evidence to suggest that mitochondrial donation, whether it be PNT or MST, has the potential to reduce the risk of mitochondrial DNA disease. The human data demonstrate that the procedures are compatible with onward embryo development and can result in good quality blastocysts likely to establish a pregnancy if transferred to the uterus, a prerequisite of any IVF treatment. Furthermore, the amount of karyoplast-associated mtDNA transferred with the nuclear DNA during the procedure is minimal, suggesting that mitochondrial donation will significantly reduce transmission of mtDNA mutations to a level that is well below the critical threshold for disease expression. The challenge is deciding when an adequate level of safety has been demonstrated to allow the timely application of mitochondrial donation in the clinic [40]. To address this, an independent panel of experts was convened by the Human Fertilisation and Embryology Authority (HFEA) to perform an extensive review of the available scientific evidence regarding the safety and efficacy of mitochondrial donation [38]. The conclusion of their most recent review was that MST and PNT are sufficiently safe to be offered as clinical risk reduction treatments for carefully selected patients under strict regulation (http://hfeaarchive.uksouth.cloudapp.azure.com/www.hfea.gov.uk/docs/Fourth_scientific_review_mitochondria_2016.pdf).

An important consideration with mitochondrial donation is whether the nuclear genome transferred to the donor oocyte/zygote is compatible with the mtDNA provided by the donor. Previous studies have proposed that nuclear-mitochondrial mismatch is evident in some animal models [41, 42], but this does not appear to be a consistent observation, with other animal studies reporting no negative effects despite the presence of divergent mitochondrial genomes [43–45]. Furthermore, a recent study tested the nuclear-mitochondrial mismatch hypothesis in human populations and reported that nuclear and mitochondrial genomes from divergent populations can co-exist in healthy individuals without a deleterious effect [46].

It is important to note that the studies which show potential nuclear-mitochondrial incompatibility involve highly inbred laboratory animals, which are very different to highly outbred human populations, and so the significance to mitochondrial donation continues to provoke intense discussion [47–49]. Evidence to support the view that mitochondrial donation does not disrupt human nuclear-mitochondrial interactions is provided by comparable fertilisation and blastocyst rates in MST embryos containing different mtDNA haplogroups [25] and identical OXPHOS transcript levels in PNT embryos containing either the same or different mtDNA haplogroups [24]. Taken together, these data suggest that mitochondrial donation does not affect mitochondrial gene expression during human preimplantation development. Further evidence is provided by the study of hESCs derived from blastocysts containing divergent mtDNA haplogroups, which revealed comparable mitochondrial respiratory chain enzyme activities and oxygen consumption rates when the same nuclear

DNA was combined with different mtDNA haplogroups, suggesting that mitochondrial function is not altered despite the haplotype differences [27, 50].

Regulatory Approval of Mitochondrial Donation

In 2005, when human studies began to investigate the potential of mitochondrial donation to prevent transmission of mitochondrial DNA disease, the experiments were permitted by law for research purposes but could not be offered as a clinical treatment. Therefore, to make mitochondrial donation a realistic reproductive option available to women affected by mitochondrial DNA disease, it was vital that UK legislation was amended to allow clinical application of the novel IVF treatment. An extensive policy process ensued and, with great foresight, occurred in conjunction with the scientific development of mitochondrial donation. This policy process took place over several years and comprised discussions and debates covering many scientific, ethical and legal issues around mitochondrial donation, which were subsequently used to make recommendations to the UK government [51]. This included four comprehensive reviews on the safety and efficacy of mitochondrial donation, the first of which was published in 2011 and concluded that there was no evidence to suggest that mitochondrial donation was unsafe for clinical use but proposed further experiments to support this finding. The same conclusion was reached in subsequent reviews published in 2013 and 2014, with the most recent review published in 2016 declaring both MST and PNT sufficiently safe to proceed with cautious clinical application. The ethical issues surrounding the use of mitochondrial donation were also considered at length by many in multiple contexts, including the Nuffield Council on Bioethics. Their report, published in 2012, concluded that it would be ethical for families to use mitochondrial donation provided that the technique was shown to be safe and effective (http://nuffieldbioethics.org/wp-content/uploads/2014/06/Novel_techniques_for_the_prevention_of_mitochondrial_DNA_disorders_compressed.pdf).

A key component of the policy process was public engagement, with the government keen to gauge public opinion of mitochondrial donation before proceeding with draft regulations. A public dialogue was launched in 2012, which formed part of an extensive consultation that was credited as an exemplary case of public engagement for policy purposes (http://webarchive.nationalarchives.gov.uk/20170110134326/http://www.sciencewise-erc.org.uk/cms/assets/Uploads/Mitochondria-evaluation-FINAL-2013.pdf). The public consultation revealed broad support for permitting mitochondrial donation in the UK and led to the Mitochondrial Donation Regulations being put before Parliament in 2015. Patient engagement was another crucial aspect of this, with many patients and families sharing their experiences of mitochondrial disease with the politicians who would ultimately vote on whether to allow mitochondrial donation in the UK. Patient organisations, including The Lily Foundation and Muscular Dystrophy UK, played an integral role and were very much at the forefront in terms of advocacy for the technique. This culminated in overwhelming support for mitochondrial donation in both Houses of Parliament, and regulations were approved to permit clinical application of the technique in March 2015. This saw the UK become the first country to legislate in this area, but to ensure full scrutiny of all the available scientific evidence around the safety and efficacy of the technique, it was not until December 2016 that the HFEA approved the use of mitochondrial donation. This was quickly followed by the Newcastle Fertility Centre becoming the first fertility unit to be granted a licence by the HFEA to offer mitochondrial donation to reduce the transmission of mitochondrial DNA disease. Specifically, this licence allows PNT to be offered to a select group of patients when PGD is not appropriate, or unlikely to reduce the risk of mitochondrial disease, with individual applications considered on a case-by-case basis. The regulatory approval in the UK provides a template for potential regulation of mitochondrial donation in other countries, although every country has a different regulatory system.

Developing the Clinical Service

Following a collaborative process with the HFEA to develop regulations that will govern the use of mitochondrial donation in the UK, Newcastle has established the Mitochondrial Reproductive Advice Clinic as part of the innovative new clinical service offered. This clinic has a dual purpose, the first being to assess fitness for pregnancy, which is important given the intending mother could be affected by mitochondrial disease. The second purpose is to discuss the reproductive options available for women who carry mtDNA mutations so that the decision to proceed with a particular option is well informed. It is important that women are made aware of these options early in reproductive life, which will increase the likelihood of having a child irrespective of the option chosen. Not every reproductive choice will be suitable for every individual, and given that each has its own limitations, it is crucial that the options are discussed with mitochondrial experts who can tailor the information and provide advice to each patient. The clinic aims to convey the complex features of mitochondrial genetics in a simple and concise way, with several different resources used to achieve this goal. This includes a short animation which clearly explains all the reproductive options available to couples, with time to discuss these further during the consultation.

For those patients who wish to consider an IVF-based reproductive option, there are opportunities to discuss this in the Mitochondrial IVF Clinic overseen by both mitochondrial and fertility experts. This clinic will establish if patients are suitable for an IVF-based treatment and provide a comprehensive overview of what an IVF cycle will entail. Information will also be provided on managing expectation, which is important given that IVF treatments can fail at any stage and establishing a pregnancy is not guaranteed. Consequently, couples may require multiple IVF cycles before a pregnancy is achieved, with emotional support provided throughout.

As highlighted in the HFEA regulations, long-term follow-up of any children born through mitochondrial donation will be crucial to confirm the safety and efficacy of the technique. Patients and their families will be informed of the benefits of this follow-up and encouraged to participate. Patient focus groups have been integral in defining the overall structure of this care pathway, which comprises antenatal checks during pregnancy through to a detailed neurodevelopmental assessment of the child at 18 months old. Feedback from multiple focus groups revealed that parents are keen to participate in follow-up but reluctant to 'medicalise' a healthy child and so hospital visits should be minimal. Taking this into account, the follow-up pathway utilises the health professionals that are seen as part of routine assessments and check-ups for babies and young children in the UK NHS, with only a small amount of additional information collected during these appointments. The outcome of this follow-up is important to inform the HFEA, patients and the public on the longer-term safety of mitochondrial donation.

References

1. Gorman GS, Chinnery PF, DiMauro S, Hirano M, Koga Y, McFarland R, Suomalainen A, Thorburn DR, Zeviani M, Turnbull DM. Mitochondrial diseases. Nat Rev Dis Primers. 2016;2:16080.
2. Frazier AE, Thorburn DR, Compton AG. Mitochondrial energy generation disorders: genes, mechanisms and clues to pathology. J Biol Chem. 2017; https://doi.org/10.1074/jbc.R117.809194.
3. Wortmann SB, Koolen DA, Smeitink JA, van den Heuvel L, Rodenburg RJ. Whole exome sequencing of suspected mitochondrial patients in clinical practice. J Inherit Metab Dis. 2015;38(3):437–43.
4. Pickett SJ, Grady JP, Ng YS, Gorman GS, Schaefer AM, Wilson IJ, Cordell HJ, Turnbull DM, Taylor RW, McFarland R. Phenotypic heterogeneity in m.3243A>G mitochondrial disease: the role of nuclear factors. Ann Clin Transl Neurol. 2018;5(3):333–45.
5. Smeets HJ, Sallevelt SC, Dreesen JC, de Die-Smulders CE, de Coo IF. Preventing the transmission of mitochondrial DNA disorders using prenatal or preimplantation genetic diagnosis. Ann N Y Acad Sci. 2015;1350:29–36.
6. Ferlin T, Landrieu P, Rambaud C, Fernandez H, Dumoulin R, Rustin P, Mousson B. Segregation of the G8993 mutant mitochondrial DNA through generations and embryonic tissues in a family at risk of Leigh syndrome. J Pediatr. 1997;131(3):447–9.
7. Harding AE, Holt IJ, Sweeney MG, Brockington M, Davis MB. Prenatal diagnosis of mitochondrial DNA8993 T----G disease. Am J Hum Genet. 1992;50(3):629–33.

8. Steffann J, Gigarel N, Corcos J, Bonniere M, Encha-Razavi F, Sinico M, Prevot S, Dumez Y, Yamgnane A, Frydman R, Munnich A, Bonnefont JP. Stability of the m.8993T->G mtDNA mutation load during human embryofetal development has implications for the feasibility of prenatal diagnosis in NARP syndrome. J Med Genet. 2007;44(10):664–9.
9. Nesbitt V, Alston CL, Blakely EL, Fratter C, Feeney CL, Poulton J, Brown GK, Turnbull DM, Taylor RW, McFarland R. A national perspective on prenatal testing for mitochondrial disease. Eur J Hum Genet. 2014;22(11):1255–9.
10. Sallevelt SC, de Die-Smulders CE, Hendrickx AT, Hellebrekers DM, de Coo IF, Alston CL, Knowles C, Taylor RW, McFarland R, Smeets HJ. De novo mtDNA point mutations are common and have a low recurrence risk. J Med Genet. 2016;54(2):73–83.
11. Heindryckx B, Neupane J, Vandewoestyne M, Christodoulou C, Jackers Y, Gerris J, Van den Abbeel E, Van Coster R, Deforce D, De Sutter P. Mutation-free baby born from a mitochondrial encephalopathy, lactic acidosis and stroke-like syndrome carrier after blastocyst trophectoderm preimplantation genetic diagnosis. Mitochondrion. 2014;18:12–7.
12. Monnot S, Gigarel N, Samuels DC, Burlet P, Hesters L, Frydman N, Frydman R, Kerbrat V, Funalot B, Martinovic J, Benachi A, Feingold J, Munnich A, Bonnefont JP, Steffann J. Segregation of mtDNA throughout human embryofetal development: m.3243A>G as a model system. Hum Mutat. 2011;32(1):116–25.
13. Sallevelt SC, Dreesen JC, Drusedau M, Hellebrekers DM, Paulussen AD, Coonen E, van Golde RJ, Geraedts JP, Gianaroli L, Magli MC, Zeviani M, Smeets HJ, de Die-Smulders CE. PGD for the m.14487 T>C mitochondrial DNA mutation resulted in the birth of a healthy boy. Hum Reprod. 2017;32(3):698–703.
14. Sallevelt SC, Dreesen JC, Drusedau M, Spierts S, Coonen E, van Tienen FH, van Golde RJ, de Coo IF, Geraedts JP, de Die-Smulders CE, Smeets HJ. Preimplantation genetic diagnosis in mitochondrial DNA disorders: challenge and success. J Med Genet. 2013;50(2):125–32.
15. Steffann J, Frydman N, Gigarel N, Burlet P, Ray PF, Fanchin R, Feyereisen E, Kerbrat V, Tachdjian G, Bonnefont JP, Frydman R, Munnich A. Analysis of mtDNA variant segregation during early human embryonic development: a tool for successful NARP preimplantation diagnosis. J Med Genet. 2006;43(3):244–7.
16. Treff NR, Campos J, Tao X, Levy B, Ferry KM, Scott RT Jr. Blastocyst preimplantation genetic diagnosis (PGD) of a mitochondrial DNA disorder. Fertil Steril. 2012;98(5):1236–40.
17. Sallevelt S, Dreesen J, Coonen E, Paulussen ADC, Hellebrekers D, de Die-Smulders CEM, Smeets HJM, Lindsey P. Preimplantation genetic diagnosis for mitochondrial DNA mutations: analysis of one blastomere suffices. J Med Genet. 2017;54(10):693–7.
18. Vandewoestyne M, Heindryckx B, De Gheselle S, Lepez T, Neupane J, Gerris J, Van Coster R, De Sutter P, Deforce D. Poor correlation between polar bodies and blastomere mutation load in a patient with m.3243A>G tRNALeu(UUR) point mutation. Mitochondrion. 2012;12(4):477–9.
19. Cimadomo D, Capalbo A, Ubaldi FM, Scarica C, Palagiano A, Canipari R, Rienzi L. The impact of biopsy on human embryo developmental potential during preimplantation genetic diagnosis. Biomed Res Int. 2016;2016:7193075.
20. Mitalipov S, Amato P, Parry S, Falk MJ. Limitations of preimplantation genetic diagnosis for mitochondrial DNA diseases. Cell Rep. 2014;7(4):935–7.
21. Hellebrekers DM, Wolfe R, Hendrickx AT, de Coo IF, de Die CE, Geraedts JP, Chinnery PF, Smeets HJ. PGD and heteroplasmic mitochondrial DNA point mutations: a systematic review estimating the chance of healthy offspring. Hum Reprod Update. 2012;18(4):341–9.
22. Richardson J, Irving L, Hyslop LA, Choudhary M, Murdoch A, Turnbull DM, Herbert M. Concise reviews: assisted reproductive technologies to prevent transmission of mitochondrial DNA disease. Stem Cells. 2015;33(3):639–45.
23. Gorman GS, Grady JP, Turnbull DM. Mitochondrial donation—how many women could benefit? N Engl J Med. 2015;372(9):885–7.
24. Hyslop LA, Blakeley P, Craven L, Richardson J, Fogarty NM, Fragouli E, Lamb M, Wamaitha SE, Prathalingam N, Zhang Q, O'Keefe H, Takeda Y, Arizzi L, Alfarawati S, Tuppen HA, Irving L, Kalleas D, Choudhary M, Wells D, Murdoch AP, Turnbull DM, Niakan KK, Herbert M. Towards clinical application of pronuclear transfer to prevent mitochondrial DNA disease. Nature. 2016;534(7607):383–6.
25. Kang E, Wu J, Gutierrez NM, Koski A, Tippner-Hedges R, Agaronyan K, Platero-Luengo A, Martinez-Redondo P, Ma H, Lee Y, Hayama T, Van Dyken C, Wang X, Luo S, Ahmed R, Li Y, Ji D, Kayali R, Cinnioglu C, Olson S, Jensen J, Battaglia D, Lee D, Wu D, Huang T, Wolf DP, Temiakov D, Belmonte JC, Amato P, Mitalipov S. Mitochondrial replacement in human oocytes carrying pathogenic mitochondrial DNA mutations. Nature. 2016;540(7632):270–5.
26. Tachibana M, Amato P, Sparman M, Woodward J, Sanchis DM, Ma H, Gutierrez NM, Tippner-Hedges R, Kang E, Lee HS, Ramsey C, Masterson K, Battaglia D, Lee D, Wu D, Jensen J, Patton P, Gokhale S, Stouffer R, Mitalipov S. Towards germline gene therapy of inherited mitochondrial diseases. Nature. 2013;493(7434):627–31.
27. Yamada M, Emmanuele V, Sanchez-Quintero MJ, Sun B, Lallos G, Paull D, Zimmer M, Pagett S, Prosser RW, Sauer MV, Hirano M, Egli D. Genetic drift can compromise mitochondrial replacement by nuclear transfer in human oocytes. Cell Stem Cell. 2016;18(6):749–54.
28. Ma H, O'Neil RC, Marti Gutierrez N, Hariharan M, Zhang ZZ, He Y, Cinnioglu C, Kayali R, Kang E, Lee

Y, Hayama T, Koski A, Nery J, Castanon R, Tippner-Hedges R, Ahmed R, Van Dyken C, Li Y, Olson S, Battaglia D, Lee DM, Wu DH, Amato P, Wolf DP, Ecker JR, Mitalipov S. Functional human oocytes generated by transfer of polar body genomes. Cell Stem Cell. 2016;20(1):112–9.
29. Craven L, Murphy J, Turnbull DM, Taylor RW, Gorman GS, McFarland R. Scientific and ethical issues in mitochondrial donation. New Bioeth. 2018;24(1):57–73.
30. McGrath J, Solter D. Nuclear transplantation in the mouse embryo by microsurgery and cell fusion. Science. 1983;220(4603):1300–2.
31. Meirelles FV, Smith LC. Mitochondrial genotype segregation in a mouse heteroplasmic lineage produced by embryonic karyoplast transplantation. Genetics. 1997;145(2):445–51.
32. Meirelles FV, Smith LC. Mitochondrial genotype segregation during preimplantation development in mouse heteroplasmic embryos. Genetics. 1998;148(2):877–83.
33. Neupane J, Vandewoestyne M, Ghimire S, Lu Y, Qian C, Van Coster R, Gerris J, Deroo T, Deforce D, De Sutter P, Heindryckx B. Assessment of nuclear transfer techniques to prevent the transmission of heritable mitochondrial disorders without compromising embryonic development competence in mice. Mitochondrion. 2014;18:27–33.
34. Sato A, Kono T, Nakada K, Ishikawa K, Inoue S, Yonekawa H, Hayashi J. Gene therapy for progeny of mito-mice carrying pathogenic mtDNA by nuclear transplantation. Proc Natl Acad Sci U S A. 2005;102(46):16765–70.
35. Craven L, Tuppen HA, Greggains GD, Harbottle SJ, Murphy JL, Cree LM, Murdoch AP, Chinnery PF, Taylor RW, Lightowlers RN, Herbert M, Turnbull DM. Pronuclear transfer in human embryos to prevent transmission of mitochondrial DNA disease. Nature. 2010;465(7294):82–5.
36. Tachibana M, Sparman M, Sritanaudomchai H, Ma H, Clepper L, Woodward J, Li Y, Ramsey C, Kolotushkina O, Mitalipov S. Mitochondrial gene replacement in primate offspring and embryonic stem cells. Nature. 2009;461(7262):367–72.
37. Paull D, Emmanuele V, Weiss KA, Treff N, Stewart L, Hua H, Zimmer M, Kahler DJ, Goland RS, Noggle SA, Prosser R, Hirano M, Sauer MV, Egli D. Nuclear genome transfer in human oocytes eliminates mitochondrial DNA variants. Nature. 2013;493(7434):632–7.
38. Greenfield A, Braude P, Flinter F, Lovell-Badge R, Ogilvie C, Perry ACF. Assisted reproductive technologies to prevent human mitochondrial disease transmission. Nat Biotechnol. 2017;35(11):1059–68.
39. Zhang J, Liu H, Luo S, Lu Z, Chavez-Badiola A, Liu Z, Yang M, Merhi Z, Silber SJ, Munne S, Konstantinidis M, Wells D, Tang JJ, Huang T. Live birth derived from oocyte spindle transfer to prevent mitochondrial disease. Reprod Biomed Online. 2017;34(4):361–8.
40. Herbert M, Turnbull D. Progress in mitochondrial replacement therapies. Nat Rev Mol Cell Biol. 2018;19(2):71–2.
41. Holmbeck MA, Donner JR, Villa-Cuesta E, Rand DM. A Drosophila model for mito-nuclear diseases generated by an incompatible interaction between tRNA and tRNA synthetase. Dis Model Mech. 2015;8(8):843–54.
42. Ma H, Marti Gutierrez N, Morey R, Van Dyken C, Kang E, Hayama T, Lee Y, Li Y, Tippner-Hedges R, Wolf DP, Laurent LC, Mitalipov S. Incompatibility between nuclear and mitochondrial genomes contributes to an interspecies reproductive barrier. Cell Metab. 2016;24(2):283–94.
43. Battersby BJ, Shoubridge EA. Selection of a mtDNA sequence variant in hepatocytes of heteroplasmic mice is not due to differences in respiratory chain function or efficiency of replication. Hum Mol Genet. 2001;10(22):2469–79.
44. Cannon MV, Dunn DA, Irwin MH, Brooks AI, Bartol FF, Trounce IA, Pinkert CA. Xenomitochondrial mice: investigation into mitochondrial compensatory mechanisms. Mitochondrion. 2011;11(1):33–9.
45. Gregorova S, Divina P, Storchova R, Trachtulec Z, Fotopulosova V, Svenson KL, Donahue LR, Paigen B, Forejt J. Mouse consomic strains: exploiting genetic divergence between Mus m. musculus and Mus m. domesticus subspecies. Genome Res. 2008;18(3):509–15.
46. Rishishwar L, Jordan IK. Implications of human evolution and admixture for mitochondrial replacement therapy. BMC Genomics. 2017;18(1):140.
47. Chinnery PF, Craven L, Mitalipov S, Stewart JB, Herbert M, Turnbull DM. The challenges of mitochondrial replacement. PLoS Genet. 2014;10(4):e1004315.
48. Eyre-Walker A. Mitochondrial replacement therapy: are mito-nuclear interactions likely to be a problem? Genetics. 2017;205(4):1365–72.
49. Reinhardt K, Dowling DK, Morrow EH. Medicine. Mitochondrial replacement, evolution, and the clinic. Science. 2013;341(6152):1345–6.
50. Ma H, Folmes CD, Wu J, Morey R, Mora-Castilla S, Ocampo A, Ma L, Poulton J, Wang X, Ahmed R, Kang E, Lee Y, Hayama T, Li Y, Van Dyken C, Gutierrez NM, Tippner-Hedges R, Koski A, Mitalipov N, Amato P, Wolf DP, Huang T, Terzic A, Laurent LC, Izpisua Belmonte JC, Mitalipov S. Metabolic rescue in pluripotent cells from patients with mtDNA disease. Nature. 2015;524(7564):234–8.
51. Craven L, Herbert M, Murdoch A, Murphy J, Lawford Davies J, Turnbull DM. Research into policy: a brief history of mitochondrial donation. Stem Cells. 2016;34(2):265–7.
52. Craven L, Alston CL, Taylor RW, Turnbull DM. Recent advances in mitochondrial disease. Annu Rev Genomics Hum Genet. 2017;18:257–75.

The manufacturer's authorised representative in the EU is Springer Nature Customer Service Centre GmbH, Europaplatz 3, 69115 Heidelberg, Germany. If you have any concerns regarding our products, please contact ProductSafety@springernature.com

Printed and bound by CPI Group (UK) Ltd, Croydon, CR0 4YY
22/09/2026
02221056-0010